COMPLICATIONS IN
PEDIATRIC
SURGERY

COMPLICATIONS IN PEDIATRIC SURGERY

Edited by

MICHAEL G. CATY, M.D.
State University of New York at Buffalo
Women and Children's Hospital of Buffalo
Buffalo, New York, USA

Associate Editors

Philip L. Glick, M.D., M.B.A.
State University of New York at Buffalo
Women and Children's Hospital of Buffalo
Buffalo, New York, USA

Marc A. Levitt, M.D.
University of Cincinnati School of Medicine
Cincinnati Children's Hospital Medical Center
Cincinnati, Ohio, USA

Jeffrey H. Haynes, M.D.
Medical College of Virginia
Virginia Commonwealth University Health System
Richmond, Virgina, USA

informa
healthcare

New York   London

Informa Healthcare USA, Inc.
52 Vanderbilt Avenue
New York, NY 10017

© 2009 by Informa Healthcare USA, Inc.
Informa Healthcare is an Informa business

No claim to original U.S. Government works
Printed in the United States of America on acid-free paper
10 9 8 7 6 5 4 3 2 1

International Standard Book Number-10: 0-8247-2836-X (Hardcover)
International Standard Book Number-13: 978-0-8247-2836-6 (Hardcover)

Library of Congress Cataloging-in-Publication Data

Complications in pediatric surgery / edited by Michael G. Caty.
      p. ; cm.
   Includes bibliographical references and index.
   ISBN-13: 978-0-8247-2836-6 (hardcover : alk. paper)
   ISBN-10: 0-8247-2836-X (hardcover : alk. paper)
   1. Children–Surgery–Complications.   I. Caty, Michael G.
   [DNLM: 1. Surgical Procedures, Operative.   2. Child.   3. Infant.
   4. Intraoperative Complications.   WO 925 C737 2008]

RD137.C586 2008
617.9'8 – dc22   2008035269

For Corporate Sales and Reprint Permissions call 212-520-2700 or write to: Sales Department, 52 Vanderbilt Avenue, 16th floor, New York, NY 10017.

Visit the Informa Web site at
www.informa.com

and the Informa Healthcare Web site at
www.informahealthcare.com

Foreword

Drs. Caty, Glick, Levitt, and Haynes have produced a different kind of book on *Complications in Pediatric Surgery*. They have divided this book into two sections: the first section is devoted to systematic issues, as they relate to complications and the second section deals with specific organ systems and operations. Most textbooks on surgical complications are organized in the same way as the second section of this book, namely, along organ systems and operations.

The first section of this book provides a unique and innovative addition to the literature on patient safety. In the current era, hospitals and medical centers are intensely focused on safety and error prevention, spending a huge amount of their resources and money on these problems. This becomes immediately obvious when we see the introduction of electronic medical records and order entries in most medical centers in the United States. It impacts on surgeons more specifically with regards to the "time outs" we all go through in the operating room before each surgical procedure. Site marking is another example of these efforts in the operating room. Medical centers are looking to the aviation industry's experience with error reduction as a template for medical error reduction. Thus, the chapter by John Nance on this subject is a welcome addition to the book.

The second section of the book, as mentioned above, represents a more traditional approach to complications in surgery, being organized along organ systems and specific diagnoses and operations. The authors have again been innovative in this section by having experts on various operations answering a specific list of questions about the technical details of the various operations. As we all know, one cannot learn to do an operation from a textbook or atlas because all the small details of the operation, which can make the difference between success and failure, cannot all be illustrated through drawings or photographs. The saying "the devil is in the details" is applicable to a complex operation. However, the approach the editors have taken by asking a list of detailed questions about the procedure to the expert comes as close as possible to watching the expert actually do the operation.

In summary, this new textbook of *Complications in Pediatric Surgery* offers both traditional and innovative approaches to pediatric surgical error reduction and management, and will be a significant addition to any pediatric surgeon's library.

Arnold G. Coran, M.D.
Professor of Surgery, Section of Pediatric Surgery
University of Michigan Medical School
Ann Arbor, Michigan, U.S.A.

Preface

As pediatric surgeons, our goal is to achieve optimal surgical outcomes. In order to attain success, it is imperative that we avoid complications. The phrase *primum non nocere* (first do no harm) is known to all who practice medicine. This mandate has been central to the practice of medicine and demands that physicians avoid medical error. The publication of "To Err Is Human" by the Institute of Medicine in 1999 crystallized the problem of medical error in the United States, demonstrating that within hospitals each year approximately 100,000 patients died due to medical error. This was a sentinel event in health care, calling for improved medical safety both in and out of hospitals. The report emphasized not only individual physician error, but also the significant role "systems" errors play.

Our textbook attempts to balance a perspective between systems issues and the more traditional organ based complication avoidance strategies. In the first part of the text, systems approaches to medicine are explored from several points of view, including aviation, the legal system, medication safety, and evidence-based medicine. The second part of the text follows an organ-based approach to complication recognition and avoidance. Contained within the second part of the text is a series of discussions with experts on complication avoidance and management. Each expert responded to a series of questions pertaining to an operation with which they had considerable experience and expertise. These responses come from years of experience in the management of these problems and should prove useful to all pediatric surgeons.

Complications in Pediatric Surgery is the authors' and editors' contribution to improve the practice of pediatric surgery. It is our hope that the medical community, and in turn all patients, will benefit from the information contained within this text.

Michael G. Caty, M.D.

Contents

Contributors

Jennifer Hall Aldrink, M.D. Fellow in Pediatric Surgery, The Ohio State University, Nationwide Children's Hospital, Columbus, Ohio, U.S.A.

Richard J. Andrassy, M.D. Denton A. Cooley Professor and Chairman, Department of Surgery, University of Texas Medical School at Houston, and Executive Vice President of Clinical Affairs and Associate Dean for Clinical Affairs, University of Texas at Houston, Houston, Texas, U.S.A.

Nikolai A. Bildzukewicz, M.D. Resident in Surgery, Department of Surgery, Thomas Jefferson University Hospital, Philadelphia, Pennsylvania, U.S.A.

Anthony A. Caldamone, M.D. Chief, Pediatric Urology, Hasbro Children's Hospital, and Professor of Surgery (Urology) and Pediatrics, Alpert School of Medicine, Brown University, Providence, Rhode Island, U.S.A.

Michael G. Caty, M.D. Professor of Surgery and Pediatrics, Program Director in Pediatric Surgery, State University of New York at Buffalo, and John E. Fisher Professor of Pediatric Surgery and Surgeon-in-Chief, Women and Children's Hospital of Buffalo, Buffalo, New York, U.S.A.

Venita Chandra, M.D. Resident in Surgery, Stanford Hospitals & Clinics, Stanford, California, U.S.A.

Mary Ellen Connolly, M.S., CPNP Division of Pediatric Surgery, University of Maryland School of Medicine, Baltimore, Maryland, U.S.A.

Roshni Dasgupta, M.D. Assistant Professor of Surgery, University of Cincinnati School of Medicine, and Attending Surgeon, Cincinnati Children's Hospital Medical Center, Cincinnati, Ohio, U.S.A.

Stephen P. Dunn, M.D. Professor of Surgery, Thomas Jefferson School of Medicine, and Director of Pediatric Transplantation, Alfred I. DuPont Hospital for Children, Wilmington, Delaware, U.S.A.

Sanjeev Dutta, M.D., M.A. Assistant Professor of Surgery and Pediatrics, Associate Director, Goodman Stimulation Center, Stanford Hospitals & Clinics, and Attending Surgeon, Division of Pediatric Surgery, Lucile Packard Children's Hospital, Stanford, California, U.S.A.

Mauricio A. Escobar, M.D. Chief Resident in Pediatric Surgery, State University of New York at Buffalo, Women and Children's Hospital of Buffalo, Buffalo, New York, U.S.A.

Richard A. Falcone, Jr., M.D., M.P.H. Assistant Professor of Surgery, University of Cincinnati School of Medicine, and Attending Surgeon, Cincinnati Children's Hospital Medical Center, Cincinnati, Ohio, U.S.A.

Steven J. Fishman, M.D. Associate Professor, Harvard Medical School, and Stuart and Jane Weitzman Family Chair in Surgery, Co-Director, Vascular Anomalies Center, Senior Associate in Surgery, Children's Hospital Boston, Boston, Massachusetts, U.S.A.

Philip L. Glick, M.D., M.B.A. Professor of Surgery, Pediatrics, and Obstetrics and Gynecology, State University of New York at Buffalo, and Attending Surgeon, Women and Children's Hospital of Buffalo, Buffalo, New York, U.S.A.

Arin K. Greene, M.D., M.M.Sc.   Instructor in Plastic Surgery, Harvard Medical School, Children's Hospital Boston, Boston, Massachusetts, U.S.A.

Jeffrey H. Haynes, M.D.   Associate Professor of Surgery and Pediatrics, Medical College of Virginia, and Attending Surgeon, Virginia Commonwealth University Health System, Richmond, Virginia, U.S.A.

Ronald B. Hirschl, M.D.   Professor of Surgery, Division of Pediatric Surgery, Department of Surgery, University of Michigan Health System, and Surgeon-in-Chief, C.S. Mott Children's Hospital, Ann Arbor, Michigan, U.S.A.

Karen Iacono, M.S.   Pediatric Nurse Practitioner, Women and Children's Hospital of Buffalo, Buffalo, New York, U.S.A.

Frederick M. Karrer, M.D.   Professor of Surgery and Pediatrics, University of Colorado School of Medicine, and Chief, Division of Pediatric Surgery, The Children's Hospital, Colorado, Aurora, Colorado, U.S.A.

Robert E. Kelly, Jr., M.D.   Associate Professor of Clinical Surgery and Pediatrics, Eastern Virginia Medical School, Children's Hospital of the King's Daughters, Norfolk, Virginia, U.S.A.

Lucille Kingston, R.N., PNP-BC, CORLN   Pediatric Ear Nose & Throat Associates, Women and Children's Hospital of Buffalo, Buffalo, New York, U.S.A.

M. Ann Kuhn, M.D.   Assistant Professor of Surgery and Pediatrics, Eastern Virginia Medical School, Children's Hospital of the King's Daughters, Norfolk, Virginia, U.S.A.

Linda C. Laing, J.D.   Partner, Notaro, Laing, & Navarro, P.C., Buffalo, New York, U.S.A.

Jacob C. Langer, M.D.   Professor of Surgery, University of Toronto, and Chief and Robert M. Filler Chair, Pediatric and General and Thoracic Surgery, Hospital for Sick Children, Toronto, Ontario, Canada

Stanley T. Lau, M.D.   Chief Resident in Pediatric Surgery, State University of New York at Buffalo, Women and Children's Hospital of Buffalo, Buffalo, New York, U.S.A.

Lucian L. Leape, M.D.   Adjunct Professor of Health Policy, Department of Health Policy and Management, Harvard School of Public Health, Cambridge, Massachusetts, U.S.A.

Michael S. Leonard, M.D., M.S.   Pediatric Quality & Safety Officer, Associate Director, Pediatric Hospital Medicine, Golisano Children's Hospital at Strong, University of Rochester Medical Center, Rochester, New York, U.S.A.

Marc A. Levitt, M.D.   Associate Professor of Surgery, University of Cincinnati School of Medicine, and Associate Director, Colorectal Center, Cincinnati Children's Hospital Medical Center, Cincinnati, Ohio, U.S.A.

Carmel A. McComiskey, M.S., PNP-BC, CPNP-AC   Clinical Instructor in Surgery and Nursing, University of Maryland School of Medicine and Nursing, Division of Pediatric Surgery, Baltimore, Maryland, U.S.A.

Kimberly W. McCrudden, M.D.   Clinical Assistant Professor of Surgery, Division of Pediatric Surgery, Department of Surgery, University of Michigan Health System, and Co-Director, Extracorporeal Life Support, C.S. Mott Children's Hospital, Ann Arbor, Michigan, U.S.A.

John J. Nance, J.D.   Southern Methodist University, Dallas, Texas, and Founding Member, National Patient Safety Foundation, Tacoma, Washington, U.S.A.

Kurt D. Newman, M.D.   Professor of Surgery and Pediatrics, George Washington University, and Executive Director, Joseph E. Robert Jr. Center for Surgical Care, Children's National Medical Center, Washington, D.C., U.S.A.

Oluyinka O. Olutoye, M.B.Ch.B., Ph.D.   Associate Professor, Departments of Surgery, Pediatrics, and Obstetrics and Gynecology, Baylor College of Medicine, and Co-Director, Texas Children's Fetal Center, Texas Children's Hospital, Houston, Texas, U.S.A.

Kyriacos Panayides, M.D. Pediatric Surgeon, Pediatric Subspecialty Clinic, Des Moines, Iowa, U.S.A.

Richard H. Pearl, M.D. Professor of Surgery and Pediatrics, University of Illinois College of Medicine, Peoria, and Director of Pediatric Trauma, Surgeon-in-Chief, Children's Hospital of Illinois, Peoria, Illinois, U.S.A.

Alberto Peña, M.D. Professor of Surgery and Pediatrics, University of Cincinnati College of Medicine, and Director, Colorectal Center for Children, Cincinnati Children's Hospital Medical Center, Cincinnati, Ohio, U.S.A.

Todd A. Ponsky, M.D. Assistant Professor of Surgery, Division of Pediatric Surgery, Case Western Reserve University, and Attending Surgeon, Rainbow Babies and Children's Hospital, Cleveland, Ohio, U.S.A.

Shawn J. Rangel, M.D. Clinical Instructor in Surgery, Harvard Medical School, and Attending Surgeon, Children's Hospital Boston, Boston, Massachusetts, U.S.A.

Sara K. Rasmussen, M.D., Ph.D. Resident in General Surgery, Medical College of Virginia, Virginia Commonwealth University Health System, Richmond, Virginia, U.S.A.

Nicholas C. Saenz, M.D. Division of Pediatric Surgery, Rady Children's Hospital, San Diego, and Voluntary Assistant Clinical Professor, Department of Surgery, University of California, San Diego, San Diego, California, U.S.A.

Michael A. Skinner, M.D. Edwin Ide Smith M.D. Professor of Pediatric Surgery, University of Texas Southwestern, Children's Medical Center of Dallas, Dallas, Texas, U.S.A.

Steven Stylianos, M.D. Professor of Surgery, University of Miami Leonard M. Miller School of Medicine, and Chief, Department of Pediatric Surgery, Regional Pediatric Trauma Program, Miami Children's Hospital, Miami, Florida, U.S.A.

Michael G. Vitale, M.D. Herbert Irving Assistant Professor of Orthopaedic Surgery, Columbia University College of Physicians and Surgeons, and Director, Pediatric Outcome Studies, International Center for Health Outcomes and Innovation Research, Children's Hospital of New York, New York, New York, U.S.A.

Sani Z. Yamout, M.D. Research Fellow in Pediatric Surgery, Division of Pediatric Surgery, Women and Children's Hospital of Buffalo, Buffalo, New York, U.S.A.

Jennifer K. Yates, M.D. Section of Pediatric Urology, Hasbro Children's Hospital, and Resident in Urology, Division of Urology, Alpert School of Medicine, Brown University, Providence, Rhode Island, U.S.A.

Garret Zallen, M.D. Assistant Professor of Surgery, Oregon Health Sciences University, Attending Surgeon, Doernbecher Children's Hospital, Portland, Oregon, U.S.A.

Expert Contributors

Craig T. Albanese, M.D.   Professor of Surgery, Pediatrics, and Obstetrics and Gynecology, Chief, Division of Pediatric Surgery, Stanford Hospitals & Clinics, and John A. and Cynthia Fry Gunn Director of Surgical Services, Lucile Packard Children's Hospital, Stanford, California, U.S.A.

R. Peter Altman, M.D.   Professor of Surgery, Columbia University College of Physicians and Surgeons, and Surgeon-in-Chief, Morgan Stanley Children's Hospital of New York Presbyterian, New York, New York, U.S.A.

Richard G. Azizkhan, M.D.   Professor of Surgery and Pediatrics, Lester Martin Chair of Pediatric Surgery, and Vice Chair, Department of Surgery, University of Cincinnati School of Medicine, and Surgeon-in-Chief, Cincinnati Children's Hospital Medical Center, Cincinnati, Ohio, U.S.A.

Charles E. Bagwell, M.D.   Professor and Chairman, Division of Pediatric Surgery, Medical College of Virginia, and Attending Surgeon, Virginia Commonwealth University Health System, Richmond, Virginia, U.S.A.

Arnold G. Coran, M.D.   Professor of Pediatric Surgery, University of Michigan Medical School, Ann Arbor, Michigan, U.S.A.

Andrew M. Davidoff, M.D.   Associate Professor, Department of Surgery and Pediatrics, University of Tennessee School of Medicine, and Chief, Division of General Pediatric Surgery, St. Jude Children's Research Hospital, Memphis, Tennessee, U.S.A.

Sigmund H. Ein, M.D.   Associate Professor of Surgery, Adjunct Clinical Faculty, University of Toronto, Faculty of Medicine, and Honorary Staff Surgeon, The Hospital for Sick Children, Toronto, Ontario, Canada

Jay L. Grosfeld, M.D.   Lafayette Page Professor and Chairman Emeritus, Department of Surgery, Indiana University School of Medicine, Surgeon-in-Chief and Director of Pediatric Surgery Emeritus, Riley Hospital for Children, Indianapolis, Indiana, U.S.A.

Carroll M. Harmon, M.D., Ph.D.   Associate Professor of Surgery, University of Alabama at Birmingham School of Medicine, and Attending Surgeon, Children's Hospital Birmingham, Alabama, U.S.A.

George W. Holcomb, M.D., M.B.A.   Katherine Berry Richardson Professor of Surgery, University of Missouri-Kansas City School of Medicine, and Surgeon-in-Chief, Children's Mercy Hospital, Kansas City, Missouri, U.S.A.

Michael D. Klein, M.D.   Arvin I. Phillipart Chair and Professor of Surgery, Wayne State University School of Medicine, and Surgeon-in-Chief, Children's Hospital of Michigan, Detroit, Michigan, U.S.A.

Kevin P. Lally, M.D., M.S.   Professor of Surgery, Chairman, Department of Pediatric Surgery, University of Texas Medical School, Houston, and Surgeon-in-Chief, Children's Memorial Hermann Hospital, Houston, Texas, U.S.A.

Jacob C. Langer, M.D.   Professor of Surgery, University of Toronto, and Chief and Robert M. Filler Chair, Pediatric and General and Thoracic Surgery, Hospital for Sick Children, Toronto, Ontario, Canada

Thom E. Lobe, M.D.   Professor of Pediatrics, University of Tennessee Health Science Center, Memphis, Tennessee; Adjunct Clinical Professor of Surgery, Iowa University, Iowa City; and Adjunct Professor of Pediatric Surgery, Des Moines University College of Medicine, Des Moines, Iowa, U.S.A.

Dennis P. Lund, M.D.   Chairman, Division of General Surgery, University of Wisconsin-Madison, Surgeon-in-Chief, University of Wisconsin Children's Hospital, Madison, Wisconsin, U.S.A.

Kurt D. Newman, M.D.   Professor of Surgery and Pediatrics, George Washington University, and Executive Director, Joseph E. Robert Jr. Center for Surgical Care, Children's National Medical Center, Washington, D.C., U.S.A.

Donald Nuss, M.B.Ch.B.   Professor of Clinical Surgery and Pediatrics, Eastern Virginia Medical School, and Attending Surgeon, Children's Hospital of the King's Daughters, Norfolk, Virginia, U.S.A.

Alberto Peña, M.D.   Professor of Surgery and Pediatrics, University of Cincinnati College of Medicine, and Director, Colorectal Center for Children, Cincinnati Children's Hospital Medical Center, Cincinnati, Ohio, U.S.A.

Frederick J. Rescorla, M.D.   Professor of Surgery, Indiana University School of Medicine, and Surgeon-in-Chief, Riley Hospital for Children, Indianapolis, Indiana, U.S.A.

Frederick C. Ryckman, M.D.   Professor of Surgery, University of Cincinnati College of Medicine; and Director, Liver Transplantation, and Surgical Director, Intestinal Transplant Surgery, Cincinnati Children's Hospital Medical Center, Cincinnati, Ohio, U.S.A.

Robert Sawin, M.D.   Professor of Surgery, University of Washington School of Medicine, Surgeon-in-Chief, Children's Hospital and Regional Medical Center, Seattle, Washington, U.S.A.

Felix Schier, M.D.   Professor and Head, Department of Pediatrics Surgery, University Medical Center, Mainz, Germany

Charles J. Stolar, M.D.   Professor of Surgery and Pediatrics, Columbia University College of Physicians and Surgeons, and Chief, Pediatric Surgery, Morgan Stanley Children's Hospital of New York-Presbyterian, New York, New York, U.S.A.

Steven Stylianos, M.D.   Professor of Surgery, University of Miami Leonard M. Miller School of Medicine, and Chief, Department of Pediatric Surgery, Regional Pediatric Trauma Program, Miami Children's Hospital, Miami, Florida, U.S.A.

Brad W. Warner, M.D.   Apolline Blair Professor of Surgery, Washington University School of Medicine, and Surgeon-in-Chief, Saint Louis Children's Hospital, Saint Louis, Missouri, U.S.A.

Pierre Williot, M.D.   Clinical Associate Professor of Surgery, State University of New York at Buffalo, and Attending Surgeon, Women and Children's Hospital of Buffalo, Buffalo, New York, U.S.A.

SECTION I | Scope of the Problem/Systems Approach

1 | Errors in Medicine

Lucian L. Leape, M.D.

INTRODUCTION

The subject of medical error has seldom been discussed, either privately or publicly, until quite recently (1). Physicians and nurses have been reluctant to discuss their mistakes, feelings exacerbated by the adversarial climate produced by the threat of malpractice litigation. The public also preferred to believe that errors in medical practice were rare, and seldom questioned their care.

On the other hand, surgeons have a long tradition of examining their mistakes in weekly morbidity and mortality conferences. Surgery requires both pragmatism and honesty. One learns early not to continue to do things that do not work, to do what does work, and to be analytical about mishaps. Complications occur and cannot be ignored or wished away. For example, you cannot ignore the postoperative patient with persistent fever or increasing abdominal distension. Surgeons have experience in admitting mistakes. Our response to them, however, has not been as successful as it could be.

EXTENT OF THE PROBLEM OF ERROR AND ACCIDENTAL INJURY

In 1991, the Harvard Medical Practice Study (MPS) reported the results of a large and comprehensive study of accidental injury of patients in hospitals. It evaluated the incidence, cause, and consequences of adverse events (AEs). AEs were defined as unintended injuries caused by medical treatment that result in a measurable disability (including death) or a prolongation of hospital stay. In this randomly selected sample of 30,000 patients hospitalized in acute care hospitals in the state of New York, the investigators found 1133 AEs, which represented an injury rate of 3.7 per hundred admissions. This worked out to an estimated 98,609 AEs a year in the state of New York. Fourteen percent of patients died as a result of their injuries (2,3).

If these results are extrapolated to the nation as a whole, it is estimated that nationwide 1.3 million people are injured annually by treatment intended to help them, and that 180,000 people die each year as a result of medical accidents. Further analysis revealed that more than two-thirds of these injuries were due to errors (defined as an unintended act, either of omission or commission, or one that does not achieve its intended outcome) and thus were preventable (4). In 1991, Bedel reported that 64% of cardiac arrests at a teaching hospital were caused by errors. Misuse of medications was the leading cause (5).

Medication errors have been studied most extensively, and numerous studies have found them to be common: nursing dosing errors have been reported as high as 20% (6). Fortunately, most of these are minor, such as giving a medication late or failing to observe the patient actually take the dose. However, a study of adverse drug events in two Harvard teaching hospitals found that serious errors in the use of medications, those that caused injuries, occurred in nearly 2% of patients, while an additional 5.5% experienced "near misses," errors with potential for injury that were intercepted or by luck failed to cause harm (7).

In late 1999, the Institute of Medicine (IOM) released an analysis of the problem of medical error, entitled "To Err is Human" (8). This publication provided an updated extrapolation from the MPS and a subsequent study in Utah and Colorado, from which it estimated that 44,000 to 98,000 people die annually in the United States as a result of medical errors.

The report stimulated a swift response among policy-makers. Within 2 weeks of its release, Congress began hearings and the President ordered a government-wide study of the feasibility of implementing its recommendations. Subsequently, the President directed governmental agencies and departments, including the Department of Defense, Department of Veterans Affairs, and the Health Care Financing Agency to implement the IOM recommendations.

Meanwhile, professional societies and health care organizations intensified their efforts in patient safety.

Some have questioned the validity of the IOM/MPS estimates. Unfortunately, these were probably underestimates because they were based on record reviews, which are incomplete sources, and confined to inpatients, who receive only a fraction of all medical treatments. Later studies of specific injuries (such as adverse drug events or nosocomial infections) have invariably come up with higher numbers.

Many physicians, nonetheless, find the numbers hard to believe because they are not consistent with their personal experience. There are several reasons why this is so. First, observational studies reveal that most errors are unknown to the one making them. Even when they result in injury, the antecedent errors are often not recognized. Second, normal psychological defense mechanisms lead us to rationalize, repress, or forget mistakes, so they are not carried as mental "data" unless they are particularly bad and embarrassing. Third is the problem of rates versus actual numbers. The estimate that nearly 100,000 patients die annually from medical errors results, on average, in only one preventable death per physician every 6 years. Given that at least half would not be recognized, the number of preventable deaths *perceived* by a physician might be only one per 12 years, which does not seem bad to most of us. Yet this low individual rate results overall in 100,000 deaths per year. Similarly, a 1% prescribing error applied to the over 3 billion prescriptions written annually can cause a large number of adverse drug events, even if only one in 100 errors results in harm.

RELUCTANCE TO DEAL WITH ERRORS

Traditionally, health professionals—doctors, nurses, and pharmacists in particular—have had a great deal of difficulty in dealing with human error. One of the reasons is the emphasis during training on the need for error-free practice (9). In everyday hospital practice, the message is equally clear: mistakes are unacceptable. Because doctors, nurses, and pharmacists are expected to function without error, they feel ashamed and inadequate when they make mistakes, as they inevitably do (1). This is the downside of a laudable goal of professional training: developing a sense of responsibility for the patient. If you feel personally responsible for a patient, you also feel personally responsible for anything that goes wrong.

These high standards of practice are reinforced in hospital practice by an unforgiving system of censure and discipline. We strive to eliminate errors by requiring perfection, and respond to failure (error) by blaming individuals. Errors are assumed to be someone's fault, caused by a lack of sufficient attention or, worse, lack of caring enough to do it right.

Not surprisingly, this "blame and train" approach to medical error creates strong pressure on individuals to cover up mistakes rather than to admit them (10). Even if punishment is not overt, the realization that their colleagues will regard them as incompetent or careless makes many health professionals reluctant to admit or discuss their errors. For physicians, the ever-present threat of malpractice litigation provides an additional incentive to keep silent about mistakes. Even a minor error can place the physician's whole career in jeopardy if it results in a serious bad outcome.

Students of error and human performance reject the "blame and train" approach to error prevention. While the proximal error leading to an accident is, in fact, usually a "human error," the causes of that error are often well beyond the individual's control. Systems that rely on perfect performance by individuals to prevent errors are doomed to fail, for the simple reason that humans are incapable of perfect performance. If doctors, nurses, pharmacists, and administrators are to succeed in reducing errors in hospital care, they will need to fundamentally change the way they think about errors and why they occur. Fortunately, a great deal has been learned about error prevention in other disciplines, information that is relevant to the hospital practice of medicine.

CAUSES OF ERRORS

To reduce errors, we need to understand why people make them. Two disciplines, cognitive psychology and human factors engineering have studied errors intensively for the past half century or more. While a review of these activities is beyond the scope of this chapter, several insights are particularly helpful in developing an approach to error reduction in health care.

The most important lesson from this research, which should come as no surprise, is that human error is common. We all make mistakes every day. Second, errors are not "accidents," but occur because of well-known mechanisms, such as loss of attention due to interruptions or distractions. In a real sense, errors are "normal" pathology. Third, error is often a byproduct of useful attributes of human cognition, such as the ability to relegate complex but routine tasks to automatic function, which frees our minds for other functions, but also "sets us up" for slips and lapses when attention is diverted. The ability to change focus of attention rapidly lets us react promptly to multiple stimuli, but it also allows us to become distracted easily. The ability to generalize from prior experience helps us to understand new situations, but it also causes biased memory and oversimplification.

A common cause of errors is being required to perform activities—tasks and processes— that rely on mental functions that are known to be weak, such as short-term memory. For example, physicians rely on their memory for determining the dose of a drug; nurses rely on their memory to give a medication on time, and to the right patient. To a human factors specialist, it is not surprising that many errors occur in these common functions. The corollary of the observation that errors are caused by reliance on weak cognitive functions is that errors can be prevented by designing tasks and processes that minimize dependency on these functions.

Latent Errors and Systems Failures

Cognitive psychologists and human factors experts have taught us that errors often happen because of conditions beyond the individual's control—defects in the systems in which we work that lead us to make mistakes. Reason (11) has called these *latent* errors, errors whose effects are delayed—"accidents waiting to happen"—in contrast to *active* errors, whose effects are felt immediately. Reason and Perrow (12) believe these systems failures are the "root causes" of errors. They are failures in the design of processes, in the management of the conditions of work, and in training of individuals for their jobs. These are proximal errors that become manifest when individuals "at the sharp end" make an error that directly results in patient injury.

An important type of latent error has been labeled *psychological precursors* by Reason. These are working conditions that predispose to errors. Inappropriate work schedules, for example, can result in high workloads and undue time pressures, conditions that induce errors. Poor training can lead to inadequate recognition of hazards or inappropriate procedures that lead to accidents. A precursor can be the product of more than one management or training failure. For example, excessive time pressure can result from poor scheduling, but it can also be the product of inadequate training or faulty division of responsibilities. Because they can affect all cognitive processes, these antecedent errors can cause a diverse group of unsafe acts that in turn result in an immense variety of errors.

Successful error prevention efforts must focus on *underlying causes*—errors in design and implementation of processes and systems, not on the errors themselves. If this theory is correct, and most thoughtful students of error prevention believe that it is, then to prevent errors it is these *systems failures* we must correct.

SYSTEMS FAILURES

Which are the most serious systems failures? Where can remedial efforts be most profitably targeted?

Systems failures can be grouped into two broad categories: design failures and organization and environmental failures. Both types of failures are common in health care organizations.

Design Failures

Many hospital systems were never "designed" in the true sense, but just grew. As a result, errors are often induced simply because the processes have not been thought out and basic human factors principles have been disregarded in their design. Design failures can be classified into three categories: process design, task design, and equipment design.

Process design failures result from failure to analyze the purposes of the system and how best to achieve them, for example: What are objectives of the system? How can it best meet users' needs? What are the potential hazards of this process? What are all the ways something can go wrong? "What ifs?" (Thinking through the consequences of actions that can go wrong).

For example, what is the system for making sure that perioperative antibiotics are administered to every patient who needs them (and none who do not), in the right dose, at the right time? The science behind their use is well established, and the objectives are clear. But how fail-safe are the methods for ensuring 100% on-time performance? Most hospital systems fall woefully short. Similarly, methods for ensuring no-fail identification of the surgical site in two-sided situations are inadequate in most hospitals. Methods for tracking and positively identifying drug, dose, and patient are often primitive when compared to the systems in common use in industry. Every day patients get drugs intended for others and drugs to which they are known to be allergic. Supermarkets do a better job of keeping track of their products than many hospitals do in keeping track of their drugs!

Task design failures result from failure to incorporate *human factors principles* in design. A human factors principle is a concept of designing a task so it is easy to do it correctly and difficult to do it wrong. Some examples of human factors principles:

- *Reduce reliance on memory*. Work should be designed to minimize the requirements for human functions that are known to be particularly fallible, such as short-term memory and vigilance (prolonged attention).
- *Standardization* reinforces pattern recognition that humans do well. It is one of the most effective ways to prevent errors—witness the aviation checklists, maintenance protocols, etc. The advantages, in efficiency, as well as in error reduction, of standardizing drug doses and times of administration are obvious. Is it really acceptable to ask nurses to follow six different "K-scales" (directions for how much potassium to give according to patient serum potassium levels) solely to satisfy different physician prescribing patterns? Other candidates for standardization include information displays, methods for common practices (such as surgical dressings), and the geographic location of equipment and supplies in a patient care unit.
- *Simplification* reduces errors by reducing the number of opportunities for error. If a single task can be performed flawlessly 99% of the time, the overall success rate for a sequence that included 10 such tasks would be only 90% (0.99 to the 10th power). For a 40-step process (such as the medication system in most hospitals), the overall error-free rate at the 0.99 level would be 67%. Merely reducing the number of steps from 40 to 10 would dramatically reduce the overall error rate.
- *Constraints and forcing functions*. A constraint is the design of a task to make it *difficult* to do it wrong. A "forcing function" is a design feature that makes it *impossible* to do it wrong (such as the lock that prohibits release of the parking gear of a car unless the brake pedal is depressed.). Removal of concentrated KCl from nursing units was a forcing function that eliminated the accidental (lethal) intravenous injection of concentrated KCl that occurred several times every year in U.S. hospitals. Similarly, if a computerized system is used for medication orders, it can be designed so that a physician cannot enter an order for a lethal overdose of a drug, nor prescribe a medication a patient is known to be allergic to.
- *Protocols and checklists*. Physicians should not have to rely on their memories to retrieve a laboratory test result, nor remember every medication that a patient should receive, nor what all the steps in a complicated treatment consist of. Nor should nurses have to remember the time a medication dose is due. The evidence is clear: reliance on memory is a prescription for failure. Predictable, inevitable failure—and, with modern methods, no longer excusable. Checklists, protocols, and computerized decision aids are effective methods for assisting in these chores. Computers are even better and much more reliable than humans.

Equipment design failures result from failure to apply basic human factors principles in the design of display and controls so that they are readily understood (13). It is truly astonishing that most people using most of the equipment in hospitals do not understand how the equipment works. This is primarily a design problem—manufacturers often have not seen to it that the complicated and vital equipment that we use (such as anesthesia machines, ventilators, cardiac assist devices, etc.) presents the users with information and controls that can be readily understood. It is incredible that in most hospitals it is still possible to connect to an epidural catheter a syringe with medication prepared only for intravenous use (such as vincristine) with lethal results. A simple forcing function design (such as has long been used with oxygen and nitrous oxide connections in anesthesia machines) could prevent this error.

Organizational and Environmental Failures

The most profound systems failures, understandably, occur at the organizational and environmental level. Health care organizations are particularly dysfunctional. Lack of commitment to safety, a punitive environment that inhibits reporting and discussion of errors and AEs, and lack of leadership are common systems failures that prevent creation of a safe environment in many hospitals and practices.

The contrast of most health care organizations with "high reliability" organizations (HRO) is instructive. These are intrinsically hazardous industries that have succeeded in becoming amazingly safe (such as aviation, nuclear power, and aluminum manufacturing) (14,15). The characteristic that sets HRO apart from the rest is a fierce commitment to prevention of injury. Safety is truly "Job 1." It is the CEO's primary responsibility. The safety program has a budget, a plan, and accountability. Goals are set and progress is monitored.

HRO are "learning" organizations, to use Senge's term (16). When mishaps occur, they respond with concern, curiosity, and action. Messengers are rewarded, not punished. A serious accident is not covered up or discounted, but is looked upon as an opportunity for improvement. It is promptly and intensively investigated to uncover the underlying causes and correct them. The objective is to prevent recurrence, not prevent embarrassment, which is so often perceived by the public to be the objective for hospitals when things go wrong. Safety is recognized as a systems problem. Safety is also everyone's responsibility.

HRO also recognize the importance of working conditions and managerial style in creating a safe and supportive work place. By contrast, in many hospitals excessive workloads and long working hours are commonplace. Witness the recent struggles for nurses to eliminate mandatory overtime and excessive staffing ratios, and of housestaff to achieve humane working hours.

Finally, HRO recognize the value of teams. When individuals work well with one another they help each another avoid mistakes, intercept errors, and reduce psychological precursors. In general, hospitals have been poor team builders because doctors and nurses have traditionally functioned semi-autonomously, and autocratically, at times in actual conflict.

OBSTACLES TO SYSTEMS RE-DESIGN

Like any established institution, the modern hospital presents significant barriers to those who seek to change its practices. While these appear to both extensive and daunting, their recognition is the first step in designing methods to overcome them. The following major obstacles are found in most hospitals:

1. *A culture of shame and blame.* In most hospitals, there are strong sanctions (overt or covert) against those who make mistakes. Because errors are thought to be due to carelessness, workers are punished when they make mistakes. For physicians, such "punishment" is more likely covert—disapproval or shunning. As a result, most failures are not reported (17). Failures are also not discussed, which makes improvement, i.e., systems redesign, impossible.
2. *Infrequent occurrence of events.* Despite the alarming statistics that have been reported, serious errors are not common events in the experience of most hospital professionals. We hear about sensational errors—the lethal dose of potassium, etc.—but most doctors, pharmacists, and nurses do not see that kind of error even once a year. The low frequency of errors leads to complacency; it also means that a change targeted at a low frequency problem can increase work for a low yield.
3. *Complexity and lack of ownership.* Hospital systems are complex, involving a wide variety of personnel and interlocking flows of materials and information. Many individuals have interests in multiple operations, and each system and subsystem has multiple stakeholders, but none of the stakeholders has complete control of any of the systems—there are no owners. The system for ordering, dispensing, and administering medications is a good example of

the challenges posed by complex systems. This system is characterized by multiple actors (physicians, nurses, pharmacists, clerks, and technicians), multiple choices (drugs, names, routes, and doses), multiple hand-offs that are frequent and fragile, no ownership, no natural team, and no one with hospital-wide authority to make changes and insure quality.

4. *Information nonavailability.* Because of the complexity of processes, information transfer can pose a major challenge to knowledge-based problem solving. In a study of systems analysis of adverse drug events, lack of information about the patient and lack of knowledge of drugs were found to be the most common systems failures, accounting for 40% of the serious, injury-producing errors (18). Modern medicine is complicated—it is difficult to remember everything one needs to know to diagnose, treat, and monitor care in all kinds of patients. It is also difficult to insure that all the pertinent information about each patient is readily available to all who are involved in decisions about care. Doctors, nurses, pharmacists, and others need to have information available when it is needed, where it is needed, and in a form that can be readily used.

5. *Physician resistance.* Physicians have been reluctant participants in the modern safety movement. Why? An obvious, and oft-cited, reason is the fear of inciting malpractice litigation. Many do not believe that state peer review statutes provide adequate protection. Although there are no studies demonstrating that internal review of mishaps increases malpractice risk, and those hospitals that are making major strides in safety do not have higher suit rates, many physicians choose not to take the chance.

   A second reason is that many do not accept the systems concept. It seems like a vague and complicated solution to a simple problem: you made a mistake—take your punishment. It goes against everything we have been taught—if we are careful and do our homework, we won't make mistakes. And, it smacks of irresponsibility: "Don't blame me, it's the system." Finally, as indicated above, many do not believe the numbers: the high rates of injury and death do not jibe with their personal experience.

6. *Lack of leadership.* It is not just doctors who have not signed on to the safety movement, neither have the CEOs of most hospitals and health care systems. They also do not believe the numbers, they also are caught in the blaming approach to safety and they, too, are not sure they believe the systems approach. CEOs are leery of getting ahead of their doctors since they have limited control over their practices. Finally, they do not feel much pressure, from the public or from their boards to change.

7. *Tolerance of stylistic practices.* One manifestation of lack of leadership is the long tradition of hospitals catering to the idiosyncrasies and special demands of individual physicians. In drug prescribing, for example, tolerance of illegible orders, nonstandard orders, and catering to prescribing differences all contribute to the likelihood of error. Noncompliance with safety practices, such as hand disinfecting and "sign your site" policies, is also tolerated. No other business or industry would tolerate such flagrant disregard of its policies. Following rules is basic. Safe practice cannot be achieved in such an environment. Clearly, changing such long-standing practices can be a formidable challenge.

The evidence is indisputable. Medical errors result from a complex interplay of multiple factors. Yet, rather than addressing those underlying system design faults, error prevention has traditionally relied almost exclusively on the carefulness and dedication of individual caregivers, reinforced by punishment for failure. But punishment drives reporting of errors underground, preventing the very systems examination that is needed to discover the underlying causes.

CREATING SAFE HEALTH CARE

Achieving a high level of accident-free care requires a total institutional commitment. Safe care cannot be accomplished by individuals alone, however careful they may be or however hard they try. It is the systems that must be changed. Hospitals that wish to utilize a systems analysis approach to error reduction need to have a substantial commitment of leadership and be willing to provide necessary resources. In hospitals that are serious about safety, progress in system redesign is the subject of every meeting of the executive committee and every meeting of the Board of Directors. Safety is truly "Job 1."

Changes must occur at the organizational/environment level and in specific practices. At the organization level, institutional policies must reflect a commitment to a nonblaming supportive environment: prohibition of punishment for making errors, limitations on work hours and workloads, training for safety, honesty and openness in dealing with mistakes, and a genuine interest in understanding and correcting the underlying failures behind serious events. Both management and staff must accept the idea that errors are inevitable everyday occurrences, and personnel need to be convinced that information generated by error reporting and investigation will not be used against them. In the current climate in most hospitals, this may prove to be the most challenging task.

"High-reliability" organizations have found that training personnel to work in teams significantly reduces errors. In addition, they find that attention to worker safety (injury rates in health workers are higher than in many manufacturing industries) improves overall performance. Attention to these considerations, in addition to providing humane workloads and duty hours, almost certainly will pay off in health care as well.

At the practice level, hospitals need to proceed on two levels simultaneously. First, any hospital that is serious about safety should have a "crash" program to implement all known safe practices. The National Quality Forum (NQF) has identified 30 such proven practices. Beginning in 2003, the Joint Commission required that hospitals implement some of these safe practices (e.g., positive methods for identification of the patient and the site of surgery) (19), and they become part of the standards for the accreditation inspections. New practices from the NQF list are added each year. Second, hospitals must work at redesign of systems that are known to be inadequate. These are easily identified by frontline workers (nurses, doctors, pharmacists, etc.) if they are asked to be involved in the process. Continuing problems in failure to administer perioperative antibiotics on time, inadequate protocols for dealing with wrong sponge counts, recurring episodes of hypoglycemia in diabetics, failure of prompt and adequate anticoagulation, mix-ups of intravenous solutions, and wound infections are common problems in most hospitals. Personnel should be empowered to work on the problems that they find most pressing—and given the resources (time, expertise) to redesign their systems.

Creating a safe process, whether it be redesigning care plans or performing surgery, requires attention to methods of error reduction at each stage of system development: design, construction, maintenance, allocation of resources, training, and development of operational procedures. Responsible individuals at each stage need to think through the consequences of their decisions and to reason back from discovered deficiencies to re-design and re-organize the process.

In addition to this agenda, the manner by which hospitals respond to errors and accidents is revealing. In an organization that truly seeks to create a culture of safety, serious mishaps are treated as opportunities for learning and improvement, not as embarrassments to be concealed. Reporting is safe and worthwhile. Strenuous efforts are made to uncover the multiple underlying contributing factors (there is never a single "root cause") and correct those that can be corrected. The importance of the presence of psychological precursors as causes should not be minimized. Changes in the work environment to reduce stress, equalize workloads, and insure appropriate training of personnel are as important methods of error reduction as technically dazzling innovations such as computerized order entry.

SYSTEMS VERSUS PERSONAL RESPONSIBILITY

Not uncommonly, when they first hear about the systems approach to error prevention, doctors will respond with concern that not punishing a person for making an error relieves him of responsibility. Actually, the converse is true. The person who makes an error is the one who has the most responsibility—to try to identify the underlying systems failures and do something about them to prevent someone else from making the same mistake later. While systems investigation and analysis require expertise, the individual who has made an error has more information than anyone as to what the underlying factors might be; he must be an active participant in the investigation. In a safety-oriented organization, every employee also feels a personal responsibility to identify unsafe conditions before an accident occurs, report them, and work toward their elimination. This is much more difficult than just reporting errors.

On the other hand, if a doctor or nurse has injured a patient through an error caused by carelessness, egregious misconduct, neglect, or criminal activity, he or she must be accountable. Often, however, that person had a prior history of reckless behavior and disregard of safe practices. Why was he or she permitted to continue working? That is the management question. Responsibility does not begin when accidents occur. Simply put, management must "manage" for patient safety just as they manage for efficiency and profit maximization.

IMPLICATIONS OF THE NONPUNITIVE SYSTEMS APPROACH TO PREVENTION OF SURGICAL COMPLICATIONS

Most surgeons tend to think of complications as being of two types: preventable and unpreventable. The former are caused by errors, the latter by factors we do not understand. In spite of (apparently) flawless technique, some patients bleed or have wound infections. But *all* "un preventable" surgical complications are ultimately preventable. They await advances in science. And those advances will come. The complications of today are very different from those of 30 or 40 years ago: heart block, bleeding, and heart failure in the early days of heart surgery, newborns who died of respiratory failure before there were adequate ventilators, or those who died following neonatal intestinal surgery before the development of total parenteral nutrition. These complications yielded to the advance of scientific understanding. Our current crop will also disappear with time as we learn more.

Preventable complications, on the other hand, occur not because of lack of scientific knowledge or understanding, but because of failures of execution—because of errors or other defects in care. These we can do something about right now. And many people are. There are care units that have succeeded in getting 100% of patients to receive indicated perioperative antibiotics on time. Some have virtually eliminated ventilator-associated pneumonia; others have had no line sepsis for 6 months. We all can—and should—learn from these models of excellence.

Actually, the two types of complications are not that different once one accepts the notion that human errors are caused by systems failures. There is a system's cause behind every failure, whether caused by an error or not, and recognizing that cause is the first step in its correction. But the secret in every case is to focus on the process, not the person. Safety by design.

The challenge in patient safety is immense. We need to make major changes in our culture—away from shaming and blaming to supporting and collaboration, away from focus on the individual to focus on the system, away from defensiveness and concealment to openness and inquiry. Not only do we have the major immediate task of implementing known safe practices, we must embark on an aggressive search for hazards—"accidents waiting to happen"—and redesign our systems before accidents occur, not afterward.

The important challenge for physicians is not just to think beyond individual performance to systems, but also to expand our focus beyond the individual to the care team. Teams provide better and safer care. Physicians need to be full members of teams—leaders, not commanders. Leaders who respect the expertise and commitment of nurses, pharmacists, technicians, and others, and show that respect in how we treat them and in our concern about their hours, work loads, and working conditions. Safety is a team sport, and everyone has to be on the team.

REFERENCES

1. Leape L. Error in medicine. JAMA 1994;272:1851–1857.
2. Brennan TA, Leape LL, Laird N, et al. Incidence of adverse events and negligence in hospitalized patients: Results from the Harvard Medical Practice Study I. New Eng J Med 1991;324:370–376.
3. Leape LL, Brennan TA, Laird NM, et al. The nature of adverse events in hospitalized patients: Results from the Harvard Medical Practice Study II. New Eng J Med 1991;324:377–384.
4. Leape LL, Lawthers AG, Brennan TA, et al. Preventing medical injury. Qual Rev Bull 1993;19:144–149.
5. Bedell S, Deitz D, Leeman D, et al. Incidence and characteristics of preventable iatrogenic cardiac arrests. JAMA 1991;265:2815–2820.
6. Barker KN, Flynn EA, Pepper GA, et al. Medication errors observed in 36 health care facilities. Arch Intern Med 2002;162:1897–1903.
7. Bates DW, Cullen DJ, Laird N, et al. Incidence of adverse drug events and potential adverse drug events. JAMA 1995;274:29–34.
8. Kohn KT, Corrigan JM, Donaldson MS, eds. To Err is Human: Building a Safer Health System. Washington, DC: National Academy Press, 1999.

9. Hilfiker D. Facing our mistakes. New Eng J Med 1984;310:118–122.

10. McIntyre N, Popper K. The critical attitude in medicine: The need for a new ethics. Br Med J 1989;287:1919–1923.

11. Reason J. Human Error. Cambridge: Cambridge University Press, 1990.

12. Perrow C. Normal Accidents. Living with High-Risk Technologies. New York: Basic Books, 1984.

13. Norman DA. The Design of Everyday Things. 1st Doubleday/Currency ed. New York: Doubleday, 1990.

14. Weick KE, Sutcliffe KM, Obstfeld D. Organizing for high reliability. Res Organizat Behav 1999;21:81–123.

15. Weick KE. Organizational culture as a source of high reliability. Calif Manage Rev 1987;29:112–127.

16. Senge P, Kleiner A, Roberts C, et al. The Fifth Discipline Fieldbook: Strategies and Tools for Building a Learning Organization. New York: Currency and Doubleday, 1994.

17. Cullen DJ, Bates DW, Small SD, et al. The incident reporting system does not detect adverse drug events. J Qual Improv 1995;21:541–548.

18. Leape LL, Bates DW, Cullen DJ, et al. Systems analysis of adverse drug events. JAMA 1995;274:35–43.

19. JCAHO. Joint Commission announces national patient safety goals. 2002; http://www.jcaho.org/news+room/latest+from+jcaho/npsg.htmv: Accessed 12/03/02.

2 | A Systems Approach to Error Reduction: Lessons from the Aviation Industry

John J. Nance, J.D.*

Over the last decade, health care professionals have been told repeatedly that lessons learned by the aviation industry regarding the maximization of operational safety in a complex human system are, in fact, directly applicable to medical practice. Many practitioners, however, have assumed that those parallels between aviation and medicine were too broad and general to be useful, accepting the erroneous allegation that the lessons from aviation were limited to recommendations for checklists, extreme regimentation, standardization of procedures, and practices which would allegedly reduce life in the OR and the ED to the procedural efficiency of a commercial cockpit (thus embracing what some physicians have derisively referred to as "cookbook medicine").

The reality, however, is that the lessons and discoveries derived from aviation's steep human factors learning curve spanning the past 20 years are startlingly applicable and unexpectedly relevant to medical practice, especially with respect to the safety-critical role of human communications. Given the critical need to improve the perceived patient safety record of health care in general, and the apparent failure of traditional methods of safety improvement to provide more than incremental advances so far, the logic of a deeper examination of the lessons aviation might offer is inescapable.

THE NATURE OF THE EMERGENCY

Following the issuance of a pivotal report from the Institute of Medicine in 1999, *To Err Is Human* (1), there has been growing alarm within the medical community that the public perception of health care and the relative safety of using the American health care system in particular have dropped to unacceptable levels. Indeed, there is increasing print and broadcast attention being paid to various horrifying medical mistakes around the nation. In addition, the corresponding failure of journalists to grasp the systemic nature of medical failures commonly results in shrill reports focusing on guilt and blame rather than causation and systemic correction. The overall result is driving a disturbing perception among Americans that our medical system is dangerous and becoming more so with time. When you couple this slide in public confidence with the increasing Internet availability of medical information to the layman and blend in alarmed patients and families who have been too long systematically excluded from medical decisions and informational interaction, the crisis in confidence, sometimes delivered in a less-than-friendly fashion, becomes a daily challenge to medical practitioners. To make matters worse, add the volatility of the liability insurance crisis and myriad other pressures of practice in all forms of medicine, and the resulting potential for catastrophic misunderstandings with angry parents (whether reasonably so or otherwise) becomes obvious. And, as all understand, such misunderstandings and anger often translate to legal action. At the very least, these extraordinary burdens on health care professionals have created a new, unprecedented need for a vastly improved liaison between patient/family and practitioner, and for pediatric surgeons, that means a major challenge to become both a superlative and an effective communicator when dealing with patients and parents alike.

Correspondingly, within the transparent fishbowl that such increased scrutiny and suspicion creates, the necessity to immediately and fully disclose any error or misadventure affecting the patient, however minor, is exceeded only by the emergency need to vastly improve the safety levels of the practice in the first place.

It is to this latter overarching need—the common quest to significantly minimize the possibility of mistakes impacting patients—that this chapter is primarily addressed.

*Also the author of *Why Hospitals Should Fly* (Second River Press, 2008).

THE FIRST AXIOM—HUMAN ERROR IS INEVITABLE

One of the most difficult lessons that aviation in general and aviators in particular had to learn was based on a reversal of a major cultural assumption: That professional aviators who had the "right stuff" and were appropriately diligent and competent and current and qualified could, when they had acquired sufficient experience, achieve perfect performance, and fly without committing errors. In fact, the entire structure of aviation, whether military, airline, civilian/corporate, or private, has been built on this assumption of attainable infallibility.

So, too, has the training of physicians and nurses been predicated on precisely the same foundation: the assumption of attainable infallibility.

Human beings, however, are not even capable of achieving the reliability rates reached by much of the mechanical and computational equipment we build. While a silicon-based computer may well approach a status of perfect performance (although through the use of complicated algorithms of checking and rechecking), we carbon-based creatures have analog brains with superior cognitive reasoning but grossly inferior error rates.

What does this translate to? The very uncomfortable reality that every pilot is subject to misunderstanding a critical radio call, misreading a critical instrument at a critical moment, permitting fatigue or emotion to cloud his or her good judgment, and in the process, forge a link in what may become a causal accident chain. Standing before the senior airmen in the aviation community to inform them of the sad inevitability of human *fallibility* along these lines has been an unpleasant experience at best for everyone, but despite a temporary period of denial and resistance, the results of this cultural revelation have sparked a revolution of safety improvement.

In medicine the challenge is identical. Physicians and professional pilots (as well as professional military men and women) have traditionally been expected to not only achieve an unattainable state of infallible performance, but to be extremely hard on themselves if they ever slip from that impossible standard. Since slippage (and mistake) is inevitable, the resulting inner dynamic tension and personal performance pressure is a constant agony.

For surgeons—and especially the exceptionally demanding world of pediatric surgical practice—these personal pressures and vulnerabilities to disappointment with one's own performance are magnified (Surgeons, in fact, are closest in temperament to professional military fighter pilots in their very legitimate need for maintaining a high level of personal self-confidence in their professional abilities, a self-confidence easily damaged or shattered by a single mistake in hurting a patient.)

But what do we make of this depressing news that professionals—surgeons in particular—are incapable of avoiding error? Does this fly in the face of attempts to improve overall medical safety by essentially guaranteeing that the underlying error rate that apparently drives the number of adverse patient injuries and deaths reported by the IOM must continue? In other words, is the entire discussion of reducing medical injuries moot?

In a word, no.

There are *two* parts to this equation. The first part—that humans cannot be perfect even if they are the best and the brightest in their profession—is the starting point. But in terms of safety, the end point is the corresponding truth that once human *fallibility* has been acknowledged, it becomes obvious that the way to reduce or eliminate the potential impact of inevitable human mistake—and thus reduce patient injury—is by building safety buffers into the medical system to safely absorb otherwise unavoidable medical mistakes before they can cause injury or dire harm. The even better news arising from this is the fact that once we begin to ask the question "How do we, will we, and can we fail?" The potential hazards start to emerge from the shadows and we can go about the task of constructing systems to safely absorb them.

For instance, acceptance of the reality that any drug or chemical solution kept in an OR will eventually be injected, without alteration, into a patient by mistake leads directly to the urgent need to prevent potentially fatal compounds from ever entering the OR in the first place.

The prime example is undiluted KCl. If KCl cannot be accessed in its undiluted state, it cannot be accidentally injected and cannot, therefore, accidentally cause an unwanted coronary arrest.

Correspondingly, since there will always be a potential of operating on the wrong limb of a child who cannot otherwise assist in identifying the impending disaster, there is no choice but to construct a carefully conceived and *always* adhered-to series of steps to reduce that propensity to nearly zero (preinterview, chart review by at least three separate people at separate times, clear marking of the surgical site with indelible ink, and a standard, checklist-driven set of terms that everyone adheres to, etc.).

Aviation knows this problem well. The propensity of even the most experienced captains to misread an instrument approach procedure and attempt to fly a perfectly good airplane into the ground could not be countered effectively before everyone wholly acknowledged that propensity. Once that happened, a combination of "fixes," including new electronics, standard callouts, in-cockpit approach briefings, and an unprecedented willingness to listen to one's subordinates was incorporated as a defense system to vastly reduce, if not eliminate, the catastrophic potential for repeat.

DECIPHERING THE LESSONS FROM OTHER CATASTROPHES

In medical practice, as in the business of aviation, the process of preventing future accidents and injuries depends as much on the rapid application of costly lessons from actual practice as on a complex structure of carefully considered preventative measures. In medicine, that is extremely difficult in an atmosphere of apprehension over potential litigation and corresponding "discovery" motions seeking to ferret out even the most innocuous close call or mistake. The adverse interaction of the medical and legal worlds has driven a vast reservoir of clinical knowledge of noncatastrophic misadventures and mistakes underground and has seriously retarded the ability of health care to communicate lessons from even the most publicized and exposed medical disasters. In this vein, aviation and health care could not be more different. Aviation has not only a central, national reporting system capable of disseminating crucial warnings and cautions based on immediate experience to prevent future harm, but also individual reporting systems within airlines and a vast network of connections among aircraft manufacturers and owners worldwide. The Aviation Safety Reporting System (ASRS) was established in 1975 under a Memorandum of Agreement between the Federal Aviation Administration (FAA) and the National Aeronautics and Space Administration (NASA). The FAA provides most of the program funding; NASA administers the program and establishes its policies in consultation with the FAA and the aviation community. NASA has chosen to operate the program through a contractor selected via competitive bidding. The current contractor is Battelle Memorial Institute. The ASRS collects, analyzes, and responds to voluntarily submitted aviation safety incident reports to lessen the likelihood of aviation accidents. ASRS provides a protected, de-identified, and fully protected means for any aviation professional to immediately insert vital safety information into the mainstream, with such information (such as a new air traffic control procedure which is essentially dangerous) being evaluated by highly trained recipients who have the ability to pick up a phone and insert it at the top levels of the FAA.

Health care has virtually nothing like that in effect as of this writing, although massive efforts are underway to create a medical version of the ASRS NASA system and to establish full protection for systems within hospitals and health care systems.

Clearly, daily practice produces untold lessons that can be used to improve patient safety. The problem is collecting those lessons, intelligently interpreting them, and immediately disseminating them to the widest clinical audience possible.

Aviation in particular has paid dearly for many of its lessons and corrections made in the safety system, and many times that price has been expressed in a catastrophic crash of an airliner costing hundreds of lives. But aviation did not come naturally to this ability to learn lessons as an industry. The ability to extract the majority of the salient cautions from such mishaps is, in fact, a markedly contemporary skill most clearly expressed in the methodologies of the National Transportation Safety Board (NTSB), which is charged with investigating every aviation accident in the United States.

The traditional method of probing an aviation mishap (when human failure was a concern) used to center around simply identifying who had failed and the precise nature of the performance failure (i.e., the pilot failed to follow the appropriate procedure, or failed to turn on or off a particular switch, etc.). The *reason* for the human failure was essentially ignored as being undiscoverable, even though later evolution of the process showed that repair of the system to prevent endless repeats of the same mistake absolutely required discovery of the nature, quality, and causation of that human failure. Moreover, the concept that there was a single, identifiable cause of an accident had even been embodied during the creation of the NTSB by Congress when it mistakenly mandated that the NTSB discover and announce the "probable cause" of every investigated accident.

Slowly, however, two major facts became apparent to the NTSB: (1) There is never a single "probable cause" to any accident, and in fact there is always a chain of contributing causes; and (2) Any *contributing* causes not addressed systemically and prevented from recurring in aviation will inevitably become part of some similar causal chain in the future leading to another accident.

For instance, the worst aviation accident in history in terms of number of deaths occurred on March 27, 1977, on the Canary Island known as Tenerife, when two Boeing 747s collided on a fog-shrouded runway as one attempted to take off without a takeoff clearance from the control tower. While the obvious primary triggering cause of the accident was the senior captain's decision to begin takeoff roll without the clearance, there were dozens of serious contributing causes, including the significant cultural problem in commercial cockpits of excessive respect for a senior captain leading to copilot or flight engineer unwillingness to speak up when something seemed wrong or dangerous. Essentially unaddressed worldwide as a contributing cause, the dysfunctional, traditional cockpit culture was doomed to bring down other crews, and on the night of December 29, 1979, the same dangerous dynamic led to a fatal crash of a United Airlines DC-8 in a Portland, Oregon, neighborhood after an otherwise experienced copilot and engineer refused to challenge the dangerous decision of their captain to burn off too much fuel. The DC-8, having run out of gas while still airborne and circling in leisurely preparation for a precautionary emergency landing (one of the main landing gear was not indicating down and locked), was unable to reach the airport.

Not only with respect to the cultural problems in airline cockpits, but equally in relation to the fact that wildly dissimilar contributing causes could and would reappear in later accidents, if not addressed and cured, the aviation industry had no choice but to begin to treat every identified incapacity of the *system* as a stand-alone problem to be dealt with and corrected. Indeed, the dramatic improvements in commercial aviation safety in the past 20 years flow in part from that one, single alteration in accident investigation philosophy.

How does this apply to the demanding and complex practice of pediatric surgery?

Because a corresponding truth is that in health care, just as in aviation, there is also no incident, mistake, or close call that results from a single cause. That truth, in fact, is an axiom.

The recognition that there is no single-point causation is important, because physicians are essentially taught otherwise by a culture which demands accountability, but deals with it, not as a declaration of concurrent responsibility, but as a personal indictment of blame and admission.

Take the current example provided by the February 17, 2003, tragedy at Duke University Medical Center when a failure to catch a blood-type mismatch in a set of donated organs (heart/lung) led to catastrophic rejection and the death of a 17-year-old Mexican girl named Jesica Santillan. The surgeon in that case, Dr. James Jaggers, MD, appeared on national television following her death, squared his shoulders, and took "full responsibility" for the fatal error as the head of the surgical team. He, in other words, accepted the blame as well as the accountability for an assumption that the entire system made (that the blood types were compatible). To the credit of both Duke and the surgeon involved, there was never a protracted attempt to shirk accountability or a reluctance to disclose the error. But in the minds of far too many Americans who saw or heard that statement, the case was closed because the *surgeon* was now identified as being responsible for the death, rather than the medical center's *system*.

The surgeon, in other words, had in essence been tarred with the appearance of being a bad doctor, despite his previous record of superlative performance that proved the contrary. The utter failure of the media, the medical center, and the medical profession in general to properly explain in a timely fashion that the tragedy was, in fact, the result of a failed system and many other contributing factors served to worsen the American public's false impression that patient safety problems stem from negligent doctors, not flawed systems. Aside from the fact that Duke was already hard at work repairing the systemic insufficiencies, the public saw none of those efforts, and understood less.

In fact, the underlying mistake made by the surgeon would have been patently impossible without systemic enabling. As Don Berwick, founder and head of the Institute for Health care Improvement in Boston, and Dr. James Reason on of the University of Manchester in Britain both teach, systems get the results they are designed to achieve. In other words, errors are literally hard-wired into the medical system. At Duke, it was painfully clear that what also failed were whatever checks and balances existed to make certain that there was no tissue mismatch, and that failure in both system design and execution occurred long before the surgeon ever walked into the OR. In other words, insofar as their system was *not* specifically designed to catch an error that was not only possible but also, over time, probable, the system was essentially designed to create a catastrophic mismatch sometime in the future. It worked precisely as [inadvertently] designed.

Repair, reform, or complete overhaul of those procedures (or in their absence, the creation of reliable procedures) would be required at minimum to eliminate the possibility of a repeat tragedy. Yet, the public—and the medical community—were left to believe that the single-point failure of a surgeon wholly disconnected from any of the systems around him that forged, loaded, and cocked the gun of major error and resulting injury whose trigger he pulled was all that needed to be considered in the emotional aftermath.

No patient injury arising from medical mistake ever results from a single-point failure. Conversely, no medical system can become significantly safer and better insulated from permitting a mistake from causing an injury unless the entire system is examined for defects that can contribute to a future injury. The system is culpable even in the rare case of an incompetent practitioner appearing to be the single-point cause of a terrible injury (i.e., due to liquor consumption and progressive physical incompetence, a surgeon performing a routine circumcision accidentally amputates a baby's penis.). Why was not the misbehaving individual identified before? Why were not there subsystems that could have identified alcoholism, or deteriorating skills, or any other personal/professional shortcoming before it resulted in an injury? These are system questions, and they will always be required if we are to correctly respond to any discovered system incapacities.

In aviation, the discovery that there is never a single cause to an accident or near-accident began by the 1980s to drive a massive and significant shift in both the NTSB and the FAA's methods of requiring the airline industry to make needed changes. No longer were human failure accidents merely written off as human failures that could not be understood. Instead, multiple elements of causation, from pilot fatigue to distraction to poor performance, began to be traced back to failures in the airline to properly monitor, hire, train, or support such personnel. Today it would be virtually unsupportable, from the point of view of potential legal liability as well as from a moral requirement to maintain the highest levels of safety, for an airline (or the FAA) to ignore problems that have been cited as contributing factors in an accident. While the performance of the airline industry is still far from perfect or uniformly stellar (especially in light of increasing financial pressure), airlines that ignore these factors place themselves in the crosshairs of potential ruin.

For instance, consider the plight of Alaska Airlines following the crash in 2000 of Flight 261 (an MD-80 had developed a major flight control problem involving the pitch trim on the horizontal stabilizer). One of the contributing causes of the accident was the culture of excessive cost control that had developed in their major maintenance facility in Oakland, California. The philosophy of being extremely cognizant of cost control had begun to lead to nonconservative decisions on when to replace certain parts that while not overtly illicit or illegal, nevertheless warped the airline's traditional emphasis on maintaining safety standards far above any identified acceptable or legal minimums. That atmosphere led to the overruling of a senior mechanic when he determined over a weekend that a so-called jackscrew assembly vital to pitch control in that particular MD-80 needed replacement. Broadly stated, the regular supervisor on the following day forced his crew to repeatedly re-test the worn jackscrew until it had passed a wear test several times, then ordered the worn part kept on the doomed aircraft. That decision alone did not cause the crash. Contributing factors included a lack of grease from another mistake, a system-wide misunderstanding of the vulnerability of the jackscrew to repeated manipulation by the pilots in the event of a jammed condition, and a massive failure of both the manufacturer and the FAA in designing and certifying a major flight control component that was subject to what aviation calls a "single-point failure mode." In other words, once the threads on the jackscrew were stripped on that fateful day in January of 2000 and the "nut" holding the horizontal stabilizer in place had literally slammed to the bottom flange of the jackscrew assembly shaft, there should have been no physical way the nut could have gone further and pulled loose altogether. There should have been, in other words, a fail-safe component that would have permitted a safe emergency diversion to Los Angeles International. Unfortunately, without that fail-safe component, the nut pulled free allowing the stabilizer to flip up almost 90° to the relative wind, rendering the aircraft completely unflyable. But that failure became an important part of the *causal chain*, since the aircraft would not have been lost had a new jackscrew been installed as originally ordered three years before the accident.

It is true that a wide gulf divides the mechanically based disciplines of aeronautical engineering/maintenance and pediatric surgery, but the basic facts that causation is always a chain of connected occurrences is axiomatic and true in either area.

How do we apply this truth? By realizing that regardless of the discipline, if an injury results from a specific causal chain, then removing a single link will prevent the injury. Therefore, identifying the scope and breadth of the various possible links in a causal chain of systemic vulnerabilities provides a significant chance to prevent the sort of tragedy that ultimately and wrongly fell on the shoulders of the devastated surgeon at Duke.

RECOGNIZING THE ONSET OF A CAUSAL CHAIN BEFORE IT CAN KILL—THE VITAL ROLE OF TEAM COMMUNICATIONS

Flight crews are now being taught to be alert for *patterns* of occurrences, stress factors, or even behavioral patterns which have been identified in past accidents as often leading to disaster. In the middle of a difficult instrument approach to a mountainous airport, for instance, the realization that a captain is pushing too hard and becoming inordinately frantic to get on the ground should spark a copilot or flight engineer to speak up and make that exact point to keep the captain's deteriorating behavior from becoming a link to an accident. "Sir, I think we should go around. I'm not comfortable with this," has become a respectful warning that no airline captain dare ignore, since he or she has been taught that to disregard such a warning may well result in a downgrade to copilot, or firing altogether.

In surgical practice there are also many times when, as in aviation, an event seems to be driving the participants instead of the other way around, and such moments are very commonly seen when we carefully examine cases of patient injury or death which resulted from mistakes in the OR. If all surgeons were trained to be very alert for the telltale patterns found in other patient injury causal sequences, and were trained to immediately break that sequence, there would be a heightened ability to purposefully stop a slide toward injury. Questioning the status and condition of the patient, questioning the procedure or any component thereof, or just calling a momentary time-out to take stock of where you are, is a powerful way of breaking a causal chain.

It took many ruinous airline accidents before the airline industry began to understand that even if a frightening slide toward an accident were recognized in time, a captain who could not or would not allow subordinate communication would stubbornly maintain that slide until a disaster did, in fact, result. The response was the development of a course called Crew Resource Management, a major cultural change which involved teaching and directing captains to "lead with participation" of subordinate crewmembers, and directing copilots and flight engineers to be "assertive with respect."

In fact, airline captains today are flight checked in the air and periodically in simulators not only on their ability to fly the aircraft to which they are assigned, but on how well they create and maintain a cooperative and communicative culture under their command. Twenty years ago an airline captain evaluated him or herself—and was in turn evaluated *as* a commander— by how well he or she could demonstrate ironclad control and absolute knowledge of every required fact and procedure. Today, a captain is evaluated primarily as a leader whose abilities depend on how well he or she can extract and use all the human talent entrusted to him or her. That is a radical change in philosophy, and yet it has been precisely what was needed. There are a frightening number of major accidents in recent aviation history resulting, in part, from an iron-willed captain essentially flying solo in an airliner and disregarding or intimidating his or her subordinates along with any safety information they might possess.

In the Tenerife accident, if either subordinate crewmember had been empowered to turn to the chief pilot and say, "Sir, something's wrong! Let's abort the takeoff," the collision would not have occurred. In Portland, Oregon, had either the copilot or the flight engineer leaned over and told the captain to get the aircraft on the ground immediately, they would not have run out of fuel in the air. In other words, the subordinate crews' silence in both cases forged a link in the causal chain that could have been broken—and the accident stopped—if they had been trained to recognize the danger of the behavioral vector they were on.

These cautionary principles are equally applicable to medical practice in general, and pediatrics—especially pediatric surgery—in particular. Why? Because no physician is capable of perfect, flawless performance one hundred percent of the time, yet a culture that allows only one-way communication from a commander (the traditional role of the physician, and especially the surgeon) is essentially depending on the infallibility of that practitioner/commander to protect the patient. Since we know that such dependency is both misguided and ineffective in achieving the higher levels of assurance that no human mistake can imperil a patient, just as in the airline industry, we are forced by both the pressures of a concerned public and a knowledgeable plaintiff's bar (medical malpractice lawyers) to add new safety precautions. This, then, is the point: Those "new" safety precautions have been in the OR and in the ED and ICU all along. They are the knowledge base of the scrub nurse, the anesthesiologist, the infusionist, the circulating nurse, the resident observing the procedure, the attending pediatrician, and anyone else with even a modicum of medical training engaged with any part of the process of caring for the patient and the family. In other words, just as was the case with the most senior and experienced and superlative of the airline captains, surgeons must realize that, although an imperfect source of clinical advice, those medical professionals who are on their team when trained and allowed to communicate in real time, provide an extra margin of safety which we have no right to deny any patient.

Instead of thinking of a copilot leaning over and asking whether the captain would like to "... do it with the rollers out this time?" (meaning landing with the landing gear extended), think in terms of an experienced pediatric surgical scrub nurse gently nudging you and pointing out something that could be dangerous to a patient, a perceived problem which you may not have seen.

But how should a professional respond when challenged? Doesn't this "process" severely undermine the professional image and authority you have spent years perfecting?

Senior airline captains often thought so in the mid-1980s when training in these new methods of fostering team communications and the instant availability of critical information to the leader. Protests such as: "You're taking all my authority and leaving me with all the responsibility!" were rampant at first, until the brighter among our captains began to understand that, far from taking their authority, these new methods added to their ability to do the job safely by providing more information and by providing alternate points of view in sometimes critical situations demanding careful decisions made in short periods of time. With this cultural change, these senior commanders realized, they no longer had to worry that a decision they were about to make might be wrong or that asking the copilot or flight engineer their thoughts would appear to be an act of weakness. Suddenly seeking all the professional information and balanced feelings from the highly paid professionals under their command became not only a requirement, but also a comfort, in that the additional information or point of view the commander might not have considered or even remembered was made available before a bad decision could be made and set in motion. The critical point here is that far from being an irritating challenge, respectful, assertive, and timely information from copilots, and flight engineers became an invaluable tool for the captains, and the resulting need to drop the false facade of omnipotence and infallibility became a huge relief.

In addition, the seismic change in communicative culture began to amass a startling record of averted airline accidents. Two of the more spectacular "saves" which, in the absence of "crew resource management" principles, would have resulted in the loss of all passengers and crew, are those of United Air Lines Flight 811 south of Honolulu on February 12, 1989, in which a main cargo door blew off the aircraft killing nine passengers and knocking out two of the four engines; and the near-disaster of United Air Lines Flight 232 near Sioux City, Iowa, on July 19, 1989, in which amazing crew coordination resulted in the saving of two-thirds of the passengers and crew in a crash landing most Americans have seen replayed endlessly on television.

So, too, in medical practice and especially in the subjective pressure cooker of surgery, the culture has to change from one in which the surgeon essentially forces the otherwise helpless patient to accept the surgeon's carbon-based, analog brain as the only source of knowledge, skill, information, and protection against human error, and an enlightened environment in which the surgeon not only welcomes, but demands, that those professionals around him or her provide real-time information on anything they see, hear, feel, perceive, or even intuit might be threatening the welfare and the safety of the patient. In this safer OR environment, the surgeon becomes a leader, not a blind commander hanging his or her self-worth on the false presumption of the attainment of infallibility.

But what happens when we create "Attila the Nurse," someone who takes this new and somewhat frightening ability to speak up whenever he or she feels it's appropriate and then overuses it, correcting the surgeon until it appears the nurse is trying to *be* the surgeon? Is not this a manifest danger of empowering those who do not have an MD and a surgical residency to their name?

> Yes, but guess who's responsibility it is to correct such behavior in an enlightened way. Yours, as the leader.

Again, we have well and truly learned these lessons the hard way in aviation, and while it is entirely true that pediatric surgery is vastly more complex and demanding than flying a 747, again the principles being outlined here of command versus leadership are the same. If "Attila the Nurse" shows up in your OR, your responsibility is to refrain from rebuking that person until the procedure is complete, and then take him or her aside to say the following: "I appreciate very much your willingness to speak up and be an interactive team member, but we need to fine-tune the way you're doing it. You're misusing your responsibility here by *over* using it." In other words, it is the responsibility and the task of the leader to encourage the participation of subordinate members of the team while molding that participation to fit what is needed during a procedure, and to train team members to fit their comments and warnings beneficially within the framework of the OR team environment. Severely admonishing such a nurse (just as we learned with copilots and flight engineers) will accomplish two undesired things: (1) Intimidate her or him to complete silence in the future; (2) Transmit through the grapevine to all other nurses that your stated intention to establish teamwork and communication within your practice is insincere and should be disregarded. In other words, you can destroy a careful and beneficial program promoting the creation of a finely tuned OR team with just one outburst of disapproval.

Is this really the task of the overburdened pediatric surgeon?

Consider how you would explain in a deposition a refusal to adopt methods that we know significantly improve patient safety by markedly reducing the chance that an individual error could metastasize to a patient injury. That is just what happened in the early days of this cultural revolution when some senior captains had to be reminded to "Please consider how what you just said about not speaking unless you invite it is going to sound at the hearing."

THE NATURE OF TEAMWORK

Another of the many axioms and truths discovered through costly experience by aviation is the reality that teamwork, which absolutely requires the presence of a functional team, is impossible if the members of that team have not been identified.

Consider the Boeing 727 crew landing at DFW airport in the mid-1980s for a quick change of passengers, cabin crew, and flight attendants. The pilots were to continue on to Chicago from Dallas. The flight attendants were to go to another flight, while a new set of flight attendants were to get aboard and work the flight to Chicago. In the boarding lounge, a lone gate agent was working hard to check in 144 passengers. Two gate agents were normally required, and all the agents were graded and retained—or not—based on their ability to get the flights out of the gate on time. The agent was, in effect, in charge of the flight while at her gate, and in this case was maintaining a "situational awareness" track of the events around her, including the fact that the arriving flight attendants had left the aircraft, and at least one flight attendant had boarded the aircraft, presumably from the new cabin crew, which was coming in from Tulsa.

After nearly 50 minutes on the ground, the gate agent completed boarding the passengers, handed the paperwork to the pilots, saw that all the passengers had taken their seats, and closed the door in time to push back the 727 on schedule.

Some 20 minutes later, the Boeing 727 crew was climbing through 10,000 feet in a clear blue sky when a man in a three piece business suit knocked on the cockpit door to ask the startled pilots if someone up front could come back and ". . . show me how to make coffee."

"Ah, sir, we're the pilots," the flight engineer said through a partially cracked cockpit door. "The flight attendants will do that for you."

"That's what I thought you'd say," the man replied. "Son," he continued, "I don't know how to break this to you, but there *are* no flight attendants."

In fact, the outbound flight attendants were still in Tulsa, and the fact that they'd been delayed had not been passed to the gate agent or the pilots in Dallas. Possessed of an iron-clad federal requirement not to fly passenger flights without the appropriate number of flight attendants, the flight was forced to return to Dallas with considerable embarrassment. The FAA imposed a $10,000 fine as well. But the lesson for the industry was the fact that despite a revolution in the degree of teamwork in the cockpits, the pilots did not even seem aware that there were fellow crewmembers in the back, let alone know who they were or whether or not they were even aboard. The hidden part of the story was the reality that most airline personnel, regardless of their airline, winced with the knowledge that the hapless flight-without-attendants in Dallas could just have easily been theirs.

When you apply the cautionary aspect of this occurrence to surgical practice, the salient point is the admonition that we need to ask the question: Who is, in fact, on the team? At first blush, it would seem that the right answer is encompassed by the OR itself. But on more careful reflection, everyone who has a hand in preparing, screening, dealing with, or interacting with the patient from preadmission through discharge and follow-up is a fully vested part of the team. Forging new lines of instant communication among and between the members of that vastly extended professional family is also a new prerequisite demanded by the findings of many medical accident probes.

All too many times, misunderstandings, misdiagnoses, and other presurgical processing breakdowns progress to a patient impact because the assumption is made institutionally that all the presurgical work has been done correctly. Just as there is need for a surgeon to seek and welcome the participatory input of his immediate team members, the other members of the team need to be given the benefit of oversight and double-checking as well, and for the very same reason: Human error is constant and insidious, and the propensity for an individual error to metastasize to a patient injury increases in direct proportion to the degree of confidence that no error has been made. Devising a system for checking and re-checking virtually everything that could bloom into a serious problem is no longer an option for safe practice and, correspondingly, a standard of care, it is a requirement. And central to that requirement is the presence of a nurtured, energized, empowered team, all of whom are both respected and listened to when information needs to be passed.

The responsibility for creation and maintenance of such a team is once again the responsibility of the leader, and more often than not, that means the surgeon.

An additional and very vital element of team creation is the establishment of a common goal. On the surface, this should be obvious. The common goal of health care professionals is to provide quality and effective care for the patient, and in the process, provide a satisfying professional environment. But if the only personnel identifying that common goal are the leaders, it becomes a barren exercise. Instead, the members of the team must believe that they *are* that hospital, or medical center, or clinic. The motivation should be spread equally over all ranks and strata, whether the people working there are the product of nearly a decade of medical training or simply the janitorial staff. Motivated people practicing together in an energized, mutually determined quest to reach a common goal can accomplish wonders, and their leader's professional life becomes progressively easier. Certainly, with respect to patient safety, the seamless communication abilities of a unified and energized team cannot be overstated.

COOKBOOK MEDICINE AND THE MINIMIZATION OF VARIABLES

A senior pilot sitting in a complex cockpit with nothing but gray outside the windscreens is obviously flying by reference to instruments alone. Robbed of the ability to "see" the attitude reference of the horizon and external references, he or she interfaces with the myriad displayed information on instrument panels to control the aircraft's flight path safely and get to destination. In this process, it appears that the pilot is multitasking, or to shift from the vernacular, is processing many different inputs simultaneously. The prevailing belief in the medical community appears to be that if a pilot can do that, so can surgeons.

But this is a wholly incorrect assumption. In fact, even the most accomplished humans cannot truly multitask if the definition of multitasking is *simultaneous* monitoring of items necessary for situational awareness. Rather, pilots and surgeons process things *in sequence*, one item at a time, stitching it all together in a continuous and intensive mental orchestration that gives the appearance of multitasking.

This is important to understand in the context of surgical practice, because accomplished surgeons, just like accomplished pilots, begin to believe that their capacity for simultaneously dealing with myriad inputs is infinite, and this is generically untrue.

Pilots, in reality, manage multiple channels of information by minimizing the number of channels they have to actively deal with at any one time, thus reducing the number of dynamic variables (such as altitude, airspeed, bank angle, heading, etc) to better concentrate their cognitive abilities on the most critical variables. The proof of this resides in numerous NTSB accident reports that cite "task saturation" as a contributing factor. Humans, in other words, whether surgeons or pilots, can be overwhelmed by too many active channels of variable information competing for immediate decisional or interactive attention.

The immediate symptomology of incipient task saturation can manifest irritation, nonresponsive communicative behavior, or other telltale indications that the professional being inundated is losing control of the situation. The immediate cure—in both aviation and medicine—is to unload the saturated professional, by either slowing the pace of the procedure or assigning some tasks to others (such as the cockpit procedure of assigning the active flight control of the aircraft to the autopilot or the copilot to permit an unloaded mind to focus on other important decisions).

Even when a surgical procedure is not becoming problematic or intense, or an aerial challenge is not speeding up or increasing in decisional intensity, the principle that variables should be minimized at all times is sound. To that end, there is a central element of aviation safety that needs to be adopted by medical professionals, and especially surgeons and surgical teams: standardization and the use of checklists for those elements of preparation, procedure, and postoperative practice which can be reduced to a predictable routine.

This does not presume that most of a surgical procedure can be, or should be, reduced to a checklist. But it does recognize the fact that in many cases of patient injury from medical mistake, variables which could have been reduced to nonvariables became one of the prime links in the causal chain. The prime point stated as succinctly as possible is this: Aviation, NASA, industry in general, and any highly complex human endeavor with potential injury or death as the penalty for system failure have learned that the best use of human capability results from focusing the skilled professional on those elements of practice variables which most need his or her analog cognitive skills. Thus, reduction of unnecessary variables (such as excessive physician preference variables in OR setup when a standard layout could be agreed to and implemented for standard procedures) correspondingly reduces not only the chance and opportunity for human error, but also reduces the degree of cognitive attention a surgeon has to divert from the most difficult elements of surgical practice.

The resistance of the surgical community—including the pediatric surgical community—to the use of checklists and standardization principles is well recorded, but the reality is that the world has changed, standards of practice have and are changing, liability exposure is correspondingly changing, and we can no longer afford to indulge unnecessary variability in practice, when the record is very clear that unnecessary variables are indefensible in the quest for greater patient safety.

CONCLUSIONS

The challenges of pediatric surgery used to be limited to the intelligent application of surgical and medical skills to the patient. Unfortunately, the world has changed, and along with it the challenges to the pediatric surgeon have burgeoned to include worries about patient/family communication, liability exposure, liability insurance, public perception, as well as the ongoing challenges of keeping current on procedures, practice standards, the growing tide of evidence-based practice consideration, technological advances affecting practice, and the substantially important necessity of maintaining one's practice as something fulfilling and enjoyable. Central to the contemporary considerations which cannot be dismissed is what some have called the

"Patient Safety Revolution," and in dealing with this entirely new set of challenges and changes, the logic of learning from another technologically complex human endeavor, such as aviation, is irrefutable. Thus, the lessons derived from aviation regarding the invaluable nature of establishing a broader-based team, invigorating seamless communication of vital information without rank among the members of the team, instituting the well-established benefits of minimizing variables and standardizing what can be standardized and the necessity of learning the valuable lessons from past mishaps and tragic mistakes through examination of the entire causal chain linking these events to the exclusion of useless emphasis on blame are all immediately accessible routes to a safer medical practice.

REFERENCE

1. Kohn LT, Corrigan JM, Donaldson MS, eds. To Err is Human: Building a Safer Health System. Washington, D. C.: Committee on Quality of Health Care in America, Institute of Medicine, 1999.

3 | A Legal Perspective on Errors in Medicine

Linda C. Laing, J.D.

INTRODUCTION: A LEGAL PERSPECTIVE ON MEDICAL ERRORS

Health care in the United States is plagued by a bad record for safety and a medical malpractice crisis. It is the author's belief that reforming the medical liability system and improving patient safety are two sides of the same coin. This chapter explores the prevalence and increased public awareness of medical error, patient safety, and other initiatives to promote disclosure of medical error and perceptions in the medical community that discourage reporting of medical error. The chapter will also discuss the interface between the existing medical liability system and medical error, the medical malpractice crisis, and limited effect of first generation medical malpractice reforms. In particular, the chapter will focus on the current challenge of structuring a new accountability system that will link patient safety to risk management toward the goal of preventing patient injury in the first instance and improving the manner in which injury caused by medical error is fairly compensated and addressed.

PREVALENCE OF MEDICAL ERRORS

With the issuance of its now legendary report, To Err is Human: Building a Better Health System, the Institute of Medicine (IOM) brought into sharp focus and into the public eye the reality and prevalence of medical error. The well-publicized results of this 1999 study faulted America's health system for causing more than one million medical errors during hospitalizations annually, of which between 44,000 and 98,000 resulted in death as well as hundreds of thousands of avoidable injuries and extra days of hospitalization (1). The IOM based its conclusions on two large retrospective epidemiologic studies published in the 1980s and early 1990s, specifically, the 1991 Harvard Medical Practice Study (which reviewed medical records of patients hospitalized in New York State in 1984) (2) and a study conducted in Colorado and Utah using 1992 data (3). The IOM noted that, even assuming the lower estimate, deaths due to medical error exceeded the number attributable to the eighth leading cause of death. While some researchers have challenged the accuracy of the IOM's numbers (4), there appears to be general agreement that the problem of medical errors is serious and one that, while highlighted and publicized by the IOM 1999 report, has long existed. Indeed, the NY (1984) and Colorado (1992) studies were preceded by one in California where it was demonstrated that 4.65% of people hospitalized suffered an adverse event and that 0.7% suffered an adverse event for which the provider would likely be found liable (5).

The 1999 IOM report noted that the addition of nonhospital errors may drive the numbers of errors and deaths much higher, since hospital patients represent only a small proportion of the total population at risk and many patients increasingly receive complex care in ambulatory settings such as outpatient surgical centers, physicians' offices, and clinics.

The IOM's now-familiar 1999 projections have been enlarged by more recent analyses including a HealthGrades analysis of Medicare data which projected a casualty rate more than twice the IOM figures, of approximately 247,000 deaths per year attributable to adverse medical events in patients studied between 2003 and 2005 with medical errors increasing 3% from 2003 to 2005 in all of the nation's 5000 hospitals. The authors of the HealthGrades Study concluded that 1.16 million medical errors occurred nationwide (6). Six years after the IOM's initial report, the IOM released a report entitled "Preventing Medication Errors," which revealed that a hospitalized patient could expect to experience, on average, one medication error per day. The Centers for Disease Control has estimated that, if ranked as a disease, medical errors would be the sixth leading cause of death in the United States, outranking deaths due to influenza, pneumonia, Alzheimer's disease, and renal disease (7). Others rank health care, more generally defined, as the third leading cause of death in the United States (8). According to the World Health Organization, health care errors affect 1 in every 10 patients around the world. Additionally, new technologies and surgical techniques, an aging population, the ability to handle more complex conditions, and a society that hungers for new treatments and cures all set the stage for a higher rate of errors in the future (9). In "Internal Bleeding: The Truth Behind America's Terrifying Epidemic of Medical Mistakes" (10), the problem of medical errors is stated to be of epidemic proportions.

In addition to mortality and other patient harm, medical errors in American hospitals also have a financial cost. The 2005 HealthGrades Study found that medical errors cost Medicare $8.6 billion in more than 3 years. In an apparent attempt to reverse this trend, the Centers for Medicare and Medicaid Services (CMS) has designated certain events "never events" and, starting October 1, 2008, will deny payment for what they view as preventable hospital errors (11).

It is unlikely that the precise frequency of the occurrence of medical errors in health care settings will be known due to the need to rely on people to recognize that errors were made, distinguish them from bad outcomes of appropriate treatment, and then report them. A true understanding of the causes, frequency, severity, preventability, and impact of medical errors on patient outcomes appears to be complicated by the lack of standardized definitions of medical error, the lack of coordination and integration of systems to report and monitor errors, and the difficulty in distinguishing preventable errors from unavoidable adverse events. Notwithstanding, the available data make a strong case for changes to reduce the prevalence of medical error. In a recent update of an analysis that compared international rates of "amenable mortality," defined as deaths that are potentially preventable with timely health care, researchers from the London School of Hygiene and Tropical Medicine found that, of the 19 countries included in the study, the United States ranked last in reductions in amenable mortality in the study period from 2002 to 2003. Not only were the U.S. rates among the worst but also the rate of improvement in between the first study period from 1997 to 1998 and the second from 2002 to 2003 was smallest in the United States. The authors blame the "comparatively poor performance of the U.S. health care system" as one factor (12). These statistics suggest that current efforts to reduce medical error require a shift in focus.

THE SYSTEMS APPROACH TO MEDICAL ERROR

The majority of quality experts appear to agree that one of the most common causes of medical errors is the medical system itself, not the individuals functioning within the system. System failures account for the vast majority of harmful errors in hospitals (1). The IOM's second report on quality of care, *Crossing the Quality Chasm*, includes rules for health care in the 21st century, one of which is "safety is a system property" (13). Thus, it is not surprising that recent reports on medical errors emphasize the need to move away from a search for individual culprits to blame for medical errors. The individual approach, sometimes referred to as the "name, shame and blame game," has been criticized for its judgmental focus. This view is premised on the belief that medical errors result from inadequate training or from a few "bad apples" in the system. Under this belief, it is assumed that medical errors can be reduced or minimized by identifying the individuals and disciplining them. Just as our "culture of blame" fuels litigation and needs to be remedied, a "culture of shame" based on unrealistic expectations that health care is always safe fuels the tendency for practitioners to hide or disregard errors. Hesitation of health care workers to report errors over fear of reprisal is a major drawback of this judgmental attitude as is the resultant inability to comprise an accurate picture of the frequency of occurrence of some types of medical errors (14).

The individual approach to medical error also falls victim to "hindsight" bias. Hindsight bias tends to attribute causation to individuals' actions according to information available after the event, which may not have been evident or available to the person who took the initial action. When all factors are considered in a retrospective review, the complexity and other circumstances of the real time situation faced by the health care provider at the time the decision was made are vulnerable to discounting. Such evaluations fail to provide the information and recommendations necessary to improve those aspects of the system that contributed to the error. The IOM's 1999 report urges that a more useful approach to medical errors can be borrowed from an industry model based on systems analysis such as has been successfully employed in the aviation industry. The nuclear power industry likewise focused on human error and the systems approach to addressing same following the accident at Three Mile Island in the last 1970s (15). This model advocates making an entire system safer rather than punishing individuals, assumes that most errors result from problems with procedures and work processes rather than bad or incompetent people, and analyzes all parts of the system in order to improve them. According to the IOM, making headway requires seeing the flaws in how the health care system itself is organized. Since "to err is human," the answer lies in buttressing the systems in which people work in, so the mistakes they are bound to make do not snowball into actual harm.

There are lessons to be learned from the successful track record with which high reliability systems have been employed in aviation. First, aviation has developed an atmosphere in which everyone is preoccupied with safety. Part of this preoccupation has included, at least in part, the adoption and adherence to safety reporting systems. The Aviation Safety Reporting System, for example, is funded by the Federal Aviation Administration but administered by National Aeronautical and Space Agency. The point of this arrangement is to focus on the prevention of accidents, not on the punishment of individuals. The Federal Aviation Administration is the regulatory body in aviation, while National Aeronautical and Space Agency is considered a neutral but knowledgeable bystander.

The Aviation Safety Reporting System entails the collection, analysis, and response to voluntarily submitted aviation safety incident reports. This includes reports on near misses, where an error or safety violation has occurred but did not result in an accident. In fact, reporting and analysis of near misses is considered to be invaluable for safety improvement because it allows people to focus on the interactions between system elements, identify design flaws, and fix the problem before anyone is harmed by a system failure.

It is the systems approach to error that is the hallmark of the patient safety movement. Patient safety advocates promote disclosure as fundamental to the detection of error and prevention of future errors. The goal of the patient safety movement is to prevent iatrogenic injury, or injuries caused by medical management, and to reduce errors through systemic changes (16).

As was noted in the IOM's 1999 report, the system approach to errors has a proven track record of success in the medical field as demonstrated by the success with which the systems approach to error reduction was employed in the anesthesia patient safety movement which commenced in early 1980s. Anesthesiologists were then victim to a high incidence of malpractice lawsuits and some of the highest insurance premiums. Then, in the late 1980s, the American Society of Anesthesiologists launched a project to analyze every claim brought against its members and developed new ways to reduce medical error with a systems approach. In a seminal 1978 publication, Jeffery B. Cooper, Ph.D., described the use of the aviation-inspired "critical incident analysis" technique to understand the causes of anesthesia-related mishaps and injuries (17). In 1985, the Anesthesia Patient Safety Foundation was launched as the first independent (allowing organizational agility and the freedom to tackle openly the sensitive issue of anesthesia accidents) multidisciplinary organization (practitioners, equipment and drug manufacturers, and many related professionals) with the mission of assuring that no patient shall be harmed by anesthesia. Around the same time, the American Society of Anesthesiologists inaugurated the Closed Claim Study, which continues today as an ongoing project which has yielded important discoveries through the study of anesthesia mishaps. By 2002, anesthesiologists had one of the highest safety ratings in the medical profession and the number of anesthesia-related deaths had been reduced from 1 in 100,000 to about 1 in 200,000. Improvements in anesthesia safety have also brought an important benefit to anesthesiologists, who have enjoyed a decrease in their malpractice insurance premiums (18). The success of the anesthesia patient safety movement was recognized in 1996 when the American Medical Association ("AMA") and corporate partners founded the National Patient Safety Foundation, which was based on the Anesthesia Patient Safety Foundation model.

The success of the systems approach to error in the anesthesia context raises the question as to why this approach has not been embraced by other medical specialties. In considering this question, it is important to note several fundamental differences between health care and other high reliability systems like aviation. Health care has unacceptably high incident rates, as demonstrated in patient safety research and as set forth in the IOM reports on medical errors. Another difference is that most adverse events in health care are less visible than those in aviation and nuclear plants. Although some high-profile cases get media coverage such as operative procedures at the wrong site, an adverse event that occurs in one patient does not attract the same kind of attention as an airplane crash or a nuclear accident. Yet another difference is that medical errors often go undetected, especially when there's a near miss that does not result in an adverse event. By contrast, errors in routine aviation and nuclear operations set off alarms that call attention to the error (19).

Health care also differs in that the interactivity between system elements is far less standardized than in high reliability systems like aviation. The human element and susceptibility to human error is far more pervasive in health care. This is especially evident in outpatient care, when individual patients or their caregivers need to manage their own care when they go home. This places a premium on the value of communication, collaboration, and education—activities that must be individualized to help each patient get safe and effective care. While communication is important on several levels, it is particularly important in the patient–physician relationship.

PRACTICE POINTER

This author's experience is consistent with the studies discussed elsewhere in this chapter, which evidence a strong correlation between a physician's malpractice experience and the physician's ability to effectively communicate with one's patients, establish rapport, and provide care and treatment consistent with what the patient expects. Teaching effective communication should become a part of medical education curriculum not only at the training level but also as part of continuing medical education. Further, and particularly given that the vast majority of health care providers practice alone or in small groups, it is recommended that physicians support efforts to correctly and comprehensively manage patients and information as they are handed off from one part of the system to another. For example, successful management of pediatric asthma requires health educators to instruct the child's family how to medicate the child and avoid behavior and allergens that can trigger asthma attacks, look for effective self-management, nurses to handle emergency phone calls, and long-term home visits. As has been noted by David M. Lawrence, M.D., a member of the IOM's report committee, physician autonomy is an outmoded notion that exists only in isolated settings serving an isolated population without referring many patients to other physicians (20).

An additional salient difference between the work environment of airline pilots and that of clinicians and patients is the level and sophistication of the information technology infrastructure that supports their work. While pilots have immediate access to the information required to make informed decisions, no comparable information technology infrastructure is widely available in the health care industry at present. While electronic medical records (EMRs) are being used in some areas of medicine, only a handful of communities have established a community-wide, secure Internet-based platform to facilitate access to clinical information by multiple providers, not just those within a given institution, such as a hospital or group practice (21).

PRACTICE POINTER

Health care providers should support efforts to move toward an EMR-based system of recordkeeping including community-wide programs. In terms of the costs associated with same, physicians are urged to pursue from third-party payers incentive-based compensation, which exists to promote physician efforts to use EMR.

It is this author's view that the success of the systems approach is based on disclosure of medical error and that, absent the creation of a safe environment in which error information is shared and analyzed without fear of individual recrimination and a restructuring of medical liability system, the generation and exchange of data on medical errors will continue to be driven underground. Personal and organizational liability concerns must be addressed if a free exchange of information upon which system changes can be constructed is to be accomplished. Further, there needs to be a focus on improving communication as between patients and their caregivers. As was noted by Kenneth A. Kern, M.D., change must focus on a number of factors. "There is no single integrated process. There are multiple parallel patchwork systems. They all compete—the surgeon, the hospital, the residency, the legal system, the political system, the patients, and the advocacy system. This is the basis of the medicolegal system. You would have to have all this together to solve any problem" (22). In summary, it appears that the greatest gains in patient safety will come from efforts to align incentives and activities in the interactions of clinicians and patients as influenced by legal liability, purchasing and regulatory policies, the education and training of health professionals, the health literacy and expectations of patients, and the organizational arrangements or systems that support health care delivery (1).

DISCLOSURE OF MEDICAL ERROR—A CHANGING TIDE

Patient safety advocates promote disclosure as fundamental to the detection of error and prevention of future errors (16). Beyond the patient safety movement, there appears to be a broad consensus that disclosure of unanticipated outcomes is desirable and, as more fully set forth later, regulators have begun to require it. The rational is clear: The experience of other industries, such as aviation and nuclear power, suggests that openness about error is critical to development of effective prevention strategies. The following is an overview of the various approaches to error disclosure and how each is handicapped by the liability climate and other concerns that continue to drive underground efforts to admit and correct medical mistakes.

Disclosure of Errors Among Physicians

Tradition of Self-Critique in Medical Education
That physicians cannot make 100% correct treatment decisions, 100% of the time has never been a secret among physicians. Ernst Codman, a surgeon at Massachusetts General Hospital between 1911 and 1917, was a forerunner of efforts to standardize care. He devised an "End Result System" that documented each patient's diagnosis, outcome, treatment plan, and any complications from treatment. Dr. Codman urged hospitals to review cases in which errors may have occurred, pressed for the publication of results, called for transparency among colleagues, and urged disclosure to the public (23).

Despite initial resistance to Codman's efforts, physicians have regularly met in the hospital setting at morbidity and mortality conferences (dubbed "M&M"s) to review serious complications and errors since the early 20th century. Again, anesthesia appears to have led the way. An early prototype of M&M conferences was the Anesthesia Mortality Committee in Philadelphia, which was created in 1935 to educate physicians and to improve the quality of care by reviewing cases in which morbidity or mortality occurred (24). These conclaves have been considered an essential part of continuing medical education, particularly among surgeons and anesthesiologists. In these confidential settings, a physician presents a case to other attending physicians, residents, and medical students. Relevant medical literature is reviewed and avenues to prevent recurrence are discussed. Effectiveness is based upon complete candor, which is, in turn, based on confidentiality of the proceedings. M&M conferences are part of the long and strong history of self-regulation in medicine (24). M&M conferences were the forerunner of the peer review process, which has long been considered by many to be one of the medical field's most effective risk management and quality control mechanisms, as it promises to provide physicians with a safe forum in which to review the quality of care they are providing (25).

PRACTICE POINTER

When presenting cases at peer review proceedings, avoid preparing written handouts. If written materials are necessary, number each copy and collect all copies at the end of the meeting. This prevents documents from inadvertent disclosure outside the protected peer review forum.

Changes Resulting from Involvement of Third Parties in Quality Assurance
The involvement of outside agencies in the process of quality evaluation and peer review in the 1950s signaled a shift in peer review from a largely self-policing mechanism of the medical profession to a regulatory one. The Joint Commission for the Accreditation of Hospitals (JCAH) [subsequently to be renamed the "Joint Commission for the Accreditation of Health care Organizations" (JCAHO) and currently known simply as the "Joint Commission"] was formed in 1951. The Joint Commission is a nonprofit, independent organization to whom both state and federal authorities typically defer with respect to hospital oversight. The Joint Commission has been granted authority by federal and state governments to accredit hospitals with the result that hospital participation in Joint Commission Quality Assurance ("QA") programs became a mandatory requirement for certification as a Medicare provider eligible for federal reimbursement by the Health Care Financing Administration. Health care facilities do not have a choice as to whether they have a peer review system. Instead, they are required to have a peer review system in order to meet licensing obligations, to qualify for Medicare, and to be accredited by the Joint Commission. The AMA has created guidelines for the existence, function, and maintenance of peer review committees (25).

Moreover, peer review proceedings became the subject of state and federal legislation. One notable example of federal peer review law is the Health Care Quality Improvement Act of 1986 ("HCQIA") (26). The HCQIA provides qualified immunity from suit to physician peer review committees investigating the competence or professional conduct of a physician. Immunity is only afforded if the peer review is conducted in good faith, without malice and affords the subject physician with due process rights (similar to those set forth in most hospital medical staff bylaws) such as notice of charges and a fair hearing. Most states mandate hospitals to conduct ongoing peer review activities. The doctrine of corporate responsibility, the law in multiple jurisdictions including New York, holds a hospital responsible, in consultation with its medical staff, for establishing policies and procedures and monitoring the quality of care afforded to assure that physicians granted clinical privileges are competent.

"The net result was that QA developed 'teeth' in the guise of Peer Review, a process that involved outside agencies and could result in sanctions, rather than education. This paradigm can best be termed 'Adversarial QA'" (27). The corresponding increase in medical malpractice litigation and the desire for plaintiffs' attorneys to discover the documents and testimony resulting from the peer review process have led to distrust of the peer review process by physicians who are the target of it as well as liability concerns of the physicians participating in the process (27,28).

Limited Discussion of Medical Error in Peer Review Settings
The change in the focus of peer review from education to regulatory may explain the results of studies concluding that errors are infrequently discussed in M&M conferences and other peer review forums. It has been noted that, within the Anesthesia Department of a major teaching institution between 1987 and 1988, 72% of the M&M Conferences did not involve morbidity or mortality and that cases involving error with sequelae (and thus potential medical malpractice) constituted only approximately 20% of the conferences (29). As low as 10% of cases presented in internal medicine conferences discussed error (30). A study of surgical M&M conferences, which were part of a formal quality assurance program, revealed that physicians were often absent when their complication was discussed, with only 33% of the staff surgeons attending when their complications were discussed (30). Even when errors are discussed at the conferences, it is rare for participants to use language indicating that an error occurred and few acknowledge making the error at hand (31). Physicians have reported that in about half of the cases in which error was discussed, "the tough issues were not addressed" (32).

Influence of Liability Concerns on Error Discussion in the Peer Review Setting
Although the peer review process has been noted to be an effective tool in addressing medical error, there are roadblocks to its effective execution. M&M conferences have been described as integral to continuing medical education and error correction, but are hampered by concerns that colleagues cannot report errors openly because of risks of liability (33). Further, physicians taking part in the process often fear that their criticism of fellow physicians will be made public in the event that there is an investigation or result in litigation involving the colleague who is the subject of the proceeding (28). A basis for these fears can be found in case law wherein

physician peer reviewers are charged with slander, defamation, or tortuous interference with business relations (28). While there exist some federal (26) and state law (34) protections for peer review evaluation, the protection is not afforded where these activities are performed in bad faith for economic credentialing or other reasons unrelated to quality care. Further, the HCQIA immunity does not protect peer reviewers if they violate federal or state civil rights laws (26). As a result, some physicians have attempted to circumvent HCQIA immunity by alleging that the peer review committee's adverse actions were based upon their race, sex, religion, age, or national origin (35). Federal courts have likewise held that the medical peer review privilege does not apply in antitrust cases in which a plaintiff sought discovery of peer review records in order to demonstrate that the defendants used the peer review process to destroy plaintiff's medical practice and limit competition (36) and in cases where a plaintiff physician alleges that a hospital engaged in false advertising, deceptive business practices, and fraud (37).

Some have questioned whether the legal liability of statements made during peer review conferences is a reasonable concern in light of evidentiary protections that are in place to encourage physicians to speak out honestly and review their errors as afforded by the federal self-critical analysis privilege and the medical peer review privilege that has been enacted in all 50 states and the District of Columbia (38). The answer may lie in the fact that these laws are subject to judicial interpretations which have been noted to usurp legislative intentions as more fully set forth later.

Patient Safety and Quality Improvement Act of 2005—A Federal Law Aspiring to Protect the Confidentiality of Peer Review Information

It is important to note that, until the passage of the Patient Safety and Quality Improvement Act of 2005 (PSQIA) (39), there was no federal law protecting peer review information. Although the HCQIA of 1986 set forth the federal guidelines for a hospital's peer review process and provides immunity for good faith participation, it does not protect peer review documents or discussions from being disclosed to an adverse party (26).

From a patient safety perspective, the PSQIA creates a system of review organizations that encourage the voluntary sharing of information on medical error, free from concerns that such information could be used in litigation and disciplinary proceedings. In brief, the goal of PSQIA is to enable providers to contract voluntarily with Patient Safety Organizations (PSOs) to help them identify and analyze threats to patient safety and change health care structures and processes to improve health care outcomes without fear of data disclosure. From a procedural perspective, the PSQIA broadens confidentiality and legal protections for peer review and quality assurance activities that may overcome certain disincentives to error disclosure as noted earlier. The PSQIA creates extensive legal privileges for, and prohibits disclosure of, "patient safety work products" developed by or for newly created PSOs. Notably, the new law preempts state laws that are not as protective of the documentation created in the course of such activities while leaving intact state laws that afford greater legal protections.

Under the PSQIA, anything meeting the definition of "patient safety work product" will not be subject to any subpoena or administrative order (state, federal, or local), nor will it be discoverable or admissible in any civil, criminal, administrative, and/or any professional disciplinary proceeding (except proceedings alleging lack of good faith by a patient safety organization itself). In addition to the legal privilege, the law requires that patient safety work products must be kept confidential and must not be disclosed, unless one of a few exceptions applies. Civil money penalties are established for violators of the confidentiality protection.

As of this writing, there are no implementing regulations of PSQIA and, thus, no operational guidelines. Draft regulations were sent from the Department of Health and Human Services/Agency for Health care Research and Quality to the Office of Management and Budget in October of 2007 and it is expected that proposed regulations will be published in the *Federal Register* in 2008. Accordingly, physicians need to continue to rely on the existing federal and state peer review privileges discussed later in determining what peer review materials may be discoverable and in what context. Additionally, it is notable that the PSQIA may not offer the panacea envisioned by many of its champions. First, the act provides protection for patient safety work product only if it is, in fact, reported to a PSO and has been developed as part of a "patient safety evaluation system." Isolated incidents, even if reported, will not benefit from the act unless they are identified by an approved system. The structure and operational burdens of that system will have to await the drafting and implementation of regulations. Second, participation is voluntary, and it cannot be determined at this juncture whether providers will want to go to whatever effort is ultimately required to avail themselves of the protections of the PSQIA. Participation may well be limited by the reality that the act is not going to cause the malpractice crisis or the existing tort system to go away. It is notable that the act exempts from its coverage original patient and provider information, including medical and billing records. Thus, all the information currently available to patients and their attorneys will remain discoverable. Existing accreditation standards and case law mandating that patients be informed of unanticipated outcomes or deviations from professionally recognized standards will also remain and thus limit the confidentiality protections of the PSQIA.

Protection of Peer Review Materials Under the Self-Critical Analysis Privilege Under Federal Law—An Eroding Concept

The federal courts have not recognized a federal peer review privilege under Federal Rules of Evidence 501. Issues that arise in federal court proceedings about the discoverability of peer review records instead are dealt with on a case-by-base basis resulting in varying decisions as to whether the court will recognize the common law self-critical analysis privilege. "Recognition of the self-evaluative privilege is often justified based on the rationale that the confidentiality created under the privilege is in society's best interests because it will encourage (hospitals) to engage in frank assessments of their activities without fear that the results will be used against (the hospital) in litigation" (40). The three criteria needed to invoke the self-critical analysis privilege under federal law are that (1) the information sought must come from some internal investigation undertaken by the institution; (2) there must be a significant public interest in maintaining the confidentiality of that information; and (3) without such protection, it must be unlikely that the institution would engage in the self-critical activity (41). In considering the privilege, the courts have balanced the plaintiff's right to discovery and the interests of the institution in shielding its self-critical documents.

The seminal case in which the federal courts have recognized a self-critical analysis privilege under Rule 501 of the Federal Rules of Evidence for a hospital peer review conference on the treatment of patients is *Bredice vs. Doctors Hospital*, decided in 1970 (42). In *Bredice*, the plaintiff moved for production of documents of any board or committee concerning the death of the decedent. The court denied plaintiff's motion based on a public policy rationale that these meetings, performed in accordance with Joint Commission standards for encouraging quality improvement, necessitated confidentiality and protection from disclosure in the overwhelming public interest. Subsequent federal court cases followed the reasoning of the *Bredice* court in holding that the self-critical analysis privilege protected peer review materials from discovery (43).

Eroding the ability of physicians to rely on the common law self-critical analysis privilege to protect the confidentiality of peer review records (27,38) is another seminal case, *Syposs vs. United States* (44), that was decided following a series of decisions in which the federal courts rejected the privilege in nonmedical cases (45). In *Syposs*, the court held that peer review records of the Veteran's Administration Hospital concerning a physician defendant were discoverable in a medical malpractice action brought under the Federal Tort Claims Act. Interestingly, the *Syposs* court noted that congress had the opportunity to recognize a peer review privilege when enacting the HCQIA in 1986 and chose not to do so.

Thus, the viability of this common law privilege has been called into question and may be of limited value in protecting peer review information (27,38). Further, medical malpractice cases where physicians fear peer review information may be used to build a case against them are usually brought in state court where state law would govern the issue.

Protection of Peer Review Materials Under State Law—An Inconsistent Track Record

All 50 states except New Jersey and the District of Columbia have statutes that protect the work of medical review/peer review committees (46). The philosophy underlying most state law peer review privileges is that physicians must be encouraged to be candid and vigorous in the performance evaluation of their peers, without fear that those evaluations will be used to build a case against the subject physician in a medical malpractice lawsuit. Legislators create these statutes on the assumption that, absent statutory protection from disclosure (and in some cases, from liability as well), physicians would be reluctant to sit on peer review committees and engage in frank evaluations of their colleagues' peer review. Confidentiality is rooted in public policy to support physicians in their self-regulatory efforts to monitor the competency and conduct of their peers.

The 1980s were noted for the passing of statutory protection for materials and participants in peer review (27) to encourage effective peer review (36). For example, Public Health Law (PHL) § 2805-m was added to the New York laws in 1986 as part of a comprehensive package of medical malpractice reform legislation (47). Subsequently, a New York court observed that the New York State Legislature enacted PHL § 2805-m in part to combat the incidence of medical malpractice, noting that:

> physicians responsible for acts of professional misconduct should be subject to effective discipline and . . . improvement in the disciplinary process will contribute to the protection of the public health and the reduction of the incidence of malpractice . . . To permit disclosure of those reports in circumstances where their contents could lead to admissible evidence of medical malpractice would be entirely contrary to the spirit and intent of the comprehensive professional malpractice legislation adopted by the New York State legislature in 1985 and 1986. (48)

The New York legislature believed that a lower incidence of medical malpractice would ensure the continued adequacy of medical malpractice insurance for health care providers and thereby make adequate medical services available to the public (47).

The confidentiality provision embodied in PHL § 2805-m covers not only incident reports but also quality assurance committee decisions and is described in the legislative history as designed to "ensure that physicians and other health care providers and institutions are not deterred from participating in quality assurance, incident reporting and peer review programs or from complying with misconduct reporting requirements" (49).

While the state peer review laws differ both in terms of scope and in terms of strength by jurisdiction, they appear to share three common purposes: (1) to provide immunity from liability for committee members participating in good faith in the peer review process, (2) to afford confidentiality so that parties involved in peer review proceedings refrain from disclosing information regarding those proceedings to outsiders, and (3) to protect the medical review committee and its records and materials from discovery in civil actions by granting of an evidentiary privilege which allows a party to exercise the right to prevent an individual from testifying on certain matters at judicial proceedings (50).

Peer review statutes range from those that are especially broad and protecting like that of the District of Columbia (51) which protects from discovery in all medical malpractice and disciplinary hearings in which the physician is targeted, all documents prepared by the peer review committee, to those which protect peer review documents but provide an exception for statements made by a physician defendant when he or she attends a peer review committee meeting (34). In New York, records related to peer review activities are routinely available to licensing and disciplinary bodies, any statements (written or oral) made by a physician who is the target of peer review are given no protections against disclosure in a medical malpractice case when they relate to the subject matter of the litigation (52), medical peer review records are discoverable where the claim in the case does not sound in malpractice (53), and certain legal protections are not available in settings such as ambulatory surgery centers and nursing homes. Another variation is illustrated by New Jersey law which protects information and data secured by utilization review committees (as are required for hospitals to qualify under the Social Security Act and to take part in state and federally funded programs) but not medical peer review records (54). Moreover, the New Jersey courts have declined to expressly adopt as a full privilege the protections for self-critical analysis materials. Instead, the New Jersey courts favor a case-by-case weighing process in considering concerns arising from the disclosure of evaluation and deliberation materials (55).

As noted by the 1999 IOM report, the scope of peer review protection varies from state to state considerably. Questions about what constitutes a protected "committee," what materials are protected from discovery, what is "peer review activity," from what type of proceedings these materials are protected, who receives the protection and other factual issues have opened the door for plaintiffs attorneys to argue and for courts to decide that peer review materials made are not protected under state peer review laws. Further, courts tend to give narrow construction to legal privileges and immunities (25). "The net result is a 'half-hearted' privilege . . . that leaves parties twisting in the wind while lawyers determine its scope" (27). The case-by-case interpretations and ambiguity of the statutory language may contribute to the reluctance of physicians to take a chance and disclose potentially damning information (25,27,56). Further, many jurisdictions protect the participants in the peer review process but not the target (27). This is consistent with the approach in the HCQIA of 1986 which provides qualified immunity from damages only to the participants in peer review committees, not the subject physician (26). Moreover, it is important to note that state laws protecting peer review materials have no binding effect on federal courts (25). Illustrative is the case of *Salomon vs. Our Lady of Victory Hospital* in which the United States District Court for the Western District of New York permitted plaintiff to discover, in a federal case in which she alleged sexual discrimination and a misuse of the peer review process in retaliation to her complaints, the chart reviews, credentials files, quality assurance files, and administrative files for all of the physicians affiliated with the hospital department where she worked. The court was not persuaded by the objections of the hospital and other defendants that the documents were confidential pursuant to New York State law nor the self-critical analysis privilege "because they are not recognized under the federal common law" (35).

Finally, it is notable that efforts are afoot to remove the confidential status afforded to the peer review process. One notable example is a bill recently proposed to the New York State Assembly, which also strives to make failure to engage in the peer review process an act of professional misconduct. The bill proposal provides in pertinent part as follows:

> Instead of shielding patients from information and extending the 'white wall of silence', this bill presents a three-tiered resolution that opens up the peer review process and guarantees full and good faith participation. First, the confidentiality protection is removed from physicians who participate in the peer review process. Second, failing to participate fully, freely and in good faith in any peer review process constitutes professional misconduct. Third, every hospital is required to make the granting or renewing of privileges contingent upon physicians' agreement to participate fully, freely and in good faith in any peer review process. (57)

Commentators have traced the decline of the peer review privilege on both the federal and the state levels and noted the difficulty this trend presents for creating patient safety systems based on accurate medical error information (58). The erosion of the medical peer review privileges leaves physicians without adequate assurances of the confidentiality of their participation in peer review activity, thereby undermining the effectiveness of peer review. The lack of federal recognition for peer review confidentiality, coupled with narrow statutory interpretations by state courts, serves to discourage physicians from participating in peer review activities. While the quality improvement purpose of peer review is consistent with the purpose of medical error reporting systems, such collaborative efforts are unlikely to succeed in the current state of peer review jurisprudence (56).

PRACTICE POINTER

Practitioners should not assume that documents will be statutorily protected as confidential merely by being characterized after the fact as quality assurance or peer review material. It is the burden of the party invoking the privilege to demonstrate that the documents were generated as a result of a formalized quality assurance/peer review meeting conducted in accordance with an established policy. Thus, such policies and procedures should be in writing and from time to time reviewed by counsel for continued legal compliance with applicable law. Also helpful is a mechanism to clearly label such documents as "Confidential Peer Review Material" at the time they are generated and a process which ensures that these materials are consistently maintained in a fashion separate from the patient's medical record.

Influence of Professional Norms on Error Disclosure in the Peer Review Forum and Beyond
The above-noted limitations of the federal self-critical analysis privilege and the state statutory peer review privileges may, in part, explain why physicians continue to be reluctant to openly discuss their errors even among colleagues in the peer review setting. While this highlights that some further degree of legal protection may be necessary to support and enhance this important avenue of medical error disclosure, existing professional norms may render legal

changes insufficient to create an environment conducive to reporting. A landmark 1994 article by Lucian Leape "Error in Medicine" concluded that "It is apparent that the most fundamental change that will be needed if hospitals are to make meaningful progress in error reduction is a cultural one" (59).

Medical training and the culture instilled during this training has considerable strength in emphasizing autonomy and personal responsibility. It has also led to a culture of hierarchy and authority in decision making and to a belief that mistakes should not be made (1). The IOM 1999 report goes on to state that when mistakes do occur, they are typically treated as a personal and professional failure. Many physicians believe that errors arise from personal ignorance or ineptitude, and therefore mistakes are not acceptable (1).

Also important and relevant to reporting of medical errors among peers are institutional factors. The lack of an ongoing institutional commitment to provide for an environment conducive to the open, protected nonpunitive system for error reporting and collection of error-related data has been noted as a major obstacle to a successful safety patient program. Candor in reporting is essential to study the occurrence, consequence, and etiology of errors. Subsequent design and implementation of preventative measures is then required. Additionally, the organization needs to prevent error reporting from being used by one professional group against another within the hierarchy and should facilitate the development of a "colleagues in care" relationship among all providers regardless of discipline. In order for an organization to learn, it must be willing to acknowledge that errors occur then undertake a critical analysis of what contributes to this occurrence. Errors are a signal that change in practice may be necessary. An organization must view the reporting of errors as a positive contribution to the overall strength and integrity of the organization. Leadership should demonstrate an understanding that, while knowing about past errors will not prevent all future errors, knowing about past errors can and will have a positive effect on patient safety (60).

Other factors that have been noted to impede discussion of medical errors among colleagues include fear of institutional sanctions, anxiety about maintaining good relationships with peers, loss of business, and damage to reputation (61). Clinicians have been termed the "second victims" of medical errors (62). A threefold increase in depression, accompanied by a clinically meaningful increase in burnout and decrease in overall quality of life, has also been noted (63). The significance of this finding is highlighted by the fact that the baseline rates of physician distress in modern medicine are high. Another study concluded that many physicians report anxiety, loss of confidence, sleeping difficulties, and reduced job satisfaction following errors (64).

There is insufficient evidence to predict the impact that eliminating one or more of these disincentives would have on reporting behavior (65). Further, it is notable that most data on this subject involves residents in training (66), leaving a question as to whether it is appropriate to extrapolate these findings to fully trained practitioners. However, these impediments have been noted to have a negative effect on the reporting of medical errors in general (38) and thus are an important consideration in efforts to improve and promote error reporting.

PRACTICE POINTER

Serious consideration should be given to creation of an environment which supports and encourages sharing of information about medical error in which there is ongoing education and training about how and when this should be done.

Disclosure of Medical Errors to Third-Party Reporting Systems

As noted in the IOM's 2004 Report (21), clinical performance data involving medical errors is one key building block for a safe health care delivery system and can serve a full range of purposes, including accountability from a professional licensure or legal liability perspective to learning including the redesign of care processes and testing of hypotheses. Indeed, reporting systems have successfully monitored other kinds of medical events including drug reactions, vaccine reactions, and nosocomial infections (67). The IOM has called for the development of an information technology infrastructure including coordinated error reporting as essential to improve the safety of health care (1,21).

The 1999 IOM report recommended the creation of external reporting system to identify and learn from errors so as to prevent future occurrences. Two types of reporting systems were discussed, specifically, mandatory reporting systems intended to hold providers accountable for improvements and voluntary reporting systems, to detect system weaknesses before serious harm occurs. As to the first prong, the IOM recommended establishing a nationwide mandatory system for states to collect standardized information (initially from hospitals but eventually from other institutional and ambulatory health care settings) on adverse events that result in death or serious harm to hold hospitals accountable for serious medical errors. The IOM reasoned that these should be made public because the public has the right to be informed of unsafe conditions and that, in the case of serious adverse events, disclosure to the public is an appropriate and desirable practice. It was further noted that confidentiality and protection from liability might be inappropriate in the case of serious error. The requirement of public disclosure of mandatory reported errors was deemed consistent with the rationale that errors which caused death or serious patient injury would be the ones most likely to draw lawsuits any way.

Additionally, the IOM recommended the concurrent development of voluntary confidential systems for reporting errors that result in little or no harm or "near misses" (1). Voluntary systems were envisioned as confidential and existing solely to improve patient safety and quality. These systems would not necessarily be run by the state and would collect and aggregate information about a broad set of errors that result in no or minimal harm in order to detect system weaknesses before harm occurs.

The National Academy for State Health Policy (NASHP) has similarly concluded that mandatory and voluntary systems can work together to help reduce death and serious injury in the health care system (68). Such a twofold system appears to represent a balancing act to satisfy the competing objectives of the need to levy strong incentives on health care organizations to make systemic changes to protect patients and the need to encourage providers to participate in error reporting and reduction efforts by preventing misuse of the information in the court room.

While medical error reporting systems exist at the federal and state level in an attempt to build a database upon which providers can monitor patient safety and collect useful information, they suffer from underreporting, even when the reports are anonymous, voluntary and confidential (38), and the lack of a standardized format and terminology for the capture and reporting of data related to medical errors limits the usefulness of the data that is reported.

Mandatory Reporting Systems

The primary purpose of mandatory reporting systems is to hold providers accountable by ensuring that serious mistakes are reported, in most cases to state authorities; investigated; and that appropriate follow-up action is taken. Organizations that continue unsafe practices risk citations, penalties, sanctions or revocation of licenses, and possible public exposure and loss of business. The overreaching objective for mandatory reporting systems is to have the reporting analyzed and feed findings back to reporting facilities to enable them to design and implement interventions to reduce error (69). The main appeal of public reporting is to restore confidence that something is being done to restore patient safety.

The IOM recommended that state regulatory programs continue to operate mandatory reporting systems as they have the authority to investigate specific cases and issue penalties or fines. The IOM did not specify what type of data, whether aggregate or institution specific, should be made publicly available from the mandatory reporting system but does not appear to have intended that the data be specific to individual health care practitioners as such a requirement would be inconsistent with their underlying premise that only a small fraction of errors are attributable to incompetent providers, the vast majority of errors are attributable to systems issues, and that blaming or levying sanctions on individual providers is not the solution to this problem.

While states are intended to play a chief role in mandatory reporting, the IOM recommended that congress take the following steps in order to establish a nationwide mandatory reporting system: (1) designate the National Quality Forum (NQF) as the entity responsible for issuing and maintaining reporting standards to be used by states, (2) require health care institutions to report standardized information on a defined list of adverse events, and (3) provide funds and technical expertise to state governments to establish or improve their error reporting systems (1).

The NQF was established in May of 1999 following the recommendation of the President's Advisory Commission on Consumer Protection and Quality in the Health Care Industry, and is a private, nonprofit voluntary consensus standards setting organization created to develop and implement a national strategy for the measurement and reporting of health care quality. Acting on the IOM's recommendation, the NQF, in 2002, released a list of 27 serious, preventable adverse events that should be reported by all licensed health care facilities (70). The list includes standardized definitions of key terms to encourage consistent use and implementation across the county. This list was updated in 2006 and now identifies 28 adverse events that are serious and of concern to health care providers, consumers, and all stakeholders. The 28 events are organized into six categories—five that relate to the provision of care (surgical, product or device, patient protection, care management, and environmental) and one that includes four criminal events (71).

However, no nationwide mandatory reporting system has yet been enacted. Instead, and as more fully set forth later, the federal government's current approach to the reduction of medical errors appears to be through the endorsement of voluntary reporting systems with reliance on parallel efforts of private accreditation systems.

Mandatory reporting systems do exist on the state level. The NASHP recently collected information about all state adverse event reporting systems that were authorized as of October 2007. For purposes of NASHP's research, state adverse event reporting systems were defined as those systems authorized and operated by state governments to collect reports from hospitals (and in some cases other types of facilities such as ambulatory surgical centers) about adverse events with the intent of improving safety (72). According to the NASHP's 2007 report:

1. A total of 27 adverse event reporting systems are in place with the intent to improve patient safety. These states are California, Colorado, Connecticut, District of Columbia, Florida, Georgia, Illinois, Indiana, Kansas, Maine, Maryland, Massachusetts, Minnesota, Nevada, New Jersey, New York, Ohio, Oregon, Pennsylvania, Rhode Island, South Carolina, South Dakota, Tennessee, Utah, Vermont, Washington, and Wyoming.
2. Between 2005 and 2007, 15 states and the District of Columbia enacted and revised patient safety reporting systems, several of whom added well-defined reportable event lists.
3. There is a trend toward increased focus on standardization of reports. By 2007, almost half of the states with reporting systems had adopted the NQF's recommended list of standardized reportable events, including the most recently authorized systems.
4. By 2007, nine states had developed a web-based system that could be used for analysis and feedback to data reporters (as compared to 2000 when only New York had this capability).
5. All but four states require that root cause analysis (RCA) results and/or corrective action plans be submitted in response to serious adverse events.
6. In 2007, most states cited the purpose of their systems as providing regulatory and quality improvement functions as compared to 2000 when the stated purpose of most state reporting systems was to improve patient safety by holding individual health care facilities accountable for preventable adverse events and perhaps secondarily to improve quality and patient safety across facilities.
7. The current trend is toward strong comprehensive data protection with all but four of the 27 systems having some type of legal protection beyond general peer review protections to prevent unwanted disclosure of data.
8. There is a trend toward disclosure of adverse events to patients and/or families. In 2000, only one state (New York) required hospitals to disclose to patients when an adverse event occurred. In 2007, eleven of the 27 states mandated this type of disclosure likely in acknowledgment of the theory that disclosure is not tied to increased lawsuits. These states are California, Florida, Maryland, Massachusetts, New Jersey, New York, Nevada, Oregon, Pennsylvania, Tennessee, and Vermont.
9. All but three states have provided or plan to provide public reports of some of their collected data. Seventeen systems publicly release aggregate data that does not identify facilities and seven have released or plan to release facility-specific data. Examples of state initiatives include Virginia's requirement that data on complications after surgery be reported, Florida's and Illinois' release of report cards and posting them on the Internet, New York's mandated release of physician profiles, and Washington's disclosure of patient safety information to the pubic (68).

While some of these state laws were enacted in response to the IOM's 1999 report, others date back to the 1980s when they were enacted as part of a medical malpractice reform package. One notable example is New York. In 1985, the New York State Department of Health developed its first mandatory adverse event reporting system known as the Hospital Incident Reporting System (34,47). The program required reporting of preventable adverse events and a description of steps taken to address underlying deficiencies in hospital systems and/or practitioner training and capabilities. This program was created by the legislature to capture preventable events caused by human or mechanical error resulting in patient harm. The statute requires hospitals to collect and report information on negative health outcomes and incidents (34,47), protects the confidentiality of the reports, and prevents disclosure of incident reports under the Freedom of Information Law (73). The New York system is a good example of one that has evolved from a report-only process primarily focused on accountability when it was first enacted to one that currently also seeks to improve quality and patient safety across facilities. The critical elements of the current New York State Patient Occurrence Reporting Tracking System enacted in 1998 are making the system legally required, protecting reported information from discovery, clear and objective definitions of reporting criteria, a secure Web-based system, providing feedback to users relative to their own performance, and analyzing data at both the facility and statewide levels with dissemination of lessons learned (74).

Like New York, most of these state mandatory reporting laws impose a legal obligation to report, require reports of data concerning medical errors that result in serious injury or death, require use of the reported data to verify data to ensure consistency with reporting definitions and attribution to error, require analysis of data, require identification of ways to avoid recurrence of the error, and mandate oversight and evaluation of corrective actions taken (75).

One of the two top problems with mandatory reporting systems is insufficient funding which limits the ability of state regulators to ensure compliance with reporting guidelines, to follow up with facilities, and to conduct analysis and feedback of data (68,75). The second problem is underreporting of adverse events (76). Physician surveys indicate that a majority of physicians believe that fear of malpractice exposure is a barrier to adverse event reporting (77). A survey of hospital leaders indicates that many have serious reservations about a mandatory error reporting system; believe that existing state reporting standards fail in some cases to provide clear guidance on what should be reported; and that mandatory reporting with public disclosure may actually discourage internal reporting, lead to lawsuits and impart little benefit to public safety (78).

The patchwork nature of the state mandatory reporting system has also generated criticism. The 1999 IOM report observed that few states aggregate the data or analyze them to identify general trends with analysis with follow-up instead of occurring on a case-by-case basis (75). One commentator laments that "State mandating reporting systems, in place in 22 states, may also cause inconsistencies and result in confusing procedures and inaccurate data or no data collected at all" (79).

Lack of coordinated follow-up of information mandatorily reported has also generated criticism. New York's mandatory medical error reporting system was the subject of such criticism in a 2005 report of the New York Public Interest Research Group which concluded that the New York State Department of Health (NYDOH) had failed to follow up on findings from 5 years earlier that thousands of patients in New York State were dying from medical errors and certainly had not met its stated goal of reducing medical errors by half (80).

Reporting to Private Accreditation Systems

The Joint Commission is a private accreditor, which granted authority by federal and state governments to accredit hospitals. The Joint Commission's Sentinel Event Policy, promulgated in 1996, lies somewhere in between state-mandated reports of medical errors and voluntary reporting systems. The Joint Commission's policy focuses on "serious" or "sentinel" events defined as "an unexpected occurrence involving death or serious physical or psychological injury, or the risk thereof" including unanticipated death or major loss of functioning unrelated to the patient's condition, patient suicide, wrong-site surgery, infant abduction/discharge to the wrong family, rape, and hemolytic reactions (81).

The hallmark characteristic of the Sentinel Event Policy is the production of a credible intensive analysis following the occurrence of a serious event commencing with a no-holds-barred vetting of all the potential causes underlying the event or what the Joint Commission refers to as "root causes." The Joint Commission's use of the term "root cause analysis" (RCA) evidences that their policy is, like the engineering world from which the term was borrowed, focused on a system approach to solving problems and producing desired outcomes. RCA focuses primarily on the organization's systems and processes as opposed to individual performance. Events are called "sentinel" because they signal the need for immediate investigation through the RCA process and response. The Joint Commission observed that the terms "sentinel event" and "medical error" are not synonymous, not all sentinel events occur because of an error and not all errors result in sentinel events. The stated goals of the Sentinel Event Policy are to positively impact patient care, prevent sentinel events, focus the attention of an organization on understanding the causes of a sentinel event and changing systems and processes to prevent recurrence, and maintain the confidence of the public in accredited organizations (81).

Although they were initially required, the Joint Commission now only "encourages" Sentinel Event Reports. To encourage reporting of Sentinel Events, the Joint Commission has established a policy of not penalizing the accreditation status of an organization that reports such events and performs a RCA. However, reporting is not entirely voluntary if an institution wants to maintain its accreditation status. In cases where a hospital fails to report serious events to the Joint Commission and the Joint Commission learns about it from a third party, the hospital must conduct a RCA or risk loss of accreditation (81). Thus far, the Joint Commission has been able to maintain the confidentiality of all sentinel event information. However, the major protection against information discovered under the Sentinel Event Policy cited by the Joint Commission is the peer review privilege, which, as discussed earlier, is in danger of being eroded.

Voluntary reports under the Sentinel Event Policy have been low. Peter B. Angood, M.D., Vice President and Chief Patient Safety Officer for the Joint Commission, estimates that the Joint Commission's database represents only 1% to 2% of sentinel events actually occurring across the country (82).

Voluntary Reporting of Medical Errors

As a complement to the mandatory reporting of serious errors, the IOM recommended establishing voluntary reporting systems to collect information on less serious mistakes that result in little or no harm or what have been termed "near misses." Information gathered by voluntary reporting systems may be used to identify vulnerabilities and weaknesses in health care systems and to make improvements to prevent serious errors from occurring (1).

It has been suggested that voluntary reporting to a neutral third party may elicit greater participation as has been the experience in the airline industry. Aviation incident reports originally went to the Federal Aviation Administration, an entity with punitive power and few reports resulted. Reports increased dramatically when the system was changed so that reports were directed instead to the National Aeronautics and Space Administration, a neutral entity without such power (1). A focus on voluntary reporting of near misses to a neutral third party until legal issues are addressed may be the most effective in gaining participation and making safety progress given that the focus of this alternative is in keeping with the nonpunitive systems-based philosophy inherent in effectively reducing error (83). This is the approach that appears to have been adopted in the Patient Safety and Improvement Act of 2005 (PSQIA) described earlier (39).

PRACTICE POINTER

Institutions may wish to consider developing an incident reporting system that includes the reporting of near miss events. These can be reviewed by a committee of individuals including, but not limited to, physicians; nurse managers; risk managers; quality assurance professionals; and hospital administrators. Incidents involving real and near miss events should be discussed. Those needing further investigation through RCA or failure mode analysis can be identified and these tools are implemented to determine if there are any system failures. If system failures are identified, patient safety strategies can be implemented and monitored.

Impact of Reporting to Third Parties on Patient Safety—A Concept in Need of Redress
The disparate element of the existing patchwork of third-party reporting systems on the state, federal, and accreditation levels is aptly illustrated by the following example:

> "The following 'real world' example further illustrates the problem with numerous disparate data elements for documenting an adverse event. If an individual suffered a serious adverse drug event (ADE) while in a New York hospital, the clinician would first file a report internally for review by the designated hospital representative. A second report would be filed with the New York State Department of Health through NYPORTS. Another third report could be voluntarily submitted to the Food and Drug Administration (FDA), either through the FDA MedWatch reporting system or through private-sector organizations such as the United States Pharmacopia (USP), to inform the FDA of potential serious problems with the drug. Adding further to the burden of disparate and multiple methods for representing an ADE are the voluntary reporting requirements of the hospitals' accrediting organization, the Joint Commission for Accreditation of Health care Organizations (JCAHO), whose proposed taxonomy provides yet another dataset for classifying and reporting such events. Already this example involves four different reports with varying data elements for the same ADE." (84)

In addition to the practical complexities of reporting and the need for a uniform system that involves common definitions of medical errors, there are other considerable barriers to the development of a useful system of reporting medical errors. All existing systems, even those that are voluntary nonpunitive and confidential, appear to suffer from underreporting. There is nothing to suggest that new systems such as one under the PSQIA of 2005 will be any more successful in inducing physicians to report errors (38) unless changes are made to the liability systems that appear to underlie the pervasive resistance by physicians to speak about error notwithstanding their verbal endorsement that disclosure is important (82). It is unlikely that physicians will discuss, identify, and accurately report medical errors when the data may be divulged and may be used to support litigation against them. The threats to confidentiality appears to stand in the way of a national database of errors that could lead to systems-based solutions in patient care (58). Others have noted that the blame element of reporting needs to be eliminated before it can be consistent with a systems approach to error.

> "In the current medical systems analysis, voluntary reporting or reporting of any kind is simply going to assign blame. This is the absolute opposite of what you are supposed to do in a systems approach. You never assign 'blame'. It only serves to defragment the system again." (22)

Other commentators have observed that no reporting mechanism will be successful in the absence of a serious and systematic attempt to link performance (or lack of it) to reimbursement (79). The shortcomings of the current third-party reporting systems have been summarized as follows by one commentator:

> "Reporting of adverse events and near misses is an essential part of information infrastructure, yet efforts to obtain good data on performance continues to flounder on the shoals of systems and provider resistence … Providers are confronted with varying regulatory forces that relate to medical errors and their discovery. No coordination of reporting is currently mandated in our complex state-federal system, with its market driven insurance component and its powerful civil litigation system existing in parallel." (79)

While the third-party reporting systems have the challenges, noted earlier, to overcome, it is clear that the incentives for health care providers to move in the direction of error disclosure are mounting.

> "Although many continue to debate the efficiency and reliability of such reporting systems, it is clear to even the casual observer that government and private regulators are demanding increased reporting and disclosure of patient outcomes, whether voluntary or mandatory." (85)

Disclosure to Patients
While the reporting systems previously discussed govern a provider's duty to report errors to governmental authorities, other third parties, or colleagues, this section of the chapter will focus on disclosure based on a direct dialogue between provider and patient—the newest focus in the changing tide of medical error disclosure. As described later, accreditation agencies,

trade associations, and government regulators are encouraging a national mandate for direct provider–patient disclosure of medical errors.

Patients Expect Disclosure

This mandate comes in the wake of increasing public awareness about the prevalence of medical error since the issuance of the IOM report as well as consumer access to an ever-increasing amount of quality-related information about medical providers. Readily available on the Internet is information compiled by CMS (86), the Leapfrog Group (87), the National Quality Foundation, and a host of other data clearinghouses that patients can access to make their own determinations about provider quality. At the same time, patients have made clear their expectation that their own treating hospitals and physicians provide them with truthful detailed information about their own care including disclosure of medical errors (88–91). Such disclosures are expected by patients who assume a trust-based relationship with their physicians. Patients trust their physicians to make appropriate care and treatment decisions including those involving difficult and uncomfortable intervention. This trust is violated when an error occurs, an injury that is compounded when the physician fails to acknowledge the error and apologize.

> "Patients generally desire (in order of diminishing unanimity): 1) a clear statement that an error has occurred; 2) an explanation of the full detail of the error; 3) a sincere apology; 4) reassurances that the something is being done to make sure the error does not happen again; and 5) financial compensation for injury, pain or suffering; and 6) accountability on the part of the responsible physician." (38,87)

Another study concluded that 98% of patients desire to be informed of even a minor error and that this desire to be informed increases with the severity of the outcome (90).

Further, patients and families have banded together to push for full disclosure of medical errors, along with apologies, by establishing patient advocacy groups. Grassroots organizations such as Sorry Works!, Patients United Limiting Substandards and Errors in Health care, Medically Induced Trauma Support Services, Consumers Advancing Patient Safety, and others are raising the awareness of political leaders, legislators, and the medical community about the urgent need for change.

Physicians Agree with the Concept of Disclosure But Face Barriers

Physicians appear to support disclosure in principle if not in practice (82,88). This is not surprising in view of the fact that physicians have long been subject to ethical mandates requiring disclosure of medical errors. Physicians have always been responsible for communicating honestly with patients about treatment plans, prognosis, and outcomes; however difficult it may be for the patient and/or the physician. Ethical standards of physicians have mandated disclosure of errors by physicians to patients for more than 20 years. The Code of Ethics of the AMA requires disclosure when "a patient suffers significant medical complications that may have resulted from the physician's mistake or judgment." Section 8.12 of the AMA's "Opinions of the Council on Ethical and Judicial Affairs" states in plain and unambiguous terms all physicians' ethical duty to fully disclose the truth to their patients whenever medical mistakes arise.

> "E-8.12 Patient Information. It is a fundamental ethical requirement that a physician should at all times deal honestly and openly with patients. Patients have a right to know their past and present medical status and to be free of any mistaken beliefs concerning their conditions. Situations occasionally occur in which a patient suffers significant medical complications that may have resulted from the physician's mistake or judgment. In these situations, the physician is ethically required to inform the patient of all the facts necessary to ensure understanding of what has occurred. Only through full disclosure is a patient able to make informed decisions regarding future medical care.
>
> Ethical responsibility includes informing patients of changes in their diagnoses resulting from retrospective review of test results or any other information. This obligation holds even though the patient's medical treatment or therapeutic options may not be altered by the new information.
>
> Concern regarding legal liability which might result following truthful disclosure should not affect the physician's honesty with a patient. (I, II, III, IV) Issued March 1981; Updated June 1994 (92)."

Similarly, the American College of Physicians Ethics Manual states that physicians should tell patients about "procedural or judgment errors" if such information is "material to the patient's well-being" (93). In keeping is The American College of Obstetricians and Gynecologists Code of Medical Ethics which states: "The obstetrician-gynecologist should deal honestly with patients and colleagues (veracity). This includes not misrepresenting himself or herself through any form of communication in an untruthful, misleading or deceptive manner" (94).

However, a notable flaw in these ethical mandates is that they merely identify disclosure as a mandate and provide health care professionals with no guidance regarding how or when to disclose. These standards have been criticized as lacking adequate specificity, as being ill suited to the complex nature of errors, and as narrow in scope.

> "Also, the standards do not tackle common but complex, questions: How much physician contribution to an error creates the duty to disclose? Is a physician obligated to disclose a systems error? What are the obligations of a physician who witnesses a colleague's harmful error?" (38)

Notwithstanding the seemingly clear and long-standing ethical mandate, surveys of physicians found that disclosure of errors to patients occurred in less than one-third of cases (95–97).

A reported in 2007 study demonstrates that this trend of infrequent disclosure continues. Ninety percent (90%) of faculty and residents surveyed about disclosure of unanticipated outcomes responded that they would disclose a minor or major harm to a patient. Yet, in practice, only 41% actually disclosed an outcome involving unanticipated minor harm, and only 5% disclosed an actual major error (98).

Even when patients are told of medical errors, there appears to be a disconnect between the amount of information patients expect to be told and what the physician believes to be sufficient disclosure. Illustrative is a 2002 study of disclosure practices reported from more than 200 hospitals, which concluded:

> "More than half of respondents report that they would always disclose a death or serious injury, but when presented with actual clinical scenarios, respondents were much less likely to disclose preventable harms than to disclose nonpreventable harms of comparable severity. Reluctance to disclose preventable harms was twice as likely to occur at hospitals having major concerns about the malpractice implications of disclosure." (99)

Other research has found that

1. While 92% of patients believed they should always be told about complications, only 60% of the physicians believed that patients should always be told;
2. While 81% of the patients believed they should be advised of the possible future adverse outcomes of the complications, only 33% of the physicians believed that patients should be told about possible future adverse outcomes (100).

Disclosing errors is challenging for both physicians and health care institutions (101). One study suggests that physicians see several barriers to disclosure including difficulty defining errors, the need for training in handling errors, and the threat of malpractice litigation (102). Another cites confusion about the parameters of disclosure tied to vagueness in existing standards and policies, a lack of institutional commitment to the cultural change needed to support disclosure, cautionary legal advice, and physician reticence due to inadequate disclosure training as among the factors impeding disclosure (103).

Further barriers appear to be related to the psychological impact of medical error on the provider. Studies evidence that physicians, drawn to the profession to help and not harm patients, experience guilt; shame; diminished self-confidence; agony over the harm caused; concern about loss of patient trust; and concerns about career impact following medical error (104). The anxiety of guilt is heightened around the people connected to the event and thus people avoid people who may judge or remind them of their past wrong (105). This helps explain why physicians avoid patients after mistakes and have reduced empathy and compassion for the patient (106) when the patient needs it most. Silence harms both the physician and the patient as well as the relationship between the two.

An additional barrier that may influence physician disclosure of a medical error to a patient may flow from a risk manager, insurance company, and/or attorney perspective, specifically the requirements of a physician's or hospital's malpractice insurance policy. Liability insurers generally require immediate reporting of an event that may invoke the insurer's responsibility. A standard insurance contract clause requires that the insured make no statements and/or take no actions that could compromise the insurer from defending the claim. A common stipulation in such "cooperation clauses" forbids the insured from "admitting liability" to an injured party (83,85,107).

PRACTICE POINTER

Whether a disclosure should include an apology and in what terms is a decision best made by a physician with the benefit of risk management and legal advice. When a disclosure is coupled with a fault-admitting apology, also known as an apology of responsibility or full apology (as distinct from an apology of sympathy—"I'm sorry this happened to you."— also known as a partial apology), same should be made in coordination with a physician's liability carrier so that the physician does not jeopardize coverage on the grounds that the physician violated the cooperation's clause of his or her malpractice insurance policy. Additionally, legal advice can assist the physician in weighing the potential evidentiary risks of a disclosure coupled with a fault-admitting apology.

Patient Disclosure Initiatives
Attempting to bridge the gap between the patient's expectation that medical errors be disclosed and actual clinical practice of physicians in disclosing errors to patients are a number of standards and programs that are being promulgated on a number of levels in the United States (108).

Joint Commission—Patient Standard for Error Disclosure to Patients
In 2001, the Joint Commission issued new Sentinel Event Policies and Procedures, the most controversial of which was the requirement that patients or survivors be told of the occurrence of error that lead to harm or death. Hospitals accredited by the Joint Commission are required to inform patients of any "unanticipated" outcomes that significantly differ from their expected outcome (109). The Joint Commission's standard, which is likely the most widely disseminated physician to patient disclosure standard, has been described as "groundbreaking" to the extent it heralded a shift from mere endorsement of the importance of disclosure to a requirement with teeth because it is linked to the accreditation status of hospitals (108). While the Joint Commission is heralded as having issued the first nationwide standard regarding disclosure of medical errors to patients (108), several things are notably lacking about the Joint Commission's requirement of error disclosure to patients. First, the term "unanticipated outcomes" is undefined, a fact that may result in confusion about whether an event is reportable and thus lead to underreporting (110). This terminology has led to debates over whether the fact that certain complications of treatment, such as postoperative infections, are well known to occasionally occur means that they are "anticipated" and therefore do not require disclosure. Second, the disclosure required is an explanation of the outcome amounting to a disclosure of facts and not an admission of an "error" or "mistake" partly out of a concern that the standard not force admissions of liability (96). One commentator has observed that the Joint Commission standards, like the ethical mandates, are notably silent on whether the physician should issue an apology, expression of regret, assumption of responsibility, or reassurance that changes will be made to prevent recurrence. "One suspects, particularly given patient expectations, that the duty to disclose and responsibility to one's patient include much more than a factual release—that physicians have an obligation to repair the broken trust in some deeper way" (38). Third, the Joint Commission is focusing on whether the required disclosures are taking place in connection with a "sentinel event" defined as "an unexpected occurrence involving death or serious physical or psychological injury, or the risk thereof". Accordingly, the Joint Commission standard would presumably not apply to other less clear-cut types of medical error such as minor error which does not cause harm or have the potential to do so and near misses defined as errors that could have caused harm but did not reach the patient because it was intercepted. As noted in the IOM

1999 report, disclosure about errors all along this continuum is necessary to improve patient safety (1).

Not encouraging is a survey of hospital administrators conducted a year after implementation of the Joint Commission requirement which found that, although nearly all hospitals reported that they sometimes informed patients or their families when an adverse event occurred, only about half did so routinely. Fear of malpractice litigation was the most commonly cited barrier to disclosure (99).

A 2002 survey of institutional risk managers revealed that 36% of health care organizations had established disclosure policies (99). By 2005, this fraction had apparently increased to 69% (111). There is little systematic evidence available regarding the impact of these policies on the practice of disclosure (111).

Notwithstanding, the Joint Commission's standard has been a force in pushing the health care community to reevaluate attitudes about what information is appropriate to share with patients. Further, it serves to highlight the shifting focus from the traditional assumption that the caregiver's role is to decide what might be good for the patient both in terms of treatment and in terms of action as well as what scope of information should be disclosed to or withheld from a patient, to a recognition that the patient is the arbiter of how information that pertains to him or her should be conveyed and used (112).

2006 NQF Safe Practice Guidelines on the Disclosure of Serious Unanticipated Outcomes to Patients

The NQF is a not-for-profit, public–private partnership created to develop and implement a national strategy for health care quality measurement and reporting including endorsing national consensus standards for measuring and publicly reporting on performance according to expert opinion and consensus among major quality-of-care organizations such as the Joint Commission, the Institute of Health care Improvement, the Agency for Health care Research and Quality, and the CMS (113). As noted earlier, the NQF was charged with and did issue, in 2002 and 2008, lists of serious, preventable adverse events that should be reported by all licensed health care facilities. In November of 2006, the NQF endorsed a new safe practice guideline on the disclosure of serious unanticipated outcomes to patients (114). The key elements of this safe practice are as follows:

1. Content to be disclosed to the patient
   I. Provide facts about the event
      a. Presence of error or system failure, if known
      b. Results of event analysis to support informed decision making by the patient
   II. Express regret for unanticipated outcome
   III. Give formal apology if unanticipated outcome caused by error or system failure
2. Institutional requirements
   I. Integrate disclosure, patient-safety, and risk-management activities
   II. Establish disclosure support system
      a. Provide background disclosure education
      b. Ensure that disclosure coaching is available at all times
      c. Provide emotional support for health care workers, administrators, patients, and families
   III. Use performance-improvement tools to track and enhance disclosure (108).

PRACTICE POINTER

Immediately following an incident, a patient or his or her family may ask questions. The initial explanation should be free of speculation. Patients and their families can be advised that the physician and/or hospital is not sure about the details of the "how" and "why" an incident occurred and that the incident needs to be carefully analyzed to determine the cause of the incident. It is important to note that disclosure is a sequential and factual communication that should take place in stages as information is known and not in a hurried, defensive, one-shot fashion. Following such an initial conversation, and particularly where a patient's medical picture is complex and/or involves multiple medical specialties, a multidisciplinary team consisting of risk management; attending physician and consulting physicians; social work, if applicable; and legal should be convened to discuss what occurred and what further investigation may be necessary. How and what is disclosed to the patient/family will also be affected by whether what occurred was a preventable unanticipated outcome or an outcome that was not preventable. While both disclosures are best made with transparency and empathy (as even an adverse outcome caused by a known complication is distressing to a patient), an apology of responsibility is not advisable relative to an outcome that was not preventable as may be appropriate to an outcome that was preventable. When it is unknown whether the outcome was preventable, providers are cautioned to communicate only known facts. A disclosure in either case should also include an explanation of how the injury occurred and what steps are being taken to prevent recurrence. When disclosure calls for a fault-admitting-responsibility-accepting disclosure, legal guidance will assist the provider in negotiating the insurance issues discussed earlier as well as in weighing the potential evidentiary risks (115).

Finally, disclosure impacting multiple stakeholders, for example, hospitals and physicians that may be insured by different carriers with different and/or competing interests, should take into consideration the respective interests of each and avoid finger pointing.

The enforcement mechanism of the safe-practice guidelines is related to use of the NQF safe practices as standards in the pay-for-performance programs of Leapfrog Group. The Leapfrog Group is a coalition of 29 large health care purchasing coalitions which publishes information regarding compliance with NQF safe practices submitted to them by the more than 1300 hospitals representing more than half of the nation's hospital beds (108).

The voluntary nature of compliance with NQF's disclosure safe practice, the lack of external validation of data submitted to NQF and the nonparticipatory status of many providers in NQF, and/or Leapfrog programs have been cited as a basis to question whether NQF's disclosure safe practice will promote substantive change. Nonetheless, it has been noted to incorporate several elements that will advance disclosure.

1. Presenting disclosure as a patient safety challenge rather than merely a risk management program and encouraging hospitals to integrate their risk management, patient safety, and quality problems;
2. Recognizing that disclosures are complex exchanges that require training and institutional support;
3. Outlines a framework for the disclosure discussion including apology where appropriate;
4. Encourages application of performance-improvement tools to the disclosure process, beginning with the tracking of disclosure outcomes (108).

2006 Consensus Statement of Harvard Hospitals

Similar to the NQF standard in its attempt to more clearly define what should be disclosed to a patient involved in a medical error is the March 2006 Consensus Statement of Harvard Hospitals entitled "When Things go Wrong: Responding to Adverse Events" (110). Dr. Lucian Leape, a national specialist on patient safety, lead a group of physicians, patients, and hospital administrators in drafting this policy for physicians to acknowledge and apologize for medical errors to their patients. The policy creates a roadmap for uniform response to some of medicine's most difficult situations at Massachusetts General Hospital, Brigham and Women's Hospital, Beth Israel Deaconess Medical Center, Dana-Farber Cancer Institute, Children's Hospital of Boston, and the rest of Harvard's teaching hospitals. The consensus statement indicates that Harvard's 16 teaching hospitals are hoping that a policy of routine disclosure and apology after preventable adverse events can begin to address the emotional scars both patients and physicians endure in such cases. The statement outlines the reasoning and evidence for every step in the process of communicating with patients and their families in the aftermath of an unexpected outcome including the importance of disclosing, taking responsibility, apologizing, and discussing the prevention of recurrences.

Although noting the promising results of programs which combine disclosure and apology with a compensation scheme such as the Veteran's Affairs (VA) and other programs discussed later, the Harvard Consensus Statement stopped short of adopting a model for providing compensation outside the court system. These programs are addressed later, including what is presently known about their impact on the traditional tort liability systems whereby patients typically seek redress for the damages caused by medical error attributable to preventable events.

Disclosure Programs Designed to Decrease Malpractice Liability

There is a growing movement that disclosure of medical errors to patients, when properly managed and controlled, has the potential for lessening the frequency and severity of medical malpractice litigation (89,116–119). Evidence is emerging that disclosure may actually reduce the likelihood of lawsuits and positively influence the outcome of lawsuits already filed (86,88,114,118–121). However, it is also notable that most studies of the effect of disclosure on malpractice lawsuits involve the retrospective assessment of patients or family members that they would have been less likely to sue if the physician provided full disclosure (90).

Illustrative on how disclosure may impact the outcome of medical malpractice litigation is a 2000 study of a multimillion dollar malpractice judgment performed by a jury selection research firm. The study consisted of the same case presented to two juries except that the facts in one included disclosure of the underlying event to the patient by the physician. The jury's verdict in the scenario including disclosure was millions of dollars less than the other nondisclosure version. Post-trial discussions with the jurors revealed that, in the case of no disclosure where the verdict was higher, the jury felt the anger of the patient, concurred in the plaintiff's theory that there was a conspiracy by the health care organization to hide information and punished the organization by awarding more than pecuniary damages. By contrast, the jury hearing the case with disclosure felt their duty was to compensate only for genuine losses and thus yielded a lower verdict (122).

Advocates of patient disclosure as a means of lessening malpractice risk also cite the studies evidencing that patients are motivated to sue because they felt the physician was not honest and/or they were unable to find out information about the incident from those involved (123–125).

The concept of "full disclosure/early offer" has been embraced by a number of hospital systems and insurers across the United States and received national attention in 2005 when Senators Hillary Rodham Clinton (D. NY) and Barack Obama (D. Ill.) teamed up to introduce the National Medical Error Disclosure and Compensation (MEDiC) Act of 2005 (126,127). Based, in part on state and private sector initiatives, the legislation aimed to reduce liability-related costs by heading off expensive lawsuits with apologies and financial compensation from doctors. While the MEDiC Act was not passed by Congress, its proposed provisions are notable and indicate the rising profile of this issue on the national level. Under the proposed act, physicians, hospitals, insurers, and others who choose to enroll in the voluntary program would set up a system for identifying safety lapses and informing patients. The patients then could choose to participate in a negotiation process in which they would review compensatory offers from the physician or entity at fault. If someone rejects the offers and sues the doctor anyway, he or she would be unable to use the negotiation proceedings as an evidence in court. The proposal embraces the concept that early acceptance of responsibility by physicians who make mistakes often results in decreased litigation.

Significantly predating MEDiC was the "full disclosure/early offer" program established in 1987 by the Veterans Affairs Medical Center in Lexington, Kentucky and which was extended to all Veterans Affairs medical centers in 2005 (128). The VA program consists of patient notification of negligence, a face-to-face meeting of hospital administrators and the patient and/or family and assisting patients with filing claims. The VA's program, described as a "radical policy of full disclosure," was the subject of an analysis which compared the number and cost of malpractice payments made by the VA Medical Center in Lexington, Kentucky, with those of 35 other VA medical centers and found that liability payments made by the Lexington VA Medical Center were "moderate" compared to those of similar facilities. The authors attributed the result to transparency about substandard care and timely compensation, although they noted that the analysis "suggests but does not prove the financial superiority of a full disclosure program" (114). A subsequent study evidenced that the VA approach appears to have mitigated the financial repercussions of inevitable adverse events that result in injury to patients (129).

As more fully set forth later, the success of the VA's program in minimizing claims and malpractice payouts has been an impetus for other medical centers and insurers to adopt similar policies of disclosure and early resolution. While it has been noted that the VA's experience may not translate into the private sector because of certain immunity and other benefits enjoyed by the VA as an arm of the federal government (130), the trend toward these programs continues.

Similar programs incorporating varying degrees of full error disclosure and/or provision of financial compensation without patients having to file a malpractice claim have been developed by the University of Michigan Health System in Ann Arbor, which instituted its program in 2002 (127,131), Baltimore's Johns Hopkins Medicine which instituted its program in 2003 (132), Minneapolis-based Allina Hospitals and Clinics (132), the University of Illinois Medical Center (117), Virginia Mason Medical Center (117), Kaiser Permanete (119), Gesinger Health System (119,133), facilities subject to the Catholic Health Initiatives (119), Brigham and Women's Hospital (119), and Stanford University (134,135).

The University of Michigan Health System reported that the cost and frequency of litigation decreased under their program, with annual litigation expense reduced from three to one million and the number of claims decreasing by more than 50% (127). The results of the Michigan program highlight that actual monetary payments to a patient are only a fraction of a provider's total litigation costs. Other "hidden" expenses include defense attorney fees, time spent by physicians and other staff preparing for and attending depositions and trial proceedings, fees charged by expert witnesses who will testify on the defendant's behalf, travel costs, and other incidental expenses that can far exceed the amount of any verdict or settlement. By meeting with a patient soon after an incident and taking steps to encourage early settlement, virtually all of these costs can be avoided (85).

According to Richard C. Boothman, Chief Risk Officer for the University of Michigan Health System, the program's emphasis is on improving patient safety and physician–patient communication and specifically educating a patient as to the nature of his or her claim and why it may or may not be a compensable error rather than on medical malpractice (132).

Insurers with similar programs include COPIC Insurance Co. of Denver and West Virginia Mutual Insurance Co. of Charleston, W. Va (132). Insuring more than 6000 physicians, COPIC is the largest liability insurer in Colorado. In 2000, this physician-directed insurer developed the "3Rs" program to facilitate transparent communications about injuries and expedite compensation in selected circumstances. The key features of COPIC's 3Rs program are disclosure linked to a no-fault compensation of up to $30,000.00 for a patient's out-of-pocket expenses, disclosure training and coaching for physicians, payments not being reported to the National Practitioner Data Bank and exclusion of cases involving death, clear negligence, attorney involvement, complaint to state licensure board, or written demand for payment. In reviewing the 2000 to 2006 program results, COPIC found that, of the 3200 events managed through the program, 25% involved payments to patients in an average amount of $5400.00 per case, 7 cases where payment was made were subsequently litigated and resulted in tort compensation, and 16 cases where no payment was made resulted in subsequent litigation with awards of tort compensation in 6 (108). In addition to cost savings potential, early finding also include improved physician–patient communication and improved satisfaction of all parties involved (110).

Many of these programs cite resistance of physicians and other stakeholders as an issue at least initially complicating the implementation of such programs (117), an issue that was mitigated with education and training. Stanford's closed system, in which its hospitals, physicians, and medical staff are all insured by one entity, is cited as a factor that its originators hope will facilitate implementation of its Process for the Early Assessment and Resolution of Loss (PEARL) program. PEARL is both a disclosure program and an early intervention program that allows a preventable unanticipated outcome to be quickly identified, assessed, and resolved (115).

However, it is important to note that these disclosure initiatives are relatively new (110,121). While all have, in fact, experienced a decline in lawsuits, the organizations will not directly link the new policies to the decline (117). Further, little is known about the effectiveness and the results of the relatively small number of entities involved. Accordingly, it has been observed that extrapolation of these results systemwide might not be appropriate (108).

These programs have also been criticized as improbable risk management strategies by researchers who found that forecasting of reduced litigation volume or cost do not withstand close scrutiny and conclude that the more pressing question is whether moving toward routine disclosure will expand litigation and to what extent. "Disclosure is the right thing to do; so is compensating patients who sustain injury as a result of substandard care. Continuing moves toward transparency about medical injuries will expose tensions between these two objectives.

That severe injuries are prevalent and that most of them never trigger litigation are epidemiological facts that have long been evident. The affordability of the medical malpractice system rests on this fragile foundation, and routine disclosure threatens to shake it. Movement toward full disclosure should proceed with a realistic expectation of the financial implications and prudent planning to meet them" (136).

"I'm Sorry" Laws

Recent legislation may afford health care providers an opportunity to test the effect of informing patients when a mistake has been made without the consequences of the admission being revealed to a jury. Part of the movement in the medical industry to encourage doctors to promptly and fully inform patients of errors and, when warranted, apologize, is state legislation that allows physicians to apologize when things go wrong without having to fear that their words will be used against them in court. These laws seek to address concerns that, under evidentiary law, prior out-of-court statements of defendant physicians may be used against them as a way of providing expert testimony that establishes a prima facie case of malpractice.

Twenty-nine (29) states have enacted evidentiary rules that make expressions of sympathy, apologies, or other benevolent gestures following an accident or error inadmissible in civil court to prove liability (137). While a complete analysis of these laws is beyond the scope of this chapter, it is important to note that they vary in scope. Some are broad in scope like Colorado's law, which specifically excludes statements by a health care provider admitting fault as well as those expressing sympathy (138). Arizona, Connecticut, Georgia, and Oregon also give protection to full apologies or apologies of responsibility (139). Others, like those enacted in California, Florida, Texas, and Washington, provide that, while an apology or expression of sympathy after an incident cannot constitute an admission of liability, clear statements of fault are still admissible (140). Although Massachusetts was the first state to adopt a physician apology law in 1986, the current statute protects only a narrow set of physician apologies. The Massachusetts statute protects benevolent gestures of sympathy as inadmissible as evidence of an admission of liability in a civil action, but it does not protect a physician who takes responsibility for medical error (141).

There is also variation from state to state as to the form of protected expression ranging from statements, affirmations, and gestures to statements, writings or action, and any expression. While most of the statutes apply to expressions by a health care provider or employee, there are variations as to whom a protected apology can be made. Expressions made to anyone are covered in some states while other states limit the scope to one or some combination of the patient and the patient's family members, friends, or legal representative(s). Only one state, Illinois, requires the expression to be made within a specified time period (72 hours). It is thought that this time restriction was intended to limit protection to "genuine" apologies made immediately after an adverse event and before litigation is contemplated (142).

The broad protections of the Colorado's law are notable in that this is the same state where COPIC's disclosure and early settlement program was comprised. The importance of Colorado's broad tort reform to the existence of COPIC's 3Rs program has been noted (108).

In states with no or limited evidentiary protections like those described earlier, providers need to be mindful that while courts have held apologies or admissions of error in malpractice cases are not proof of a departure from the standard of care and thus are insufficient evidence of liability, other courts have held that similar admissions of error are proof of the standard of care, breach thereof, or both (38,85).

It is also notable that there are evidentiary rules beyond those enacted by "I'm Sorry" laws to be considered in weighing whether an apology will be admitted as evidence. These are the evidentiary rules regarding inconsistent statements and admissions against interest. As a general rule, any statement, written or not, made by or on behalf of a party which is inconsistent with his or her present position may be introduced as evidence against them. An admission against interest such as "I'm sorry that I made a mistake" is a statement made against one's own interest or a statement made by a party on his or her own behalf which is relevant to a trial issue. A judge may use these alternative evidentiary rules to deem a statement admissible.

Finally, providers need to be aware that tort reform initiatives including "I'm Sorry" laws may be overturned. In November of 2007, Illinois' 2005 tort reform legislation which included safeguards to protect certain apologies and expressions of grief from a health care provider to a patient was overturned by Cook County Circuit Court Judge Diane Larson who declared the law unconstitutional. As with changing protections for peer review materials, apology law is in a state of flux that leaves providers on uncertain ground as courts are asked to consider its validity (142).

PRACTICE POINTER

Health care providers would be well advised to be aware of what legal protections are available for apologies in his or her jurisdiction before engaging in a discussion with a patient about a medical error, well before such a situation presents itself. Because "I'm Sorry" may be construed as "I'm responsible," physicians need to be prepared with alternative ways of dealing with the patient's need for personal attention, time, and sympathy in view of the growing awareness that neglecting or refusing to pay attention to this in the face of a medical error may be the patient's impetus for a lawsuit. Doing so in a setting and on a timetable that the physician has control is preferable to answering the same questions in the hostile environment of a medical malpractice case.

Legal Mandates for Disclosure

A more limited number of states have gone a step beyond evidentiary exclusions by adding a mandatory requirement that imposes a duty on hospitals to inform patients of adverse medical outcomes. Between 2002 and 2007, seven states passed such laws, specifically, California, Florida, Nevada, New Jersey, Oregon, Pennsylvania, and Vermont (143). No empirical evidence is yet available with which to gauge compliance with those laws. However, knowledgeable experts in the field have expressed skepticism about the suitability of disclosure practices for regulatory oversight. "Without comprehensive adverse-event reporting systems and the substantial resources needed to audit charts and contact patients, it is extremely difficult for regulators to monitor the occurrence of disclosures, much less their quality. To our knowledge, none of the states that have enacted mandates have attempted serious enforcement and only Pennsylvania actually specifies the sanctions for noncompliance" (108). It has been noted that content of disclosure "is an especially elusive target for regulation" citing research suggesting that a key barrier to disclosure is the uncertainty of health care workers regarding how much information to share with patients after adverse events (108).

Fear that Disclosure of Medical Errors to Patients Will Increase Medical Malpractice Claims

The IOM 1999 report highlighted the fact that a substantial number of medical errors go undetected by the system and unreported. Thus, the concern has arisen that, while disclosure might quell some patients' interests in litigating as earlier noted, it will "ignite interest in others, particularly those who would never have known of their injury in the absence of the disclosure" (108). Moreover, a recent study of the litigation consequences of disclosure found that forecasts of reduced litigation volume or cost do not withstand close scrutiny and that a policy question more pressing than whether moving toward routine disclosure will expand litigation is the question of how large such an expansion might be (136).

Further, despite the innovative programs noted earlier, medical error is still largely addressed in the area of civil litigation which continues to function as it has for decades with its focus on individual blame and punishment. The next section of this chapter provides an overview of the United States torts system and how it deals with medical errors.

MEDICAL ERRORS AND U.S. TORT SYSTEM

This portion of the chapter explores the medical malpractice system and its core elements of tort law, liability insurance and the safety of medical care. It is this author's view that the current system is not adequately addressing the true crisis in health care, which is the high prevalence of error in medicine. How medical errors are dealt within the existing medical malpractice system evidences the disconnect between the tort approach to medical errors which is punitive, adversarial, and focused on the individual and the systems approach to error reduction and quality care improvement which strives to shift the focus to procedures and work processes rather than perceived "bad apples" (144).

Medical malpractice law has been justified as the means to ensure a just outcome, where there otherwise would be none, by compensating patients for harm occasioned by a physician or other health care provider who fails to exercise the degree of care and skill that a health care provider in the same specialty would use under similar circumstances. In a perfect world, this law would serve the respective goals that the medical and legal professions have in maintaining as paramount the interests of their patients and clients. However, the modern medical malpractice system is flawed, has many inconsistencies, and is negatively perceived by physicians as one which permits patients to seek compensation for outcomes clearly out of the hands of treating physicians and health care teams.

The current process promotes the trial bar's view of physicians as "conspirators of silence" to the extent that physicians served with notice of a pending medical malpractice case against them are told by their defense attorneys and by their insurance carriers to maintain silence and not discuss the case with anyone outside the protected attorney–client relationship. It is then the job of the medical malpractice defense attorney to maintain that silence, dispute fault, deflect responsibility, and make it as slow and as expensive as possible for plaintiffs to prosecute claims.

This is all in conflict with the nonpunitive systems approach to medical error reduction, which is dependent on timely and complete disclosure of medical errors. The unwillingness of physicians to participate in disclosure and other error reduction initiatives has been attributed to the disconnect between these two systems (144). While certainly not all medical errors are medical malpractice, the malpractice crisis has created an environment of distrust among physicians that frustrates efforts to improve patient safety which are premised on error disclosure and which fuels litigation brought by patients who have come to distrust a health care environment where all errors are kept secret. While this disconnect appears to have been perpetuated by the continued focus of health policy based upon tort reform and calming insurance markets, the ascendance of the patient safety movement, with its focus on enhancing the safety of medical care, presents an opportunity to explore a system focused on reducing medical error before it triggers the need for litigation and compensation and improving the efficacy of these processes where ultimately necessary and appropriate.

What Medical Errors are Actionable?

The Selection Process

The determination of which medical errors become the subject of medical malpractice litigation is subject to a long tradition of self-regulation (145). This is to say that the decision as to whether a claim is made is based on the decision of patients in consultation with their attorneys, and, in states that require filing of a certificate of merit at the outset of a case, after expert input is obtained. This system has been described as a form of cost-free regulation driven by market incentives that direct plaintiffs' attorneys to select and bring cases. Attorneys weigh the investigation and expert costs of prosecuting a case against their expected compensation (typically a contingency fee representing a percentage of the plaintiff's award) (146).

It has been noted that the involvement of an attorney specializing in medical malpractice, including the likelihood that they will consult with a medical expert at the outset of a case, may help to filter out unsubstantiated claims as do contingent fee arrangements whereby plaintiffs' lawyers recover fees only if the plaintiff obtains money through a judgment or settlement (147). However, others have noted that the contingency fee arrangement has also resulted in situations where meritorious but difficult and/or expensive cases to prove are deselected.

> "Because they were risking their own professional capital, however, lawyers have not historically concentrated on all forms of medical negligence, or even on the most intrinsically dangerous specialties. They have gravitated instead toward cases in which negligence appeared easiest to demonstrate in the courtroom, cases that most often produced payments (whether or not the bad outcomes were really the result of medical mistakes), and cases most likely to yield the largest settlements. Those dynamics have tended historically to elevate the frequency of malpractice actions in various specialties at various times (e.g., obstetrics in the 1980s), while leaving the vast majority of all patient victims as a whole outside the system and without compensation of any sort." (148)

Legal Definitions Pertaining to Medical Malpractice

Medical malpractice claims have traditionally been governed not by federal law but by state common law. Common law consists of legal rules established by the courts, as opposed to statutory law which is legislated. The rules for handling malpractice cases vary from state to state, in part, because the legal precedents which establish case law in one state are generally given no weight in other states. However, most states recognize that medical malpractice law as part of the general body of "tort" law that deals with injuries to people or property. The concept underlying the tort known as "negligence" is that people should exercise reasonable care in what they do and should be held responsible for "reasonably foreseeable" injuries resulting from failure to exercise due care. Careless behavior that places an unreasonable risk of injury on another person is "negligence." Medical malpractice is generally considered to be a special case of negligence, where a medical professional causes unreasonable risk of harm to a patient due to his or her failure to meet an established standard of care.

Claims of medical malpractice are most typically targeted at individual physicians on the negligence-based theories noted earlier. Individual physicians are subject to suit not only based on their own conduct but can also be held liable for the conduct of others under agency law. Under the principle of respondent superior ("let the master answer"), a principal may be liable for the torts of his or her subordinate. Under the law in most states, the principal is liable for the agent when the principal has the right or obligation to control what the agent does. If, for example, an attending physician has the duty to supervise a resident, the attending can be held liable for the resident's conduct, whether or not the attending was in fact supervising the resident.

While a complete analysis of the alternative theories that can be raised in a medical malpractice care is beyond the scope of this chapter, it is important to note that hospitals and other health care facilities are not infrequently made party to medical malpractice actions both on negligence grounds and on grounds of corporate negligence and/or vicarious liability. Under the theory of vicarious liability, a hospital can be held liable for the negligent acts of nurses and other employed staff of the hospital. One increasingly popular claim of corporate negligence is that the hospital's failure to properly credential a member of the medical or allied staff subjected the patient to an incompetent practitioner (144).

Legally Required Elements of a Medical Malpractice Claim

In a medical malpractice case, the patient or plaintiff has the burden of proving by a "preponderance of evidence" that he or she received substandard medical care that caused injuries. Most states recognize that several elements are necessary to establish the tort of malpractice. Failure to prove any one element is fatal to a malpractice claim.

1. *Duty* is the first element that a plaintiff is required to prove. This element is generally established by evidencing the existence of a patient–physician relationship. For purposes of the malpractice analysis, this is a question of law, not ethics. Under the law, a duty arises because the physician agreed to assume a duty to the patient.
2. *Breach of a duty* is the second element that must be proven by a malpractice plaintiff. This requires the plaintiff to prove that his or her physician provided medical care that was negligent in that it fell below accepted standards of care. This element of proof requires testimony from an expert who has the credentials and expertise necessary to testify about the required standard of care and whether or not the defendant met that standard. Specifically, this requires expert testimony as to the degree of skill and diligence exercised by other practitioners in the same field when confronted with the same or a similar care at the time of the subject care. While practice standards and hospital policies might be relevant to the question of negligence in some states (and it certainly will assist a physician's defense to show compliance with them), a physician's failure to adhere to such practice standards and policies is generally not sufficient to demonstrate negligence. Subject to case law, which is neither uniform nor clear, is the question of whether a physician's own apology or admission of fault is sufficient to establish the standard of care or its breach (38). It is also notable that a medical malpractice plaintiff must establish departure from an accepted standard. An error in judgment does not suffice nor does a bad outcome. Further, compliance with applicable standards of care does not require the guarantee of successful outcomes. The breach of

standard element is at the heart of most malpractice cases since it involves finding fault and placing blame and is typically one of the most contentious issues in the case.

3. *Causation* is the third element that must be established by the plaintiff to support a claim of malpractice. Specifically, the plaintiff must establish that the negligent care caused injuries. As with breach, expert testimony is almost always required to prove causation. Causation is often the most scientifically complicated element of a malpractice case. It is the rare case where causation is as clear as with surgery on the wrong body part. More often, the proof on causation is complicated by factors such as the plaintiff's preexisting conditions, degree of compliance of the plaintiff with recommended treatment, and questions about the treatment of more than one health care provider, to name a few.

4. *Damages* is the final element of proof that must be established by the plaintiff. This element of proof focuses on how much money is needed to compensate the injured party for what they suffered and to "make them whole." This means restoring a claimant as nearly as can be done with money to the state of life they enjoyed before the injury, accounting for all needs and circumstances. Typical damages include what is alternatively referred to as monetary, pecuniary, or economic damages (hereinafter referred to as "economic damages"). Examples of economic damages are lost wages and medical expenses. This element of damages typically calls for payment of all documented (or projected usually established through the testimony of an expert economist) costs related to the injury for past, current, and future needs. Additionally, noneconomic damages such as "pain and suffering" and "loss of enjoyment of life" are compensable to whatever degree the fact finder deems appropriate for the injury. This aspect of damages is intended to capture the emotional or other nonmonetary values of injured status. Although rare in medical malpractice cases, damages can sometimes also include punitive damages awarded to punish the defendant for medical negligence and to deter him or her from future misconduct. Payment of damages is typically made pursuant to a negotiated settlement or court judgment at the time of resolution either as a lump sum or pursuant to a structured settlement. Funding for the system comes largely from physicians' and hospitals' liability insurance or alternative risk programs such as self-insurance funds. In the current system, decisions on damages are a province of the jury. However, it is notable that the courts do also have influence over this decision. Under New York law, the trial judge has the authority to modify awards that "deviate materially from reasonable compensation". This empowers the judge to compare a verdict with other similar cases and reduce "outlier" awards.

Litigation Impact of Never Events

An interesting issue raised by the recent CMS pronouncement that they will not pay for "never events" is the impact this may have on the medical malpractice litigation process. Some commentators have raised concerns that strict liability for health care providers may result from defining and memorializing "never events" (149).

As described earlier, the NQF published a document in 2006 entitled "Serious Reportable Events in Health care—2006 Update: A Consensus Report" (71). The 2006 list contained 28 events that it characterized as "serious, largely preventable, and of concern to health care providers, consumers and all stakeholders". The 2006 list included all those identified in 2002 (70), modified some of them, and added one concerning the wrong donor sperm or egg. While the purpose of the NQF's lists was not to describe events that were never to occur, CMS nonetheless adopted a modified list of "Never Events" in 2006.

The CMS list of never events differs substantially from the NQF list and covers objects inadvertently left in after surgery, air embolism, blood incompatibility, catheter-associated urinary tract infection, pressure ulcers, vascular catheter-associated infection, surgical site infection after coronary artery bypass graft surgery, and hospital-acquired injuries including fractures, dislocations, intracranial injuries, crushing injuries, and burns (147). In April of 2008, CMS proposed to add to the list of never events nine additional hospital-acquired conditions including surgical site infections, pneumonia caused by a specific bacteria resulting in Legionnaires' disease, extreme blood sugar derangement, iatrogenic pneumothorax, delirium, deep vein thrombosis/pulmonary embolism, staphylococcus aureus septicemia, and clostridium defficile associated with disease.

Notable from a review of CMS' present and proposed lists is that some conditions could be said to be expected complications which occur absent a breach of the standard of care. Whereas under current medical liability law a provider could defend a claim that one of these conditions was an expected complication and not a result of negligence, the inclusion of an event on the never event list could result in a form of strict liability. Illustrative is the case where a patient is admitted to a hospital following hip replacement surgery with noted mobility limitations. Notwithstanding orders to remain in bed, the patient attempts to walk to the bathroom, falls, and suffers a fracture (one of the conditions on the CMS list). In the event of a subsequent suit, the hospital would ordinarily defend on the basis of the order (assuming it was properly implemented and the patient had a call button in reach) and raise the patient's noncompliance as the cause of the fracture. Ordinarily, the hospital would present expert testimony that falls can happen in the absence of negligence and that not all falls are preventable. However, a plaintiff's attorney now has the ammunition to argue that CMS views the event as one that should never have occurred and that the facility is strictly liable for the damages caused (149). There is also concerns that the hospitals where these events occur will become virtual insurers of patient safety and also take on liability for the acts of individual nonemployed physicians who are involved in never events. The full impact of this remains to be seen.

PRACTICE POINTER

Hospitalist physicians who may be involved in the care of patients with compromised immune symptoms and thus more susceptible to one of the CMS "never events" may be well advised to obtain indemnity and defense from the hospitals in which they work.

Stages of a Malpractice Case

Medical malpractice cases are typically required to be commenced, which happens upon service of a pleading called a Summons and Complaint, within a specified time period after the subject care known as the "statute of limitations." In New York, for example, this period is two and one-half years with the exception of death cases and cases involving minors. Virtually all states allow longer limitations periods for disability, incompetency, minority, foreign objects left in the body or fraudulent concealment preventing earlier discovery. In some states, like New York and Pennsylvania, a certificate of merit is required to be filed at the outset of the case to certify that an appropriately licensed professional has reviewed the case and concluded, "to a reasonable degree of medical certainty," that the care fell outside accepted standards and caused damages.

The next stage of a malpractice case is discovery, which is usually the longest phase in the case. This phase involves the taking of party depositions (and in some states not including New York, expert depositions) and the exchange of medical records and other relevant documents. Disclosure is the legal mechanism whereby one party in a lawsuit may compel the other to provide relevant information not protected by some legal privilege. It is in this stage of the case that battles are fought about the discoverability of peer review records, reports of any governmental investigations, and incident reports.

Cases not settled or resolved by summary judgment or other dispositive motions next proceed to trial. In most states, medical malpractice trials are presided over by a state court judge and decided by a jury predominantly composed of laypersons.

The journey down the tort pathway is long and medical malpractice cases proceed slowly from stage to stage. Delay is a hallmark of the existing system with the average malpractice claim taking 2 years to resolve and with larger claims, particularly those involving multiple defendants, taking 5 years or longer. As noted by one commentator, delay has negative consequences for all of the parties:

> Delay withholds information from patients for prolonged periods while defense lawyers position their cases strategically for settlement or trial, denies compensation to legitimate claimants, diminishes learning opportunities for health care providers, imposes high psychic costs on all parties, and increases uncertainty for malpractice insurers when pricing coverage. (150)

Proof: Importance of Documentation

The importance of documentation, specifically medical records in a medical malpractice case, is often summed up in the phrase "If it isn't documented, it wasn't done." Often formidable is the challenge faced by the defense attorney in a medical malpractice case by medical records that are illegible, incomplete, lack dates or times and/or do not contain a description of what was done, and communicated to the patient. Documentation done contemporaneously (and before the patient has a bad outcome) is effective and influential in at least three settings: prior to the suit for the attorney reviewing a potential case, for the judge deciding a pretrial motion for summary judgment and dismissal, and the jury deciding the case at trial (151).

PRACTICE POINTER

For the specialist, proper documentation in the medical record can be an effective instrument for communicating his or her respective involvement in a patient's case. In the case of a seriously ill patient whose care involves multiple physicians, the note by a consulting specialist which describes the limited nature of his or her involvement and communicates their opinions for plan for future care, if any, to the patient, nursing staff, and fellow physicians, especially the attending doctor, may avoid entanglement in a malpractice claim (151). However, in doing so it is important to be mindful of the equally important risk management edict that the medical record should never be used by one health care provider to level criticisms against or blame another as such concerns are more appropriately addressed in confidential peer review forums.

Key Role of Expert Witnesses

As described earlier, expert testimony is needed in a medical malpractice case to prove a number of elements including that the defendant physician provided medical care that was negligent in that it fell below accepted standards of care. The testimony of a medical expert is not only required at trial as a necessary part of both the plaintiff's and the defendant's proof, but, in states with certificate of merit requirements such as New York, expert input is required to attest that medical records have been reviewed and that, in the expert's opinion, there is support for the allegations of negligence being made.

The scope of expert testimony needed will vary depending on the requirements for proving standard of care and causation in the jurisdiction where the claim is brought. In general, however, courts permit the plaintiff to establish the standard of care using the opinion of a physician who testifies on the basis of his or her professional experience and judgment. Some jurisdictions require that the expert be certified in the relevant medical specialty and/or that the expert have practice or teaching experience. It is up to the court and the jury to determine whether the expert has the requisite credentials and whether the testimony is credible (152). This task can be formidable when the testimony is technical and esoteric and hence difficult to refute in terms intelligible to judges and jurors, such as is customarily involved in a medical malpractice case.

In states that permit pretrial depositions of the party's respective experts, the expert's credentials or lack of them can be explored prior to the trial. In states like New York where pretrial knowledge of experts is limited to a name-redacted outline of credentials and opinions to be offered at trial which is only received shortly before trial, the first opportunity to challenge an expert's credentials may be when the witness takes the stand to testify.

The credibility of expert testimony is traditionally an issue resolved on a case-by-case basis with the court and the jurors each weighing in. However, notable are recent efforts to interject an element of peer review to the expert testimony process toward the goal of reducing frivolous or dishonest expert testimony. Such efforts stem from the 2001 case of *Austin vs. American Association of Neurological Surgeons* in which the Seventh Circuit Court of Appeals upheld the right of medical specialty societies to police their own members (153). Many of these societies, including the American Association of Neurological Surgeons (AANS) at issue in the *Austin* case, have panels to review the quality of medical malpractice testimony. If an expert's testimony is contrary to what a majority or respectable minority in the field would state, the expert may be subject to discipline for an ethical violation, an occurrence that could diminish the expert's credibility in future cases. In the *Austin* case, Dr. Austin unsuccessfully challenged the AANS' suspension of his membership which he claimed was in "revenge" for having testified as an expert witness for the plaintiff in a medical malpractice suit brought against another member of AANS. In upholding the suspension, the court found that there is a great deal of skepticism about expert evidence, that more not less policing of expert testimony is required and that associations have a right to police their members.

PRACTICE POINTER

Health care providers who are defendants in medical malpractice cases should take an active role not only in identifying an expert supportive of the care at issue (with the best possible credentials and without a personal connection to the defendant that could be raised on cross-examination as a test of impartiality and thus credibility) but also in assisting defense counsel in being armed with specialty-specific guidelines and peer reviewed materials that can be used to challenge plaintiff's expert. This has been noted to be a form of "Do-It-Yourself Tort Reform" (154).

Better Physician–Patient Communication May Avoid Selection

There is evidence to support that the quality of the patient–physician relationship and particularly the quality of ongoing communication is an important factor in determining who gets sued in a medical malpractice case (145). One study that analyzed the audiotapes of conversations between physicians and patients found that the physicians with the best communication skills were also the physicians who had not been sued. The study showed that the physicians not sued tended to ask more questions and encourage patients to talk about their feelings and spent more time with the patients compared to those physicians who had been sued (123). Similarly, a study at Vanderbilt University School of Medicine concluded that a physician's malpractice experience is mostly closely related not to patient volume or specialty of medicine, but rather to the physician's ability to effectively communicate with their patients, establish rapport, and provide care and treatment consistent with what the patient expects (155).

The view that a better bedside manner helps physicians avoid complaints and litigation is further supported by research done at McGill University in Montreal (156). Researchers tracked more than 3400 physicians who, between 1993 and 1996, took the clinical skills examination administered by the Medical Council of Canada, and then went on to practice medicine in the provinces of Ontario and Quebec. The results showed a strong correlation between the doctors' ability to communicate well with patients and the number of complaints filed against them in their first 2 to 12 years of practice. Physicians with the highest numbers of patient complaints registered against them were, more often than not, found among those who scored low when their communication skills were tested (actors portrayed patients) in the clinical skills examination (156).

PRACTICE POINTER

While managed care can present a challenge as to how much time physicians have to spend with their patients, a factor that can impede effective and quality communication, providers are encouraged to place an emphasis on effectively communicating with patients so that lawsuits are not filed for the wrong reasons. This is another type of "do-it-yourself tort reform".

The Role of Liability Insurance in the Medical Malpractice System

"The medical malpractice system consists of three activities: medical care to keep patients safe, a legal process to air and resolve complaints and liability insurance to pay compensation when appropriate" (150). This section of the chapter discusses the third element including the impact of medical malpractice crises on the medical malpractice system.

Insurance Requirements and Their Genesis

Medical malpractice insurance has two main purposes: to compensate the injured patient for sub-standard care of negligent health care professionals and protection of the negligent health care professional's practice in order for them to continue to serve the medically needy. Liability insurance distributes the cost of the liability system which, in turn, reflects societal values.

Society, through the courts and the legislative process, decides what injuries should be compensated, in what circumstances and in what amounts. Interestingly, the advent of liability insurance was occasioned by physicians who pioneered it at the end of the 19th century as an accommodation to the system of malpractice litigation that had arisen in the United States in the 1840s (148).

Medical malpractice insurance is another area of the medical system subject to state law. Under current law, nearly all states require physicians to have liability insurance (147). Physicians typically must have insurance coverage to not only practice but also as a condition of hospital privileges, as a condition of participation on the provider panels of third-party payers, and, in some states like Pennsylvania, as a condition of licensure. As a standard primary layer, physicians were historically required to obtain and pay for $1 million in coverage per incident and an aggregate of $3 million per year. However, these requirements have been increasing to $1.3 million and $3.9 million, respectively. Due to rising awards, excess-layer insurance has become increasingly important to physicians and hospitals. Physicians typically buy their insurance from a commercial company or a physician-owned mutual company. Traditionally, rates for physicians are not experience based, but are dependent on the degree of risk involved in the provider's specialty as well as expected litigation costs in the local area in which the provider is located and the profit rate sought by the insurer. This is distinct from the fact that the cost of coverage for hospitals is typically linked to the history of claims from year to year and thus is experienced rated (147). Rate increases are subject to approval by the relevant state insurance authority.

Medical malpractice insurance can be occurrence based, which covers all incidents in the policy year regardless of when the claim is filed, or of a claims-made variety, which covers only claims filed in the policy year. Coverage is more meager under a claims-made policy which leaves a long "tail" of exposure for incidents that have not yet become claims. While claims-made policies are generally less expensive than occurrence policies, most physicians purchase costly tail policies to cover these incidents in addition to paying for a claims-made policy.

PRACTICE POINTER

When moving from group to group or hospital to hospital, physicians are well advised to get the new group to assume the cost of tail coverage to cover any gap caused by claims-made coverage supplied by the old group as a term and condition of joining the new group. They are further well served by negotiating terms of any new arrangement to include the group's agreement to pay for tail if the physician leaves, regardless of the terms of departure. A "drop-down" position the physician could negotiate is that the group pays full cost of tail if it terminates the physician without cause and that tail be at the physician's expense only if he or she voluntarily leaves.

Recurrent Medical Malpractice Insurance Crises

Since the 1980s, one hallmark of the medical malpractice system has been recurrent periods of escalating liability insurance premiums for physicians, sometimes accompanied by difficulty in obtaining insurance coverage at any price. A medical malpractice crisis is a period of volatility in the medical professional liability insurance market in which deterioration in insurance carriers' financial ratios is followed by higher-than-historical increases in insurance premiums and/or decreased supply of insurance (150). As noted by one commentator:

> "volatility in the medical malpractice insurance market results from the interaction between the cyclical nature of the insurance business generally and the comparatively high and concentrated nature of the uncertainties involved in predicting future medical liability losses in particulars." (157)

While there were periodic upsurges in medical malpractice claims in the 1840s to 1850s, 1870s, 1920s to 1930s, and 1950s, medical malpractice litigation received little national attention until the late 1960s, the same time medical care came into increased scrutiny of the then U.S. Department of Health, Education and Welfare (145). The first medical malpractice insurance crisis, 1968 to 1969, signaled a shift in focus in health care delivery from a largely self-regulated industry based on professional decisions to one involving political decisions of the government and other third-party stakeholders (145,158).

During this time, several private liability insurers left the market because of rising claims and inadequate rates, resulting in an availability crisis and an affordability issue for those physicians and hospitals who could find insurance. The growing "menace" of malpractice suits was decried in 1975 when claims frequency and severity rose in the fragile investment climate of the post-oil shock recession. Illustrative of the spike in claims frequency and severity is California's experience where, between 1968 and 1974, the number of medical liability claims doubled and the number of losses in excess of $300,000.00 increased 11-fold, from 3 to 34. Loses amounting to $180.00 for each $100.00 of premium led most commercial insurers to conclude that the practice of medicine was uninsurable and they refused to provide medical liability insurance at any price (159). Physicians demanded relief, highlighting the implications for patient access (145). In response, states began enacting legislation aimed at reforming the tort system in which malpractice litigation was played out and/or toward the goal of increasing insurance availability. One of the most prominent reforms at this time, and one which would prove to be a template for reforms enacted in response to subsequent malpractice crisis periods, was California's Medical Injury Compensation Reform Act (MICRA) enacted in 1975. The principal provisions of MICRA, which has since been included in the category of what are referred to as "first generation reforms" (144) included a $250,000.00 cap on noneconomic malpractice damage awards, change in the collateral source rule such that prior payments by medical and/or disability insurers could be introduced by defendants as evidence entitling them to an offset against any verdict, scheduled as opposed to lump sum payment of jury awards and a sliding scale limit to contingency fees of plaintiff's lawyers (144).

The second crisis in the 1980s has been described as one of affordability in that insurers continued to write policies but charged premiums that many physicians could not afford to pay. The key sequence of events that occurred in the previous crisis recurred. "Physicians in multiple states encountered a sudden spike in malpractice insurance premiums, difficulties in securing coverage followed, prompting concerns about effects on access to certain services such as obstetrical and trauma care" (160).

The ensuing 10 years witnessed another wave of state malpractice policymaking, beginning around 1985 and continuing into the mid-1990s. Most of the reforms in this period were first generation reforms which continued to focus on the tort system like shortened statutes of limitation, expert witness requirements, and pretrial tribunals to prescreen liability cases (144).

The current malpractice insurance crisis has been described as one involving both availability and affordability (160). Availability has been affected by exodus from the market of a number of insurers including St. Paul Companies which stopped writing policies in 2001. At this time, St. Paul was the second largest malpractice carrier in the country. As in prior periods of crises, the exodus was triggered by an upward trend in claims frequency and severity (158).

The affordability aspect of the current crises is illustrated by recent developments in New York including a 14% increase in rates (which results in New York physicians paying 55% to 80% more for their liability insurance in 2008 than they were in 2003) as approved by the Department of Insurance in July of 2007 followed by a proposal that each physician be surcharged $50,000.00 to lower medical liability insurance to keep insurance companies from going bankrupt (161).

Like the two previous crises, the current one also appears to be one that is affecting access to care. Again, the New York experience is illustrative. Following the rate increase in July of 2007, 215 gynecologists and 2000 obstetricians in New York stopped delivering babies, according to the New York Chapter of the American College of Obstetricians and Gynecologists (162). Data from the American College of Obstetricians and Gynecologists (ACOG) indicates that the current crisis has similarly impacted OB/GYNs throughout the county. Specifically, a survey conducted by ACOG evidences that the lack of affordable liability insurance forced 70% of OB/GYNs to make changes to their practices (163). A survey conducted by the American Hospital Association evidences the negative impact of the current crises on the availability of hospital physicians with 45% of hospitals reporting that the professional liability crises resulted in the loss of physicians or reduced coverage in emergency departments (164).

In response, state legislatures have again gone to work, once more primarily focusing on first generation reforms like damage caps. Forty-four states introduced bills between 2004 and 2005 seeking to cap noneconomic damage while 2005 saw 48 states introducing more than 400 bills on medical liability and malpractice with more than 80% consisting of first generation reforms (144).

At the height of the recent crises, the AMA identified 22 states as being in crisis including New York. While a complete analysis of the symptoms and scope of the current crises and its predecessors is beyond the scope of this chapter (165), the foregoing indicates that the current problems are not new and have recurred even in the face of tort reform designed to address them. Further, the question of what reforms are necessary to resolve the problem remains unsolved as the stakeholders who have driven the crisis continue to debate the cause of the crises. Competing hypotheses are offered by the insurance carriers, health care providers, and trial attorneys: the three leading interest groups in the debate.

Insurers blame plaintiff's attorneys for their aggressive pursuit of clients and capitalizing on the public's enhanced awareness of and concern over medical errors and argue that increased premiums are driven by the significant increases in the size (or severity) of payouts to successful plaintiffs as well as the noticeable increase in frequency of claims (160). In pointing the finger at the trial bar, insurers are joined by physicians and hospitals who also attribute a role to what they perceive as the public's expectation of perfection in medicine (160).

Trial attorneys have responded to these criticisms by pronouncing themselves as champions of patient safety and patient safety crusaders whose role is to use the legal system, specifically the threat of litigation, to make providers practice more safely. They further attribute rising malpractice premiums to insurance underwriting cycles and practices (160,166) and, in some cases, to insurer price gouging.

As to the responsibility borne by malpractice insurers, it is notable that premiums continued to rise in California after passage of the initial reform package (MICRA) in 1975, until the passage of proposition 103 in 1988, which contained insurance reform. Proposition 103 rolled back the insurance rates in effect at the time of its enactment 20%, statutorily froze rates for 1 year, created "prior approval" regulation on newly submitted increases, allowed consumers to challenge insurer's rate increase proposals, ended the insurance industry's exemption from state and federal antitrust laws, and made the Insurance Commissioner an elected position. Within 3 years, the total medical malpractice premiums had dropped by 20.2% from the 1988 high (167). Thus, it appears, at least in California, that insurance reform which sought to regulate the rate setting freedom of the insurers was needed over and above the tort reform package.

Beyond the scope of this chapter is an analysis of the evidence supporting each of these divergent explanations other than to state that a wealth of literature can be found to support each position. It is this author's view that any effort to address the problem will involve addressing all the concerns, moving beyond reform efforts focused primarily on first generation tort reform and recognizing that the tort system is highly deficient in the prevention of injuries due to medical errors.

Performance of the Medical Liability System

In theory, the malpractice system functions efficiently:

> "... the courts step in to provide compensation and deterrence in cases in which self-regulation has failed to prevent a breach of accepted standards of care; plaintiffs' attorneys serve as gatekeepers, separating meritorious from unpromising claims; and liability coverage ensures that providers are not bankrupted by a single large payout and that resources are available to compensate patients." (147)

Several goals of medical malpractice litigation have been articulated both by advocates of the economic function of tort law, who assert that liability rules are justified by their promotion of deterrence or insurance (168), and by those who advocate tort law as a means of corrective justice (169).

Following are a number of criteria which can be used to evaluate the performance of the medical liability system:

1. compensation of patients injured by negligence,
2. deterrence of negligent physicians,
3. vehicle of corrective justice, and
4. promotion of economic efficiency.

As more fully set forth later, there is evidence that the current medical liability system functions in a way that departs significantly from these goals and that it is not effective either in decreasing the rate of medical error or in effectively compensating those who are harmed by medical error.

Compensation

There are several studies which show that the system does not perform well either in compensating eligible patients or in avoiding claims by those who are not eligible (170). The New York and California studies cited in the 1999 IOM report (1) evidence that tort law performs its compensation function relatively poorly because most patients injured by negligence do not bring malpractice claims. The California study found that a physician who committed an error leading to injury had only a 4% chance of having to compensate the patient (1). Based on the New York sample, Harvard Medical Practice Study researchers found a poor fit between negligent injuries and claims with the total number of malpractice claims filed being approximately 14% of the total number of injuries caused by negligence (2). A validation study in Utah and Colorado similarly concluded that only 2.5% of patients who were injured because of negligence filed a malpractice claim (3). A 10-year follow-up of the Harvard data from New York shows that the key predictor of payment was the plaintiff's degree of disability, not the presence of negligence (171). These studies point to a medical malpractice liability system that is flawed in terms of its ability to direct compensation to its intended beneficiaries (144,147).

Deterrence

The rationale behind the deterrence goal of the medical liability system is that providers threatened with the economic and psychological costs of litigation will be motivated to take safety precautions. Importantly, one of the assumptions on which this goal rests is that health care providers are faced with the costs of their own negligence. This assumption is called into question by the role of medical malpractice insurance in the medical liability system, which insulates physicians from the settlement or verdict economic costs of a malpractice claim. Additionally, the few studies on this subject do not show that the medical liability system actually deters negligence in medicine (144,172). Because most safety problems in medicine have system-based causes and solutions not within the control of individual physicians, malpractice pressures do not typically enhance the deterrent effect of liability but rather result in misdeterrence, which is commonly called defensive medicine (144). This is the practice of physicians taking actions that may not be necessary yet because of the fear of litigation. The defensive practice of medicine is the deviation from sound medical practice that is induced primarily by a threat of liability (173). The goal of defensive medicine is to ensure that, in the event the patient sues, the physician has gone above and beyond what is required.

While defensive medicine may on its face appear to enhance the quality of care by supplementing necessary care, it is important to note that it increases spending on health care and has the potential for imposing physical and psychological harm on the patient. Unnecessary invasive procedures come with a risk of physical harm and unnecessary diagnostic tests impose a risk of psychological harm from false positives and anxiety resulting from delayed results.

As with most topics impacting the medical liability system, there is a debate about the scope and cost of defensive medicine with some claiming it to be "virtually impossible" to measure it accurately (144,173). However, there appears to be anecdotal evidence that defensive medicine is being practiced (174).

Anecdotal evidence suggests that, in periods of "tort crisis", fear of being sued and the unaffordability or unavailability of liability insurance may have a different deterrent effect in that it may deter physicians from remaining in practice or continuing to provide high-risk services (146).

Corrective Justice

The medical liability system may be viewed as meeting its goal of corrective justice in that those injured persons who file claims are involved in a process that allows them to discover what happened, demonstrate to the defendant the result of his or her behavior, and impose payment and other penalties on a defendant. Although the tort system may thus be seen as performing its corrective justice function fairly well for those who enter the system, it is a narrow and punitive conception of corrective justice (144). Further, while the system does induce negative emotions in physicians sued, it rarely inspires genuine remorse or feelings that justice has been done. Instead, most physician defendants find little merit in the suits brought against them and feel they are the victims of a random event (146). It is also notable that the punishment goal is wastefully administered in that defendants who are subsequently exonerated as well as those held liable are forced to endure the negative aspects of the process.

Efficiency

Operational efficiency is also not a goal well served by the medical liability system. This is evidenced by studies showing that, of every dollar spent on malpractice insurance premiums, only 40¢ is paid to patients as compensation with 40¢ of the rest paid in legal fees and 20¢ for insurance overhead (175,176). A recent study concludes that the vast majority of expenditures go toward litigation over errors and payment of them and that the overhead costs of malpractice litigation are exorbitant (177). Further, efficiency is frustrated by the significant amount of time it takes for a medical liability case to resolve. Under our current system, there is a median wait of more than 2 years between the time of an incident and the time the claim is filed, followed by litigation during an average of another 2 years for a total of 4 years.

The inefficiency of the justice system is illustrated by the fact that similar cases are not decided alike, particularly when it comes to damages. While the concept of compensatory damages is a well-entrenched aspect of the liability system, there is little guidance as to how damages awards are to be calculated. Whereas most legal decisions are affected by precedent, none exists for the computation of compensatory loss. Instead, each decision is independent and individualized to fit its circumstances.

Impact of Caps and Other First Generation Reforms

As noted earlier, the recurrent medical liability insurance crises have triggered legislative reform, most of it focused on reforming the medical liability system. Tort reform is essentially an attempt to control the frequency and severity of claims. Common provisions of tort reform include measures that make it more difficult for an injured patient to get into the courts and/or to win a suit and that limit the amount that can be awarded in a successful suit. Common tort reform measures that were passed by states in the 1970s, again in the 1980s, and continuing are as follows:

1. Caps on noneconomic damages awarded to a plaintiff for unqualifiable losses such as pain and suffering, emotional distress, or loss of consortium. These damages involve no direct economic loss and have no precise value. It is difficult for juries to assign a dollar value to these losses, given the minimal guidance they customarily receive from the courts. As a result, these awards tend to be erratic and, because of the highly charged environment of personal injury trials, excessive.
2. Periodic payment of damages which allows a defendant to pay a damages award over time as opposed to one lump sum payment. The rationale for this reform is that it will prevent bankrupting providers who lose malpractice suits.
3. Abolition of the collateral source rule. The collateral source rule of the common laws provides that evidence may not be admitted at trial to show that plaintiff's loses have been compensated from other sources, such as health insurance or Workers' Compensation.
4. Limiting attorney contingency fees. Attorneys for plaintiffs in tort cases almost always work on a contingency fee basis, receiving a percentage of the damage award. This arrangement makes it possible for people of all economic levels to bring suit for injuries resulting from negligence. Reformers argue that attorneys' fees are often excessive, take away from the victim's compensation, and encourage attorneys to bring frivolous suits.
5. Abolition of joint and several liability. Joint and several liability is a theory of recovery that permits the plaintiff to recover damages from multiple defendants collectively, or from each defendant individually. In a state that follows the rule of joint and several liability, if a patient sues three defendants, two of whom are 95% responsible for the defendant's injuries, but are also bankrupt, the plaintiff may recover 100% of her damages from the solvent defendant that is 5% responsible for her injuries.

The rule of joint and several liability is neither fair nor rational, because it fails to equitably distribute liability. The rule allows a defendant only minimally liable for a given harm to be forced to pay the entire judgment, when the codefendants are unable to pay their share. The personal injury bar's argument in support of joint and several liability—that the rule protects the right of their clients to be fully compensated—fails to address the hardship imposed by the rule on codefendants that are required to pay damages beyond their proportion of fault.

Recent studies that take a retrospective look at the malpractice reforms of the 1970s and 1980s are casting serious doubt upon the efficacy of tort reform in addressing the problem of high malpractice insurance rates. One study of reforms in Wyoming revealed that Wyoming's tort reforms had been only minimally effective in reducing either claim frequency or claim severity (178).

A study of the effect of tort reform nationally on medical malpractice insurance over the period from 1984 to 1991 showed that although reforms had little effect on insurance premiums, they did succeed in enhancing insurance profitability and diminishing uncertainty which in turn helped stabilize the malpractice insurance market (179).

Even when tort reforms do become law, they often face constitutional challenges in state courts. Many of the reforms passed following the malpractice crises of the 1970s and 1980s were substantially found to violate state constitutional provisions (180).

It has also been questioned whether these reforms are fair to patients who have been injured (181). For example, caps on damages are often criticized as setting arbitrary limits on what medical malpractice victims may receive for injuries suffered and harming those who are the most seriously injured by malpractice.

The shortcomings of first generation reform have been noted as follows:

"They are irrelevant or counterproductive, however, to other shortcomings of malpractice litigation: that too many avoidable injuries occur; that compensation is frequently inadequate; that litigation is too slow, too costly, too uncertain, and too unpleasant; that premiums for primary coverage are too volatile and, for some physicians, too expensive; and that excess coverage and reinsurance are currently too costly for hospitals and other health care institutions. Put differently, MICRA-style reform perhaps yields somewhat less of a bad system, but it does not create a better system." (150)

Systems Reform

Tort reforms are not designed to remedy the fundamental failings of the malpractice system and more sweeping reform of the system is needed. Efforts need to focus on getting the medical liability system and patient safety mechanism working hand in hand. While a discussion of the second generation reforms that might accomplish this are beyond the scope of this chapter, it is notable that a number of alternatives have been proposed in the wake of a growing sense that the tort system is broken. The leading recommendations can be divided into three approaches. The first involves using alternative mechanisms to resolve disputes such as the early offer programs described earlier and which were patterned on the VA model (182). Other reforms in this category, which are likewise focused on ways to resolve cases more consistently and more quickly, include administrative law hearings, mediation, and specialized medical courts (147). The distinguishing feature of special health courts, a concept advanced by the national legal reform coalition Commons Good (183), would be trained judges, selected for their expertise in health care. Dedicated solely to addressing medical liability cases, these judges would develop standards of care with the help of neutral experts, hired by and accountable to the court and not by a party to the dispute.

The second approach is premised on dispensing with negligence as the basis for compensation. While some have termed this a "no-fault" system, this is misleading in that a pure no-fault system covers any injury as in automobile accidents and is focused merely on compensating the needy. A better description is a nonjudicial insurance system covering preventable injuries with a standard of avoidability (147,184).

The third approach is aimed at locating responsibility for errors on the institutional level. This has been termed "enterprise liability" and is premised on establishing hospitals or integrated delivery systems as the sole locus of legal responsibility. It has been observed that an organization approach to compensation and deterrence along these lines would be in keeping with the systems approach to quality improvement (147).

CONCLUSION

Disclosure is the right thing to do from a variety of perspectives but so is compensating patients who sustain injury as a result of substandard care. The continued push for transparency of medical errors has exposed the tension between these two objectives and the difficulty in moving toward error prevention in a heated malpractice environment. Needed is a move beyond the traditional approach of tort reform to system reform. The current system is inadequate as a deterrent to substandard practice or as a fair method for patient compensation and as a means of reducing preventable error and calls for change.

ACKNOWLEDGMENT

The author gratefully acknowledges Kathleen A. Posenjak, RN, BSN for her risk management perspective on the chapter and Michael G. Caty, MD, for extending the invitation to write the chapter.

REFERENCES AND NOTES

1. Institute of Medicine. To Err is Human: Building a Safer Health System. Kohn LT, Corrigan JM, Donaldson MS, eds. Washington, DC: National Academics Press, 2000 (hereinafter referred to as the "IOM's 1999 report").
2. Brennan TA, Leape LL, Laird NM, et al. Incidence of adverse events and negligence in hospitalized patients: Results of the Harvard Medical Practice Study I. NEJM 1991; 324(6):370–376.
3. Thomas EJ, Studdert DM, Burstin HR, et al. Incidence and types of adverse events and negligent care in Utah and Colorado. Medical Care 2000; 38:261–271.
4. Hayward RA, Hofer TP. Estimating hospital deaths due to medical errors: Preventability is in the eye of the beholder, JAMA 2001; 286;415–420. Also see McDonald CJ, Weiner M, Hui SL. Deaths due to medical errors are exaggerated in Institute of Medicine Report. JAMA 2000; 284(1):93–95. Also see Brennan TA. The Institute of Medicine Report on medical errors—Could it do harm? NEJM 2000; 342(15):1123–1125.
5. Mills DH, Boyden JS, Rubsamen DS. Report on the Medical Insurance Feasibility Study. San Francisco, CA: Sutter Publication, 1977.
6. Health Grades, Health Grades Quality Study: Second Annual Patient Safety in American Hospitals Report 3, 2005. At http://www.healthgrades.com/media/DMS/pdf/patientsafety in American Hospital Reports FI.
7. Centers for Disease Control and Prevention, National Vital Statistics System, 2000. At http://www.cdc.gov/nchs/nuss.htm.
8. Spitz B, Abramson J. When health policy is a problem: A report from the field. J Health Politics, Policy and Law 2005; 30(3):327–366.
9. For an excellent discussion of the manner in which the culture of technology drives medical liability, see: Jacobson PD. Medical liability and the culture of technology. In: Sage WA, Kersh R, eds. Medical Malpractice and the U.S. Health Care System. New York: Cambridge University Press, 2006.
10. Wachter RM, Shojanni KG. Internal Bleeding: The Truth Behind America's Terrifying Epidemic of Medical Mistakes. New York: Rugged Land, 2004.
11. 42 U.S.C. § 1395ww(d)(4)(D)(i)(2007).
12. Nolte E, McKee CM. Measuring the health of nations: Updating an earlier analysis. Health Affairs 2008; 27(1):58–71.
13. Institute of Medicine. Crossing the Quality Chasm: A New Health System for the 21st Century. Washington, DC: National Academy Press, 2001.
14. Reason J. Human error: Models and management. Br Med J 2000; 320:768–770. Also see Reason J. Human Error. Cambridge, UK: Cambridge University Press, 1990.
15. Bates DW, Cohen M, Leape LL, et al. Reducing the frequency of errors in medicine using information technology. J Am Med Inform Assoc 2001; 8(4):299–308.
16. Mello MM, Kelly CN, Brennan TA. Fostering rational regulation of patient safety. J Health Polit Policy Law 2005; 30(3):375–426.
17. Cooper JB, Newbower RS, Long CD, et al. Preventable anesthesia mishaps: A study of human factors. Anesthesiology 1978; 49:399–406.
18. Guadagnino C. "Improving Anesthesia Safety" (an interview with Ellison Pierce M.D.) Physicians's News Digest, 2000.

19. "Medical Errors and Perspectives on Patient Safety," Massachusetts Medical Society; available to www.mass.med.org/cme.

20. Guadagnino C. Impacts of Error Reduction Initiatives. Physician's News Digest, 2000.

21. Institute of Medicine. "Patient Safety: Achieving a New Standard of Care." Aspden P, Corrigan JM, Wolcott J and Erickson SM, eds. Washington, DC: National Academics Press, 2004.

22. Tracy TF, Crawford LS, Krizek TJ. When medical error becomes medical malpractice: The victims and the circumstances. Arch Surg 2003; 138(4):447–454. At www.archsurg.com.

23. Codman EA. A Study in Hospital Efficiency, As Demonstrated by the Case Report of the First Five Years of a Private Hospital. Boston, MA: Todd Company Printers, 1917. Reprinted by The Joint Commission on Accreditation of Health care Organization Oakbrook Terrace, Illinois, 1996.

24. Orlander JD, Barber TW, Fincke BG. The morbidity and mortality conference: The delicate nature of learning from error. Acad Med 2002; 77(10):1001–1006.

25. Nijm LM. Pitfalls of peer review: The limited protections of State and Federal peer review law for physicians. J Legal Med 2003; 24(4):541–556.

26. 42 U.S.C. § 1110-1 et. seq.

27. Knoll AM. Mea culpa, mea culpa: A call for privilege for self-disclosure of error in the setting of primary medical education. J Health Law 2002; 35(3):419–438.

28. Mulholland DM, Zarone P. Waiver of the peer review privilege: A survey of the law. S D Law Rev 2004; 49:424–428.

29. Biddle C, Oaster TR. Investigating the nature of the morbidity and mortality conference. Acad Med 1990; 65(6):420–421.

30. Thompson JS, Prior MA. Quality assurance and morbidity and mortality conference. J Surg Res 1992; 52:97–100.

31. Pierluissi E, Fischer MA, Campbell AR, et al. Discussion of medical errors in morbidity and mortality conferences. JAMA 2003; 290(21):2838–2842.

32. Wu AW, Folkman S, McPhee SJ, et al. Do house officers learn from their mistakes? Qual Saf Health Care 2003; 12:221–226.

33. Moore FD. A Miracle and a Privilege: Recounting a Half Century of Surgical Advances. Washington, DC: Joseph Henry Press, 1995.

34. New York State Public Health Law § 2805-m(2) and New York Education Law 6527(3) are an example of state law. McKinney, 2002.

35. See *Salamon vs. Our Lady of Victory Hospital*, et al. 1999 WL 955513 (W.D.N.Y.), 2002 WL 436766 (W.D.N.Y.), 2006 WL 625839 (W.D.N.Y.) (in which the court held that New York State peer review protections did not preclude plaintiff's access to the chart reviews, credentials files, quality assurance files, and administrative files for all physicians affiliated with the gastroenterology department which plaintiff complained had used peer review to retaliate against her when she complained about sexual harassment by the department chief.); *Franzon vs. Massena Memorial Hospital*, 189 F.R.D. 220 (W.D.N.Y. 1999) (in which the court held that state law privileges afforded physician peer review and the quality assurance process did not preclude discovery of hospital's peer review materials and quality assurance files by a physician who alleged that the hospital used the peer review process to retaliate against him for exercising First Amendment Rights); *Johnson vs. Nyack Hospital*, 169 F.R.D. 550 (S.D.N.Y., 1996) (in which the court held peer review records were discoverable by a physician who claimed that the hospital had denied his application for staff privileges based on race discrimination). Also see *Christie vs. Adkins*, No. 06-13107 (11th Cir., 2007) cert. denied No. 07-538 (U.S. Jan. 7, 2008) and *Virmani vs. Novan Health Inc.*, 259 F.2d 284 (4th Cir., 2001).

36. *Memorial Hospital vs. Shador*, 664 F.2d 1058 (7th Cir., 1981) and *Benson vs. St. Joseph Regional Health Center*, No. 11-04-04323 (May 1, 2006).

37. *Ryan vs. Staten Island University Hospital*, No. 04-DV-2666 (April 13, 2006).

38. Wei M. Doctors, apologies, and the law: An analysis and critique of apology laws. J Health Law 2007; 40(1):107–159. At http://ssrn.com/abstract = 955668.

39. Patient Safety and Quality Improvement Act of 2005, S. 544, 109th Congress, § 923 (2005); Public Law 109–141.

40. Brown LM, Gruner RS, Kandel AO, eds. The Legal Audit: Corporate Internal Investigation. St. Paul, Minnisota. Thomson West Publishers, 2006.

41. See *Brem vs. DeCarlo*, 162 FRD 94, CD. Md. (1995).

42. *Bredice vs. Doctors Hospital, Inc.*, 50 F.R.D. 249 (D.D.C., 1970), aff'd. 479 F.2d 920 (D. C. Cir., 1973).

43. *Weekoty vs. US*, 30 F.Supp.3d 1342 (D.N.M. 1998); *Spinks vs. Children's Hospital National Medical Center*, 124 F.R.D. 9, 12 (D.D.C. 1989); *Utterback vs. Yoon*, 121 F.R.D. 297 (W.D., Ky. 1987).

44. *Syposs vs. United States*, 63 F.Supp.2d 301, 306 (W.D.N.Y. 1999).

45. *In Re Crazy Eddie*, 792 F.Supp. 197 (EDNY 1992) (rejecting the privilege in a case involving audit documents in a securities case), *University of Pennsylvania vs. EEOC*, 493 U.S. 182 (1990) (a United States Supreme Court case in which the court declined to recognize the privilege to protect peer review documents generated during tenure considerations of an associate professor at the Wharton

School of Business) and *Spencer Savings Bank vs. Excell Mortgage Corp.*, 960 F.Supp 835, 843–844 (DNJ 1997) (wherein the court rejected the privilege as to mortgage loan documents).

46. The state laws are: Ala. Code § 34-24-58 (2003); Alaska Stat. § 18.23.030 (Michie 2003); Ariz. Rev. Stat. § 36-445.0 (2003); Ark. Code Ann. § 20-9-503 (Michie 2003); Cal. Evid. Code §§ 1156, 1157 (West 2003); Colo. Rev. Stat. §§ 12-36.5-104, 25-3-109 (2002); Conn. Gen. Stat. § 19a-17b (2003); Del. Code Ann. Tit. 24 § 1768 (2003); D.C. Code Ann. § 44-805 (2003); Fla. Stat. Ann. § 395.0193 (West 2003); Ga. Code Ann. § 31-7-15 (2002); Haw. Rev. Stat. Ann. §§ 671D-10, 624-25.5 (Michie 2002); Idaho Code §§ 39-1392b, 39-1392e (Michie 2003); 735 Ill. Comp. Stat. 5/8-2102 (2003); Ind. Code Ann. § 34-30-15-1 (West 2003); Iowa Code § 147.135 (2003); Kan. Stat. Ann. § 65-4915 (2003); Ky. Rev. Stat. Ann. § 311.377 (Michie 2003); La. Rev. Stat. Ann. § 13:3715.3 (West 2003); Me. Rev. Stat. Ann. Tit. 32 § 2599 (West 2003); Md. Code Ann. Health Occ. § 1-401 (2003); Mass. Ann. Laws Ch. 111 § 204 (Law. Co-op 2003); Mich. Comp. Laws Ann. § 333.20175 (West 2003); Minn. Stat. Ann. §§ 145.61, 145.64 (West 2002); Miss. Code Ann. § 41-63-9 (2003); Mo. Rev. Stat. § 537.035 (2003); Mont. Code Ann. § 37-2-201 (2002); Neb. Rev. Stat. Ann. § 71-2048 (Michie 2002); Nev. Rev. Stat. Ann. § 49.265 (2003);N.H. Rev. Stat. Ann. § 151.13-a (2002); N.M. Stat. Ann. § 41-9-5 (Michie 2002); N.Y. Pub. Health Law § 2805-m and Education Law 6527 (McKinney 2003); N.C. Gen. Stat. § 131E-95 (2003); N.D. Cent. Code § 23-34-03 (2002); Ohio Rev. Code Ann. §§ 2305.24, 2305.251, 2305-252 (Anderson 2003); Okla. Stat. Ann. Tit. 63 § 1-1709-1 (West 2002); Or. Rev. Stat. § 41.675 (2001); Pa. Stat. Ann. Tit. 63 § 425.4 (2002); R.I. Gen. Laws § 23-17-25 (2002); S.C. Code Ann. § 40-71-20 (Law. Co-Op 2002); S.D. Cod. Laws § 36-4-26.1 (2005); Tenn. Code Ann. § 63-6-219 (2003); Texas Occupational Code § 151.002 (formerly Texas Revised Civil Statutes Article 4495); Utah Code Ann. § 58-67-701 (2003); Vt. Stat. Ann. Tit. 26 § 1443 (2003); Va. Code Ann. § 8.01-581.17 (Michie 2003); Wash. Rev. Code Ann. § 4.24.250 (West 2003); W. Va. Code § 30-3 C-3 (2003); Wis. Stat. Ann § 146.38 (West 2002). Wyo. Stat. Ann. § 35-17-105 (Michie 2003). Also see *Virmani vs. Novan Health Inc.*, 259 F.3d 284 (4th Cir., 2001) which contains references to these laws.

47. Medical and Dental Malpractice and Professional Conduct,1986 New York Laws, Ch. 266, § 31.

48. *White vs. New York City Health and Hospital's Corporation*, No. 88 CIV 7536, 1990 WL 33747, at *10 (S.D.N.Y. March 19, 1990).

49. *Lizotte vs. New York City Health & Hosps. Corp.*, No. 85 CIV 7548, 1989 WL 260217, at 2 (S.D.N.Y. Nov. 28, 1989); *Brazinski vs. New York Chiropractic Coll.*, 284 A.D.2d 647, 725 N.Y.S.2d 456 (2001); *Logue vs. Velez*, 92 N.Y.S.2d 13, 677 N.Y.S.2d 6 (1998).

50. While a complete discussion of the pros and cons of each state statutory peer review privilege, the interjurisdictional variations, and the interpretive case law is beyond the scope of this chapter, the reader is referred to Creech CD. The medical review committee privilege: A jurisdictional survey. North Carol Law Rev 1988; 67:179–184; Cate MJ. Physician peer review. J Legal Med 1999; 20:479–484; Scheutzon SO, Gillis SL. Confidentiality and privilege of peer review information: More imagined than real. J Law and Health 1993; 7:169–179; and Scheutzow SO. State medical peer review: High cost but no benefit—is it time for a change? Am J Law Med 1999; 25(1):7–60.

51. District of Columbia D. C. Code Ann § 44-802 (2001).

52. *Koithan vs. Zornek MD*, 22 A.D.2d 1080, 642 NYS2d 115 (4th Dept., 1996); *Bryant vs. Bui MD*, 265 A.D.2d 848, 695 NYS2d 790 (4th Dept., 1999); *Kraus vs. West*, 184 Misc.2d 539, 708 NYS2d 836 (2000). It is also notable that, in New York, the courts have held that the findings of the New York State Department of Health (DOH) following investigation of a complaint were admissible in a subsequent medical malpractice case when the DOH's findings related to the conduct at issue in the malpractice lawsuit. See *Cramer vs. Bendeditire Hospital*, 190 Misc.2d 191 (Sup. Ct. Ulser Co. 2002) (in which the court held admissible a redacted copy of the DOH's report of its investigation of the incident at issue in the subsequent medical malpractice lawsuit); also see *Smith vs. Delago*, 2 A.D.2d 1259, 730 N.Y.S.2d 445 (3rd Dept., 2003) (in which plaintiff obtained a copy of the DOH's investigation of a complaint about the hospital medical care of plaintiff via a Freedom of Information Law request. The DOH report included redacted interviews with hospital staff and the DOH's independent review of the medical care was provided. The Appellate Court found that the plaintiff was entitled to the DOH's statement of deficiencies, redacted to remove conclusions of law and the opinions of the DOH.)

53. *White vs. New York City Health and Hospitals Corp.*, No. 88 CIV 7536, 1990 WL 33747 (S.D.N.Y., 1990); *Lizotte vs. New York City Health and Hospitals Corp.*, No. 85 CIV 7548, 1989 WL 260217 (S.D.N.Y., 1989); *Tartaglia vs. Paul Revere Life Ins. Co.*, 948 F.Supp. 325 (S.D.N.Y., 1996); *Kristen K. vs. Children's Hospital of Buffalo*, 204 A.D.2d 1007, 614 N.Y.S.2d 89 (4th Dept., 1994).

54. N.J.S. 2a:84A-22.8(a).

55. *Payton vs. New Jersey Turnpike Authority*, 148 N.J. 524 (1997). Also see *Reyes vs. Meadowlands Hosp. Med. Ctr.*, 355 N.J. Super. 226, 236 (Law Div. 2001). In *Reyes*, a malpractice case, the court refused to permit the hospital to assert a self-critical privilege and rejected the implication in two earlier cases that medical professionals would not agree to take part in a process to improve patient care without a "cloak of confidentiality."

56. Kohlberg KR. The medical peer review privilege: A linchpin for patient safety measures. Mass Law Rev 2000; 86(4):157–162.

57. Bill Summary—A07840. At http://www.assembly.state.ny.us/legal?bn = A07840.

58. Brennan TA. Hospital peer review and clinical privileges actions: To report or not report. J Am Med Assoc 1999; 282(4):381–382; Liang BA. Promoting patient safety through reducing medical error: A paradigm of cooperation between patient, physician and attorney. South Ill Univ Law J 2000; 24;555–556; Liang BA. Error in medicine: Legal impediments to U.S. reform. J Health Polit Policy Law 1999; 24;40–41.

59. Leape LL. Error in medicine. JAMA 1994; 272(23):1851–1857.

60. Lehman AG. Medical culture and error disclosure. Virtual Mentor 2008; 10(5):282–287.

61. Milstein A, Adler NE. Out of sight, out of mind: Why doesn't widespread clinical quality failure command our attention? Health Aff 2003; 22(2):119–127.

62. Wu AW. Medical error: The second victim. The doctor who makes the mistake needs help too. Br Med J 2000; 320:726–727.

63. West CP, Huschka MM, Novotny PJ, et al. Association of perceived medical errors with resident distress and empathy; a prospective longitudinal study. JAMA 2006; 296:1071–1078.

64. Waterman AD, Garbutt J, Hazel E, et al. The emotional impact of medical errors on practicing physicians in the United States and Canada. Jt Comm J Qual Patient Saf 2007; 33(8):467–476.

65. Mariner WK, Miller FH. Medical error reporting: Professional tensions between confidentiality and liability. Massachusetts Health Policy Forum Issue Brief No. 13, 2001. At http://masshealthpolicyforum.brandeis.edu/forums/all.html.

66. Newman MC. The emotional impact of medical errors on family physicians. Arch Fam Med 1996; 5:71–75.

67. Within the federal government, there are eight major patient safety reporting and surveillance systems. From a reporting perspective, these include two systems managed by the Centers for Disease Control and Prevention (CDC), specifically the National Nosocomial Infections Surveillance (NNIS) system and the Dialysis Surveillance Network (DSN). The Food and Drug Administration (FDA) manages MedWatch, which handles reporting of medical device, biologic and blood product, and special nutritionals events. For a discussion on the specifics of these systems, see IOM 2004 Report Appendix C: Examples of Federal, State and Private Sector Reporting Systems, pp. 341–426 at Note 21. Also see Harrington MH. Revisiting Medical Error: Five Years After IOM Reports, Have Reporting Systems Made a Measurable Difference? Health Matrix 2005; 15(2):329–377.

68. Flowers L, Riley T. State-based mandatory reporting of medical errors. Nat Acad State Health Pol. 2001:1–61; available @ www.nashp.org.

69. Brennan TA, Mello MM, Studdert DM. Liability, patient safety and defense medicine: What does the future hold? In: Sage WM, Kersh R, eds. Medical Malpractice and the U. S. Health Care System. New York, New York: Cambridge University Press, 2006:97.

70. Serious Reportable Events in Health care. Washington, DC: National Quality Forum, 2002. At www.qualityforum.org/publications/reports. At www.qualityforum.org/publications/reports.

71. Serious Reportable Events in Health care 2006 Update. Washington, DC: National Quality Forum, 2006. At www.qualityforum.org/publications/reports.

72. 2007 Guide to State Adverse Event Reporting Systems. Portland, ME: National Academy for State Health Policy. At http://www.nashp.org/files/shpsurveyreport_adverse 2007.pdf.

73. New York State Public Officer's Law Article 6, § 87 (Added L. 1977, c. 933).

74. Flink E, Chevalier CL, Ruperto A,et al. Lessons learned from the evolution of mandatory adverse event reporting systems. Agency for Health care Research and Quality, 2005. At http://www.ahrg.gov/downloads/pub/advances/vol3/flink.pdf. Also see Tuttle D, Panzer R, Baird T. Using administrative data to improve compliance with mandatory state event reporting. J Qual Improv 2002; 28(6):349–358.

75. Redhead CS. Health Care Quality: Improving Patient Safety by Promoting Medical Errors Reporting. CRS Report for Congress, 2005. Order Code RL31983. At opencrs.com/document/RL31982.

76. State Reporting of Medical Errors and Adverse Events: Results of a 50-State Survey. Portland, ME: National Academy for State Health Policy, 2000. At http://www.nashp.org.

77. Robinson AR, Hahmann KB, Rifkin JI, et al. Physician and public opinions on quality of health care and the problem of medical errors. Arch Internal Med 2002; 162(19):2186–2190.

78. Weissman JS, Annas CL, Epstein AM, et al. Error reporting and disclosure systems: Views from hospital leaders. JAMA 2005; 293(11):1359–1366.

79. Furrow BR. Regulating patient safety: Toward a federal model of medical error reduction. Widener Law Rev 2005; 12(1):1–33.

80. Horner B, Levin A, Marx R. Empty Promises: The Failure of the New York State Health Department to Monitor Medical Errors. New York: Public Interest Research Group, 2005. At www.nypirg.org.

81. Sentinel Event Policy and Procedures. Joint Commission on Accreditation of Health care Organizations, 2005. At http://www.jointcommission.org.

82. By the Numbers Part I: Medical error data collection and reporting. Joint Commission Benchmark, 2008; 10(2):1–10. At http://www.jcrinc.com.

83. Liang BA. Risks of reporting sentinel events. Health Aff 2000; 19(5):112–120.

84. IOM 2004 Report, Chapter 9 "Standardized Reporting," pp. 280–281. See Note 21.

85. Schroder JC. Disclosing medical errors: Practical, ethical and legal considerations. Health Law Weekly 2004; 2(26). At www.ahlaweb.healthlawyers.org.
86. The Prescription Drug, Improvement and Modernization Act of 2003 [42 USC § 1395 ww(b)(3)(B)(vii)] requires hospitals to submit quality reports for 10 quality indications developed by the National Quality Foundation and, via the Medicare Compare Program, this information is available on the Internet.
87. http://www.leapfroggroup.org.
88. Mazur KM, Simon SR, Yood RA, et al. Health plan members' views about disclosure of medical errors. Ann Int Med 2004; 140(6):409–418.
89. Gallagher TH, Waterman AD, Ebers AG, et al. Patients and physicians' attitudes regarding the disclosure of medical errors. JAMA 2003; 289(8): 1001–1007.
90. Witman AB, Park DM, Hardin SB. How do patients want physicians to handle mistakes? A survey of internal medicine patients in an academic setting. Arch Int Med 1996; 156(22):2565–2569.
91. Duclos CW, Eichler M, Taylor L, et al. Patient perspectives of patient-provider communications after adverse events. Int J Quality Health Care 2005; 17(6):479–483.
92. Available on AMA's website: www.ama-assn.org.
93. Snyder L, Leffler C. Ethics Manual: Fifth Edition Annals of Internal Medicine, 2005; 142(7):560–582.
94. Available on ACOG website: www.acog.org/from_home/acogcode.pdf.
95. Blendon RJ, DesRoches CM, Brodie M, et al. Views of practicing physicians and the public on medical errors. NEJM 2002; 347(24):1933–1940.
96. Gallagher TH, Waterman AD, Garbutt JM, et al. US and Canadian physicians' attitudes and experiences regarding disclosing errors to patients. Arch Int Med 2006; 166(15):1605–1611.
97. Schoen C, Osborn R, Huynh PT, et al. Taking the pulse of health care systems: Experiences of patients with health problems in six countries. Health Aff 2005; suppl. Web Exclusives: November 3, 2005; 16:
98. Kaldjian LC, Jones EW, Wu BJ, et al. Disclosing medical errors to patients: Attitudes and practices of physicians and trainees. J Gen Int Med 2007; 22(7):988–996.
99. Lamb RM, Studdert DM, Bohmer RM, et al. Hospital disclosure practices: Results of a national survey. Health Aff 2003; 22(2):73–83.
100. Hingorani M, Wong T, Vafidis G. Patients' and doctors' attitudes to amount of information given after unintended injury during treatment: Cross-sectional, questionnaire survey. Brit Med J 1999; 318(7184):640–641.
101. Gallagher TH, Levinson W. A time for professional action. Arch Int Med 2005; 165(16):1819–1824.
102. Robinson AR, Hohmann KB, Rifkin JI, et al. Physician and public opinions on quality of health care and the problem of medical errors. Arch Int Med 2002; 162(19):2186–2190.
103. Gallagher TH, Denman CR, Leape LL, et al. Disclosing unanticipated outcomes to patients: The art and practice. J Patient Saf 2007; 3(3):158–165.
104. Delbanco T, Bell SK. Guilty, afraid and alone—Struggling with medical error. NEJM 2007; 357(17):1682–1683.
105. Gawande A. Complications: A Surgeon's Notes on an Imperfect Science. New York: Metropolitan Books, 2002.
106. West CP, Huschka MM, Novotny PJ, et al. Association of perceived medical errors with resident distress and empathy: A prospective longitudinal study. JAMA 2006; 296(9):1071–1078.
107. Banja JC. Persisting problems in disclosing medical error. Harv Health Policy Rev 2004; 5(1):15. At www.hhpr.org. Also see Banja JD. Does medical error disclosure violate the medical malpractice insurance cooperation clause? Advances in Patient Safety 2004; 9:371–38.
108. Gallagher TH, Studdert D, Levinson W, et al. Disclosing harmful medical errors to patients. NEJM 2007; 356(26):2713–2719.
109. Joint Commission on Accreditation of Health Care Organization, Revision to Joint Commission Standards in Support of Patient Safety and Medical Health Care Error Reduction, 2001. At http://www.premiermc.com/all/safety/recourses/patient_safety/downloads/12_JCAHO_stdrs_05-01-01.doc.
110. When Things Go Wrong: Responding to Adverse Events. A Consensus Statement of the Harvard Hospitals. Burlington, Massachusetts: Massachusetts Coalition for the Prevention of Medical Errors, 2006.
111. Gallagher T, Brundate G, Bonmarito KM, et al. Risk managers' attitudes and experiences regarding patient safety and error disclosure: A national survey. ASHRM J 2006; 26:11–16.
112. "Disclosure: What works now and what can work even better," Monograph Prepared by the Task Force of the American Society of Health care Risk Management, 2004. At www.ashrm.org.
113. At www.qualityforum.org.
114. Safe Practices for Better Health care. Washington, DC: National Quality Forum, 2007. At http://www.qualityforum.org/projects/completed/safe_practices.
115. Taft L. Disclosing unanticipated outcomes: A challenge to providers and their lawyers. Health Law News 2008; 12(5):11–16.

116. Kraman SS, Hamm G. Risk management: Extreme honesty may be the best policy. Ann Int Med 1999; 131(12):963–967.

117. Wu AW, Cavanaugh TA, McPhee SJ, et al. To tell the truth: Ethical and practical issues in disclosing medical mistakes to patients. J Gen Int Med 1997; 12(12):770–775.

118. Wojcieszak D. The Sorry Works! Coalition: Doctors, Insurers, Lawyers, Hospital Administration, Patients and Researchers Joining Together to Provide a "Middle Ground" Solution to the Medical Malpractice Crisis. At http://www.sorryworks.net/ WhatIs.phtml.

119. Shapiro E. Disclosing medical errors: Best practices from the "leading edge." 2008 unpublished paper contracted by the Robert Wood Johnson Foundation. Available at www.IHI.org.

120. COPIC: COPIC's 3R Program. At http://www.callcopic.com/resources/custom/PDF/3rd-newsletter/vol-3-issue-1-jun-2006.pdf.

121. Kachalia A, Shojania KG, Hofer TP, et al. Does full disclosure of medical errors affect malpractice liability? The jury is still out. Jt Comm J Qual Saf 2003; 29(10):503–511.

122. Popp PL. How will disclosure affect future litigation? Journal of Health care Risk Management 2003; 5–9.

123. Levinson W, Roter DL, Mullooly JP, et al. Physician-patient communication: The relationship with malpractice claims among primary care physicians and surgeons. JAMA 1997; 277(7):553–559.

124. Hickson GB, Clayton EW, Githens PB, et al. Factors that prompted families to file medical malpractice claims following perinatal injuries. JAMA 1992; 268(11):359–363.

125. Vincent C, Young M, Phillips A. Why do people sue doctors? A study of patients and relatives taking legal action. Lancet 1994; 343(8913):1609–1613.

126. The National Medical Error Disclosure and Compensation Act 2005; S. 1784, 109th Congress, 2005.

127. Clinton HR, Obama B. Making patient safety the centerpiece of medical liability reform. NEJM 2006; 354(21):2205–2208.

128. Department of Veterans Affairs, Disclosure of Adverse Evens to Patients, VHA Directive 2005. At http://www.1va.gov/vhaethics/download/AEpolicy.pdf.

129. Kraman SS, Cranfill L, Hamm G, et al. John M. Eisenburg Patient Safety Awards. Advocacy: The Lexington Veterans Affairs Medical Center. Jt Comm J Qual Improv 2002; 28(12):646–650.

130. It has been noted that the VAs are government hospitals that benefit from much stronger barriers to lawsuits because their physicians are immune from personal liability as government employees under the Federal Tort Claims Act (FTCA), they enjoy the shield of presuit administrative requirements and have more options for resolution outside of litigation (the government-based system has the ability to compensate those who have suffered an adverse event through remedial treatment or even disability payments without going through a lawsuit). See notes 38 and 121.

131. The U-M System Approach to Malpractice Claims. At http://www.med.umichsedu/news/umhsm.htm.

132. Geier P. Emerging Med-Mal strategy: "I'm Sorry.". National Law Journal. July 24, 2008.

133. Note that Gesinger began to communicate errors and adverse outcomes to patients when it became the law in Pennsylvania. In 2002, the Pennsylvania State Legislature passed Act 13, the Medical Care Availability and Reduction of Error (MCARE) Act which provides that "A person who has sustained injury or death as a result of medical negligence by a health care provider must be afforded a prompt determination and fair compensation." and "Every effort must be made to reduce and eliminate medical errors by identifying problems and implementing solutions that promote patient safety."

134. It appears this program is under development as reported by the co-designer of the program, Lee Taft, JD, Taft Solutions, Dallas, Texas. See Note 115.

135. Process for Early Assessment & Resolution of Loss (PEARL) White Paper published as collaboration between Taft Solutions, Stanford University Medical Center Office of Risk Management, and the Office of General Counsel of the Stanford University, September 2007.

136. Studdert DM, Mello MM, Gawande A, et al. Disclosure of medical injury to patients: An impossible risk management strategy. Health Aff 2007; 26(1):215–226.

137. Sorry Works Coalition. At http://sorryworks.net/files/states_with_apology_laws.ppt.

138. 2003 COLO. LEGIS. SERV. Ch. 126 (H.B. 03-1232), approved 4/17/03.

139. Liebman CB, Hyman CS. Disclosure and fair resolution of adverse events. In: Sage, WM, Kersh R, eds. Medical Malpractice and the U.S. Health Care System. New York, New York: Cambridge University Press, 2006.

140. CAL. EVID. CODE § 1160; FLA. STATE. ANN. § 90.4026; TEX. CIV. PRAC. & REM. CODE ANN. § 18.0612; WASH. REV. CODE ANN. § 5.66.010.

141. Mass. Gen. Laws, Ch. 233, § 23D.

142. Stuart JK, Fernandez DE. Don't be sorry—preventing your apologies from becoming admissions. Smith Amundsen Health Care Quarterly Winter 2007.

143. California Evidence Code § 1160 (2000); Florida Stat. § 395 1051 (2004); Nevada NRS § 439.855 (2004); New Jersey Stat. § 26:2 H-12.25 (2005); Oregon Rev. Stat. § 677.082 (2003); Pennsylvania 40 P. S. § 1303.308(b) (2004); Vermont § 310 (2006).

144. Mello MM, Studdert DM. The medical malpractice system. In: Sage WM, Kersh R, eds. Medical Malpractice and the U.S. Health Care System. New York, New York: Cambridge University Press, 2006:11–29.
145. Kersh R. Medical malpractice and the new politics of health care. In: Sage WM, Kersh R, eds. Medical Malpractice and the U.S. Health Care System. New York, New York: Cambridge University Press, 2006:43–67.
146. Brennan TA, Mello MM. Patient safety and medical malpractice: A case study. Ann Int Med 2003; 139(4):267–273.
147. Studdert DN, Mello MM, Brennan TA. Medical malpractice. NEJM 2004; 350(3):283–292.
148. Mohr JC. American medical malpractice litigation in historical perspective. JAMA 2000; 283(13):1731–1737.
149. Brown CD, Mitchell N, Scott KP. Litigation impact of never events. Health Law News 2008; 12(2):26–30.
150. Sage WM. Malpractice reform as a health policy problem. In: Sage WM, Kersh R, eds. Medical Malpractice and the U.S. Health Care System. New York, New York: Cambridge University Press, 2006:30–42.
151. Higgins TJ. Communication breakdowns that lead to lawsuits: A Plaintiff's attorney's view toward reducing malpractice claims. NYSBA Health Law J Winter 2008; 13(1):23–26.
152. Strove CT. Expertise and the legal process. In: Sage WM, Kersh R, eds. Medical Malpractice and the U.S. Health Care System. New York, New York: Cambridge University Press, 2006:173–190.
153. *Austin vs. American Association of Neurological Surgeons*. 253 F.3d 967, 57 Fed. R. Evid. Sev. 385 (United States Court of Appeals, Seventh Circuit, 2001).
154. Segal J, Sccopulos M. Do-It-Yourself Tort Reform. Wall Street Journal. July 12, 2007.
155. Hickson GB, Federspiel CF, Pichert JW. Patient complaints and malpractice risk. JAMA 2002; 287(22):2951–2957.
156. Volpp KG, Rosen AK, Rosenbaum PR, et al. Physician scores on a national clinical skills examination as predicators of complaints to medical regulatory authorities. JAMA 2007; 298(9):984–992.
157. Baker T. Medical malpractice insurance reform: 'Enterprise Insurance' and some alternatives. In: Sage WM, Kersh R, eds. Medical Malpractice and the U.S. Health Care System. New York, New York: Cambridge University Press, 2006:267–290.
158. Sage WM. The forgotten third: Liability insurance and the medical malpractice crisis. Health Aff 2004; 23(4):10–21.
159. Anderson R. Commentaries—defending the practice of medicine. Arch Int Med 2004; 164(11):1173–1178.
160. Mello MM, Studdert DM, Brennan TA. The new medical malpractice crisis. NEJM 2003; 348(23):2281–2284.
161. Pawlak S. Debate over malpractice crisis comes to capital. *Legislative Gazette*. March 10, 2008. At www.legislativegazette.com.
162. Solomont EB. Doctors fear malpractice disaster. *The New York Sun*. May 14, 2008. At www2.nysun.com.
163. The American College of Obstetricians and Gynecologists. At http://www.acog.org.
164. American Hospital Association, Professional Liability Insurance Survey (2003).
165. For this, see "Medical Liability Reform—Now!" American Medical Association, 5/2/08. At http://www.ama-assn.org/go/mlrnow.
166. Marchev M. The medical malpractice insurance crisis: Opportunity for state action. National Academy for State Health Policy, July 2002.
167. How Insurance Reform Lowered Doctors' Medical Malpractice Rates in California and How Malpractice Caps Failed. Foundation for Taxpayer & Consumer Rights, March 7, 2003.
168. Landes WM, Posner PA. The Economic Structure of Tort Law. Boston, Mass. Harvard University Press, 1987.
169. Coleman JL. Moral Theories of Torts: Their Scope and Limits: Part II. Law Philos 1983; 2(1):5–36. Coleman JL. Moral Theories of Torts: Their Scope and Limits: Part I. Law Philos 1982; 1(3):371–380.
170. Weiler PC, Hiatt H, Newhouse JP, et al. A Measure of Malpractice Cambridge. Boston, Mass. Massachusetts Harvard University Press, 1993.
171. Brennan TA, Soc CM, Burstin HR. Relation between negligent adverse events and the outcomes of medical malpractice litigation. NEJM 1996; 335(26):1963–1967.
172. Mello MM, Brennan TA. Deterrence of medical errors: Theory and evidence for malpractice reform. Tex Law Rev 2002; 80:1595–1638.
173. Studdert DM, Mello MD, Sage WM, et al. Defensive medicine among high risk specialist physicians in a volatile malpractice environment. JAMA 2005; 293(21):2609–2617.
174. Sage WM. Regulating for patient safety: The law's response to medical errors: Malpractice reform as a health policy problem. Widener Law Rev 2005; 12:107–119.
175. Danzon PM. Liability for medical malpractice. In: Culyer AJ, Newhouse JP, eds. Handbook of Health Economics. Amsterdam, The Netherlands: Elsevier, 2000.

176. Towers Perrin 2007 report on tort costs available at www.towersperrin.com. This study also evidences the inefficiency of the tort system in its report that the system returns less than 50% on the dollar to claimants with the breakdown as follows: 22¢ to the litigant for economic damages; 24¢ to the litigant for noneconomic damages; 19¢ to the plaintiff's attorney; 14¢ for defense costs and 21¢ for administrative costs. The high administrative costs of the medical liability system need to be compared to those in the Workers' Compensation system (20–30%) and Social Security disability insurance (5%) to fully appreciate their impact.

177. Studdert DM, Mello MM, Gawande AA. Claims, errors and compensation payments in medical malpractice litigation. NEJM 2006; 354(19):2024–2033.

178. Shuck BC, Martin S. Wyoming tort reform and the medical malpractice insurance crisis: A second opinion. Land Water Law Rev 1993;28:593–600.

179. Viscusi WK, Born P. The national implications of liability reforms for general liability and medical malpractice insurance. Seton Hall Law Rev 1994; 24:1743–1766.

180. Alabama, Florida, Illinois, New Hampshire, South Dakota, Texas and Washington Abolishment of the collateral source rule was found unconstitutional in Alabama (in part), Kansas and Kentucky. Abolishment of joint and several liability was found unconstitutional in Illionois and Montana. In November of 2007, Cook County Circuit Court Judge Diane Larson overruled Illinois landmark 2005 legislation on the basis that she found its cap provisions unconstitutional and inappropriately disregarding the jury's role of determining appropriate compensation. In April of 2008, in *Park vs. Wellstar* (No. 07-CV-135208), a Georgia judge in Fulton County Supreme Court ruled that Georgia cap on non-economic damage was unconstitutional.

181. Mehlman MJ. Promoting fairness in the medical malpractice system. In: Sage WM, Kersh R, eds. Medical Malpractice and the U.S. Health Care System. New York, New York: Cambridge University Press, 2006.

182. Sack K. Doctors say "I'm Sorry" before "See You in Court," New York Times. May 18, 2008.

183. www.cgood.org.

184. Kachalia AB, Mello MM, Brennan TA. Beyond negligence: Avoidability and medical injury compensation. Soc Sci Med 2008; 66(2):387–402.

4 | A Nursing Perspective on Errors in Medicine: Pediatric Surgery

Mary Ellen Connolly, M.S., CPNP., Karen Iacono, M.S.,
Lucille Kingston, R.N., PNP-BC, CORLN, and Carmel A. McComiskey, M.S., PNP-BC, CPNP-AC

INTRODUCTION AND HISTORY

In 1965, Dr. Henry Silver and Loretta Ford developed the role of the advanced practice nurse (APN) at the University of Colorado, after recognizing a need for nurses to perform duties previously considered within the role of the physician. Nurse practitioners were initially trained to provide primary health care to patients in rural underserved areas. Since then, the role of the APN has evolved to include the care of chronically ill children, management of hospitalized children, specialty care, and, most recently, the daily delivery of acute care. Pediatric nurse practitioners are registered nurses who have earned masters degrees in pediatric advanced practice.

During the same time period, physicians elsewhere were developing physician assistant programs: mid-level, two-year provider programs targeting corpsman, who could assist in underserved areas as well.

ROLE OF THE APN IN PEDIATRIC SURGERY

The APN role in pediatric surgery has varied from region to region, state to state, and program to program, but over time, it has evolved to include care of the child with a surgical diagnosis in the neonatal intensive care unit (NICU), in the pediatric intensive care unit (PICU), in the operating room, in case management departments, on general pediatric floors, and in private practices. In addition, with the Residency Review Committees' recommendation mandating the reduction of work hours by residents, APNs are well positioned to provide inpatient care. Roles of the APN in error/complication avoidance in the pediatric surgical patient will be addressed (1).

ACUTE CARE

One model of the pediatric surgery service uses APNs to provide daily care to children admitted to inpatient units. APNs have developed different strategies to facilitate this care. Most provide daily management of complex patients including admission orders, history and physical examinations, laboratory monitoring, discharge planning, education, and visit documentation. Many have admitting and discharge privileges. At some centers, APNs provide consultation in the Emergency Department, triaging surgical emergencies, and expediting the process for admission or operative intervention.

Nurses with extensive experience in pediatric surgery provide expert tertiary management, develop computerized order sets, participate in both surgical and pediatric resident and medical student education, and provide advice regarding holistic care to the chronically ill pediatric surgery patient.

APNs provide continuity of care in a health care system where students and residents rotate through specialty units without the necessary experience to provide optimum care in a timely fashion. Establishing an inpatient nurse practitioner role increases the quality of care, the timeliness of responses to care-making decisions, and the consistency of the care; it minimizes the risk for potential errors or complications. This role contributes to decreased cost of care by eliminating redundant work efforts, increases revenues, by substituting a skilled surgical care provider, so that the attending surgical staff can spend more time in the operating room generating revenue.

APNs contribute to the quality of care. Those trained at the tertiary level of a pediatric facility provide support in the areas of pain management, fluid and electrolyte management, wound care, maintenance of special lines and tubes, and identification and prompt response to perioperative complications. The APNs' ability to establish and utilize relationships with community resources allows for prompt intervention when specialty needs arise. This is an advantage as surgeons are often unavailable for long periods of time, and unable to involve themselves in complex social or societal issues that impact the discharge outcome. Facilitating communication expedites the plan of care, preventing conflicting recommendations from multiple services. Communication between surgeons, parents, and staff is enhanced by the daily presence of a nurse practitioner.

Teaching family members how to care for their children is vital to the well-being of the child, improves the parent's confidence, the long-term outcome, the family's satisfaction, and the stability of the home-care environment. Simple postoperative instructions are equally important in facilitating complex critical care at home. APNs develop home-care teaching tools on a variety of topics: gastrostomy use and care, feeding routines, bowel management, enema preparation, and pain management. Parents report greater satisfaction when they receive teaching materials in writing and when they know whom to call should they need help. The APN supports the child when transitioning back into the school setting.

DISCHARGE OF THE CHILD WITH COMPLEX CHRONIC HOME-CARE NEEDS

Babies born with congenital anomalies require complex care immediately after repair. Most times, children with complex needs can be cared for at home with meticulous planning, discharge education, and coordination of home-care benefits to support complex home care.

The collaborative approach of assembling multiple providers to agree upon the care needed at home, and communicating this care to case management is a complicated process. Identifying service planning, monitoring its delivery, evaluating service outcomes and cost-effectiveness of home care is often done by case management nurses with pediatric surgery experience. In addition, collaboration with nutrition, social work, home health nursing, durable medical equipment providers, and pharmacies requires communication. The APN knows the diagnoses, the expected care, and the expected needs. Having the necessary equipment and resources available at the time of discharge for a smooth transition from hospital to home.

Planning the discharge and home care requires an organized approach to assure a safe transition to a well-equipped environment. Parents want to take care of their children and most times, when given the tools, exceed our expectations. Coordinating the key elements listed below assists the family with this objective:

Parent education
Skilled nursing visits
Durable medical equipment
Enteral/parenteral feedings and equipment
Coordination of insurance and community services
(Physical therapy (PT)/occupational therapy (OT)/Speech)
Subspecialty follow-up care
Support groups

Often, despite our best effort, these children become the 'frequent flyers' of our pediatric units, spending many days with us. It is often the APN who becomes the primary care provider for this population.

MANAGEMENT OF THE COMPLICATED SURGICAL PATIENT AT HOME

The APN manages the home care of the complicated surgical patient. For example, those patients with total parenteral nutrition, central venous lines, tracheostomies, feeding tubes, or complicated wounds often require intensive follow-up to direct the care delivered at home. The

APN orders and reviews weekly laboratory work as well as frequent reviews of the fluid and nutritional balances and feeding tolerance. Feeds are advanced; orders written and communicated to various home-care providers to facilitate the child's long-term recovery (2–4).

PROCEDURAL CARE

Across the country, APNs are providing assistance with procedures. For example, at Miami Children's Hospital, specially trained APNs are providing nitrous oxide/oxygen inhalation as an alternative to conscious sedation for painful procedures for the pediatric surgical service. This has enhanced the care patients receive, decreasing pain and anxiety, facilitating procedures that can be done without anesthesia personnel and optimizes the use of operative areas and operative time (5).

OUTPATIENT CARE

Several models of APN care exist for outpatient care. They assist pediatric nurse practitioners facilitate preoperative preparation of the surgical population, in anesthesia preoperative evaluation, providing perioperative education regarding postoperative care and pain management at home; and thereby streamlining and improving outpatient care but also increasing patient satisfaction. In addition, APNs follow those patients with indwelling tubes, complex enteral feedings, and complex wounds.

All pediatric surgical practice includes long-term bowel management of children with complicated anorectal malformations. This requires effort, consistent teaching, and sometimes, daily contact with parents and patients. Bowel management programs are staffed by APNs, who are well trained to provide this care; often tailoring enema and laxative therapies, teaching behavior modification, and providing nutritional counseling.

TELEPHONE TRIAGE

Answering telephone calls in a pediatric surgery practice is a time-consuming practice. There are three main types of advices: emergent, routine, and chronic.

APNs develop tools to train the ancillary staff to answer routine questions by developing telephone standards of care with regard to routine preoperative advice (need for laboratory testing, npo orders, time of surgery, referrals, etc.), postoperative advice (dressings, baths, diet, return to school/work notes, etc.), strategies to route more urgent calls, and finally triaging themselves, those calls requiring higher level assessment and advice (calls regarding complicated long-term patients or calls from referring providers). APNs also develop prescription refill protocols.

APNs are expert in assisting ancillary staff in the standardization of a decision-making strategy:

- Type of symptom
- Age of patient
- Duration
- Child's behavior
- Caller's anxiety
- Presence of underlying disease.

At the time of the call, the APN must decide if the patient should be seen now (ED, office), later at an appointed clinic visit, or cared for at home. Decision making focuses on complete assessments of all clues. The APN uses the telephone relationship to continue to teach and to promote autonomy and patient/parental assurance and security (6). In addition, APNs possess communication skills and can adapt their history-taking ability to collect data by telephone to compile a potential differential diagnosis, initiate the treatment plan, and document the condition as well as plan of care in the record (7,8).

WOUND CARE

The nurse practitioner with advanced training in wound management is an instrumental member of the pediatric surgery team. The APN is frequently consulted by other departments for guidance regarding skin management and wound healing. Fortunately, most postoperative pediatric patients are in good health and have wounds that heal by primary intention. Approximately 2 to 4 weeks before surgery, the child and family meet and discuss the care of the surgical wound with the APN. This discussion addresses dressing changes, suture removal, home nursing visits, bathing, swimming, sports, physical education, and extra-curricular activities. Incisional pain is also discussed, along with specific pain relief interventions. Postoperative pain is an important preoperative discussion topic; parents and children want to be actively involved in pain management strategies. At this time, the APN submits to the case manager any requests for home care or rehabilitative services. This early communication between the APN and discharge coordinator assists in avoidance of delay in discharge from the hospital. At discharge, patients/families are given the following set of instructions for routine postoperative wound care:

- Avoid alcohol, iodine, and peroxide, which are cytotoxic and may prevent wound healing.
- Cleanse incisions with soap and water after 48 hours.
- Apply dry gauze dressing and paper tape if there is drainage or friction from clothing; otherwise leave the suture line open to air.
- Leave steri-adhesive strips in place; these usually fall off after 1 to 2 weeks.
- Avoid creams and ointments.
- Avoid prolonged soaking or swimming while strips are still in place.
- Notify the APN immediately if there are signs of infection such as fever, purulent drainage, redness, or tenderness at incision (9).

Parents frequently call concerned that their child has a wound infection. Since the majority of postoperative wounds in pediatric patients heal without infection or delay, wounds require antibiotic treatment only if two or more of the above noted signs and symptoms of infection are present. The APN triages these concerns from parents. The APN assesses and plans the timing of a visit to the surgery practice.

The APN is the consultant for management of wounds that heal by secondary intention and for the occasional chronic wound. These wounds are often seen in children with systemic illness (sepsis, cardiac failure, and cancers). The APN recommends strategies for the management of excessive exudates, maceration of skin around the wound bed, and cost-effective choice of dressing materials (10). The APN collaborates with the bedside nursing staff in the assessment and routine care of complicated wounds. The nurses' observations of changes in the patient condition allow for early intervention and correction of problems, avoiding complications. Educational offerings to the nursing staff improve their ability to assess pediatric skin and wounds. The APN encourages the family to become involved in wound care early on in the child's postoperative course. This early involvement of the family aids in early discharge of the patient to home and provides the family and child with a sense of responsibility and control over the child's care. The APN identifies a family member to be responsible for home care of the complicated wound and ensures the appropriate patient education. Once discharged home, the APN follows the child with a complicated wound through frequent phone discussions and follow-up visits (11).

The APN is responsible for coordinating the home management of the pediatric surgery patient with a wound. Ideally, the wound care at home should be designed to be as simple as possible while embracing the principles of wound care. The APN makes recommendations for wound dressings that can be changed as frequently as once a day or as infrequently as once a week. The use of modern wound dressings that keep the wound bed warm and moist and require minimal dressing changes is encouraged (10). Less frequent dressing changes reduce procedural stress and pain. This schedule is also much easier for a busy parent to manage at home.

PRESSURE ULCERS

The Braden Q Scale for pediatric assessment of risk for pressure ulcer development is an easy scale to use. This tool incorporates mobility, neuro-sensory perception, friction/sheer forces, nutrition, and tissue perfusion issues into a succinct scale for the bedside practitioner. The tool is frequently incorporated into daily nursing flow sheets. The "Q" scale is the appropriate tool for the child less than 5 years old. The adult Braden scale can be used for children older than 5 years. The APN collaborates with the nurse at the bedside to complete the scale, and uses scores to guide decisions regarding appropriate pressure relieving devices/beds. The nurse practitioner is able to make cost-effective decisions and ensure quality patient care through the use of the Braden scales (12).

Pressure ulcers are frequently treated on an outpatient basis in the pediatric population. The primary risk factors for pressure ulcer development in children are paralysis, insensate areas, high activity, and immobility. Pressure ulcers occur most frequently in the lower extremities or feet. The wheelchair-dependent child is more likely to develop pressure ulcers in the sacral areas (13). Education and prevention of pressure ulcers is emphasized. The APN reinforces strategies to reduce pressure on sacral areas while in the wheelchair and the need to do "push ups" every hour to relieve pressure on the sacral area. Parents are taught how to assess the skin for early signs of pressure ulcer development and initial home treatment as well as which specific areas are at high risk for pressure ulcer development. The APN collaborates with the physical therapist or occupational therapist to ensure proper fitting orthotics that do not cause skin breakdown. Assessment of the wound for infection, stage of development, undermining, tunneling, and slough occurs at each visit. Best practice recommendations for wound care include moist, warm wound healing environments. The APN chooses dressings that are easy to use and cost effective. Referrals for home nursing visits complete the process by promoting ongoing wound assessments, family education, and compliance to the treatment plan (13).

STOMAS

The APN plays a crucial role in collaborating and managing the preoperative, operative, and postoperative care of a pediatric surgical patient. The surgical placement and management of the various types of stomas (colostomy, ileostomy, gastrostomy, cecostomy or jejunostomy) involve a preoperative discussion between the surgeon, nurse practitioner, patient, and family.

While great advances have occurred regarding stoma formation and management, both early and late complications are common. Many surgical practices have found reduced complications when a team approach occurs between the surgeon, APN, patient, and family. This requires an understanding of enterostomal construction and physiology to prevent and treat complications.

Many potential complications may occur in the placement of a stoma. The role of the APN in the reduction and management of complications should focus on all aspects of surgical therapy. Collaboration of care among the surgical team, family, patient, and nursing staff includes education and counseling throughout the surgical course including follow-up care.

PREOPERATIVE COURSE

The creation of a stoma occurs both on an elective and on emergent basis. It is imperative to initiate a collaborative plan in either case. The surgeon and APN counsel and educate the family. This eases anxiety and facilitates postoperative management. Education includes a clear and concise definition of a stoma, identification of potential postoperative complications, and review of the plan of care including stoma management.

Selection and marking of a potential stoma site should take place preoperatively whenever feasible. Upon marking a site selection, careful consideration is made in regards to patient positioning, size, skin folds, beltline, and bony prominences. When use of an ostomy pouch is necessary, measurements should be made to ensure a good fit and seal of the appliance. When ostomies require tubes, patient accessibility should be considered. For example, in a patient undergoing placement of a cecostomy, the stoma and device should be placed above the beltline avoiding skin folds and be visible to the patient for easy access.

INTRAOPERATIVE COURSE

When creating a stoma, the surgeon should consider potential postoperative complications associated with stoma location. The surgeon may place a stoma within the laparotomy incision if time is of the essence. However, multiple disadvantages exist when a stoma is placed within the incision including the risk of wound infection, dehiscence, evisceration, and difficulty with stoma pouching. The ideal location of a stoma is away from the incision with enough skin exposure to create full contact with a proper fitting flange.

POSTOPERATIVE COURSE

The APN is to be involved immediately postoperatively to assist in stoma management and to initiate patient and family teaching. Stoma care instructions are individualized and visible at each patient's bedside. This allows for consistent management and reduces the potential for complications and confusion.

FOLLOW-UP MANAGEMENT

Follow-up care consists of patient and family education about stoma care and the recognition and management of complications. Some of the most common stoma complications include altered body image, skin irritation, wound infection, and appliance malfunctions.

Skin irritation is common when managing a pediatric stoma. Improper location of the stoma, poor stoma care, lack of education, and improper appliance usage lead to skin breakdown. Various skin care products are available. A skin care consult initiated postoperatively prevents and manages skin breakdown.

Patient, family, and staff education is the key to effective postoperative stoma management. Telephone triage and outpatient visits offered by the APN can manage complications. This allows for consistent patient management and increased patient satisfaction.

GASTROSTOMY TUBES

The APN is the expert in the management of gastrostomy tubes and complications. The APN is adept at identifying common complications related to gastrostomy tube feedings such as skin breakdown, stoma fit, granulation tissue, feeding intolerance, and tube dislodgement. The APN possesses skills to educate families in the recognition and management of these complications and to foster independence in the child's gastrostomy care. The APN accomplishes this through frequent teaching sessions with families (14). Written information is provided preoperatively. The family is encouraged to manipulate G-tubes preoperatively and to view gastrostomy teaching videos. Teaching continues postoperatively. Self-care principles promote independence and autonomy of the families and the child. New skills are introduced slowly based on each family's needs. Parents are given the direct line to the nurse practitioner so that assistance and encouragement is readily available once discharged home. The APN coordinates postoperative follow-up around the family's schedule of appointments with other specialists within the tertiary care facility. Families of children with complex health care needs appreciate this respect of their time.

Potential complications seen in the postoperative Nissen fundoplication patient are gas bloat, persistence of gastroesophageal reflux disease (GERD), and feeding intolerance (15). The APN teaches parents to cue into their child's physical examination. Thorough parental teaching about signs and symptoms of distress ensures accuracy and allows the APN to partner with parents and facilitates parental autonomy. Together the APN and family solve feeding, skin care, or mechanical troubleshooting issues. Families are taught signs and symptoms of gas bloat and remedies to vent the gastrostomy device and/or administer feeds more slowly, or the use of a Farrell valve during continuous feeds. Peristomal skin care and granulation prevention are highlighted. Parents are encouraged to change the gastrostomy device after the APN has demonstrated and offers encouragement and feedback. Family-centered care allows parents to provide their child's care and be true partners with the health care team. Parents who are actively involved in their child's routine care are more likely to cope and feel less uncertainty and loss of control (16).

JEJUNOSTOMY TUBES

Surgically placed jejunostomy tubes are useful for children who are unable to tolerate gastric feeds. Feedings are administered continuously to avoid "dumping" syndrome, requiring care-givers to be adept in the use of home feeding pumps. The APN collaborates with the discharge planner to order appropriate equipment for home use once the child is discharged from the hospital. Families are given information about dumping syndrome, diarrhea management, and perineal care. Once home, the APN manages the child with a jejunostomy tube. Families are encouraged to cleanse the skin around the tube with soap and water. Granulation tissue occurs rarely at jejunostomy sites, and skin care is simple. The importance of keeping the tube secure is reinforced (17).

TRACHEOSTOMY TUBES

Infants and children with airway problems requiring tracheostomy present unique challenges to the clinicians involved in their care. Tracheostomy placement and vigilant airway management keep the child healthy and prevents complications. The APN contributes to the continuum of care throughout the hospitalization and after discharge to ensure a safe and healthy airway for as long as the child has the tracheostomy.

The APN teaches patients, family, nurses, physicians, and other team members about tracheostomy care and the prevention, early identification, and treatment of complications. The APN is the patient and family advocate and she/he coordinates the necessary resources for a safe transition from hospital to home.

Once a tracheostomy is planned, the nurse practitioner meets with the family members to help them understand the benefits of the tracheostomy and its effects on the child's life. She/he provides them with written teaching materials. Postoperatively, the nurse practitioner continues to monitor the family's educational progress to ensure safe tracheostomy care. As appropriate skills and concepts are acquired by the family, the nurse practitioner coordinates resources needed in the home-care setting, including durable medical equipment and skilled nursing agencies.

Discharge care is coordinated by the nurse practitioner and the attending surgeon. The nurse practitioner continues to foster the relationship with the family through regularly sched-uled follow-up visits to reinforce and evaluate tracheostomy care and assess their coping skills. These visits also ensure that the home-care agency and nursing agency are providing services to maintain a safe environment for the child.

Tracheostomy complications include tube obstruction, accidental decannulation, tracheal infection, and stoma problems. The APN's role to prevent complications begins by providing families with the ability to assess the status of their child's tracheotomy and to provide the appropriate care. The ability to accurately assess the child's respiratory status and proper techniques in suctioning reduces the most serious complications such as tracheal tube plugging and accidental decannulation. Families are taught to assess and provide adequate hydration as well as provide humidification to minimize mucous plugging of the tracheostomy tube.

Accidental decannulation occurs if the tracheostomy tube is not secured with the tra-cheostomy tie. By thorough and effective teaching, the APN assures that parents are skilled in securing the tube and appropriately evaluating the tracheostomy tie tension, so that when the child's neck is flexed, the parent can fit only one finger comfortably between the tracheostomy tie and the child's neck. The tie is secured with a square knot.

Families are taught to care for their child's tracheostomy stoma. The daily use of 1% Hytone® and Lotrimin® prevents skin breakdown and fungal overgrowth. Early treatment of stoma infections and the use of antifungal/antibacterial powder effectively manage peristomal skin complications.

Ongoing evaluation and treatment of speech and language needs are critical for children with tracheostomies. Engaging a speech/language pathologist to address the child's communication needs and promote feeding and swallowing is necessary.

The APN's ongoing coordination of multidisciplinary care ensures that the child receives all necessary support to promote normal growth and development.

CONCLUSION

APNs possess the education and skills to direct care, decreasing complications and errors in the pediatric surgical patient. With advanced knowledge of nursing and hospital protocols, they pay close attention to patient care, concerns, education, and overall safety. Families express ease in discussing concerns with the APN. The staff nurses, parents, and patients know the APN is readily available, and rounding often to assess the patient's condition and family needs and concerns. This patient-focused, time-sensitive care promotes early intervention when a problem arises, thus meeting safety goals and decreasing complications. Their broad nursing and medical education provides a holistic approach to optimal health care delivery.

REFERENCES

1. Wise BV, McKenna C, Garvin G, et al. Nursing Care of the General Pediatric Surgical Patient. Gaithersburg, MD: Aspen Publications, 2000.
2. Torowicz DL. Maximizing services along the continuum of care from inpatient to home. Sem Nurse Manag 2000; 8(1):16–19.
3. Smith L, Daugherty H. Weaving the seamless web of care: An analysis of parents' perceptions of their needs following discharge of their child from the hospital. J Adv Nurs 2000; 31(4):12–20.
4. Lundblad B, Byrne MW, Hellstrom AL. Continuing nursing care needs of children at time of discharge from one regional medical center in Sweden. J Pediatr Nurs 2001; 16(1):73–78.
5. Burnweit C, Diana-Zerpa JA, Nahmad MH, et al. Nitrous oxide analgesia for minor pediatric surgical procedures: An effective alternative to conscious sedation. J Pediatr Surg 2000; 39(3):495–499.
6. Leprohon J, Patel VL. Decision making strategies for telephone triage in emergency medical services. Med Decis Making 2005; 15(3):250–253.
7. Wheele SQ, Siebelt B. Calling all nurses-how to perform telephone triage. Nursing 1997; 27(7):37–41.
8. Alexander M. Two important lessons: Caution with telephone triage and believing the caregiver. J Emerg Nurs 1996; 22(2):149–150.
9. Wound Care Education Institute. Skin and wound management course. 2003.
10. Cameron J. Exudate and care of the peri-wound skin. Nurs Stand 2004; 19:62–66.
11. Lindeke LL, Karajicek M, Patterson DL. PNP roles and interventions with children with special needs and their families. J Pediatr Health Care 2001; 15:138–143.
12. Curley M, Razmus I, Roberts K. Predicting pressure ulcer risk in pediatric patients: The Braden Q scale. Nurs Res 2003; 52:22–23.
13. Samiengo I. A sore spot in pediatrics: Risk factors for pressure ulcers. Pediatr Nurs 2003; 29:278–282.
14. London F. How to prepare families for discharge in the limited time available. Pediatr Nurs 2004; 3:212–214.
15. Orenstein S, Dilorenzo C. Post fundoplication complications in children. Curr Treat Opt Gastro 2001; 4:441–449.
16. Dudley S, Carr J. Vigilance: The experience of parents staying at the bedside of hospitalized children. J Pediatr Nurs 2004; 19:267–275.
17. Vanderhoof J, Young R. Enteral nutrition in short bowel syndrome. Sem Pediatr Surg 2001; 10:65–71.

5 | Virtual Reality and Simulation: Reducing Complications Through Emerging Technology

Venita Chandra, M.D. and Sanjeev Dutta, M.D., M.A.

INTRODUCTION

There is an old surgical saying that there is no such thing as a postoperative complication. The implication is that complications arising after an operation have their origins in errors committed during the operation. While not the entire truth, this wisdom draws attention to the idea that preventing intraoperative surgical errors can improve patient outcomes. Historically, surgeons looked to their errors as a source of learning through such activities as "morbidity and mortality conference." Similarly, surgical trainees were thrown into a "trial by fire" environment in which they also learned from their mistakes. Unfortunately, in all instances the errors through which this learning occurred had already resulted in adverse patient outcomes.

The spotlight on medical errors came to a focus in 1999 with the Institute of Medicine's publication of *To Err is Human* (1) which brought to public attention the nearly 100,000 American deaths that result from medical error yearly. Surgery, with its procedure-rich environment, complex team interactions, and dependency on advanced technologies, is highly susceptible to sequential errors that may culminate in an adverse event. It is no wonder, then, that surgeons are in the spotlight for error analysis, and greater focus is being placed on identifying methods by which error in the operating room can be avoided.

Much of our understanding of error, particularly in complex team situations, comes from the aviation industry. Concepts such as preoperative checklists find their origin here. Aviation places great emphasis on effective communication and leadership within crisis situations. While these concepts seem almost common sense for prevention of error, the difficulty remains as to how these processes can be taught to the surgical team.

Role playing is recognized as a powerful training tool. The addition of a realistic environment and carefully constructed scenario to induce a "suspension of disbelief" comprises a *simulation*. Recognized in other "high-risk" industries as an important adjunct to professional skills, teamwork, and safety training, simulation nonetheless has yet to be widely adopted in the field of surgery. Tradition dictates that bedside observation and graduated involvement in operative cases is adequate preparation for even technically challenging procedures. Thus, it remains an open question as to what extent a simulated environment should be used in a surgeon's training.

This chapter discusses the major factors believed to contribute to surgical error and how advances in medical simulation, including the use of virtual reality, may be used to reduce surgical error and potentially improve patient outcomes.

UNDERSTANDING SURGICAL ERROR

The Institute of Medicine's report sparked a flurry of publications in both the medical literature and the popular press, many of which emphasized the "systemic" nature of medical error; i.e., that error is not always the fault of a single individual, but rather arises from several contributing factors originating at many levels of the health care system (2–7).

Although clearly an important aspect of error, this "systems model" of medical error, according to thought leader James Reason, may not be the end of the story (3). In surgical cases and other interventional procedures, often a specific action is in and of itself the error. Termed "coal-face" error, an example would be the inadvertent transection of the ureter during a bowel resection (8,9). Although associated factors such as fogged glasses, team miscommunication, or equipment malfunction may contribute, it is difficult to overlook that the surgeon performed the error, and thus must bear at least some responsibility (9,10).

Cognitive skill, technical skill, and surgical judgment are three components identified as targets for combating coal-face surgical error. The development of cognitive skill mainly involves acquiring medical knowledge, learning the steps of procedures, and gaining spatial familiarity with the relevant anatomy (11). Technical skill requires the development of psychomotor competencies and muscle memory (11,12). Overall surgical competence, however, requires good judgment and the ability of a surgeon to assess situations and make sound conclusions, such as when to convert a laparoscopic procedure to an open one (8,13,14).

Using technology to simulate real operative conditions may allow us to teach and refine each of these vital components and thus minimize the incidence of coal-face error. Taken to the next level, integrated simulations involving multiple individuals may be used to address the complex systems-level errors which ultimately contribute to poor patient outcomes.

SIMULATION AND SIMULATORS, AND VIRTUAL REALITY

While the terms simulator and simulation are often used interchangeably, it is important to clarify the difference between them. *Simulators* are the physical objects or representations of the task to be replicated; i.e., the "tools." *Simulation* is a technique involving the application of simulators to re-create aspects of the real world, typically to replace or amplify actual experiences for education or training (15–17). A common assumption is that simulators or simulations are always coupled with a computer, but this is not a requirement. Simulators can range from low-fidelity role-playing exercises, to part-task trainers to complex high-fidelity simulations. A simulator might be something as basic and inexpensive as the back of a chair on which a suture tie can be looped to practice knot-tying, to something complex and costly, such as the mannequin-based patient simulator, a computer-controlled body form from which one may elicit several interesting physiologic and motor responses, or which can support certain technical skills such as direct laryngoscopy and endotracheal intubation. A proper simulation involves not only a simulator, but also an environment that places the simulator in a wider cognitive and circumstantial context through careful re-creation of real-world scenarios. Although the simulator may train a particular technical skill, the simulation teaches deeper thought processes (e.g., judgments) that account for the context in which the technical skill is being performed.

In most cases, the word simulator in the current surgical literature has come to mean technologically intensive computer-generated interactive virtual reality environments (VR-Sims). A VR-Sim is composed of a high-fidelity computer-generated graphical representation of a real-life scenario and an interface that mimics real-life instruments (18). The interface typically allows for interaction with the graphical environment using pressure/force feedback (haptics), and the computer is able to generate an objective set of metrics that assesses performance on the simulator. The ultimate goal of VR-Sims is to achieve an immersive, interactive state that engages the learner to behave as they would in the equivalent real-life situation. Various forms of VR-Sims are already used to facilitate training for aviation, heavy machinery operation, and space and military operations. Surgery is an excellent focus for VR-Sim technology, because the discipline represents a high-stakes environment in which discrete measurements of performance can be made.

BACKGROUND AND HISTORY OF SIMULATORS

Simulation was used as early as 1910 to train both individuals and teams to reduce errors and improve safety. For many years, industries where errors carry a high cost such as commercial aviation and nuclear power have used simulated environments to successfully reduce accidents and improve safety (19–22). The replication and modeling of real-life situations offer participants a chance to practice skills and techniques in a realistic and safe environment, consistently and repetitively, with objective and quantifiable performance assessment.

In the field of aviation, pilots of both military and commercial planes must achieve a certain level of proficiency in simulators before they fly a particular aircraft. The airline industry has achieved an impressive safety record through a process of standardized education, repetitive practice, and simulator-based proficiency testing. In fact, the industry has seen a nearly 50%

reduction in the rate of human error-related airline crashes since the 1970s, for which they credit virtual reality-based education as a major contributor (23,24).

The first medical simulator was developed by Asmund Laerdal in the early 1960s. Resusci® Anne (Laerdal Medical Corporation©) was a part-task model trainer consisting of a mannequin designed to train mouth to mouth ventilation (25,26). Soon after, Abrahamson and Denson (27) produced SimOne, the first computer-controlled mannequin simulator for anesthesia training. Far ahead of its time, SimOne garnered immediate attention but failed to gain widespread acceptance due to its complexity and cost. Nonetheless, this achievement marked the beginning of computer-based simulators in medicine. Twenty years later, a group from Stanford University School of Medicine led by David M. Gaba (28) continued this effort by capitalizing on the rapid advancement in computing ability. Their system, called the comprehensive anesthesia simulation environment (CASE), involved a "hands-on" simulator that re-created the operating room environment, including manual and cognitive tasks of anesthesia administration, patient monitoring, and intervention. The efforts of these early leaders were instrumental in the advance of increasingly sophisticated simulators and simulation. As a result, medical and surgical educators today have access to an ever-growing selection of simulation tools (25).

Despite advances in technology, however, simulation will never completely replace interaction with real patients, and proponents of simulation do not view this as a desirable goal. Medicine is intrinsically more complex and requires more human empathy than do other high-risk professions. Nonetheless, applying the technology and methods that have proven effective in aircraft pilot training may significantly improve surgical procedure training and have a positive effect on patient outcomes.

CLASSIFICATION OF SIMULATORS

Surgical simulators can be classified into those that are based on physical models, those that involve computer-generated environments, and those that combine both of these approaches (hybrids). It is important to note, however, that materials as simple as a pig's foot from the butcher to practice suturing, or rubber tubing to mimic bowel, are in fact simulators that can be useful in surgical training.

Model-Based Simulators

Model-based simulators use physical representations of a body part for the purposes of training. Sophisticated advances in materials technology have allowed dramatic improvement in the realism of physical simulation, allowing many human tissues to be realistically replicated. Model-based simulators allow the learner to focus on an isolated task, and thus are useful in the development of specific technical, procedural, or psychomotor skills. Procedures commonly taught in this way include urinary catheterization, central line placement, and wound closure (11,25,29). Models of surgical procedures also exist for relatively simple operations such as removal of cysts, diagnostic peritoneal lavage, and appendectomies. In addition, some simple simulators are used for honing laparoscopic skills often termed "box-trainers"; cardboard or plastic boxes with ports for the insertion of endoscopic tools. These self-contained, occasionally video-based simulators are relatively inexpensive and highly versatile tools that enable the training of basic laparoscopic techniques such as grasping and knot tying on inanimate models.

Although model-based trainers have the advantages of being relatively inexpensive and simple to use, they do have limitations. By simulating only isolated parts of the body, a complete illusion of reality is not possible, thus the very important aspect of context in which the procedure would actually be performed is lost. Moreover, they are unable to give feedback or provide objective measures of performance, both important parameters for effective learning. In order to be used successfully, they require extensive support from expert tutors.

Computer-Based Simulation

Computer technology has the potential to deal with many of the limitations of model-based trainers. As a result, a growing number of medical simulators are computer-based. These systems provide three-dimensional (3D)-rendered images of anatomy for practice of surgical tasks (30). The computer interface enables immediate error feedback along with the capability of presenting a range of pathologies and varying degrees of difficulty, to augment learning. In addition, they are often capable of motion tracking, which can be used to objectively assess technical skill and competence (31,32)

VR-Sims, originally developed at NASA in the early 1990s, have emerged as a powerful adjunct to technology in health care and now have applications in many branches of medicine (11,33,34). VR-Sims provide more realistic representations of organ systems as compared to traditional computer graphics, combined with the means to interact with these images (35,36). Such interaction can include manipulating, slicing, cutting, and "flying through" systems of the body. As such, VR-Sims have had a significant impact in improving the realism of surgical simulators.

As a general rule, the more complex a simulated procedure, the greater the computing power it requires. Until recently, most computer-based simulations were found only in specialist research institutions to accommodate the enormous computing power that is necessary. In the last few years, however, advances in computer technology have dramatically changed the simulation industry, even bringing highly sophisticated programs within the reach of desktop computers (37).

Computer-based simulators today can be used to practice a wide range of procedures. These include simple precision-based tasks such as lumbar punctures (18,38,39), more complex tasks such as suturing, ultrasound, basic minimally invasive techniques such as instrument navigation, and tissue grasping (40–45), endoscopic procedures (45–48) and simulations of full surgical procedures including laparoscopic cholecystectomies, various ENT procedures, and management of limb trauma (49–60). These simulations, however, are limited in their realism (61). Surgical dissection, while "second nature" to surgeons, is difficult to program into a computer system. Accurately simulating deformable tissues and providing tactile feedback to augment VR images have high computational costs (62,63). While some completely virtual interactive scenarios have been produced (18,64), significant development still needs to occur before these are used in a day-to-day environment.

Hybrid Simulation

As the name implies, hybrid simulators are a combination of computer-generated displays that provide visual feedback with authentic interfaces such as actual endoscopes or laparoscopic instruments. One sophisticated example of a hybrid simulator is the previously mentioned CASE system developed by Gaba and colleagues (28,65). This system reproduces a realistic operating room environment by combining a high-tech mannequin with a computer program. The computer interface regulates the mannequin's responses to manipulation of physiological variables, including vital signs, breath sounds, pupil size, etc. In addition, a variety of procedures can be performed on the mannequins such as chest-tube insertion, arterial or venous line placements, and intubation. Although full surgical procedures cannot be done, these systems provide operating room teams with entire clinical scenarios that allow practice of crisis management, and help us to better understand the nature of communication and leadership in an operating room environment. The next evolution of hybrid simulators will allow a surgical trainee to perform a simulated procedure within a mannequin that gives an appropriate physiologic response, and requires response from an anesthesiologist trainee. Such a simulator will allow a contextually rich assessment of teamwork ability.

HOW SIMULATION TECHNOLOGIES CAN HELP REDUCE ERROR

Simulators provide the means to improve competence and performance in a variety of domains including clinical skills, technical skills, teamwork, patient management, and decision-making (judgment), all in a safe environment free from risk to the patient (16,66). They have the advantage of being consistent, repeatable, quantifiable, precise, available, and objective. The Joint Commission on Accreditation of Health care Organizations (JCAHO) has recognized these advantages and has concluded that the health care community can gain from the use of simulation-based training to reduce errors and improve patient safety when designed and delivered appropriately, and has developed guidelines for doing so (19). Simulators are playing an increasingly important role in education and training, preoperative planning, and, on an experimental basis, in an intraoperative environment.

Surgical Trainee Education

Historically, surgical education has been based on an apprenticeship model, introduced at the turn of the century by Halsted (67). Residents gain experience through supervised training on patients, taking incrementally more active roles in patient care or the operative procedure as their experience increases. Error and risk to patients are inherent in this traditional method of education, and there is significant variability of education as teaching is based on random opportunity of patient flow (18). Despite potential flaws, this model has successfully trained generations of surgeons throughout the world.

Recently, this traditional method of training has been challenged by a number of factors. There has been significant development of new technologies such as laparoscopic and robot-assisted surgery. These techniques require novel and unique motor skills that are quite different from those needed to perform open surgical procedures. In addition, regulations restricting resident work hours, the growing variety of surgical procedures being performed, and the increasing costs of operating room time all raise concerns about the ability to provide adequate direct clinical experience for the acquisition of such skills.

In light of these challenges to surgical education, the case has been made to use simulators as an alternative and complementary method of clinical exposure and skills acquisition (68). Surgical simulators have a number of advantages as compared to traditional training. They have the capacity to provide task repetition, graduated increases in task complexity, and immediate performance feedback, factors known to both improve the quality of practice and also reduce the quantity of practice required to obtain expertise in a specific area (12,69). Proper training agendas can be determined based on the specific needs and learning styles of the trainees, allowing them to focus on whole procedures or specific components and practice these as often as necessary. In addition, some simulators contain built-in tracking functions to map a learner's trajectory in detail, facilitating objective evaluation of performance and ability (32).

The greatest advantage of simulation is that, unlike the traditional paradigm of learning by operating on real patients, it separates practice from performance. Learning on simulators allows participants to fail at tasks without consequence. The trainee can reflect on the failure and restart the procedure with carefully determined changes in approach as many times as they want. Most importantly, there is no unrealistic pressure to perform at a high level from the outset, and no risk to the patient. There is considerable evidence demonstrating the benefit of this type of experiential learning (20,22,30). Simulators allow trainees to practice extensively and often climb the steepest part of a procedure's learning curve prior to touching a patient. At the least, simulator training will acquaint the trainee with the general materials and workflow of a procedure so as to later avoid problems with inefficiency when working with real patients.

Experienced Physician Education

Simulation supports lifelong learning and is applicable to physicians throughout their careers. For example, simulators can be used to maintain or refresh skills for procedures that are not often performed (16). Perhaps one of the most valuable benefits of surgical simulation, however, is the ability to train and teach new techniques to established surgeons. With the growing number of new and more complex procedures, there is a greater demand on the surgeon to achieve ever-increasing levels of proficiency and efficiency. Currently, there is substantial interest in how physician experience is related to surgical error (7,70,71). There is strong evidence to suggest that a surgeon must perform a certain volume of cases to ensure adequate patient outcome (72–75). Simulators give established physicians, as they do residents and students, a safe environment to practice new techniques and achieve the repetition of cases that allows progress along the early learning curve of a procedure prior to performing it on a real patient.

Competency-Based Curriculum

Another feature enabled by simulation is that training can be performed not just for a fixed duration or number of cases, but rather to specific criterion levels of competency for key aspects of knowledge, skill, and behavior (16,76–79). Objective measurements of performance can be analyzed, and once properly validated may be able to provide precise quantification of skills. This process of skills assessment is the basis of aviation training and licensure (33). With the increased attention to surgical error and the challenges faced by traditional training, there is increasing pressure to adapt a competency-based curriculum, in which trainees are expected to demonstrate a certain level of measured skill before being allowed to operate on a patient.

It is important to recognize that simulators are merely tools used to enhance training, and alone will not lead to improved patient safety. To be effective, simulation-based training must be implemented appropriately within a comprehensive curriculum based on proven principles of learning and an understanding of training needs and requirements. Simulation must become a standard part of these curricula along with performance measurement and feedback (19).

Crisis Resource Management Training

While specific task and procedural simulators provide training in both the cognitive and technical skills required to minimize coal-face error, integrated whole patient simulations can be used to improve crisis management skills. Crew Resource Management (CRM) training involves simulation-based training of teams during crisis situations, a technique used often in the aviation industry that is now being incorporated into medical and surgical training. A variety of scenarios can be designed depending on a hospital's training needs. The simulated patient settings can be programmed to react to treatment in numerous ways, based on the age, gender, and medical conditions the scenario is meant to represent, thus creating complete clinical episodes from "average" to "worst-case" scenarios. Several team members participate in the simulations concurrently, and their performance can be viewed and analyzed by both instructors and participants. The emphasis of CRM training is not only on technical skills, but also on team skills such as communication, vigilance, and decision making. Such skills are associated with increased patient safety by minimizing systems errors in the operating room as well as in other medical environments (80).

Overall, complete surgical curricula addressing both coal-face and systems errors can enhance medical professionals' understanding of the nature and causes of mistakes, and allow them to adopt ways to lessen and cope with mistakes to improve performance and reduce error (79). The Stanford Department of Surgery's Goodman Simulation Center aims to bring together multiple disciplines and combine modalities to develop simulator systems designed to address these different elements of surgical error.

Preoperative Planning and Diagnostics

In addition to its role in education and training, simulation is being used to reduce the likelihood of error in the operating room by augmenting preoperative planning and diagnosis. Surgeons or an entire operative team can use accurate recreations of individual patients' anatomy from high-resolution imaging data (e.g., CT scan and MRI) to rehearse patient-specific operations within a virtual environment (16,18,81,82). VR techniques are used to assemble patient-specific graphical data into "before and after" images, which can be manipulated by the surgeon before the operation so that they may predict the outcome of a case. This form of preoperative planning speeds up intraoperative decision making, and potentially improves outcomes by providing the surgeon with a preplanned outline of the procedure.

Simulation-based preoperative planning has been described by a growing number of surgical disciplines, particularly in the fields of neurosurgery (83,84), orthopedic, maxillofacial, pediatric, and general surgery (85–90). Three-dimensional imaging reconstructions have proven particularly useful in planning stereotactic and minimally invasive neurosurgical procedures, as well as increasing the understanding of complex anatomical relationships for skull base surgery and congenital skeletal anomaly repairs (91–94). Modeling of deformable facial tissues has enabled tissue changes and postoperative outcomes of craniofacial surgery to be simulated (95). Another soft tissue application of these techniques is in planning liver resections. Virtual tumor resection allows the surgeon to identify the optimal resection margins within the organ parenchyma, delineate areas at risk of insufficient blood supply or blood drainage as well as estimate the organ function postoperatively (96,97).

VR has been described recently for use in preoperative diagnostics. CT and MRI data can be rendered to permit visualization of an organ of interest in a "fly-through" path, where manipulation of the data allows perspective and angles of view that cannot be obtained with standard physical techniques such as endoscopy (98). Current applications include virtual gastroscopy, colonoscopy, and bronchoscopy (99–102). While these techniques have significant potential, they are still in the early phases of development.

Intraoperative Applications

VR and simulation applications may also reduce errors in the intraoperative arena. An example of this is "augmented reality," which involves superimposing computer-generated virtual images onto real ones to aid with intraoperative navigation. This technique has been used for fighter pilots, and has recently been proposed for use in the operating room (18,39,83,85,103). One example is a program that aids facial surgeons by allowing them to see the internal anatomic structures superimposed on the surface anatomy. In effect, this allows the surgeon to see through the patient's skin (104). Such applications require enormous amounts of computer processing power and thus currently are only run on expensive graphics workstations. Any lag in rendering can result in misinterpretation of the provided data with potentially disastrous outcome (18). In addition, delayed rendering has been linked to motion sickness in some users (105). Intraoperative applications are sill in their infancy, but hold great potential for the future.

HOW EFFECTIVE IS SIMULATION IN REDUCING ERROR?

Over the past three decades, simulators and simulation of various modalities have been used in a growing number of surgical fields (22,106–108), and the body of published literature evaluating their impact has increased considerably. Basic laparoscopic skills training on simulators have been shown in a number of studies to transfer to the operating room (109–111). Seymour and colleagues (110) were the first to report a randomized controlled trial validating the role of a virtual reality simulator for the training of surgical residents by demonstrating significantly improved performance in the operating room compared to the control group. Residents who trained on the Minimally Invasive Surgical Trainer-Virtual Reality (MIST-VR) system (Mentice Medical Simulation, Gothenberg, Sweden), made fewer errors in the operating room and were more likely to make steady progress throughout the procedure (110).

Haque and Srinivasan (112) supported these claims in their meta-analysis demonstrating shorter training times and fewer errors in specific surgical tasks after VR simulator training (112). However, a more recent review of randomized control trials by Sutherland and colleagues (113) comparing the effectiveness of various types of surgical simulators to other more traditional training modalities did not show such positive results. While they did see some evidence that those trained on simulators performed better than those without any training, they did not find substantial evidence showing simulators to be better than any other forms of training. The review proposed a number of possible reasons for failing to see a clear benefit of surgical simulation for training including the generally small sample sizes, multiple and confounding comparisons, and lack of standardization and validation of most of the studies (113).

Clearly the ultimate validation for simulation training is not only to demonstrate improved motor skills, but improved patient outcomes. Unfortunately, there is a paucity of evidence in this area and many obstacles to obtaining definitive proof of such an impact of simulators. Benefits derived from the various applications of simulation are difficult to measure, safety gains in particular are intrinsically difficult to assess. Although some benefits of simulators may be immediately discernible, many probably depend on long-term applications of the technology and curricula. In addition, validation of simulators is particularly difficult because of the often-subjective criteria used to judge changes in performance after simulator practice.

While there is as yet no clear scholarly evidence to support their impact, one should be cautious of discounting the value of simulations in surgery merely for this reason. In fact, the current system of education, training, and maintenance of proficiency has itself never been tested rigorously to determine whether it achieves its stated goals. High-level reviews of the performance of the health care industry even suggest that it does not (1,114). As the airline industry would not dream of letting a pilot on a plane without going through a simulator, so too may simulation be justified among medical trainees for practical and ethical reasons alone. In the words of David M. Gaba "no industry in which human lives depend on the skilled performance of responsible operators has waited for unequivocal proof of the benefits of simulation before embracing it (115)."

CONCLUSIONS

Recognition and understanding of errors is becoming an essential component of the practice of surgery, and new methods and technologies are being used to identify, avoid, and reduce surgical complications. The application of surgical simulators and simulation in education and training provides opportunities to practice surgical skills and procedures, commit errors, and gain experience in a safe environment with no harm to a patient.

Other high-risk professions such as aviation, nuclear power, and the military have long ago instituted simulation-based training to maximize safety and minimize risk. Health care has lagged behind in simulation applications for a number of reasons, including cost, lack of rigorous proof of effect, and cultural resistance to change. If efforts are focused on thoughtful strategies for the development, assessment, and integration of simulators into the surgical community, implementation of these technologies may revolutionize medical education and fundamentally enhance the future practice of surgery.

REFERENCES

1. Kohn K, Corrigan JM, Donaldson MS. To Err Is Human: Building a Safer Health System. Washington, DC: Institute of Medicine, 1999.
2. Turnball JE. All components of the system must be aligned. Health Papers 2001; 2(1):38–43, discussion 86.
3. Reason J. Beyond the organizational accident: the need for "error wisdom" on the frontline. Qual Saf Health Care 2004; 13(Suppl 2):ii28–ii33.
4. Reason JT, Carthey J, de Leval MR. Diagnosing "vulnerable system syndrome": an essential prerequisite to effective risk management. Qual Health Care 2001; 10(Suppl 2):ii21–ii25.
5. Gawande A. When doctors make mistakes. The New Yorker 1999; 1:40–55.
6. Gawande AA, Thomas EJ, Zinner MJ, et al.. The incidence and nature of surgical adverse events in Colorado and Utah in 1992. Surgery 1999; 126(1):66–75.
7. Etchells E, O'Neill C, Bernstein M. Patient safety in surgery: Error detection and prevention. World J Surg 2003; 27(8):936–941; discussion 941.
8. Cuschieri A. Reducing errors in the operating room: Surgical proficiency and quality assurance of execution. Surg Endosc 2005; 19(8):1022–1027.
9. Satava RM. Identification and reduction of surgical error using simulation. Minim Invasive Ther Allied Technol 2005; 14(4):257–261.
10. Way LW, Stewart L, Gantert W, et al. Causes and prevention of laparoscopic bile duct injuries: Analysis of 252 cases from a human factors and cognitive psychology perspective. Ann Surg 2003; 237(4):460–469.
11. Kneebone R. Simulation in surgical training: Educational issues and practical implications. Med Educ 2003; 37(3):267–277.
12. Ericsson KA. Deliberate practice and the acquisition and maintenance of expert performance in medicine and related domains. Acad Med 2004; 79(10 Suppl):S70–S81.
13. Morgenstern L. Achilles' heel and laparoscopic surgery. Surg Endosc 1995; 9(4):383–383.
14. Putcha RV, Burdick JS. Management of iatrogenic perforation. Gastroenterol Clin North Am 2003;32(4):1289–1309.
15. Cooper JB, Taqueti VR. A brief history of the development of mannequin simulators for clinical education and training. Qual Saf Health Care 2004;13(Suppl 1):i11–i18.
16. Gaba DM. The future vision of simulation in health care. Qual Saf Health Care 2004; 13(Suppl 1): i2–10.
17. Dutta S, Gaba D, Krummel TM. To simulate or not to simulate: what is the question? Ann Surg 2006; 243(3):301–303.
18. Meier AH, Rawn CL, Krummel TM. Virtual reality: surgical application—challenge for the new millennium. J Am Coll Surg 2001; 192(3):372–384.
19. Salas E, Wilson KA, Burke CS, et al.. Using simulation-based training to improve patient safety: What does it take? Jt Comm J Qual Patient Saf 2005; 31(7):363–371.
20. Fowlkes JE, Salas E, Baker DP, et al. The utility of event-based knowledge elicitation. Hum Factors 2000; 42(1):24–35.
21. Salas E, Burke CS, Bowers CA, et al. Team training in the skies: Does crew resource management (CRM) training work? Hum Factors 2001; 43(4):641–674.
22. Gorman PJ, Meier AH, Krummel TM. Simulation and virtual reality in surgical education: Real or unreal? Arch Surg 1999; 134(11):1203–1208.

23. Vozenilek J, Huff JS, Reznek M, et al. See one, do one, teach one: Advanced technology in medical education. Acad Emerg Med 2004; 11(11):1149–1154.
24. Levin A. Fewer crashes caused by pilots. USA Today, March 2, 2004.
25. Bradley P. The history of simulation in medical education and possible future directions. Med Educ 2006; 40(3):254–262.
26. Tjomsland N, Laerdal T, Baskett P. Resuscitation great: Bjorn Lind—the ground-breaking nurturer. Resuscitation 2005; 65(2):133–138.
27. Abrahamson S, Denson JS, Wolf RM. Effectiveness of a simulator in training anesthesiology residents. 1969. Quality Saf Health Care 2004; 13(5):395–397.
28. Gaba DM, DeAnda A. A comprehensive anesthesia simulation environment: Re-creating the operating room for research and training. Anesthesiology 1988; 69(3):387–394.
29. Kneebone R, ApSimon D. Surgical skills training: Simulation and multimedia combined. Med Educ 2001; 35(9):909–915.
30. Ackerman MJ. The Visible Human Project: A resource for education. Acad Med 1999; 74(6):667–670.
31. Spitzer VM, Whitlock DG. The Visible Human Dataset: The anatomical platform for human simulation. Anat Rec 1998; 253(2):49–57.
32. Stylopoulos N, Cotin S, Maithel SK, et al. Computer-enhanced laparoscopic training system (CELTS): Bridging the gap. Surg Endosc 2004; 18(5):782–789.
33. Satava RM. Accomplishments and challenges of surgical simulation. Surg Endosc 2001; 15(3):232–241.
34. Ellis S. Nature and origins of virtual environments: A bibliographical essay. Comput Syst Eng 1991; 2:321–347.
35. Satava RM. Surgical education and surgical simulation. World J Surg 2001; 25(11):1484–1489.
36. Delp SL, Loan JP, Hoy MG, et al. An interactive graphics-based model of the lower extremity to study orthopaedic surgical procedures. IEEE Trans Bio-med Eng 1990; 37(8):757–767.
37. Leskovský P, Harders M, Székely G. A web-based repository of surgical simulator projects. Stud Health Technol Inform 2006; 119:311–315.
38. Gorman P, Krummel T, Webster R, et al. A prototype haptic lumbar puncture simulator. Stud Health Technol Inform 2000; 70:106–109.
39. Delaney B. Imaging in medicine—here's looking in you, kid. IEEE Comput Graph Appl 1998; 18:12–19.
40. O'Toole RV, Playter RR, Krummel TM, et al. Measuring and developing suturing technique with a virtual reality surgical simulator. J Am Coll Surg 1999; 189(1):114–127.
41. Taffinder N, Sutton C, Fishwick RJ, et al. Validation of virtual reality to teach and assess psychomotor skills in laparoscopic surgery: results from randomized controlled studies using the MIST VR laparoscopic simulator. Stud Health Technol Inform 1998; 50:124–130.
42. Baur C, Guzzoni D, Georg O. VIRGY: A virtual reality and force feedback based endoscopic surgery simulator. Stud Health Technol Inform 1998; 50:110–116.
43. Meller G. A typology of simulators for medical education. J Digit Imaging 1997; 10(3 Suppl 1):194–196.
44. Meglan DA, Raju R, Merril GL, et al. The teleos virtual environment toolkit for simulation-based surgical education. Stud Health Technol Inform 1996; 29:346–351.
45. Bro-Nielsen M, Tasto JL, Cunningham R, et al. PreOp endoscopic simulator: A PC-based immersive training system for bronchoscopy. Stud Health Technol Inform 1999; 62:76–82.
46. Tasto JL, Verstreken K, Brown JM, et al. PreOp endoscopy simulator: From bronchoscopy to ureteroscopy. Stud Health Technol Inform 2000; 70:344–349.
47. Müller W, Bockholt U. The virtual reality arthroscopy training simulator. Stud Health Technol Inform 1998; 50:13–19.
48. McCarthy AD, Hollands RJ. A commercially viable virtual reality knee arthroscopy training system. Stud Health Technol Inform 1998; 50:302–308.
49. Sinclair MJ, Peifer JW, Haleblian R, et al. Computer-simulated eye surgery. A novel teaching method for residents and practitioners. Ophthalmology 1995; 102(3):517–521.
50. Ecke U, Klimek L, Müller W, et al. Virtual reality: Preparation and execution of sinus surgery. Comput Aided Surg 1998; 3(1):45–50.
51. Edmond CV, Heskamp D, Sluis D, et al. ENT endoscopic surgical training simulator. Stud Health Technol Inform 1997; 39:518–528.
52. Johnston R, Bhoyrul S, Way L, et al. Assessing a virtual reality surgical skills simulator. Stud Health Technol Inform 1996; 29:608–617.
53. Satava RM. Virtual reality surgical simulator. The first steps. Surg Endosc 1993; 7(3):203–205.
54. Schijven MP, Jakimowicz JJ, Broeders IAMJ, Tseng LNL. The Eindhoven laparoscopic cholecystectomy training course-improving operating room performance using virtual reality training: Results from the first E. A.E. S. accredited virtual reality trainings curriculum. Surg Endosc 2005; 19(9):1220–1226.
55. Peugnet F, Dubois P, Rouland JF. Virtual reality versus conventional training in retinal photocoagulation: A first clinical assessment. Comput Aided Surg 1998; 3(1):20–26.

56. Berg D, Raugi G, Gladstone H, et al. Virtual reality simulators for dermatologic surgery: Measuring their validity as a teaching tool. Dermatol Surg 2001; 27(4):370–374.

57. Gladstone HB, Raugi GJ, Berg D, et al. Virtual reality for dermatologic surgery: Virtually a reality in the 21st century. J Am Acad Dermatol 2000; 42(1 Pt 1):106–112.

58. McGovern KT. Applications of virtual reality to surgery. BMJ 1994; 308(6936):1054–1055.

59. Satava RM. Virtual endoscopy: Diagnosis using 3-D visualization and virtual representation. Surg Endosc 1996; 10(2):173–174.

60. Fried MP, Moharir VM, Shinmoto H, et al. Virtual laryngoscopy. Ann Otol Rhinol Laryngol 1999; 108(3):221–226.

61. Lange T, Indelicato DJ, Rosen JM. Virtual reality in surgical training. Surg Oncol Clin N Am 2000; 9(1):61–79, vii.

62. Basdogan C, De S, Kim J, et al. Haptics in minimally invasive surgical simulation and training. IEEE Comput Graph Appl 2004; 24(2):56–64.

63. Basdogan C, Ho CH, Srinivasan MA. Simulation of tissue cutting and bleeding for laparoscopic surgery using auxiliary surfaces. Stud Health Technol Inform 1999; 62:38–44.

64. Bro-Nielsen M, Helfrick D, Glass B, et al. VR simulation of abdominal trauma surgery. Stud Health Technol Inform 1998; 50:117–123.

65. Holzman RS, Cooper JB, Gaba DM, et al. Anesthesia crisis resource management: Real-life simulation training in operating room crises. J Clin Anesth 1995; 7(8):675–687.

66. Ziv A, Ben-David S, Ziv M. Simulation based medical education: An opportunity to learn from errors. Med Teach 2005; 27(3):193–199.

67. Halsted W. The training of the surgeon. Bull Johns Hopkins Hosp 1904; 15:267–276.

68. Gorey TF. Training in minimally invasive therapy and its impact on traditional surgical education. Irish J Med Sci 1997; 166(1):1–2.

69. Guest CB, Regehr G, Tiberius RG. The life long challenge of expertise. Med Educ 2001; 35(1):78–81.

70. Hawes R, Lehman GA, Hast J, et al. Training resident physicians in fiberoptic sigmoidoscopy. How many supervised examinations are required to achieve competence? Am J Med 1986; 80(3):465–470.

71. Mishra A, Agarwal G, Agarwal A, et al. Safety and efficacy of total thyroidectomy in hands of endocrine surgery trainees. Am J Surg 1999; 178(5):377–380.

72. Cowan JA, Dimick JB, Thompson BG, et al. Surgeon volume as an indicator of outcomes after carotid endarterectomy: An effect independent of specialty practice and hospital volume. J Am Coll Surg 2002; 195(6):814–821.

73. Katz JN, Losina E, Barrett J, et al. Association between hospital and surgeon procedure volume and outcomes of total hip replacement in the United States medicare population. J Bone Joint Surg Am 2001; 83-A(11):1622–1629.

74. Cowan JA, Dimick JB, Leveque J-C, et al. The impact of provider volume on mortality after intracranial tumor resection. Neurosurgery Online 2003; 52(1):48–53; discussion 53.

75. Gordon TA, Bowman HM, Bass EB, et al. Complex gastrointestinal surgery: Impact of provider experience on clinical and economic outcomes. J Am Coll Surg 1999; 189(1):46–56.

76. Satava RM, Gallagher AG, Pellegrini CA. Surgical competence and surgical proficiency: definitions, taxonomy, and metrics. J Am Coll Surg 2003; 196(6):933–937.

77. Davis MH, Harden RM. Competency-based assessment: making it a reality. Med Teach 2003; 25(6):565–568.

78. Patil NG, Cheng SWK, Wong J. Surgical competence. World J Surg 2003; 27(8):943–947.

79. Gallagher AG, Ritter EM, Champion H, et al. Virtual reality simulation for the operating room: Proficiency-based training as a paradigm shift in surgical skills training. Ann Surg 2005; 241(2):364–372.

80. Moorthy K, Munz Y, Forrest D, et al. Surgical crisis management skills training and assessment: A simulation[corrected]-based approach to enhancing operating room performance. Ann Surg 2006; 244(1):139–147.

81. Stefanich L, Cruz-Neira C. A virtual surgical simulator for the lower limbs. Biomed Sci Instrum 1999; 35:141–145.

82. Krummel TM. Surgical simulation and virtual reality: The coming revolution. Ann Surg 1998; 228(5):635–637.

83. Shahidi R, Mezrich R, Silver D. Proposed simulation of volumetric image navigation using a surgical microscope. J Image Guid Surg 1995; 1(5):249–265.

84. Chang SD, Murphy M, Geis P, et al. Clinical experience with image-guided robotic radiosurgery (the Cyberknife) in the treatment of brain and spinal cord tumors. Neurol Med Chir 1998; 38(11):780–783.

85. Rosen JM, Soltanian H, Laub DR, et al. The evolution of virtual reality from surgical training to the development of a simulator for health care delivery. A review. Stud Health Technol Inform 1996; 29:89–99.

86. Abdel-Malek K, McGowan DP, Goel VK, et al. Bone registration method for robot assisted surgery: Pedicle screw insertion. Proc Inst Mech Eng [H] 1997; 211(3):221–233.

87. Burghart CR, Neukirch K, Hassfeld S, et al. Computer aided planning device for preoperative bending of osteosynthesis plates. Stud Health Technol Inform 2000; 70:46–52.

88. Ross MD, Montgomery K, Linton S, et al. A national center for biocomputation: in search of a patient-specific interactive virtual surgery workbench. Stud Health Technol Inform 1998; 50:323–328.

89. Pieper SD, Laub DR, Rosen JM. A finite-element facial model for simulating plastic surgery. Plast Reconstr Surg 1995; 96(5):1100–1105.

90. Cutting C, Grayson B, McCarthy JG, et al. A virtual reality system for bone fragment positioning in multisegment craniofacial surgical procedures. Plast Reconstr Surg 1998; 102(7):2436–2443.

91. Yamazaki M, Akazawa T, Koda M, et al. Surgical simulation of instrumented posterior occipitocervical fusion in a child with congenital skeletal anomaly: Case report. Spine 2006; 31(17):E590–E594.

92. Meehan M, Morris D, Maurer CR, et al. Virtual 3D planning and guidance of mandibular distraction osteogenesis. Comput Aided Surg 2006; 11(2):51–62.

93. Koyama T, Okudera H, Gibo H, et al. Computer-generated microsurgical anatomy of the basilar artery bifurcation. Technical note. J Neurosurg 1999; 91(1):145–152.

94. Auer LM, Auer DP. Virtual endoscopy for planning and simulation of minimally invasive neurosurgery. Neurosurgery Online 1998; 43(3):529–357; discussion 537.

95. Keeve E, Girod S, Kikinis R, et al. Deformable modeling of facial tissue for craniofacial surgery simulation. Comput Aided Surg 1998; 3(5):228–238.

96. Marescaux J, Clément JM, Tassetti V, et al. Virtual reality applied to hepatic surgery simulation: the next revolution. Ann Surg 1998; 228(5):627–634.

97. Fuchs J, Warmann SW, Szavay P, et al. Three-dimensional visualization and virtual simulation of resections in pediatric solid tumors. J Pediatr Surg 2005; 40(2):364–370.

98. Paik DS, Beaulieu CF, Jeffrey RB, et al. Automated flight path planning for virtual endoscopy. Med Phys 1998; 25(5):629–637.

99. Ogata I, Komohara Y, Yamashita Y, et al. CT evaluation of gastric lesions with three-dimensional display and interactive virtual endoscopy: Comparison with conventional barium study and endoscopy. AJR 1999; 172(5):1263–1270.

100. Inamoto K, Kouzai K, Ueeda T, et al. CT virtual endoscopy of the stomach: Comparison study with gastric fiberoscopy. Abdom Imaging 2005; 30(4):473–479.

101. Röttgen R, Schröder RJ, Lorenz M, et al. [CT-colonography with the 16-slice CT for the diagnostic evaluation of colorectal neoplasms and inflammatory colon diseases]. RöFo 2003; 175(10):1384–1391.

102. Vining DJ, Liu K, Choplin RH, et al. Virtual bronchoscopy. Relationships of virtual reality endobronchial simulations to actual bronchoscopic findings. Chest 1996; 109(2):549–553.

103. Hassfeld S, Mühling J. Computer assisted oral and maxillofacial surgery—a review and an assessment of technology. Int J Oral Maxillofac Surg 2001; 30(1):2–13.

104. Wagner A, Rasse M, Millesi W, et al. Virtual reality for orthognathic surgery: The augmented reality environment concept. J Oral maxillofac Surg 1997; 55(5):456–462; discussion 462.

105. Robb R. VR assisted surgery planning using patient specific anatomic models. IEEE Eng Med Bio 1996; 15(2):60–69.

106. Fried MP, Satava R, Weghorst S, et al. Identifying and reducing errors with surgical simulation. Qual Saf Health Care 2004; 13:i19–i26.

107. Rosser JC, Herman B, Risucci DA, et al. Effectiveness of a CD-ROM multimedia tutorial in transferring cognitive knowledge essential for laparoscopic skill training. Am J Surg 2000; 179(4):320–324.

108. Reznick RK. Teaching and testing technical skills. Am J Surg 1993; 165(3):358–361.

109. Grantcharov TP, Kristiansen VB, Bendix J, et al. Randomized clinical trial of virtual reality simulation for laparoscopic skills training. Brit J Surg 2004; 91(2):146–150.

110. Seymour NE, Gallagher AG, Roman SA, et al. Virtual reality training improves operating room performance: results of a randomized, double-blinded study. Ann Surg 2002; 236(4):458–463; discussion 463.

111. Hyltander A, Liljegren E, Rhodin PH, et al. The transfer of basic skills learned in a laparoscopic simulator to the operating room. Surg Endosc 2002; 16(9):1324–1328.

112. Haque S, Srinivasan S. A meta-analysis of the training effectiveness of virtual reality surgical simulators. IEEE Trans Inf Technol Biomed 2006; 10(1):51–58.

113. Sutherland LM, Middleton PF, Anthony A, et al. Surgical simulation: a systematic review. Ann Surg 2006; 243(3):291–300.

114. Crossing the Quality Chasm: A New Health System for 21st Century. Washington, DC: Institute of Medicine, 2001.

115. Gaba DM. Improving anesthesiologists' performance by simulating reality. Anesthesiology 1992; 76(4):491–494.

6 | Application of a Systems Approach to Medication Safety

Michael S. Leonard, M.D., M.S.

INTRODUCTION

Patient safety is a subject that spans the spectrum of medical specialties. In the surgical fields, much focus has been placed on ensuring that the correct procedure is performed on the correct side of the correct patient. While surgeons must be vigilant in their efforts to avoid procedure-related errors, they must be equally attentive to errors associated with medications. Surgeons commonly prescribe analgesics and antibiotics, drugs recognized as high risk for errors and adverse drug events (ADEs) (1). Medication orders must therefore be accurate and appropriate to reduce the risk of ADEs (2–4).

Children are especially vulnerable to medication errors. Young infants, particularly neonates, have a distinct physiology from that of adults and an altered ability to metabolize drugs. Dosing for these patients must be tailored and precise. The majority of pediatric dosing is based on the patient's weight. Narrow margins of error can place children at high risk for ADEs. A safe dose for an adult can be toxic for an infant. The lay press and medical literature are filled with examples of children receiving excessive dosing (5–9). Tenfold overdoses are among the commonest of these errors, e.g., "10 mg" versus "1.0 mg," often due to missed or misplaced decimal points as well as miscalculations. Conversely, an appropriate dose for an infant would likely be subtherapeutic for an adult. Underdosing, if left uncorrected, can also result in significant morbidity and/or mortality due to ineffective treatment of the patient's illness.

Adverse drug events need to be better quantified. We must be willing to acknowledge and learn from these incidents or we are destined to continue the practices that contribute to them. There are drawbacks, however, in measuring patient safety only in terms of ADEs. Adverse drug events are relatively rare in comparison to the total number of medications prescribed on a regular basis. Therefore, assessing the impact of patient safety initiatives solely by tracking ADE rates is often impractical, and demonstration of significance difficult. Once an ADE is identified, harm has already befallen the patient. Ideally, ADEs should be intercepted *before* they occur, thereby preventing harm.

Much of the efforts in patient safety have focused on preventing harm due to errors. A complementary approach is to prevent *risk* of harm (10). Potential ADEs represent risk of harm to patients. They are the "near misses," or more accurately, the "near hits." Reducing the rate of potential ADEs provides an opportunity to reduce the rate of *actual* ADEs. Risk reduction, a concept commonly used in epidemiologic studies, can be then be used to evaluate such endeavors. *Absolute risk reduction* is simply the postintervention risk subtracted from the baseline risk. *Relative risk reduction* is the difference between baseline and postintervention risks (i.e., the absolute risk reduction) divided by the baseline risk, expressed as a percentage. Incident reporting generally identifies ADEs after they have occurred and although this tracking is important, it does not adequately identify risk of events before they happen. Since potential ADEs can be tracked and measured objectively through alternative methods, they lend themselves well to risk reduction calculations.

Physician orders must be complete to reduce the risk of ADEs (11). While most of these orders are likely filled as intended without harm to the patient, the risk is undeniably present. Each time an order is written with missing information, an assumption has to be made by another participant in the medication management team, perhaps the transcribing nurse or the pharmacist. Each time an assumption is made, an *incorrect* assumption can be made. The outcome can be harmless, but can just as easily be catastrophic. The following anecdote illustrates the danger in assuming:

A patient was scheduled to go to the operating room. In anticipation, the physician wrote an order to "give all PO meds IV." The nurse therefore crushed the patient's oral tablets and administered them through his central venous line.

Fortunately, and incredibly, the patient did not suffer any ill effects, but the potential was enormous. We all know the old joke about what happens when we assume; there was nothing humorous about this scenario.

Any medication order with incomplete or incorrect information increases the risk of an ADE. Every such order is therefore a potential ADE, which if not intercepted and corrected, may cause harm to the patient. The challenge, then, is to prevent such potential events through diligent prescribing practices, and to swiftly identify and intervene with any incomplete or incorrect order *before* an adverse event can result. The section to follow provides an example of how one institution, the Women & Children's Hospital of Buffalo, reduced the risk of ADEs due to prescribing errors (10). The PEDS cycle (Process → Education → Dissemination → Surveillance) (12) was utilized to accomplish this objective.

REDUCING THE RISK

Process
In the absence of computerized physician order entry (CPOE), the Women & Children's Hospital of Buffalo developed and instituted a Forced Format Form to make sure that physicians included all key elements of a pediatric medication order. The design was simple. The essential components for a complete pediatric medication order were printed across the top of a conventional order form as reminders for the physician. These included medication name, dose, route, and interval. Two other nontraditional components were included: weight-based dosing and indication for therapy. Since most pediatric dosing is based on the patient's weight, it is logical to include this element as a prompt for this computation. It also encourages nurses and pharmacists to double-check safe dosing calculations.

Look-alike and sound-alike drug names are a significant source of medication errors (13,14). Including the indication for therapy as a required element of the medication order helps to ensure that the right drug is being prescribed for the right reason. Cerebyx® might easily be mistaken for Celebrex® or Celexa® should the penmanship of the physician be less than impeccable. Documenting the indication for therapy can help prevent this kind of error. Cerebyx is commonly prescribed for "seizures," Celebrex for "pain," and Celexa for "depression." The likelihood of confusing these drugs is decreased with this additional information present in the order itself.

The same holds true for medication names that sound alike. Zantac® and Xanax® might not be confused on a written order, but could easily be mistaken in a *verbal* order. If you have any doubts about the previous statement, think back to the last time you drove under an overpass, through a tunnel, or across a bridge while talking on your wireless phone. Error is less likely to occur if the physician communicates that the Zantac is being ordered for "gastroesophageal reflux" or that the Xanax is being prescribed for "anxiety." The following vignette shows how including indication for therapy in a medication order can avert morbidity:

A patient admitted for an elective procedure was found smoking in the bathroom. Since she could not smoke in the hospital, she was offered the nicotine patch, which she accepted. The physician wrote the order, but instead of writing "Nicoderm,®" wrote "Nitro-Dur®."

Fortunately, the indication was questioned, and the patient received the correct medication. Again, the potential for an ADE was undeniably present. Tables 1 and 2 provide more examples of look-alike and sound-alike drug names with common indications for therapy (15,16).

There is an irony to this concept. Laboratories often require an indication, in the form of an ICD-9 code, before a blood sample will be processed. Imaging centers often require an indication before a plain radiograph will be performed. This has become accepted practice. Neither of these poses significant risk of harm to patients. The value of requiring similar information for medications, which do have the potential to cause harm, has only recently been appreciated and is just starting to be accepted.

Table 1 Look-Alike Drug Names with Indications for Therapy

Drug name	Indication for therapy
Amicar[R]	Bleeding
Amikin[R]	Infection
Nalaxone	Opioid reversal
Naproxen	Pain
Zyrtec[R]	Allergic rhinitis
Zyprexa[R]	Scizophrenia

Traditional medication order forms were removed from two hospital wards, one medical and one surgical, and replaced with the Forced Format Form during the initial implementation. A one-week sample of pilot data revealed a decrease in incomplete orders by 48% on the medical ward, and 12% on the surgical ward. The cause of this disparity was not inherent to the wards; it was instead due to a difference in the education provided about the new initiative. The residents on the medical ward were instructed on the use of the new forms. The residents on the surgical ward, representing more than half a dozen surgical subspecialties, did not receive such instruction. Forms alone cannot sufficiently change behavior; proper education must also be provided.

Education

Physicians' schedules are hectic and their time is extremely valuable. It would be a near-impossible undertaking to educate an entire medical staff face-to-face about an initiative for which the value may not initially be recognized. Therefore, an educational website was created.

The website was comprised of two sections: a tutorial and a competency exam. The tutorial instructed the user in both general principles of patient safety, such as avoidance of unsafe abbreviations, as well as issues specific to pediatrics, such as weight-based dosing. The competency exam provided a brief case scenario based upon which pediatric medication orders had to be "written." The orders incorporated all of the elements described in the section above. The user was required to complete all of the orders correctly to be considered proficient.

The website was utilized not only by resident and faculty physicians, but also by registered nurses and pharmacists. Although nurses do not write medications orders, they do take verbal orders and transcribe written orders; they must therefore know the principles of safe prescribing practices. Pharmacists must also be cognizant of this information as the recipients of medication orders. The website has subsequently been used for remediation with physicians found to write incomplete or incorrect orders. It has become a requisite part of new housestaff orientation at the State University of New York at Buffalo School of Medicine and Biomedical Sciences, and has been incorporated into its third-year medical student pediatric rotation.

New forms and comprehensive teaching were necessary but still not sufficient to achieve the level of success desired with the initiative. Poor prescribing habits continued to place patients at risk of harm. Convincing physicians, particularly those in practice for many years, to document what was too often perceived as needless information remained a challenge. The attitude reflected in questions such as "Who are you to question my orders?" and comments like "So now Big Brother is watching!" was an impediment to patient safety efforts. Sharing institutional data, and even physician-specific data, did not significantly change practice, especially from

Table 2 Sound-Alike Drug Names with Indications for Therapy

Drug name	Indication for therapy
Clonidine	Hypertension
Klonipin[R]	Seizures
Diamox[R]	Glaucoma
Trimox[R]	Infection
Prevacid[R]	Gastroesophageal reflux
Probenecid	Hyperuricemia

those who were not open to the premise that their practice might require improvement. How, then, can physicians be compelled to change their behavior?

The institution had to adopt a policy of zero tolerance. Registered nurses were instructed not to accept incomplete or incorrect orders. Pharmacists were instructed not to fill incomplete or incorrect orders. The zero-tolerance policy had its drawbacks. In essence, it made nurses and pharmacists accountable for physician behavior as well as their own; this inevitably created friction. Nurses and pharmacists were required to contact physicians for clarification or rewriting of unacceptable orders. Doctors generally perceived this as an annoyance rather than an asset. The attitude of some physicians was reflected in medication orders themselves, such as the indication "to kill the germs" for an antibiotic. The policy put an enormous strain on the nurses and pharmacists who had to make phone call after phone call to irate physicians. Doctors accused nurses and pharmacists of delaying treatment to their patients. They did not recognize the value in a brief delay in medication administration versus an adverse event. Ironically, they did not appreciate that the phone call would not have been necessary had they written the order properly in the first place. Of course, nurses and pharmacists were instructed to use their clinical judgment in emergency situations.

CPOE systems can force fields to be filled before an order is accepted, thereby eliminating missing information. It was this concept that originally inspired the Forced Format Form. However, less than 10% of U.S. hospitals have a fully implemented CPOE system (17). This fact underscores the need for simple, nontechnological solutions to serve as foundation upon which to build an environment of patient safety.

In an ideal world, physicians would be 100% compliant with safe prescribing practices. In the real world, physicians' prescribing habits are less than perfect. In an ideal world, nurses and pharmacists would be 100% effective at assuring that no incomplete or incorrect order was accepted or filled. In the real world, the time and vigilance needed for such an undertaking cannot be overestimated. Education can serve as the "carrot" for compliance with patient safety initiatives, but policies are also needed to serve as the "stick." Ultimately, the zero-tolerance policy was successful at improving compliance and reducing risk beyond that achieved through education alone (10).

Dissemination

There is a Chinese proverb: "Give a man a fish and you feed him for a day. Teach a man to fish and you feed him for a lifetime." This is true only if you also provide him with a fishing pole. Participants in the process must be given appropriate tools. For the Forced Format Form, prescribing information had to be disseminated to the physicians enabling them to complete their orders properly: an up-to-date, point-of-care pediatric drug reference.

Many such references exist; each institution should choose the one which best suits its needs. The challenge is to provide the reference at the point of care, increasing the likelihood that the physician will use it when he/she writes a medication order. The Women & Children's Hospital of Buffalo chose to provide its physicians with an electronic pediatric drug reference loaded into their personal digital assistants (PDAs). Disseminating the electronic drug reference, along with the web-based education, was shown to significantly reduce the risk of ADEs due to prescribing errors (10).

Surveillance

Tracking the occurrence of ADEs has traditionally relied on incident reporting. There are many pitfalls in relying on this methodology. Incident reporting requires extra time of health care professionals who are already occupied with patient care responsibilities. The forms are often cumbersome and difficult to complete. Staff often receive little or no feedback for their efforts, and may perceive that reporting does not result in change (18).

There is a very real fear of consequences for reporting adverse events. Even in an environment of "blameless reporting," professionals may harbor legitimate concerns about disciplinary actions imposed by their employer or from licensing agencies. Legal ramifications can be a deterrent to reporting adverse events, even anonymously. There is an inherent aversion to pointing out one's own errors, and a stigma attached to the reporting of others' mistakes. Professionals may fear losing the trust and respect of colleagues, or being labeled a "whistle blower." All of these factors underscore the need to build environments of truly blameless reporting, environments in which those who report incidents are rewarded, those who err are educated, and only those who commit acts of overt negligence or willful harm are disciplined.

Observed changes in rates of ADEs as identified by incident reports can be misleading. While differences may reflect a true change, they may also reflect a change in reporting itself independent of the actual rate of ADEs. Imagine a scenario in which a new intravenous infusion pump, believed to provide safer delivery of medications, is introduced. The nurses receive appropriate instruction on the use of the new pumps. Outcome will be measured based on the number of reported adverse events involving the new pumps as compared to those involving the previous pumps. The rate of adverse events doubles over the next month. At first glance, one might infer that the new infusion pumps actually increased the rate of ADEs and caused more harm to patients. However, it is also possible that the new technology was successful, but the number of incidents reported increased because of the heightened awareness and diligence in documenting events. You decide to continue using the new pumps for another month. At the end of this time period, the rate of ADEs is half of that measured at baseline, before the new pumps were introduced. Did the pumps truly reduce ADEs, or did the nursing staff just lose vigilance in reporting events? Examples like this highlight the need to develop new, objective methodologies to identify, track and measure adverse events.

When implementing new patient safety initiatives, ADE rates may not always be a suitable endpoint to track. An ongoing challenge in assessing the effectiveness of new processes is measuring appropriate outcomes and measuring outcomes appropriately. Failing to do so risks enormous investments in time and resources without imparting any significant benefit to the institution, or worse yet, introducing additional risk into the system. The Forced Format Form was designed to reduce risk of ADEs due to poor prescribing habits. Therefore, a suitable outcome measure was utilized: the percentage of orders that due to incomplete or incorrect information placed patients unnecessarily at risk for an ADE. Ultimately, the Women & Children's Hospital of Buffalo showed an absolute risk reduction of 38 per 100 medication orders, yielding a relative risk reduction of 49% (10).

PREVENTION: A PUBLIC HEALTH MODEL

A public health model can be used as a framework to prevent ADEs. Generally, there are three levels of prevention described: primary, secondary, and tertiary (19). An additional level, called primordial prevention, has also been suggested. The "disease" in this model is prescribing errors, including those of commission (i.e., incorrect orders) and those of omission (i.e., incomplete orders).

Primary prevention refers to the prevention of disease before it occurs. In public health, immunizations are administered to prevent disease before it has the opportunity to afflict patients. In patient safety, processes such as a forced format for medication orders, educational programs that teach safe prescribing habits, and tools like point-of-care drug references can be utilized to prevent prescribing errors. *Secondary prevention* is the early detection of disease and rapid intervention. In public health, patients are routinely screened for illnesses for which early initiation of treatment reduces morbidity and/or mortality. In patient safety, secondary prevention can also be accomplished through screening. Nurses and pharmacists routinely review medication orders and must be empowered to intervene immediately when errors are identified. Screening techniques, such as trigger tools and other methodologies currently in development, may offer more systematic prevention for the future. *Tertiary prevention* aims to minimize sequelae and maximize function after a disease has presented. In public health, developmental and rehabilitation programs serve this function for a myriad of illnesses. In patient safety, tertiary prevention may be achieved through such practices as readily accessible reversal agents (e.g., nalaxone) for at-risk patients and availability of rapid response teams, also known as medical emergency teams, should an adverse event occur (20).

Primordial prevention targets environmental and societal conditions that increase the risk of disease (21). In public health, this is the goal of health promotion activities such as antismoking campaigns. In patient safety, primordial prevention entails establishing a health care environment in which safe medication practices are embedded, promoted, and expected; an environment in which safe practices are the standard and unsafe practices are unacceptable.

Ideally, ADEs would be eliminated through primordial and primary prevention strategies. The reality is that humans are a component in the medication management process, and of course, "to err is human." In addition, not all ADEs are predictable and preventable. Secondary and tertiary prevention initiatives must also be in place to prevent or at least minimize harm to patients.

SIERRA

Patient safety is a summit that every health care facility must reach. The ascent is arduous and fraught with obstacles. The reward for the journey is an environment in which we can provide the safest possible care for our patients. It is fitting, then, that the lessons learned from those who have taken the first steps of this trek can be summarized by the acronym SIERRA:

- Simple initiatives
- Interdisciplinary teams
- Early acceptors
- Rapid pilots
- Rapid feedback
- Advertise gains

Simple Initiatives

In our zeal to create a safer health care system, there is a natural temptation toward grandiosity. Avoid creating unrealistic goals and unnecessarily intricate solutions. As Miguel de Cervantes Saavedra wrote in *Don Quixote*, "Rome was not built in a day." Identify one process and implement a practical, workable solution. Once you have achieved success with such an initiative, build upon it. A well-designed, well-implemented process can serve as a solid foundation for the next.

Interdisciplinary Teams

Delivery of optimal health care relies on the synergistic interactions between medical professionals. Consequently, system changes rarely affect only one segment of the health care team. An interdisciplinary process improvement team fosters comprehensive solutions and enables identification of impediments that might otherwise go unrecognized. A physician may not truly appreciate how a new initiative will affect a nurse's daily routine. An administrator can only speculate on how a new policy will affect a pharmacist's workload. Interdisciplinary teams remove the need for conjecture and promote practicality.

Interdisciplinary teams are important not only for development of new processes, but also for implementation. A nurse may be more receptive to a proposal introduced by a fellow nurse who is similarly impacted by the change. A physician may be more amenable to new process championed by a trusted peer than an unfamiliar administrator. Interdisciplinary teams help abolish the counterproductive "us versus them" mindset.

Early Acceptors

Recruit individuals who share your goals, welcome new ideas, and support process improvement. These are the colleagues who will champion your initiatives and help spread change. Avoid the tendency to engage your most difficult opponent; initiating change is challenging enough.

Rapid Pilots

Change within a large complex system often progresses slowly. Patient safety projects, however, should be piloted swiftly to sustain the momentum and maintain the interest of the team. Baseline and postintervention periods of several days to several weeks can often be sufficient to determine if the initiative was successful in achieving the desired goals. Pilot the initiative in a well-defined area of the institution, such as a unit or department; do not try to pilot it across an entire organization at once. Choose specific, easily measurable outcome variables.

Rapid Feedback

Health care providers are incredibly busy people who do not always have the opportunity to see the fruits of their labor. Do not spend excessive amounts of time analyzing data to the detriment of dissociating your team. Provide rapid feedback to your team and any personnel involved with the pilot study. The process may not be as beneficial as anticipated; in some cases, it may even have a negative impact. Regardless of the results, rapid feedback will enable you to sustain the momentum and maintain the interest of the team so another cycle or series of cycles can be undertaken in the true spirit of process improvement.

Advertise Gains

Everyone likes good news. Share your successes, even the small ones, with the institution. Most organizations have newsletters, bulletin boards, web pages, and/or other vehicles by which information is disseminated. Take advantage of such established mechanisms, and when necessary, create your own.

Advertising gains has a number of benefits. It boosts hospital morale and instills confidence in providers that their patients are receiving care in a safe environment. It establishes credibility in the new process that can reduce resistance to implementation in other areas of the institution. It recognizes the efforts of the patient safety team, providing positive reinforcement for their continued participation and may even promote participation by previously uninvolved personnel.

CONCLUSION

The goal of this chapter was not to provide a concrete blueprint for pediatric medication safety. It was instead to offer approaches that can be adapted to a variety of settings to promote safer prescribing practices and build safer medication management systems. The first section described how the Women & Children's Hospital of Buffalo used the PEDS cycle to reduce the risk of prescribing errors. A framework for viewing ADEs using a public health model was then presented. The chapter concluded with a discussion of how the SIERRA principles can promote effective process improvement initiatives. Alexander Pope said, "To err is human, to forgive divine," but in the ongoing efforts to establish an environment of patient safety, this author would humbly suggest "To err is human, to *improve* divine."

ACKNOWLEDGMENTS

The author would like to acknowledge and sincerely thank the following individuals for their unwavering support, immeasurable dedication, and tireless efforts to improve patient safety: Sandra McDougal, RN, MSN; Michael Cimino, MS, RPh; Joann Pilliod, RN; Steven Shaha, PhD, DBA; and Linda Brodsky, MD.

REFERENCES

1. Bates DW, Cullen DJ, Laird N, et al. Incidence of adverse drug events and potential adverse drug events. Implications for prevention. ADE Prevention Study Group. JAMA 1995; 274(1):29–34.
2. Leape LL, Bates DW, Cullen DJ, et al. Systems analysis of adverse drug events. ADE Prevention Study Group. JAMA 1995; 274(1):35–43.
3. Lesar TS, Briceland L, Stein DS. Factors related to errors in medication prescribing. JAMA 1997; 277(4):312–317.
4. Fortescue EB, Kaushal R, Landrigan CP, et al. Prioritizing strategies for preventing medication errors and adverse drug events in pediatric inpatients. Pediatrics 2003; 111(4 Pt 1):722–729.
5. Goldstein A. Overdose Kills 9-Month-Old at Children's Hospital. The Washington Post, Washington, DC, 2001.
6. Rabin R. Plenty of Blame/State Says Failures Throughout Hospital Led to Baby's Death. Newsday, Long Island, NY, 2002.
7. Wong IC, Ghaleb MA, Franklin BD, et al. Incidence and nature of dosing errors in paediatric medications: A systematic review. Drug Saf 2004; 27(9):661–670.

8. Narayanan M, Schlueter M, Clyman RI. Incidence and outcome of a 10-fold indomethacin overdose in premature infants. J Pediatr 1999; 135(1):105–107.

9. Rowe C, Koren T, Koren G. Errors by paediatric residents in calculating drug doses. Arch Dis Child 1998; 79(1):56–58.

10. Leonard MS, Cimino M, Shaha S, et al. Risk reduction for adverse drug events through sequential implementation of patient safety initiatives in a children's hospital. Pediatrics 2006; 118(4):e1124–1129.

11. Prevention of medication errors in the pediatric inpatient setting. American Academy of Pediatrics. Committee on Drugs and Committee on Hospital Care. Pediatrics 1998;102(2 Pt 1):428–430.

12. Shaha SH, Brodsky L, Leonard MS, et al. Establishing a culture of patient safety through a low-tech approach to reducing medication errors. In: Advances in Patient Safety: From Research to Implementation. Rockville, MD: Agency for Healthcare Research and Quality, 2005.

13. Lambert BL, Lin SJ, Chang KY, et al. Similarity as a risk factor in drug-name confusion errors: The look-alike (orthographic) and sound-alike (phonetic) model. Med Care 1999;37(12):1214–1225.

14. Bond GR, Thompson JD. Olanzapine pediatric overdose. Ann Emerg Med 1999; 34(2):292–293.

15. Taketomo CK, Hodding JH Kraus DM. Pediatric Dosage Handbook. 13th ed. Hudson, OH: Lexi-Comp Inc., 2006

16. Physicians' Desk Reference. 61st ed. Montvale, NJ: Thomson PDR, 2007.

17. Ash JS, Gorman PN, Seshadri V, et al. Computerized physician order entry in U.S. hospitals: Results of a 2002 survey. J Am Med Inform Assoc 2004;11(2):95–99.

18. Taylor JA, Brownstein D, Christakis DA, et al. Use of incident reports by physicians and nurses to document medical errors in pediatric patients. Pediatrics 2004;114(3):729–735.

19. Turnock BJ. Public Health. 2nd ed. Sudbury, MA: Jones and Bartlett Publishers, Inc., 2004.

20. Tibballs J, Kinney S, Duke T, et al. Reduction of paediatric in-patient cardiac arrest and death with a medical emergency team: Preliminary results. Arch Dis Child 2005; 90(11):1148–1452.

21. Last JM. A Dictionary of Epidemiology. New York, NY: Oxford University Press, Inc., 2001

7 | Wading Through the Clinical Evidence: A Primer for Pediatric Surgeons

Shawn J. Rangel, M.D. and Richard A. Falcone, Jr., M.D., M.P.H.

INTRODUCTION

The field of pediatric surgery was forged on ingenuity, technical creativity, and careful clinical observation. During the early part of the century, Drs. Ladd, Gross, and others pioneered the field by characterizing the pathophysiology and early operative management of pediatric surgical diseases. Subsequent advances in surgical care hinged largely upon anecdotal experience and careful documentation of outcomes on a case-by-case basis. Over the next several decades, our understanding of these diseases improved and operative principles were further refined. From these early observational efforts, the field of pediatric surgery was born and subsequently evolved into a distinct surgical specialty.

On the heels of these remarkable advances, further improvement in the surgical care of children hinges upon our ability to critically evaluate our evolving surgical therapies. As treatments are conceptualized and put into practice, the need to rigorously evaluate these therapies as safe and efficacious has never been greater. Rising health care costs, mounting pressure from third-party payers to demonstrate therapeutic efficacy, and the ever-increasing sophistication of parents (largely due to the availability of information on the worldwide web) are just a few of the external factors which have brought the concept of "evidence-based practice" to the forefront. Above all else, however, our need to transition from anecdotal-based care to a more evidence-based approach should be fueled by our own desire to provide the best possible care for our patients. In addition, it is crucial that we are able to appropriately interpret the available literature to provide our patients and their families with the best understanding of potential complications from the treatments we provide.

How do we as a field accomplish this task and move forward to ensure our patients are receiving the best possible care? The answer lies in training the next (and current) generation of pediatric surgeons in the process of critically appraising the published clinical evidence. This involves not only the ability to recognize the different types of epidemiological studies in the literature and how each fits into the hierarchy of clinical evidence, but also having an in-depth working knowledge of the advantages, limitations, and inherent biases of each type when used to study pediatric surgical diseases. Furthermore, the clinician must be able to identify the key reporting elements in any clinical study to effectively gauge the generalizability of results and conclusions to their own patient population.

With these considerations, the objectives of this chapter are threefold: (1) To review the advantages and limitations of the most common clinical study designs encountered in the pediatric surgical literature; (2) To review the current qualitative "state" of the published clinical evidence in support of pediatric surgical practice, and (3) To provide the clinician with a systematic approach for critically appraising a published clinical study.

WHAT IS EVIDENCE-BASED MEDICINE AND HOW DOES IT RELATE TO THE LITERATURE?

Many definitions of "evidence-based medicine" (EBM) have been proposed, but perhaps the most commonly referenced is that described by Sackett as "the integration of best clinical evidence with clinical expertise and patient values" (1). In regards to what constitutes the "best" clinical evidence, several classification schemes have been developed that rank studies on their relative scientific merit such as that published by the U.S. Services Preventative Task Force (Table 1) (2). Early concepts of EBM were relatively stringent in their definition of which studies

Table 1   Hierarchy of Clinical Evidence Based of Type of Study Design (from the United States Services Preventative Task Force)

Level I	Evidence from at least one well-conducted randomized clinical trial
Level IIa	Evidence from at least one well-conducted controlled trial without randomization
Level IIb	Evidence from well-designed prospective cohort studies (preferably multicenter design)
Level IIc	Evidence from retrospective cohort and case-control studies
Level III	Evidence from case-series and cross-sectional data
Level IV	Case reports and published editorials ("expert opinion")

could be considered evidence for the purpose of setting practice guidelines. As the concept of EBM was originally conceived for the appraisal of medical therapies where prospective data were abundant, only the most rigorous of clinical studies such as randomized clinical trials (RCTs) and prospective cohort studies were considered in the development of practice guidelines.

For the study of pediatric surgical diseases, such a rigid approach is not readily applicable given that the overwhelming body of available evidence is founded in retrospective observational data (3–5). In fact, we estimate that nearly 95% of all clinical decisions in pediatric surgery could not be "evidence-based" if only RCTs and high-quality prospective cohort studies were considered (they simply are not available) (6,7). We have previously proposed a more realistic approach toward applying EBM and pediatric surgical conditions, where development of practice guidelines and patient care decisions would be based on the best available evidence from the *entire* literature pool (outside of small case-series and case report data) (4). Although this approach does expand the available literature pool for evidence-based review, the influence of retrospective data does present a particularly difficult challenge for the practitioner when wading through relatively low-quality evidence to make treatment decisions. As such, it essential that the practicing surgeon has a through understanding of the limitations and biases of the different types of study designs encountered in the surgical literature, particularly those which are retrospective. The next section is designed to introduce the reader to the basic taxonomy of epidemiological study designs and how each fits in the hierarchy of clinical evidence.

EPIDEMIOLOGICAL STUDY DESIGNS IN THE SURGICAL LITERATURE

Epidemiological studies are generally categorized as experimental or observational. In an experimental study, which is always prospective in design, patients are actively recruited by the investigator and assigned to receive one or more interventions for the purpose of the study. Controlled clinical trials are the classic example of an experimental study, and subjects can be chosen to receive an intervention from a predetermined assignment or in a randomized fashion. Furthermore, clinical pathways and study protocols are often used to ensure standardization between study groups with respect to perioperative care and follow-up. This is what is meant by a "controlled" clinical trial. In contrast, there is no artificial manipulation of treatment assignment or preoperative care when observational designs are used to study outcomes. There is no active assignment of interventions for the purpose of the study, and patients are treated in the perioperative and postoperative period as they would normally be treated. Outcomes following interventions in observational studies are therefore only "observed," and no efforts are made to "control" for potentially confounding effects between treatment groups.

Observational studies can further be categorized into descriptive and analytical studies. Descriptive studies are carried out when there is little knowledge about the state of health or frequency of a disease. The classic examples of descriptive studies in the pediatric surgical literature include the case-report and case-series study. Collectively, these studies comprise the greatest proportion of clinical data in the pediatric surgery literature (2,4). Cross-sectional studies are another example of a descriptive observational study and may be useful for characterizing prevalence rates of disease states. An example would be a study examining the seasonal variability in the prevalence of necrotizing enterocolitis (NEC). Observational studies which are analytical are designed to test the hypothesis of whether specific exposures (or operations) lead to changes in measured outcomes as they relate to the natural history of disease. These studies include cohort and case-control studies.

For the purpose of synthesizing evidence-based decisions, the pediatric surgeon should be familiar with the different types of clinical study designs encountered in the surgical literature. These include randomized trials, cohort studies, case-control studies, and case-series reports. Although other types of study designs are also prevalent in the surgical literature, these four types of studies comprise the overwhelming body of published evidence from which clinical decisions will be made. The next section will further explore the advantages and limitations of each of these studies in the order of their relative epidemiological rigor.

Prospective, Randomized, Controlled Clinical Trial

In the prospective, randomized, controlled clinical trial, patients from a defined study population with a disease of interest are enrolled into the study prior to receiving treatment. Treatment is subsequently assigned through a randomization process (into different intervention arms which may include a placebo group), and all patients are otherwise treated equally throughout the duration of the study period. Randomized trials, in theory, allow for the automatic control of clinical characteristics and biases which may explain an observed difference outside of the interventions being compared. Although in practice it is impossible to control for all such effects, the value of properly conducted RCTs is that any such biases should be equally distributed among patients in different treatment arms. This is in contrast to observational studies, where investigators must identify and characterize potential sources of bias which may have impacted patient selection, treatment allocation, and ultimately how these biases may have affected the validity of results.

Although the RCT represents the gold-standard in clinical evidence, there are several challenges with applying this design to the study of pediatric surgical diseases. Randomized trials are very expensive and take a considerable amount of time to perform. This is particularly relevant for rare pediatric surgical diseases where the incidence is exceedingly low. In this regard, the relatively low numbers of patients encountered at an individual center may mandate the use of a multicenter design to achieve the appropriate number of patients for a statistically meaningful result. Development of such infrastructure can pose substantial logistical and financial challenges to the investigator. Specific to pediatric surgical conditions, the length of time to complete the study also may affect the relevance of results when examining therapies which are relatively new or rapidly evolving (e.g., interventions in pediatric surgical oncology).

Cohort Studies

In a cohort study, two or more groups of patients with similar baseline characteristics (collectively defined as the "cohort") are followed from an exposure of interest to a predefined endpoint. In the study of surgical diseases, the exposure can either be a risk factor leading to a disease state (e.g., Indomethacin exposure and the development of NEC), or an operative intervention leading to an endpoint of interest (e.g., peritoneal drainage for the treatment of perforated NEC and survival). In the latter example, the "nonexposed" group can either be a true control (receiving no treatment), or a group receiving a different intervention (e.g., laparotomy for the treatment of perforated NEC and survival). Cohort studies can be either prospective when the investigator defines the cohort at the beginning of the study and the endpoints of interest have not yet occurred; or retrospective, where a chart review is used to identify both exposed and unexposed patients (controls) and whether the endpoints of interest have already occurred at the time the study is initiated (Fig. 1).

The validity of the cohort study is dependent upon a strict definition of the cohort, or the key elements of similarity between comparison groups outside of the exposure or operative treatment of interest. In the hierarchy of study designs, the well-designed prospective cohort study provides the most rigorous evidence for establishing causality outside of a clinical trial. The relative strength this study hinges upon the ability of the investigator to minimize potential bias when selecting patients into different comparison groups. However, even with well-designed cohort studies, it is not possible to address all potential biases with respect to why patients were assigned to different treatments at the onset of the study. The presence of these unknown and potentially confounding factors is a consequence of nonrandomization, and the primary reason these studies are considered inferior to RCTs.

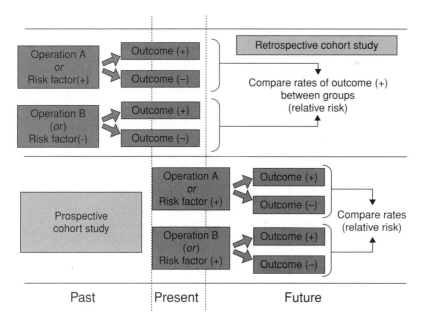

Figure 1 Schematic representation of a cohort study used to study outcomes for pediatric surgical diseases. In the classic design, patients with exposure to a risk factor of interest are identified and followed over time to determine whether an outcome (i.e., disease) develops. The rate of disease in the exposed group is then compared to the rate of disease in a similar cohort of patients who were not exposed to the risk factor of interest. For pediatric surgical diseases, outcomes of interest can also be compared for different therapeutic interventions.

There are many advantages to prospective cohort studies when used to study rare pediatric surgery conditions. These studies provide a clear temporal sequence of exposure (or operation) and outcome, therefore allowing for the calculation of incidence rates for the outcome in both exposed and nonexposed subjects. This is what is meant by defining the natural history of the exposure as it relates to the development of disease. Comparison of these rates between groups allows for the reporting of relative risk with developing an outcome based on previous exposure to a risk factor. The basic framework of the cohort design can be used to develop multi-institutional databases to characterize the natural history of pediatric surgical diseases before and following treatment. Another advantage of the cohort design is that it allows for the study of multiple outcomes of interest simultaneously. Examples of such databases currently used to study pediatric surgical diseases include the Congenital Diaphragmatic Hernia study group and the NIH-sponsored biliary atresia clinical research consortium (8,9).

There are also several important limitations with using cohort designs to study pediatric surgical diseases. Prospective cohort studies are not particularly suited for the study of rare outcomes given the large number of patients that are required to arrive at statistically meaningful conclusions. Furthermore, it is not practical to study diseases where a long temporal gap between exposure and outcome is anticipated. In this regard, the resources required to follow up on a relatively large number of patients over a prolonged time period can be both prohibitively expensive and logistically challenging. Specific to retrospective cohort studies, reliance on chart review and patient survey forms for the procurement of study data can pose significant challenges with accurate and thorough data collection. Although chart review and survey techniques are also used for prospective collection, these tools are much less effective when data are collected in a delayed fashion. Furthermore, given the fact that patients received treatment prior to the time the study was even conceived, the likelihood that there will be significant differences in covariates between groups is greater than in prospective studies.

Case-Control Studies
In the case-control design, a group of patients are initially identified with an outcome (e.g., disease) and then examined retrospectively to determine what proportion were exposed to a risk factor (or operation) of interest (Fig. 2). Controls without the outcome are then identified and the same proportions of exposed to unexposed patients are calculated and compared with

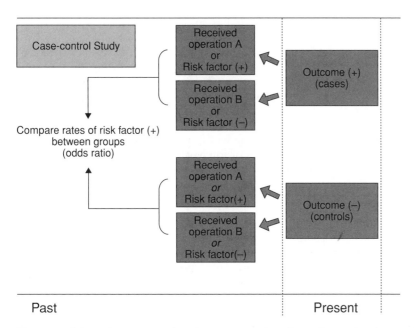

Past | Present

Figure 2 Schematic representation of a case-control study used to study outcomes for pediatric surgical diseases. In the classic design, patients with an outcome (i.e., disease) of interest are identified and compared to a similar group of patients who have not developed the outcome. The two groups are then compared with respect to their rates of previous exposure to a risk factor of interest. For the study of pediatric surgical diseases, outcomes of interest can include complications or clinically relevant endpoints (e.g., death), while exposures can be redefined as different interventional therapies.

the first group. Statistical analysis is then used to determine whether there is an association between outcome and exposure to the risk factors of interest. For example, an investigator may wish to examine whether postoperative abscesses following laparoscopic appendectomy for perforated appendicitis is associated with the use of intraoperative irrigation. They would start by identifying all patients who developed a postoperative abscess (outcome of interest) and compare them to a control group with perforated appendicitis who did not develop this complication. The proportion of patients in each group who underwent irrigations during their operation could then be compared to determine if a difference exists.

Case-control designs are useful in the study of pediatric surgical diseases for many reasons. First, they are relatively easy to perform and inexpensive compared with randomized trials and cohort studies. The case-control design also offers an efficient means to study rare conditions and infrequent outcomes as all patients with the disease are identified at the onset of the study. Although by definition case-control studies allow for the study of only one outcome at a time, the design allows for the study of multiple risk factors simultaneously (unlike cohort studies). It is this aspect of the case-control design which lends data from multiple risk factors to be analyzed with logistic regression methods.

Given that case-control studies are less expensive and easier to perform than cohort studies and RCTs, why not use this design to study all pediatric surgical diseases? The main answer lies in the inability of case-control studies to establish *causality* between exposure to a risk factor and development of disease (or other outcome). This is a subtle but important distinction between cohort and case-control data, and underlies the critical difference between these two study designs with respect to the relative strength of their reported associations. In the case of cohort studies, all exposed and unexposed patients are followed over time and the incidence of the outcome can then be determined for both groups. The risk of developing the outcome based on exposure can then be calculated and reported as a comparison with the incidence seen in the unexposed group. In case-control studies, the rate or incidence of an outcome cannot be determined as the denominator of all exposed patients leading to the observed outcomes is not known. Therefore, we can only describe relationships between exposure and outcomes data from case-control studies as an association rather than a true risk. It is this reason why comparison data from a case-control study are reported as an *odds ratio* while that from cohort study are reported as a *relative risk*.

In addition to the inability to establish causality, case-control studies are also very prone to bias due to their reliance upon retrospective data collection through chart review, surveys, and parental interviews. In this regard, recall bias can also pose a significant problem with respect to the ability to accurately collect exposure data between cases and controls. For example, mothers of children with birth defects are more likely to remember suspected risk factors (e.g., prenatal medications) than mothers with healthy children (10). Selection of representative cases may also prove challenging. The cases investigators are able to identify for inclusion into the study may not be representative of all cases with the outcome of interest. This is known as selection or sampling bias and may greatly impact the generalizability of results to the patient population with the disease as a whole.

Case Reports and Case-Series Studies

Case reports represent the most basic of clinical studies and are often used to report an experience with a new therapy or unexpected outcome. Unique to surgical diseases, investigators may also use these studies to report novel operative techniques or experience with new devices. The case-series study differs from the case report in that it reports on a number of patients treated in the same manner; usually by the same surgeon or group of surgeons at a single institution. In this capacity, case reports have played an important role in the dissemination of information regarding the evolution of operative technique for many pediatric surgical diseases. Case reports and case-series studies have come to comprise greater than half of all clinical studies reported in the pediatric surgical literature (3).

The primary weakness of case-reports and case-series data is the lack of a proper control group. These studies offer no information about outcomes in the same patient population resulting from a different treatment or the absence of treatment altogether. Furthermore, there is often no discussion of why the patients reported were chosen to undergo the procedure they did, nor why this specific series of patients were reported. Some authors have attempted to report a comparison to historical controls from their own institution or even to other published case-series data. These comparisons are seldom valid due to the potentially significant variation between groups with respect to disease severity, presence of comorbid conditions, operative technique, and perioperative care. Such comparisons should always be viewed with extreme caution, particularly if there is an attempt to use statistical analysis in the reporting of outcomes.

WHAT IS THE CURRENT STATUS OF EBM IN THE PEDIATRIC SURGERY LITERATURE?

How do we as a field compare with other areas of pediatric medicine with respect to the strength of our published clinical evidence? The most comprehensive review of this subject was undertaken by Hardin et al. in 1999, where they categorized over 9000 published clinical manuscripts from the major pediatric surgery journals over a 22-year period (3). They found that prospective clinical studies were exceedingly rare and randomized trials comprised far less than 1% of the pediatric surgery literature. In all, they found nearly 98% of all published reports were either case reports or single institutional case-series data. In a more contemporary study examining a five-year audit of the pediatric surgical literature, Rangel et al. found that over 96% of all clinical studies reporting on greater than five patients were retrospective in design (Fig. 3) (4). In a follow-up study, Rangel et al. examined the distribution of published evidence in support of commonly performed laparoscopic procedures in pediatric surgery (4). Only four randomized trials were found and 93% of all studies were retrospective, single-institutional reports. Furthermore, less than one quarter of all studies utilized a control group in the analysis of outcomes data. This would suggest that the relative paucity of high-quality prospective data is not limited to rare conditions or novel operative procedures, but rather reflects an alarming ongoing trend of how we as a field evaluate our operative interventions.

In addition to characterizing the relative distribution of study designs, other investigators have attempted to examine the methodological quality of published evidence. Moss et al. used

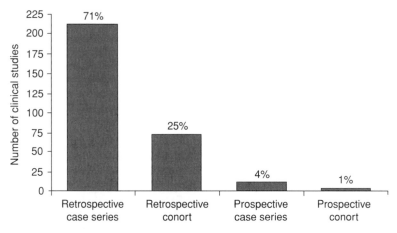

Figure 3 Distribution of clinical evidence by study design as published in the *Journal of Pediatric Surgery* during the five-year period, 1997–2002 (studies reporting five or more patients; *N* = 300 studies). *Source*: From Ref. 4.

a validated and standardized reporting checklist to examine the quality of RCTs published in the pediatric surgical literature (6). They found that the majority of these studies were plagued with significant methodological flaws in all aspects of study design and conduct, including randomization protcocols, data management techniques, and statistical analysis. Furthermore, in addition to confirming the relative paucity of RCTs in the surgical literature, they found the majority of studies were focused on comparing nonoperative therapies such as postoperative pain regimens and antibiotic usage. A much broader assessment of the quality of the clinical literature was undertaken by Rangel et al. in 2003 (4). They developed a standardized set of reporting criteria deemed essential for the nonbiased reporting surgical outcomes data. These criteria included descriptions of participating surgeons, patient characteristics, operative therapy, perioperative care, and statistical analysis. The authors used these criteria to audit a five-year cross section of all clinical studies reporting outcomes of greater than five patients published in the *Journal of Pediatric Surgery*. They found significant deficiencies in all major categories of reporting detail. In the majority of published studies, the reader could not determine how patients were chosen, who exactly performed the study, and whether any efforts had been made to ensuring all participating surgeons were performing the same operation.

The relative paucity of RCTs and other high-quality prospective studies in the pediatric surgical literature is in stark contrast to other areas of pediatric medicine. This is perhaps no better illustrated than in the field of pediatric oncology, where currently over three-quarters of all children with cancer are actively enrolled in a clinical trial. The impact of these efforts on patient care has been indisputable. Perhaps the most notable accomplishment in this regard has been in treatment of acute lymphocytic anemia, where mortality has decreased nearly 70%. This has occurred not from the development and testing of novel chemotherapeutic agents, but rather from rigorous studies examining modifications of existing multidrug regimens. Although difficult to establish, it is estimated that less than 0.1% of all children undergoing a surgical procedure are enrolled in a clinical trial of any type (6).

Why haven't RCTs had the same impact in pediatric surgery as they have had in other fields? The answer is complex and multifactorial. Pediatric surgical diseases are often quite rare, and it is difficult for even the largest childrens' hospitals to amass enough patients to come to statistically meaningful conclusions in a reasonable amount of time. Such issues require the development of multi-institutional cooperative groups such as those dedicated to pediatric oncology (11,12). Development of a multi-institutional framework to support such a large-scale study can pose significant logistical challenges and command significant financial resources. This is particularly challenging in the study of surgical diseases, where NIH funding has become relatively scarce and there is little motivation for drug companies to subsidize high-quality studies (as compared to studies comparing drugs) (13,14). In addition to financial considerations, there are several other potential challenges which are unique to studying pediatric surgical diseases (Table 2).

Table 2 Potential Barriers to using Randomized Clinical Trials and Other High Quality
Prospective Studies to Study Outcomes for Pediatric Surgical Diseases

Lack of existing infrastructure and financial resources to perform multicenter studies
Lack of equipoise among surgeons regarding standards of care and practice guidelines
Difficulty with blinding investigators and patients to surgical procedures
Challenges with standardizing operative technique and perioperative care
Reluctance of parents to randomize their children into potentially invasive treatment arms
Lack of willingness of surgeons to randomize patients into treatments they are less familiar with

HOW TO APPROACH THE CLINICAL EVIDENCE FOR THE SYNTHESIS OF EVIDENCE-BASED DECISIONS?

Now that we have an understanding of the utility and limitations of different study designs, how do we effectively and efficiently conduct a search for the best possible evidence for our clinical question? In 1995, Richardson formulated an evidence-based model for formulating a clinical question, also known as the Patient/Population/Problem, Intervention, Comparison, and Outcomes/Effects model (15). The utility of this model is the ability to use components of the structured question as key search terms for databases such as PubMed and others. This approach to results is a much more efficient and standardized method of literature search than by key word terms alone. The methodology for this strategy is beyond the scope of this chapter, but readers are encouraged to review the PICO approach from several useful sources in the references (15,16).

Approach to Reviewing RCTs

Although randomized trials are relatively rare in the pediatric surgical literature, many RCTs published in the nonsurgical literature can be of particular relevance to the practicing surgeon (e.g., advances in chemotherapy which may change the indication for operative management). As such, practicing surgeons should have a basic knowledge of proper study design if they are to effectively interpret the results of these studies and generalize results to their own patient population. Although these details are discussed below in the context of a RCT, most will be applicable to any published clinical study. The reader is encouraged to keep these concepts in mind when reviewing observational studies as well.

So what are the important elements of a published RCT to elicit? When evaluating a RCT, there are several essential attributes which need to be examined. First, it must be clear what primary question the study is designed to answer. Although properly performed subgroup analyses can be useful, the study needs to be clearly focused around a primary clinical question. Next, the therapeutic regimen (or operation) needs to be clearly described with respect to clinically relevant details as well as attempts to standardize therapy. The author should also clearly state the inclusion and exclusion criteria used in the study as well as information on the outcome of those ultimately not enrolled. This information is crucial to help the reader determine the generalizability of study subjects to their own patient population.

Another important element in the design and conduct of a clinical trial surrounds the concept of blinding. Investigators should provide information on how these steps are performed, and whether the blinding is single or double. To ensure that the placebo effect is minimized, efforts should be made to ensure patients, and preferably their family members as well, are blinded to the treatment they received. There are obvious challenges to blinding surgeons to the treatment rendered, so the design of double blinding is essentially relevant only to studies comparing medical interventions. In the absence of adequate blinding methods, it is possible that the treating (or evaluating) investigator or evaluator can influence the outcome as a result of their own bias. For example, if the patient is aware that they had a laparoscopic procedure compared to an open procedure, they may report less postoperative pain due to the increased satisfaction with cosmesis as they see this as an advantage of this approach. Alternatively, if the surgeon believes that patients treated via a laparoscopic approach will have a shorter ileus, they may feed these patients earlier than a similar patient treated by the open approach. Although bias surrounding blinding issues cannot be entirely avoided, the methods of addressing these issues must be clearly described in the methods section to best evaluate the conclusions of the study.

Understanding how patients are randomized in the study is also important to ensure that the conclusions are not potentially biased. For example, if patients are randomized based on treating surgeon or hospital, differential outcomes may simply be related to these factors and not the treatment of interest. In addition, if the surgeon is able to predict how the patient they are about to enroll in a study will be randomized, they may bias the patients' choice to enter or refuse entry into the study based on their own bias for a particular treatment.

The final area that needs to be assessed in evaluating an RCT is the statistical analysis, an area that is perhaps the most challenging for most of us to assess. Although a thorough discussion of statistical analysis methods are beyond the scope of this review, there is one basic principle that the reader should be familiar with: sample size and power. It is important that the authors report how the sample size was determined and whether the statistical power of their study was reached. If the study is underpowered, that is, there are too few patients in each arm of the study to reliably identify a difference between groups, then the results may not be valid. Utilizing an underpowered study to direct treatment choices, especially when stating that two treatments are equivalent, is a clear misinterpretation of the results.

As for attempts to standardize the reporting quality of clinical trials, the Consolidated Standards for the Reporting of Clinical Trials (CONSORT) statement was launched in 1996 (17,18). The CONSORT statement was developed by an international consortium of epidemiologists and clinical researchers who developed a checklist of 22 items to gauge the reporting quality of published clinical trials. These criteria included critical details with respect to study design, conduct, and accurate reporting. All major peer-reviewed journals have since adopted these guidelines as mandatory for publication, including the *Journal of Pediatric Surgery*, which became the first surgical journal to adopt the checklist in 2001 (19). Although the quality of RCTs has improved with wide-spread implementation of the CONSORT guidelines, the practitioner should have an understanding of the considerations behind these guidelines so that they can conduct a more knowledgeable review of a published RCT. Furthermore, this knowledge is critical for the review of less contemporary trials, as RCTs published as little as only a few years ago may not have been subjected to the CONSORT criteria.

Approach to Reviewing Nonrandomized Clinical Studies

What about the other 95% of the pediatric surgery literature? Although the CONSORT statement has had a positive impact on the quality of published clinical trials, these studies remain exceedingly rare in the pediatric surgery literature. A more generic approach is required to evaluate the remainder of the surgical literature, much of which is retrospective and potentially heavily biased. In 2003, Rangel et al. developed a set of standardized reporting criteria deemed essential for the nonbiased reporting of all clinical studies reporting on surgical conditions (4). These criteria were developed to ensure the essential details were provided so that the reader could assess the generalizability of study data to their own patient population. These criteria aimed to determine whether adequate details were furnished regarding the operating surgeons, enrolled patients, standardization of operative care, statistical analysis, and follow-up methods. The criteria were developed not to gauge the methodological quality of a published study, but rather the degree of transparent reporting. The utility in such criteria surround their role in uncovering key biases prevalent in retrospective data. In 2006, the *Journal of Pediatric Surgery* adopted these guidelines as mandatory for manuscript submission (Table 3). Readers are encouraged to use the checklist as a guide when reviewing the results of any clinical study, including RCTs.

CONCLUSION

Over the past several decades, the field of pediatric surgery has made incredible strides in the understanding of childhood surgical diseases and their operative management. On the heels of these advances, we have also witnessed the development and implementation of new, exciting and innovative operative techniques, and cutting edge technology. However, we must now face the challenge of rigorously evaluating our own operative therapies to ensure our patients are receiving the best possible surgical care. It is no longer acceptable to choose an intervention based on that fact that "we've always done it that way" or because "that's how I was trained." It is our ethical responsibility to critically evaluate these therapies to prove their safety, efficacy, and

Table 3   Checklist of Essential Details for the Reporting of Clinical Studies for Pediatric
Surgical Diseases

Reporting criteria relevant to all clinical studies
Description of participating surgeons/institutions
Can the number of participating centers be determined?
Can the practice type of participating centers be determined?
Can the number of surgeons who actually operated in the study be determined?
Can the reader determine the authors' prior experience with the reported procedure?
Is the timeline when all cases were performed clearly documented?

Description and definition of cases
Was the patient population from which the cases were selected from described?
Are the diagnostic criteria used to identify cases clearly documented?
Are selection and/or exclusion criteria for cases clearly documented?

Description of the intervention
Is the surgical technique adequately described?
Do the authors mention any attempt to standardize operative technique?
Do the authors mention any attempt to standardize perioperative care?

Analysis of outcome data
Is the mean *and* range of relevant demographic variables (e.g., age) reported?
Are outcome variables presented with appropriate measures of variability (e.g., SD)?
Are diagnostic methods for assessing outcome(s) of interest clearly described?
Do the authors address whether there is any missing data?
Is the number and nature of complications addressed?

Reporting criteria for studies using one or more comparison groups
Is the mean *and* range of relevant demographic variables (e.g., age) reported for all groups?
Are the timelines for interventions clearly documented for each treatment group?
Are actual numbers furnished along with statistical measures for demographic variables?
Are outcome variables presented with appropriate measures of variability for each group?
Do the authors describe how patients were selected into different treatment groups?
Are *Exact* type I error measurements provided for outcomes compared between groups?
Note: Reporting *P* values as <0.01 is acceptable.
Was any attempt made to blind evaluators during the analysis of outcomes data?

Source: From Ref. 4.

effectiveness for our patients. The concept of EBM provides us with a framework to accomplish this task and to gauge the relative strength of evidence in support of the different therapeutic options which are available to us. Having a firm working knowledge of how to critically evaluate the clinical evidence is essential if the pediatric surgeon is to effectively implement EBM into clinical decision making. Furthermore, this knowledge provides the clinician with framework for preparing clinical manuscripts with greater transparency and clinical utility.

REFERENCES

1. Sackett DL. Evidence-Based Medicine: How to Practice and Teach EBM. 2nd ed. New York: Churchill Livingstone, 2000.
2. Woolf SH, Battista RN, Anderson GM, et al. Assessing the clinical effectiveness of preventive maneuvers: Analytic principles and systematic methods in reviewing evidence and developing clinical practice recommendations. A report by the Canadian Task Force on the Periodic Health Examination. J Clin Epidemiol 1990; 43(9):891–905.
3. Hardin WD Jr, Stylianos S, Lally KP. Evidence-based practice in pediatric surgery. J Pediatr Surg 1999; 34(5):908–912; discussion 912–913.
4. Rangel SJ, Kelsey J, Henry MC, et al. Critical analysis of clinical research reporting in pediatric surgery: Justifying the need for a new standard. J Pediatr Surg 2003; 38(12):1739–1743.
5. Rangel SJ, Henry MC, Brindle M, et al. Small evidence for small incisions: Pediatric laparoscopy and the need for more rigorous evaluation of novel surgical therapies. J Pediatr Surg 2003; 38(10):1429–1433, review.
6. Moss RL, Henry MC, Dimmitt RA, et al. The role of prospective randomized clinical trials in pediatric surgery: State of the art? J Pediatr Surg 2001; 36(8):1182–1186.

7. Moss RL, Dimmitt RA, Henry MC, et al. A meta-analysis of peritoneal drainage versus laparotomy for perforated necrotizing enterocolitis. J Pediatr Surg 2001; 36(8):1210–1213.
8. Clark RH, Hardin WD Jr, Hirschl RB, et al. Current surgical management of congenital diaphragmatic hernia: A report from the Congenital Diaphragmatic Hernia Study Group. J Pediatr Surg 1998; 33(7):1004–1009.
9. Hoofnagle JH. Biliary Atresia Research Consortium (BARC). Hepatology 2004; 39(4):891; no abstract available.
10. Schlesselman JJ, Stolley PD. Case Control Studies: Design, Conduct Analysis. New York: Oxford University Press, 1982.
11. Lukens JN. Progress resulting from clinical trials. Solid tumors in childhood cancer. Cancer 1994; 74(9 Suppl):2710–2718; review.
12. Ross JA, Severson RK, Pollock BH, et al. Childhood cancer in the United States. A geographical analysis of cases from the Pediatric Cooperative Clinical Trials groups. Cancer 1996; 77(1):201–207.
13. Rangel SJ, Moss RL. Recent trends in the funding and utilization of NIH career development awards by surgical faculty. Surgery 2004; 136(2):232–239.
14. Rangel SJ, Efron B, Moss RL. Recent trends in National Institutes of Health funding of surgical research. Ann Surg 2002; 236(3):277–286; discussion 286–287.
15. Richardson WS, Detsky AS. Users' guides to the medical literature. VII. How to use clinical decision analysis. B. What are the results and will they help me in caring for my patients. Evidence Based Medicine Working Group. JAMA 1995; 273(20):1610–1613.
16. da Costa Santos CM, de Mattos Pimenta CA, Nobre MR. The PICO strategy for the research question construction and evidence search. Rev Lat Am Enfermagem. 2007; 15(3):508–511.
17. Altman DG. Better reporting of randomised controlled trials: The CONSORT statement. BMJ 1996; 313(7057):570–571; no abstract available.
18. Rennie D. How to report randomized controlled trials. The CONSORT statement. JAMA 1996; 276(8):649; no abstract available.
19. Moss RL. The CONSORT statement: Progress in clinical research in pediatric surgery. J Pediatr Surg 2001; 36(12):1739–1742, no abstract available.

SECTION II | Error Reduction: An Individual and Technical Approach

8 | Complications of Head and Neck Surgery

Jennifer Hall Aldrink, M.D. and Michael A. Skinner, M.D.

INTRODUCTION

Lesions of the head and neck are encountered frequently in the pediatric age group. Although these lesions often prove to be inflammatory or congenital in origin, malignant processes must always be suspected and ruled out. Malignant and benign lesions may be differentiated by the age of presentation and the physical characteristics of the lesion and its surrounding structures (1). Distinguishing between congenital, inflammatory, and malignant lesions is not always clear and may provide a significant challenge.

This chapter will review complications of head and neck lesions encountered in pediatric surgery. The discussion will include errors in diagnosis, errors in perioperative management, and technical complications of the surgical management of head and neck abnormalities.

ERRORS IN DIAGNOSIS

The most important goal in the evaluation of head and neck lesions in the pediatric population are to differentiate between benign and malignant processes. Malignant lesions of the head and neck are rarely present at birth, usually occurring later in childhood or adolescence. The majority of lesions encountered in infancy and early childhood are congenital or inflammatory in origin.

The key to making the correct diagnosis lies in the initial history and careful physical examination. When obtaining an accurate history, the age of initial presentation, duration of the lesion, changing characteristics, and associated symptoms should be sought. A history of a recent dental procedure can provide information about a subsequent inflammatory reaction in the neck. Exposure to household pets such as cats or birds can direct the search toward an infectious agent such as cat-scratch disease or toxoplasmosis. A history of exposure to radiation or even radiation therapy for benign diseases such as acne should raise the suspicion for malignancy. An acutely appearing lesion suggests one of inflammatory or infectious origin, whereas an enlarging mass over time is more likely to be malignant. Additionally, a mass present at birth or appearing shortly after is typical of congenital lesions. Other symptoms such as pain, dysphagia, hoarseness, hemoptysis, persistent cough, changes in hearing or smell, or nasal obstruction are important in determining the etiology of the mass lesion.

A thorough physical examination should seek to define the characteristics of the lesion, including its location, consistency and texture, fixation to adjacent tissues, tenderness, or associated draining sinus. Table 1 outlines the differential diagnosis for cervical masses in children.

Imaging Modalities

While diagnosing head and neck lesions is largely based on history and physical examination findings, imaging modalities play a crucial role in defining the characteristics of the lesion, determining its extension and relationship to surrounding structures, and identifying its functionality.

Ultrasonography is widely employed in the differentiation and diagnosis of various head and neck lesions. It is relatively inexpensive and is noninvasive, making it the initial study of choice in many situations (2). It is valuable in distinguishing solid masses such as thyroid nodules, lymph nodes, or tumors from cystic masses such as branchial cleft cysts or thyroglossal duct cysts. In addition, abnormalities such as hemangiomas or arteriovenous malformations (AVMs) may be characterized by ultrasound, demonstrating blood flow within these lesions. As an initial study, ultrasound may eliminate the need for further imaging studies. For example,

Table 1   Differential Diagnosis of Cervical Masses in Children

Congenital masses
Hemangioma
Cystic hygroma
Thyroglossal duct cyst
Branchial cleft cyst
Dermoid cyst
Teratoma
Foregut cyst
Laryngocele

Inflammatory masses
Cervical lymphadenopathy (bacterial or viral origin)
Abscesses
Mononucleosis
Sialadenitis
Cat-scratch disease
Tuberculosis
Sarcoidosis
Amyloidosis
Granulomatous lymphadenopathy

Neoplastic

Benign
Lipoma
Hemangioma
Thyroid nodule
Epidermoid inclusion cyst
Fibroma
Neurobibroma
Schwannoma
Paraganglioma
Salivary gland mass
Ranula
Torticollis

Malignant
Hodgkin disease
Non-Hodgkin lymphoma
Leukemia
Rhabdomyosarcoma
Neuroblastoma
Thyroid carcinoma
Salivary gland malignancy
Germ cell malignancy
Metastatic tumors

Source: From Ref. 9.

demonstrating normal thyroid parenchyma in a euthyroid patient with a thyroglossal duct cyst renders additional studies such as thyroid scintigraphy unnecessary (3).

Computed tomography (CT) provides accurate information in the evaluation of neck masses. It can demonstrate details of a mass or cyst location, the tract of a cystic lesion such as a thyroglossal duct or branchial cleft cyst, and its relationship to surrounding structures (4). CT scanning may be useful, for example, when a thyroglossal duct cyst is located off the midline, or if the diagnosis of such a lesion is in question. In addition, some congenital anomalies or malignancies of the head and neck not uncommonly extend into the mediastinum. A CT scan may be obtained to determine the extent of such a lesion and relationship to these structures (5). Figure 1(A) depicts a CT image of a lymphatic malformation, illustrating its intimate anatomic relationship with nearby structures. Likewise, contrast CT imaging is also valuable for vascular lesions such as complex hemangiomas or AVMs.

Magnetic resonance imaging (MRI) is often performed for head and neck lesions that other imaging modalities may not be able to clearly define. Like CT imaging, MRI differentiates

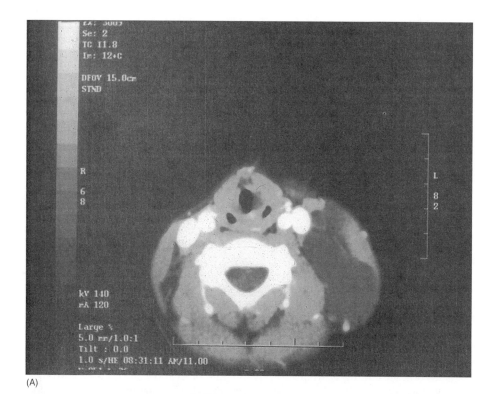

Figure 1 (A) Computed tomography scan of a lymphatic malformation illustrating anatomic relationships. (B) MRI of lymphatic malformation.

between cystic and solid lesions, determines the extent of invasion of the lesion in question, and demonstrates blood flow within a suspected vascular mass. MRI is excellent for lymphatic malformations of the head and neck region by defining lymphatic malformations in relation to neurovascular and soft tissue structures [Fig. 1(B)] (6). Disadvantages include a higher cost and requirement for sedation or anesthesia in small children.

Radioiodine thyroid scanning is useful to obtain preoperatively in anterior neck masses such as thyroid nodules or thyroglossal duct cysts, by demonstrating the presence of normal and ectopic thyroid tissue (7). Thyroid scanning is employed to determine the function of a thyroid nodule, and to define and locate the presence of normal thyroid tissue prior to surgical excision, thereby preventing the inadvertent removal of solitary thyroid tissue in a patient and rendering them hypothyroid. In the evaluation of thyroglossal duct cysts, some advocate thyroid scanning on all patients, while others advocate scanning only when the cyst is present at the base of the tongue, due to the 1% to 2% incidence of ectopic thyroid tissue in these cases (8).

Additional imaging modalities are obtained depending on the location of the lesion in question and accompanying symptoms of the patient. Chest radiographs ought to be obtained on all patients with suspected malignancy or respiratory symptoms. In particular, children with cervical adenopathy should undergo chest radiography to rule out the presence of a mediastinal mass that could complicate the induction of anesthesia. Patients who have a mediastinal mass identified should undergo a CT scan of the chest to assess for tracheal and bronchial compression. Bronchoscopy, laryngoscopy, or esophagoscopy may be necessary if warranted by the location of the lesion. Fistulography or parotid sialography may be useful in differentiating a branchial cleft remnant from other anomalies such as solid tumors, lymphatic malformations, lymphomas, or benign lymphadenopathy. Endoscopy of the upper airway may be considered for various lesions presenting with stridor, dysphagia, or cyanosis, such as a lymphatic malformation that may involve the pharynx or larynx (Fig. 2) (5). Barium contrast swallow or endoscopy may be necessary to differentiate pyriform sinus lesions from branchial cleft sinuses (1).

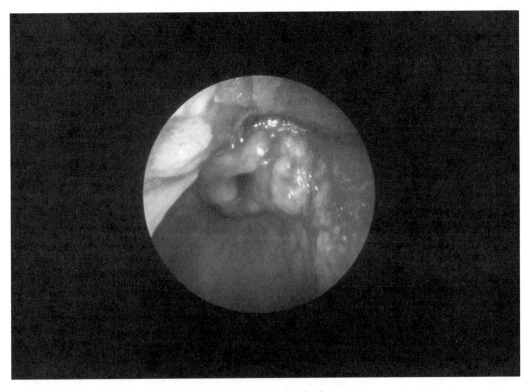

Figure 2   Endoscopic view of lymphatic malformation involving the larynx.

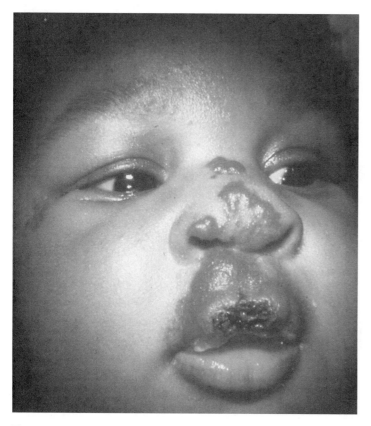

Figure 3 Hemagnioma of nose and upper lip.

Congenital Anomalies

Hemangiomas and vascular malformations account for the most frequently occurring head and neck lesions (5). They are rarely present at birth, but may appear within the first few weeks of life, gradually increasing in size over the first year of life (1). The majority of hemangiomas spontaneously regress by 3 to 4 years of age and are usually observed without intervention during this time. Exceptions to observation include lesions located in the mouth or oropharynx, potentially interfering with adequate nutritional intake or resulting in respiratory difficulties, and those located in close proximity to the eye, affecting visual development. Hemangiomas are commonly located on the scalp, occiput, preauricular area, base of the nose, and angle of the jaw (Fig. 3). They may also involve the subglottic areas and thus are invisible to the examiner (1). These types of internal hemangiomas may present with stridor or other signs of respiratory obstruction. Hemangiomas can be classified as capillary, cavernous, or combined, with the capillary variation having the typical appearance of a "flattened strawberry" (1). Cavernous hemangiomas may be associated with AVMs and may develop quite rapidly in size. These can be distinguished from simple hemangiomas by an audible bruit or palpable thrill (5). Lymphatic malformations and encephaloceles should be considered in the differential diagnosis of hemangiomas (1).

Lymphatic malformations (Fig. 4) are congenital lesions of lymphatic origin that are often found in the posterior triangle of the neck (1). Rapid enlargement of these lesions may result from hemorrhage or infection in approximately one-third of patients, leading to signs and symptoms of respiratory obstruction with stridor, dysphagia, or cyanosis (1,9).

Thyroglossal duct remnants account for approximately 75% of midline neck masses in the pediatric population (10). Other midline masses considered in the differential diagnosis are listed in Table 2. The classic presentation is a midline, nontender, palpable mass that moves with swallowing. Additional presenting symptoms are seen in Table 3 (11). The cyst is usually encountered in the thyrohyoid location (60%) within 2 cm of the midline (Fig. 5); other locations seen less frequently include submental (25%), suprasternal (13%), and intralingual (2%) (10).

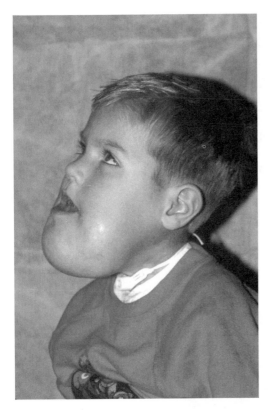 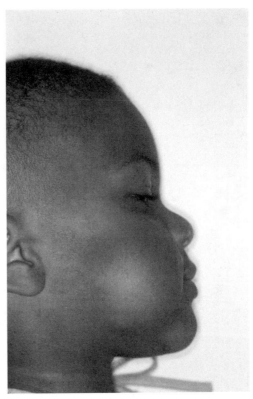

Figure 4 Lymphatic malformations involving the head and neck.

Table 2 Differential Diagnosis of Midline Neck Masses in Children

Lymphadenopathy
Pyramidal lobe of thyroid
Thyroid nodule
Thyroid adenoma
Thyroid carcinoma
Aberrant thyroid tissue
Branchial celft cyst
Dermoid cyst
Lipoma
Hemangioma
Lymphangioma
Teratoma
Laryngocele

Source: From Ref. 11.

Table 3 Presenting Symptoms of Thyroglossal Duct Cysts

Presenting Symptoms	% Patients
Midline painless mass	35.7
Midline mass fluctuating in size	30
Dysphagia	12.8
Infected fistula	10
Mid-neck tenderness	8.5
Cough	2.8

Source: From Ref. 11.

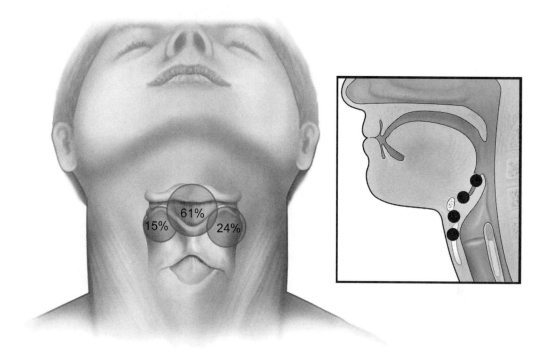

Figure 5   Variable locations of thyroglossal duct cyst.

In contrast to branchial cleft lesions, thyroglossal duct cysts typically do not drain through an external opening unless the cyst has become infected or recurs following resection or incomplete excision (Fig. 6) (1).

Lesions of the branchial clefts are far less common than those of the thyroglossal duct remnants. Second branchial cleft anomalies occur the most frequently, accounting for nearly 90%, while those of the first branchial cleft account for less than 10% (12–15). Anomalies of the third and fourth clefts are rare (9). The anomalies seen with branchial cleft remnants include cysts, fistulas, sinuses, and skin tags with cartilaginous remnants (1). They are usually located in the preauricular and submandibular areas and are intimately associated with the facial nerve (1). Congenital anomalies of the second branchial cleft are typically located along the anterior border of the sternocleidomastoid muscle.

Branchial cleft anomalies usually present with recurrent erythema, swelling, and/or mucoid discharge in the periauricular, submandibular, or anterior sternocleidomastoid regions (12). Children with these anomalies are often misdiagnosed as having recurrent cellulitis or abscesses. Although these anomalies are present at birth, several series in the literature have reported a delay in diagnosis of 3.5 to 4 years following the appearance of symptoms (12,14). In several case reviews, 25% to 50% of patients with branchial cleft anomalies had undergone multiple surgical procedures prior to definitive treatment because of errors in diagnosis (12–14). In one study, Ford found that an average number of 2.4 operations are performed per patient prior to cure (16). Unfortunately, recurrent infections and repeat operations result in fibrous tissue formation, making the definitive resection difficult with an increased chance of iatrogenic injury to surrounding structures, particularly the facial nerve (14).

Other less common congenital anomalies may present as masses in the head and neck region, and should be considered in the differential diagnosis of these presentations.

Congenital goiter, rare in the United States, is associated with maternal nutritional deficiencies and should be differentiated from thyroid malignancies (5). Ranula of the salivary gland (Fig. 7) presents as a sublingual or submental cyst. Its presentation can range from a small pea-sized swelling adjacent to the frenulum to a large cystic swelling in the submandibular or anterior midline. It is often confused with thyroglossal duct cysts, cervical dermoids, or enlarged

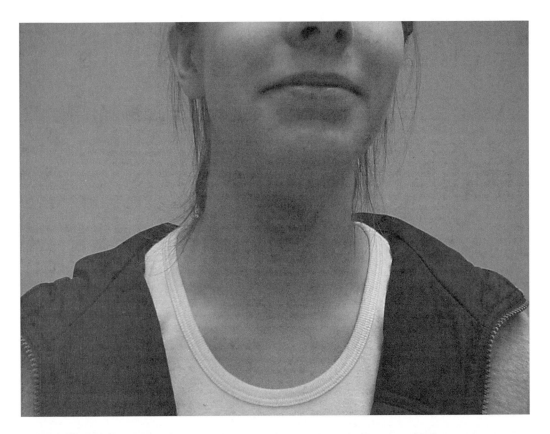

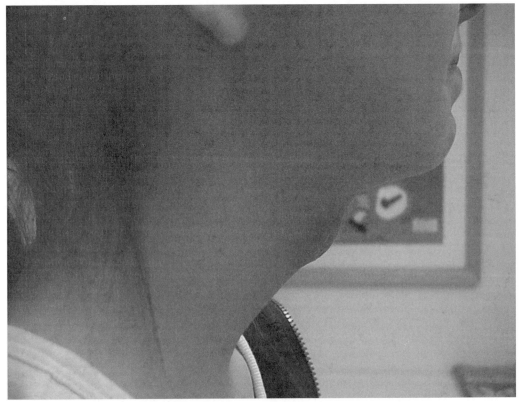

Figure 6   Appearance of a recently infected thyroglossal duct cyst.

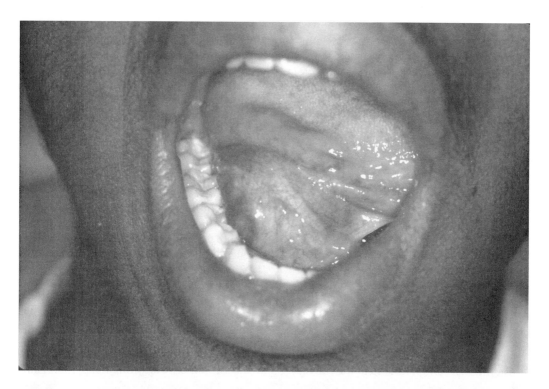

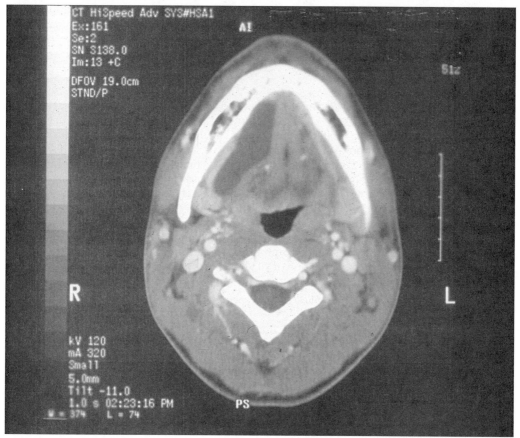

Figure 7 Sublingual cyst seen with salivary gland rannula.

lymph nodes (1). Torticollis, also known as fibromatosis colli, usually occurs in the middle to lower third of the sternocleidomastoid muscle and is associated with markedly limited range of motion of the head toward the side of the lesion (1). It presents as a fibrous mass and tightness of the sternocleidomastoid several weeks after birth, and is thought to be an idiopathic inflammatory process in the newborn period related to delivery events (9). These masses must be differentiated from neuroblastoma of the cervical sympathetic chain and rhabdomyosarcoma.

Tumors

Benign Tumors

Teratomas and dermoid cysts affect the head and neck in approximately 5% of cases (5,9). Tumors in this location are usually seen at or shortly after birth, and present with maternal polyhydramnios, respiratory obstruction, or feeding difficulties. Small lesions may not be detected until adolescence or adulthood. They are most often found in the nose, orbits, brow, forehead, and submental region of the neck (1,5) (Fig. 8). Those that overly the hyoid bone may be confused with thyroglossal duct cysts, but are generally more mobile and subcutaneous in nature.

Salivary gland tumors occur most often in the parotid, submandibular, or submaxillary salivary glands, but can arise in any of the minor glands found throughout the oral cavity as well. Hemangiomas and lymphatic malformations are the most commonly occurring benign tumors located in the salivary glands. As with other clinically apparent hemangiomas, most of these are simply observed and will spontaneously involute within 3 to 5 years. Pleomorphic or mixed tumors, Warthin tumors (papillary cystadenoma lymphomatosum) and cystadenomas are additional benign tumors of the salivary gland, most commonly affecting the parotid gland (9).

Plexiform neurofibromas are benign tumors of the peripheral nerves that occur in patients with neurofibromatosis-1 or von Recklinghausen disease. These types of neurofibromas appear early in childhood and progress in size throughout the individuals' life. They are removed due to their potential malignant degeneration and for distortion of surrounding structures.

Malignant Tumors

Rhabdomyosarcoma is the most common sarcoma occurring in children and the most common one found in the head and neck (9,17). Those arising in the head and neck region are classified into three anatomic categories: orbital, parameningeal (including the nasopharynx, nasal cavity, paranasal sinuses, infratemporal fossa, and middle ear), and nonparameningeal (17). These tumors are grouped according to the degree of resection achieved as outlined by the Intergroup Rhabdomyosarcoma Study shown in Table 4 (17). Other sarcomas are uncommon in children, but may include fibrosarcomas, liposarcomas, myosarcomas, malignant fibrous histiosarcomas, and vascular sarcomas.

Lymphomas are the third most common malignancy of children with approximately 60% of these being non-Hodgkin lymphomas (NHL) and 40% being Hodgkin disease (HD). Careful evaluation of any child with enlarged lymph nodes should be carried out, with attention to constitutional symptoms and examination of all nodal areas with measurement of any enlarged

Table 4   Intergroup Rhabdomyosarcoma Study Clinical Grouping System

Group	Definition
I	Localized disease, completely resected
	A. Confined to organ of origin, nodes not involved
	B. Contiguous involvement, nodes not involved
II	Compromised or regional resection
	A. Grossly resected disease
	B. Regional disease completely resected, nodes involved, may extend into adjacent organs
	C. Regional disease with grossly involved nodes, resected with microscopic residual
III	Incomplete resection, gross residual disease
IV	Metastatic disease present

Source: From Ref. 17.

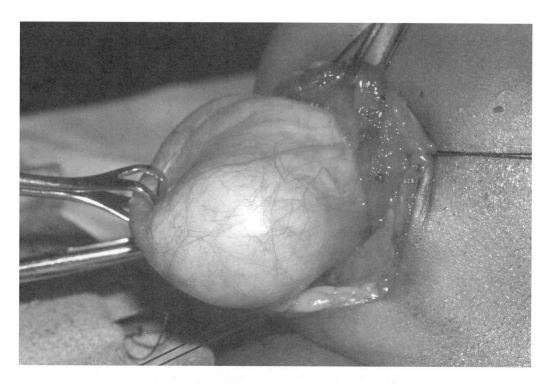

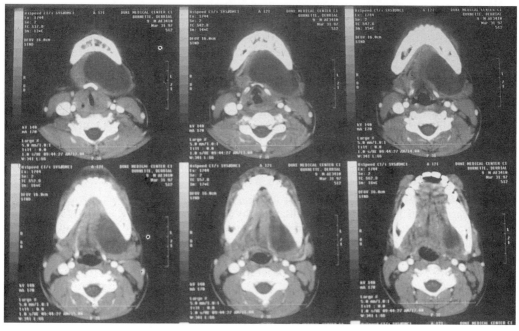

Figure 8 Teratoma arising within the neck.

nodes. Diagnosis of NHL or HD is made by histologic evaluation of surgically biopsied lymph nodes. Communication among the oncologist, surgeon, and pathologist is vital for proper specimen handling and preparation so that the combination of microscopic, molecular diagnostic, cytogenetic, and immunophenotypic studies may be performed.

Approximately 10% of all NHL in children occur in the head and neck (18). The primary sites of head and neck NHL include lymphoid tissue around the facial bones, in particular the mandible, maxillary sinus, thyroid gland, salivary glands, or lymph nodes in the neck (18).

Cutaneous lymphoma also occurs most commonly in the skin of the head and neck region. Rapidly enlarging tumors cause pain by invasion of surrounding nerves or pressure from mass effect. Those occurring in the mandible may present with a toothache or lip numbness.

Approximately half of all epithelial salivary gland tumors found in the pediatric population are malignant. These tumors often have an association with previous head and neck irradiation. The parotid gland is the most frequently affected salivary gland, while tumors occurring in the minor salivary glands are rare. The most common presentation is an asymptomatic swelling in the area of the affected gland. Fixation to skin or underlying structures, weakness, or paralysis of the facial muscles from facial nerve involvement, or lymph node enlargement indicates a high likelihood of malignancy (9). The most common salivary gland malignancy is mucoepidermoid carcinoma, accounting for approximately 50% of cases (9). Acinic cell carcinomas, adenocarcinomas, mixed, and undifferentiated carcinomas are less common primary salivary gland tumors encountered in children. Rhabdomyosarcoma and NHL have also been reported to occur in the salivary glands, most commonly the parotid (9).

Neuroblastoma is the most common solid tumor of childhood, but only rarely does the primary tumor present in the head and neck region. Enlarged nodes in the neck may represent the first sign of metastatic retroperitoneal or mediastinal disease (9). Primary neuroblastoma in the neck usually arises from the cervical sympathetic chain and presents as a painless, firm mass in the lateral neck. Occasionally, it may present as a retropharyngeal mass with symptoms of dysphagia, cough, or stridor (9). Congenital neuroblastoma is identified at birth, and must be differentiated from other congenital anomalies such as branchial cleft cysts, and tumors such as cervical teratomas that may also present as a neck mass in the newborn.

Approximately 5% of germ cell tumors occur in the head and neck region, usually presenting as a lateral or midline neck mass or rarely in the orbit, oropharynx, or nasopharynx (9). They may be congenital or present early in infancy. Congenital tumors of the oropharynx or large neck masses often present with maternal polyhydramnios, respiratory obstruction, or feeding difficulties. Germ cell tumors arising in the neck must be differentiated from benign lymphatic malformations and other malignant lesions. Tumors found in the nasopharynx must be distinguished from gliomas and encephaloceles.

Thyroid diseases of childhood are relatively rare, and tumors of the thyroid are exceedingly uncommon in this population. These diseases must still be suspected and included in the differential diagnosis of any mass lesion occurring in the neck as early diagnosis and treatment can result in excellent survival outcomes. Thyroid nodules in children have a higher likelihood of being malignant (20%) than their adult counterparts. The differential diagnosis of solitary thyroid nodules can be seen in Table 5.

Children with thyroid nodules typically present with an anterior neck mass in the setting of normal thyroid function. Examination of the neck should document the location, size, and consistency of the thyroid nodule as well as the gland itself. The presence of palpable lymph nodes increases the likelihood of a malignancy. Clinically, however, it is impossible to differentiate between a benign and malignant thyroid lesion by physical examination alone (19). Laboratory tests and imaging studies often add little to the detection of malignancy, as malignant thyroid nodules may be functional or nonfunctional, cystic, or solid. Despite the lack of reliability of radiographic studies in characterizing thyroid nodules as benign or malignant, some surgeons prefer their use to aid in preoperative localization (14,19). The role of fine needle aspiration cytology, a well-established tool to assist in the diagnosis of adult thyroid nodules is not as clearly defined in children. As outlined above, the diagnosis of a thyroid nodule in

Table 5   Differential Diagnosis of Thyroid Nodules in Children

- Carcinoma
- Adenoma
- Thyroid cyst
- Ectopic thyroid gland
- Thyroglossal duct remnant
- Cystic hygroma
- Germ cell tumor

Source: From Ref. 19.

children is far more complex than in adults. Previous studies have demonstrated that the incidence of malignancy in pediatric thyroid nodules is approximately 20% (19), and thus some surgeons advocate removal of all thyroid nodules in children less than age 13 regardless of further work up (19). The pattern of thyroid disease in adolescents is slightly different from that of younger children, and tends to follow the adult pattern of disease. In one large series, children aged 13 to 18 with thyroid nodules were found to have an incidence of malignancy of 11%, nearly half that of the younger age group (20). Therefore, adolescents with thyroid nodules should undergo more extensive evaluation in attempts to differentiate benign and malignant lesions similar to the evaluation of adults with thyroid nodules.

Thyroid carcinoma, representing 3% of all childhood malignancies, typically presents as an asymptomatic enlargement in the anterior neck with or without enlarged cervical lymph nodes. In children the cancer is usually more advanced at presentation, with lymph node metastases present in 30% to 90% of pathologic specimens (19–22). Occasionally, cervical lymphadenopathy may be the only presenting sign and must, therefore, be differentiated from other benign and malignant causes of enlarged nodes.

Infections

Benign cervical lymphadenopathy accounts for the majority of neck masses in children. Acute cervical lymphadenitis is easily identified by its inflammatory nature, but subacute or chronic infections may present with a similar picture as lymphoma. The decision to observe or biopsy an enlarged or concerning lymph node is not often clear. Generally, nodes are biopsied if they have persisted or progressed for several weeks despite appropriate antibiotic therapy, if additional affected nodal basins exist, or if the patient displays systemic signs of malignancy such as weight loss, night sweats, or fever.

Viral and bacterial etiologies account for most of the cervical lymphadenopathy encountered in the pediatric population. The diagnostic approach begins with a careful history with specific questions regarding recent upper respiratory infection, sinusitis, otitis media, pharyngitis, allergies, or constitutional symptoms. Physical examination often reveals an enlarged, mobile, fluctuant, and tender lymph node usually located in the anterior neck. The lymphadenopathy may be multiple and/or bilateral. Cervical lymphadenopathy that persists for 3 to 4 weeks is likely bacterial in origin, while viral etiologies produce a shorter, more self-limited course (1). Lymphadenopathy that fails to respond to antibiotic treatment may require needle aspiration to identify the causative organism or an alternate pathology. Although the yield of positive cultures from fine needle aspiration (FNA) of lymph nodes is only 15%, gram stain and culture (both aerobic and anaerobic) should be performed on all aspirates.

Cat-scratch disease is usually a benign, self-limiting regional lymphadenopathy following the inoculum of the gram-positive organism *Bartonella henselae*. Exposure via a lick, scratch, or bite of an animal carrier around the face can lead to subacute cervical lymphadenopathy. Salivary glands can also be infected. Early constitutional symptoms include fever and malaise, and most children have a mild, self-limited clinical course. Severe complications rarely occur, but may include encephalitis, neuroretinitis, and follicular conjunctivitis (1). Lymph node biopsy may reveal multiple microabscesses or granulomas, and the Warthin–Starry silver stain demonstrates pleiomorphic gram-positive bacilli. This disease typically resolves spontaneously in 6 to 8 weeks. If adenopathy persists or the history is unclear, a neoplastic process must be suspected and ruled out.

Mononucleosis caused by the Epstein–Barr virus is associated with cervical lymphadenopathy in the adolescent. The lymphadenopathy associated with mononucleosis is typically bilateral. Constitutional symptoms, pharyngitis, and hepatosplenomegaly generally accompany the presentation. The monospot test and/or Epstein–Barr virus titers are positive. With supportive treatment, the lymphadenopathy resolves within weeks.

Atypical mycobacteria are another cause of cervical lymphadenopathy. Lymph nodes are rubbery, firm, and nontender in their presentation, in contrast with the acutely inflamed picture typical of bacterial etiologies. If untreated, they may become matted forming a confluent mass or may be associated with a draining sinus (1,9). Constitutional symptoms in an immunocompetent child are usually absent, unless a superimposed pyogenic infection is present (9). Since cross reactivity exists between *Mycobacterium tuberculosis* and the other species, intradermal skin testing with tuberculin antigens may be valuable in achieving the correct diagnosis (23). Lymph node biopsy or needle aspiration reveals central caseating necrosis, granulomas, aggregates of histiocytes, or Langerhan giant cells (9). Incisional biopsy and FNA, however, often lead to recurrences or draining sinuses, thus complete excision is recommended for both diagnosis and definitive treatment.

Other Infections and Inflammatory Processes

Sialadenitis is a benign process occurring in the head and neck region in children. Sialadenitis can be distinguished from neoplastic processes by the presence of episodic pain and swelling in the location of the affected salivary gland. Acute suppurative sialadenitis is most commonly caused by infection with *Staphylococcus aureus* and is typically seen in infants. Other etiologic agents include mumps virus in inadequately immunized children, cat-scratch disease, atypical mycobacteria, Epstein–Barr virus, and tuberculosis. Chronic sialadenitis is often idiopathic, but may be attributable to drug sensitivity, iodine, food intolerance, poor oral hygiene, cystic fibrosis, recurrent tonsillitis, autoimmune processes, or sarcoidosis (9).

Fascial space infections most often originate from oropharyngeal, dental, or otorhinolaryngeal sites that can extend along the natural fascial planes of the neck into the deep cervical spaces (submandibular, lateral pharyngeal, retropharyngeal, and peritonsillar). These infections may also extend into compartments such as the carotid sheath and the mediastinum producing life-threatening complications.

Submandibular space infections, also known as Ludwig's angina, most commonly occur following infection of the second or third mandibular molars (9). This infection is characterized by an aggressive and rapidly spreading cellulitis involving the submandibular space. The patient may present with fever, mouth pain, tongue swelling, drooling, stiff neck, and dysphagia that can rapidly progress to airway obstruction. The submandibular area is tender to palpation and may have crepitus. Infection of the submandibular space may extend into the lateral pharyngeal space, retropharyngeal space, and occasionally mediastinum. In its course, the spreading infection may involve the epiglottis with resultant stridor and cyanosis from airway compromise.

Infections of the lateral pharyngeal space most commonly arise from dental or peritonsillar abscesses, parotitis, otitis, or mastoiditis. Clinical presentation of infections in the lateral pharyngeal space includes swelling and induration at the angle of the mandible, trismus, and systemic signs of infection (9).

Retropharyngeal space infections usually arise as a consequence of lymphatic spread from adenitis. Presentation of these infections consists of fever, drooling, dysphagia, and occasionally nuchal rigidity (9). If unrecognized, these infections can progress to airway obstruction from severe laryngeal edema.

Peritonsillar abscess or quinsy is a complication of acute tonsillitis. Fever, sore throat, dysphagia, pooling of saliva, trismus, and muffled voice are symptoms associated with its presentation. On physical examination, a swelling involving the anterior and possibly posterior tonsillar pillars is noted, and cervical lymphadenopathy is often present.

ERRORS IN PREOPERATIVE MANAGEMENT

Many lesions of the head and neck must be diagnosed rapidly, since delay or misdiagnosis may lead to catastrophic consequences such as airway obstruction, metastasis, aspiration, or sepsis. Once a diagnosis has been established, the appropriate management and timing of any intervention is determined. Errors in management may include improper perioperative nutrition and fluid management, improper timing of the surgery, and insufficient diagnostic studies prior to the procedure.

Perioperative Nutrition and Fluid Management

Preparation of the pediatric patient prior to head and neck surgery follows the same principles that apply to other body systems. Advances in knowledge about metabolism and the nutritional needs of the ill and perioperative patient have resulted in lower rates of morbidity and mortality (24). The nutritional requirements to meet the metabolic demands of a patient during an acute illness or injury are often quite different from their baseline needs. Table 6 outlines the basic age-related energy, protein, and nonprotein requirements in pediatric patients.

Table 6   Daily Nutritional Requirements of Pediatric Patients

Age	Calories (kcal/kg)	Protein (g/kg)	Electrolytes
Newborn (0—30 days)	100–120	2.5–3.0	Na 2–5 mEq/kg K 2–3 mEq/kg
1–6 mo	100–120	2.0–2.5	
6–12 mo	100–120	2.0–2.2	
1–6 yr	80–100	1.5–2.0	
6–12 yr	60–80	1.3–1.8	
>12 yr	30–60	1.0–1.5	

Source: From Ref. 24.

Careful assessment and monitoring of nutritional status constitutes part of the care of the pediatric patient. Growth patterns, weight gain, and nutritional parameters such as albumin, prealbumin, and serum transferrin should be closely followed both preoperatively and post-operatively in patients undergoing surgical interventions of the head and neck. Neoplastic processes, pharyngeal obstruction with cysts or masses, or recurrent infections of congenital cystic anomalies are all processes that may alter the nutritional status of a child and consequently affect the morbidity and/or mortality of the surgical intervention.

Euvolemia and electrolyte balance are a necessary part of the perioperative care of the pediatric patient with any surgical problem, including those of the head and neck. Patients with head and neck lesions may have difficulty with oral intake due to a mass or infection or may display anorexia as a constitutional symptom of a malignancy. Proper basal requirements and necessary replacements of fluids and electrolytes should be ensured, accounting for the usual daily losses from the respiratory, integumentary, gastrointestinal, and genitourinal systems. Adjustments must be made for changes in activity level, fever, and hypermetabolic states. Ongoing fluid losses from surgical drains, nasogastric tubes, fistulas, and open wounds must be accounted for and accurately replaced with the appropriately matched fluid.

Improper Timing of the Surgical Procedure

Optimizing a patient prior to surgical correction of a particular head and neck lesion may involve controlling infection, such as with infected congenital cystic anomalies or deep cervical fascial spaces. The proper timing of surgery in the setting of acute suppurative lesions in the head and neck may vary with the diagnosis. For example, an acutely presenting peritonsillar abscess is a surgical emergency, while a chronically draining branchial fistula may be treated with antibiotics and then excised on an elective basis.

Various other head and neck lesions dictate unique variables that affect the proper timing of surgical correction. Malignant processes may need coordination of adjuvant therapies with surgical resection. Other head and neck malignancies such as those of the thyroid or parathyroid may require additional preoperative preparation. Hyperfunctioning thyroid nodules should be controlled with antithyroid medication such as propylthiouracil or methimazole, reducing thyroid hormone production, and rendering the patient euthyroid (19). Propanolol may also be necessary perioperatively to control the hypermetabolic effects from hyperfunctioning nodules or goiters. Parathyroid adenomas or carcinomas may similarly require calcium stabilization prior to proceeding with surgical resection.

TECHNICAL COMPLICATIONS

Anatomic Structures at Risk

A thorough knowledge of the regional anatomy of the head and neck is important in avoiding injury to vital structures when performing resection or correction of lesions. The neck is divided into three main triangles: anterior, posterior, and suboccipital (Fig. 9). The anterior triangle is further subdivided into bilateral muscular triangles, bilateral carotid triangles, bilateral submandibular (also referred to as digastric) triangles, and a single midline submental triangle. The boundaries and contents of these triangles can be seen in Table 7.

Injuries to specific visceral, vascular, and nervous structures will be discussed in the following section. Figures 10 and 11 illustrate the relationship of major arterial and venous structures with other head and neck landmarks.

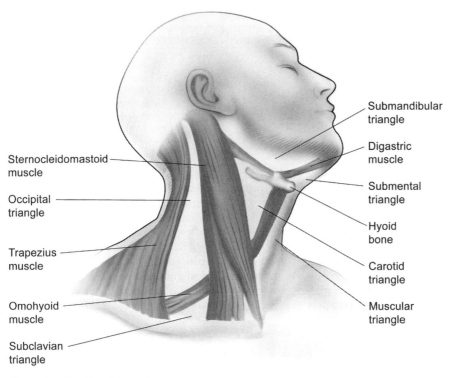

Sternocleidomastoid
muscle

Occipital
triangle

Trapezius
muscle

Omohyoid
muscle

Subclavian
triangle

Submandibular
triangle

Digastric
muscle

Submental
triangle

Hyoid
bone

Carotid
triangle

Muscular
triangle

Figure 9   Triangles of the neck.

Table 7   Triangles of the Neck

Triangle	Contents
Muscular	Thyroid gland
	Infrahyoid musculature (sternohyoid, sternothyroid, omohyoid, thyrohyoid)
	Recurrent laryngeal nerve
Carotid	Common carotid artery and bifurcation
	Internal jugular vein
	Cranial nerves X, XI, and XII
	Ansa cervicalis
	Hyoid bone
Submandibular	Submandibular gland
	Digastric muscles
	Stylohyoid muscle
	Cranial nerve XII
	Lingual artery
	Facial artery and vein
Submental	Anterior jugular veins
	Lymph nodes
	Mylohyoid muscles
Posterior	Subclavian artery and vein
	Suprascapular artery
	Transverse cervical artery
	Subclavian vein
	External jugular vein
	Brachial plexus roots
	Cranial nerve XI
	Lesser occipital, greater auricular, transverse cervical, phrenic, and supraclavicular nerves
	Anterior scalene muscle
Suboccipital	Vertebral artery
	Suboccipital nerve

Source: From Ref. 9.

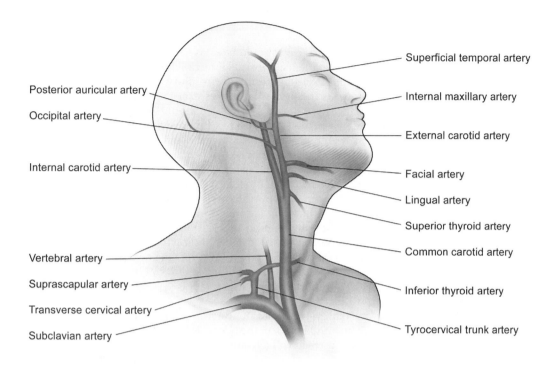

Posterior auricular artery

Occipital artery

Internal carotid artery

Vertebral artery

Suprascapular artery

Transverse cervical artery

Subclavian artery

Superficial temporal artery

Internal maxillary artery

External carotid artery

Facial artery

Lingual artery

Superior thyroid artery

Common carotid artery

Inferior thyroid artery

Tyrocervical trunk artery

Figure 10 Arterial anatomy of the head and neck.

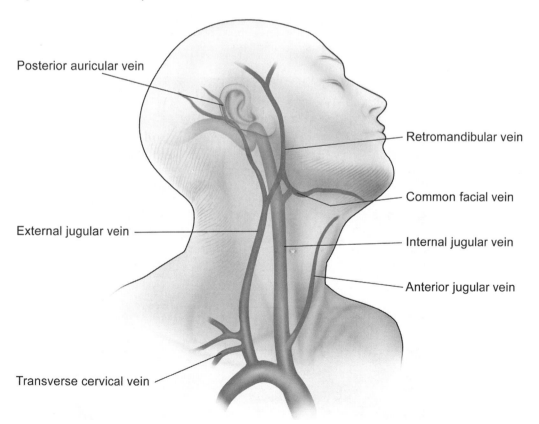

Posterior auricular vein

External jugular vein

Transverse cervical vein

Retromandibular vein

Common facial vein

Internal jugular vein

Anterior jugular vein

Figure 11 Venous anatomy of the head and neck.

Avoidance of Complications in Specific Procedures

Branchial Cleft Remnants

Remnants of the first and second branchial cleft should be excised because of their propensity to become infected. In one review of 274 patients, previous infection had occurred in 23% (1). The major morbidity from branchial cleft excisions results from injury to surrounding structures or from incomplete excision. Previous inflammation makes excision of these lesions difficult by distorting tissue planes and nearby structures. Excision should be performed soon after diagnosis, or if active infection is present, delayed until resolution. Recurrence of branchial cleft anomalies following excision has been reported to be 20% if the lesion is infected (25).

Preservation of the facial nerve is an essential component of resection of first branchial cleft remnants (12). The relationship of the anomalous tract to the facial nerve is variable (15). Intraoperatively, the branches of the facial nerve must be delineated prior to proceeding with tract excision. Several methods have been employed to assist in the adequate identification of this nerve (12). First, when anomalous tracts are identified medial to the facial nerve, a nerve stimulator may be used for verification at the time the parotid fascia is separated from the external ear canal. Second, the facial nerve can be located by following the sternocleidomastoid superiorly toward the mastoid process. A third method involves tracing a distal branch of the nerve proximally back to the main nerve trunk. The incidence of facial nerve injury following first branchial cleft fistulas has been reported to be 10% to 40%, depending on the successful identification of the nerve (13,14).

Branchial cleft cysts require total cyst and fistulous tract excision. A fine lacrimal duct probe is often inserted to identify the course and length of the tract (Fig. 12). This is a delicate maneuver requiring care to avoid penetrating the tract wall into surrounding structures. Dissection should be carried out directly on the fistulous tract, minimizing injury to the carotid sheath, and the hypoglossal and glossopharyngeal nerves (Fig. 13). If the track is found to be long, exposure may be limited as dissection proceeds cephalad. To avoid tearing the track, a separate "stepladder" incision may be made approximately 2 to 3 cm above the initial incision by using the tip of a fine clamp placed along the course of dissection as a guide (25). Using a "stepladder" incision can also minimize unsightly scar formation. Dissection should be carried out onto the wall of the cyst, minimizing injury to adjacent nerves and vessels including the vagus, spinal accessory,

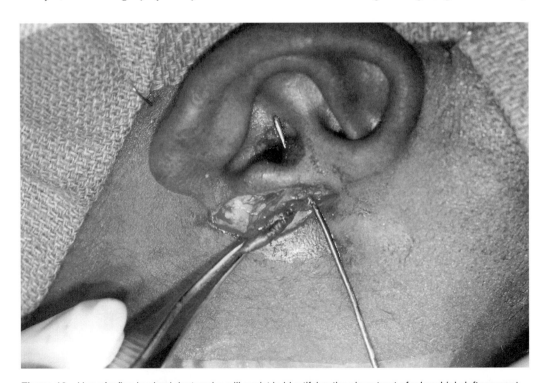

Figure 12   Use of a fine lacrimal duct probe will assist in identifying the sinus tract of a branchial cleft remnant.

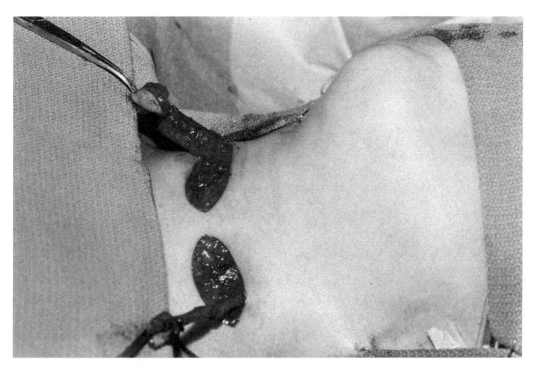

Figure 13 Dissection along the fistulous tract will reduce injuries to adjacent structures.

and hypoglossal nerves, and the carotid artery and internal jugular vein. Cyst decompression hinders dissection, and should be avoided.

Additional complications that may occur following the excision of branchial cleft remnants include fistula formation (seen often in the setting of acute infection), local seroma, and hematoma.

Thyroglossal Duct Cysts

Thyroglossal duct cysts, like branchial cleft anomalies, should be excised when diagnosed due to their risk of becoming infected. A thyroglossal duct cyst, unlike branchial cleft remnants, has no associated sinus opening unless a prior infection has resulted in spontaneous drainage, a surgical drainage procedure has been performed, or an excision has been incomplete (26). In 1920, Sistrunk first outlined the definitive procedure for thyroglossal duct cyst excision including the removal of the central portion of the hyoid bone and the duct extending to the base of the tongue (27,28). Due to the fragility of the duct and the likelihood of tearing before complete removal, he recommended that a core of tissue be excised with the duct to prevent this problem. Prior to Sistrunk's operation, thyroglossal duct cysts were treated with simple excision resulting in a recurrence rate of 50% (29). Recurrence rates with Sistrunk's procedure, when properly performed, are less than 3%, and usually present within one year following excision (29). Major complications resulting from the Sistrunk procedure can be attributed to inattention to surgical landmarks and inadequate hemostasis (29). Minor complications are largely wound related and can be seen in Table 8.

Intraoperatively, the cyst must be positively identified because ectopic thyroid tissue may mimic its appearance (1). If there is any question regarding the diagnosis, the ectopic tissue should be biopsied. Removal of solitary ectopic thyroid tissue may lead to hypothyroidism. This complication can be avoided or anticipated by use of preoperative ultrasonography or thyroid radioiodine scanning identifying normal thyroid tissue.

Inadvertent entry into the trachea can be avoided by properly identifying the thyroid cartilage and the thyrohyoid membrane. This maneuver also aids in locating the hyoid bone. Intraoperative hemorrhage is unusual, but can occur with injury to the lingual artery or vein if the dissection strays too far off the midline. Likewise, hypoglossal nerve injury can be avoided by staying close to the midline during the dissection.

Table 8 Complications of the Sistrunk Procedure

Major
Hemorrhage with airway compression

Recurrence
Abscess
Tracheotomy
Nerve injury
Hypothyroidism
Death

Minor
Seroma
Local wound infection
Stitch abscess
Dehiscence

Source: From Ref. 29.

Lymphatic Malformations
Lymphatic malformations rarely spontaneously regress and frequently develop infection or hemorrhage, so surgical excision is recommended. Although complete resection is the goal of surgical therapy, these lesions are benign, and an extensive operation with sacrifice of vital structures is not indicated (30). Several series have reported recurrence rates following complete excision between 10% and 27% (30–32). One series compared recurrence rates between complete and partially excised lesions, and found rates of 12% and 53%, respectively (30). Injection of sclerosing agents has been used as alternative treatment of lymphatic malformations. Hypertonic saline, tetracycline, bleomycin, and 50% dextrose solutions have been used in the past with occasional success (1,30). Complete success with these agents is often difficult because of the irritating nature of the agents in the presence of neurovascular tissue (1).

Nerve involvement is frequent with lymphatic malformations. In one study, neurologic impairment following excision occurred in 5% of operations and accounted for 17% of complications (30). The facial nerve, particularly the marginal mandibular and cervical branches, phrenic nerve, spinal accessory nerve, hypoglossal nerve, and recurrent laryngeal nerve are those most frequently injured (1,9,30). Figure 14 demonstrates the close relationship of the spinal accessory nerve to lesions in the posterior triangle. A nerve stimulator may be used to locate the branches of the facial nerve during dissection. Horner's syndrome has also been reported following excision in 1.4% of patients (30). Other complications following excision of cystic hygromas include local wound infections, seromas, abscesses, hematomas, and wound dehiscence.

Occasionally, dissection of large lymphatic malformations extending into the mediastinum may result in a chylothorax from disruption of lymphatics. Overall, thoracic complications occurred in 4.2% of patients in one series (30).

Lymph Node Biopsy
Biopsy of cervical lymph nodes is performed for a wide variety of infectious and malignant etiologies. Injury to surrounding structures depends on the location of the lymph node of interest. Major lymph node chains typically follow accompanying vasculature in the head and neck. Location of the node with regards to the triangles of the neck (Table 7) will assist the surgeon in identifying and avoiding specific structures at risk. An important principle to follow is to limit the dissection to the surface of the lymph node. This prevents damage to adjacent structures such as peripheral nerves. It is also important to remember that in most situations the operation is being performed to biopsy the lymph node in question, not to perform a lymph node excision. If a lymph node is small, then it is reasonable to excise the entire lymph node. Resecting large lymph nodes or chains of lymph nodes put adjacent structures at risk. This is most relevant for lymph nodes in the posterior cervical chain. The spinal accessory nerve exits from the lateral border of the sternocleidomastoid muscle and supplies the trapezius muscles. It lies in a subcutaneous position when it travels from the sternocleidomastoid process and is at risk during lymph node biopsy.

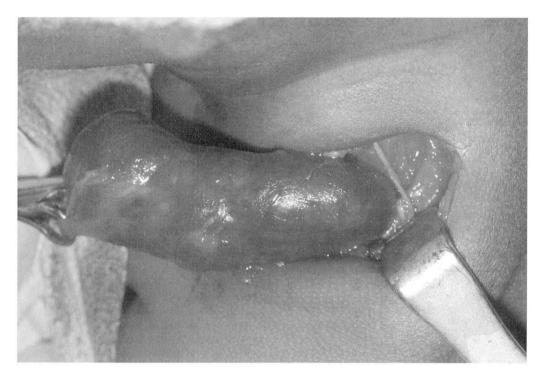

Figure 14 Spinal accessory nerve seen in close relationship to lesions of the posterior triangle.

Tracheostomy

Management of complications of tracheal surgery begins with recognizing the indications for surgery, careful attention to the technical details of the procedure, and careful postoperative management. Long-term meticulous care is necessary to prevent complications. Several series have reported complication rates between 30% and 86% (33–36). The incidence of complications following tracheostomy is related to the indication for the procedure. Children with head and neck cancer requiring tracheostomy, particularly following radiation therapy, are significantly more likely to develop a tracheostomy-related complication (37). In addition, higher complication rates in pre-term infants were attributed to gestational age, low birth weight, and medical condition of the infant (38). Mortality following tracheostomy (0.7%) likewise is often a consequence of the underlying primary disease process (33,35). Table 9 provides a list of the common indications for tracheostomy in children.

The most common complications related to tracheostomy can be seen in Table 10. The pressure exerted by the cuff on the trachea wall is one of the major contributors to the development of tracheal stenosis and granulomas (34). Excessive tube movement, use of too large a tube or overinflated cuff, devascularization at the time of surgery, cartilage excision, and tracheal infection also contribute to these morbidities (36). The incidence of stenosis is approximately 3% to 8% in most series while that of granulomas is about 10% (39,40). Routine placement of sutures on the tracheal stoma is often performed to assist with rapid replacement of the tracheostomy tube in the event that it becomes dislodged before the stoma has matured. Avoiding extensive circumferential dissection to prevent devascularization and injury to the recurrent laryngeal nerve, and preserving tissue by avoiding flap excision will also aid in the prevention of tracheostomy-related morbidities.

Lower respiratory tract infections are a common late complication in patients with tracheostomies. Pneumonia can be a serious problem in these patients, especially in those with pre-existing underlying lung pathology. Aggressive pulmonary toilet is mandatory in the postoperative care of these patients to prevent pooling of secretions and atelectasis.

Parotid Surgery

The goal of parotid surgery for both benign and malignant disease is to achieve complete excision with preservation of the facial nerve (9) (Fig. 15). This can generally be achieved unless

Table 9   Indications for Tracheostomy in Children

Congenital Abnormalities
Bilateral choanal atresia
Severe micrognathia (Pierre Robin syndrome)
Congenital airway abnormality
Craniofacial abnormality
Laryngeal papillomatosis
   Subglottic stenosis
Laryngomalacia

Lesions of the Nasopharynx and Oropharynx
Rhabdomyosarcoma
Osteogenic sarcoma
Lymphoma
Kaposi's sarcoma
Angiofibroma
Teratoma

Lesions of the Neck
   Cystic hygroma
   Carcinoma of the thyroid, parathyroid, or salivary gland
   Lymphoma
   Bilateral vocal cord paralysis
   Acquired tracheal stenosis
   Tracheal foreign body
   Laryngeal trauma

Miscellaneous
Head injury
   Chronic respiratory failure and support
   Chronic aspiration
   Central apnea
   Craniofacial trauma
   Severe burn
   Guillain–Barre syndrome
   Cardiovascular diseases

Source: From Refs. 35, 36.

Table 10   Early and Late Complications Following Tracheostomy

Early
Tube obstruction
Accidental decannulation
Stomal bleeding
Pneumonia
Pneumothorax
Pneumomediastinum
Death

Late (Major)
Tracheal granuloma
Tracheal stenosis
Tracheitis
Tracheoinominate fistula
Tracheocutaneous fistula
Accidental decannulation
Tube obstruction

Late (Minor)
Tracheomalacia
Stomal infection/cellulitis
Excessive stomal granulation

Source: From Refs. 33, 37.

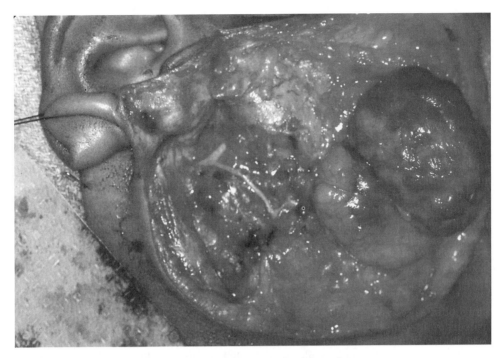

Figure 15 Preservation of the facial nerve during parotid gland dissection.

the nerve is infiltrated by tumor. Operations on the parotid gland are performed without muscle relaxants. A nerve stimulator is readily available, but with solid knowledge of the anatomy and meticulous dissection its use is unnecessary. The facial nerve is identified shortly after its emergence from the stylomastoid foramen between the digastric muscle and external auditory meatus. Identification of its branches as they course between the two lobes of the gland can be achieved by retraction of the gland superiorly and anteriorly. Facial nerve injury can occur with stretching of the fibers during this process if too much force is applied.

Although preservation of the facial nerve is the goal, malignant tumors invading the nerve and its branches require en bloc resection following the principles of oncology. If resection of the nerve is required, grafting can be performed. The facial nerve has a 90% functional success rate following nerve grafting, the highest of the peripheral nerves (9). Sural, greater auricular, and hypoglossal nerve grafts are acceptable conduits (9).

Thyroid and Parathyroid Procedures

The surgical management of thyroid carcinoma in children is controversial. Although differentiated thyroid cancer (DTC) is often advanced at the time of diagnosis, excellent cure rates can be achieved with a combination of surgical resection and radioactive iodine (RAI) administration (41). The reported 10-year survival of children with DTC is nearly 90% (42). However, long-term follow-up beyond the first decade is needed as recurrences may develop well into adulthood. One study of 99 patients with DTC followed for 25 years reported a recurrence rate of 25%, including metastatic disease (43).

Because children with thyroid carcinoma generally have better long-term outcomes compared with adults, some advocate a less aggressive surgical approach (44). They argue that DTC in children follows a relatively indolent course, and that survival is not related to the degree of gland removal. One retrospective review of 93 children with DTC found that the histologic follicular subtype and age less than 12 years at presentation were significant predictors of lower recurrence rates at 20-year follow-up (44). Based on these findings it appears that tumor factors rather than treatment factors may be more important in determining clinical outcome in children with DTC (19).

Proponents of a more conservative approach to the treatment of DTC also cite the significant incidence of major complications following total thyroidectomy and radical neck dissection in children (41,44). In the same retrospective study, major complications including permanent

Table 11   Complications Following Thyroid Surgery

Major
Permanent hypocalcemia
Permanent recurrent laryngeal nerve paralysis
Horner's syndrome
Tracheal stenosis and/or tracheostomy necessitated
Facial nerve paralysis
Major bleeding (requiring re-exploration)

Minor
Transient hypocalcemia
Transient recurrent laryngeal nerve paralysis
Wound infection/abscess
Facial edema
Lymphocele
Hypertrophic scar
Pneumothorax
Minor bleeding (hematoma, not requiring re-exploration)

Source: From Ref. 19.

hypocalcemia and recurrent laryngeal nerve injury were significantly predicted on a multi-variate analysis by the age of the patient and the type of thyroid surgery performed (45). The reported incidence of recurrent laryngeal nerve injury in children following thyroid surgery is 2.3% to 13%, while that of permanent hypocalcemia is 0.7% to 40% (42–44). Injuries to the phrenic nerve and cervical plexus are also more likely to occur in children with more extensive neck dissections (41).

Surgeons who advocate a more aggressive approach to DTC in children argue that total thyroidectomy with resection of involved regional lymph nodes is the most successful method of obtaining local control of the tumor and preventing recurrence (19,41). In addition, specimens containing papillary carcinoma reveal microscopic foci of tumor in the contralateral lobe in 30% to 85% (41). Furthermore, some have suggested that the effectiveness of RAI for detecting and treating residual disease and microscopic metastases is increased after total thyroidectomy (41). Finally, if reoperation does become necessary for recurrent disease, areas of fibrosis and scarring make the procedure more difficult, increasing the risk of complications (41).

Permanent hypocalcemia is the most common complication following thyroid surgery, with the most frequent cause being injury to the blood supply of the parathyroid glands (46). Several methods have been utilized to accomplish parathyroid preservation. First, autotransplantation of one or two of the glands may be performed in the sternocleidomastoid muscle or in the forearm of the nondominant arm (19). This method is useful when the vascular nourishment to the parathyroid glands has been compromised. Second, some advocate leaving behind the posterior aspect of the superior lobe in a less radical thyroidectomy to preserve the in situ vascular supply, usually the inferior thyroid artery (43).

Recurrent laryngeal nerve injury, the second most common complication, was found in one study to be significantly associated with failure to identify the nerve, secondary procedures of the neck, and histologic features of the thyroid (43). Anatomic variations and lack of hemostasis also contribute to a higher degree of laryngeal nerve damage. Careful hemostasis should be obtained prior to using the inferior thyroid artery as a method for identifying the recurrent laryngeal nerve, as bleeding will obscure its location (43). Secondary procedures are often more challenging due to the degree of fibrosis and scarring (41,43). In these operations, increased bleeding from scar tissue and the lack of normal anatomic relationships contribute to nerve injuries.

The external branch of the superior laryngeal nerve is also at risk during the dissection. Advanced diagnostic techniques have documented an incidence of 2% to 14% of this morbidity (47). Techniques to preserve the integrity of this nerve include isolation and individual ligation of the superior pole vessels close to the capsule of the thyroid, identifying the nerve prior to ligating these vessels, and neuromonitoring the nerve during thyroidectomy (47).

Other important complications following thyroid surgery can be seen in Table 11.

Parathyroid surgery in children is indicated for adenoma, hyperplasia, and rarely carcinoma. The surgical procedure for primary hyperparathyroidism has traditionally involved identification of all four parathyroid glands with removal of the enlarged, adenomatous gland. Since it is known that 80% to 90% of patients with primary hyperparathyroidism have a solitary adenoma, utilization of preoperative localization with sestamibi subtraction scintigraphy, and intraoperative parathyroid hormone levels has reduced the risk of postoperative hypocalcemia and nerve injury (48). If an extensive search for the remaining parathyroid glands is performed, a delicate technique is required to avoid devascularization or inadvertent removal of the glands. The technique for taking biopsies likewise is important to avoid harm to the remaining gland or biopsy specimen. The biopsy specimen is typically taken from the distal end of the gland with a small knife or scissors, and then removed with a cotton-tipped swab (49). An incorrectly performed biopsy technique may cause surgical trauma to the remaining parathyroid glands resulting in an increased number of complications (49).

Complications resulting from parathyroid surgery include permanent hypoparathyroidism, recurrent laryngeal nerve injury, wound related complications including infection, seroma, and hematoma, and recurrence of disease. Permanent hypoparathyroidism has been reported to occur in 1.4% to 7% of patients and is the result of disrupting the blood supply to the remaining glands (49). The incidence of permanent recurrent laryngeal nerve damage is 0% to 2% (49).

REFERENCES

1. Telander RL, Filston HC. Review of head and neck lesions in infancy and childhood. Surg Clin North Am 1992; 72:1429–1447.
2. Wadsworth DT, Seigal MJ. Thyroglossal duct cysts: Variability of sonographic findings. Am J Roentgenol 1994; 163:1475–1477.
3. Baatenburg de Jong RJ, Rongen RJ, Lameris JS. Ultrasound characteristics of thyroglossal duct anomalies. J Otorhinolaryngol Relat Spec 1993; 55:299–302.
4. Ward RF, Selfe RW, St. Louis L. Computed tomography and the thyroglossal duct cyst. Otolaryngol Head Neck Surg 1986; 95:93–98.
5. Guarisco JL. Congenital head and neck masses in infants and children: Part II. Ent J 1991; 70:75–82.
6. Seigel MJ, Glazen HS, St. Amour TE, et al. Lymphangiomas in children: MR imaging. Pediatr Radiol 1989; 170:467.
7. Pinczower E, Crockett DM, Atkinson JB. Preoperative thyroid scanning in the presumed thyroglossal duct cysts. Arch Otolaryngol Head Neck Surg 1992; 118:985–991.
8. Radkowski D, Arnold J, Healy GB. Thyroglossal duct remnants. Arch Otolaryngol Head Neck Surg 1991; 117:1378–1381.
9. Fallat ME. Neck. In: KT Oldham, PM Colombani, RP Foglia, eds. Surgery of Infants and Children: Scientific Principles and Practice. Philadelphia: Lippincott-Raven, 1997:835–855.
10. Dedivitis RA, Camargo DL, Peixoto GL, et al. Thyroglossal duct: A review if 55 cases. J Am Coll Surg 2002; 194:274–277.
11. Josephson GD, Spencer WR. Thyroglossal duct cyst: The New York Eye and Ear Infirmary experience and literature review. ENT 1998; 77:642–651.
12. Mounsey RA, Forte V, Friedberg J. First branchial cleft sinuses: An analysis of current management strategies and treatment outcomes. J Otolaryngol 1993; 22:457–461.
13. Agaton-Bonilla FC, Gay-Escoda C. Diagnosis and treatment of fbranchial cleft cysts and fistulae. A retrospective study of 183 patients. Int J Oral Maxillofac Surg 1996; 25:449–452.
14. Triglia JM, Nicollas R, Ducroz V, et al. First branchial cleft anomalies: A study of 39 cases and a review of the literature. Arch Otolaryngol Head Neck Surg 1998; 124:291–295.
15. D'Souza AR, Uppa HR, De R, et al. Updating concepts of first branchial cleft defects: A literature review. Int J Pediatr Otorhinolaryngol 2002; 62:103–109.
16. Ford GR, Balakrishnan A, Evans JNG, et al. Branchial cleft and pouch anomalies. J Laryngol Otol 1992; 106:137–143.
17. Daya H, Chan HSL, Sirkin W, et al. Pediatric rhabdomyosarcoma of the head and neck. Is there a place for surgical management? Arch Otolaryngol Head Neck Surg 2000; 126:468–472.
18. Duffy BA, Civin CA. Leukemias and lymphomas. In: KT Oldham, PM Colombani, RP Foglia, eds. Surgery of Infants and Children: Scientific Principles and Practice. Philadelphia: Lippincott-Raven, 1997:649–651.
19. Skinner MA. Thyroid and parathyroid. In: KT Oldham, PM Colombani, RP Foglia, eds. Surgery of Infants and Children: Scientific Principles and Practice. Philadelphia: Lippincott-Raven, 1997:860–868.
20. Yip FWK, Reeve TS, Poole AG. Thyroid nodules in childhood and adolescence. Aug N Z J Surg 1994; 64:676–678.

21. Frankenthaler RA, Sellin RV, Cangir A, et al. Lymph node metastases from papillary-follicular thyroid carcinoma in young patients. Am J Surg 1990; 160:341–343.
22. LaQuaglia MP, Telander RL. Differentiated and medullary thyroid cancer in childhood and adolescence. Semin Ped Surg 1992; 6:42–47.
23. Del Beccaro MA, Mendelman PM, Nolan C. Diagnostic usefulness of mycobacterial skin test antigens in childhood lymphadenitis. Ped Infect Dis J 1089; 8:206–210.
24. Chwals WJ. Nutrition. In: KT Oldham, PM Colombani, RP Foglia, eds. Surgery of Infants and Children: Scientific Principles and Practice. Philadelphia: Lippincott-Raven, 1997:96–98.
25. Altman RP, Hechtman DH. Congenital lesions: Thyroglossal duct cysts and branchial cleft anomalies. In: LM Nyhus, RJ Baker, JE Fischer, eds. Mastery of Surgery. 3rd ed. Boston: Little, Brown and Company, 1997:pp 383–389.
26. Mickel RA, Calceterra TC. Management of recurrent thyroglossal duct cysts. Arch Otolaryngol 1983; 109:34–36.
27. Sistrunk EW. The surgical management of cysts of the thyroglossal tract. Ann Surg 1920; 71:121–122.
28. Sistrunk WE. Technique of removal of cysts and sinuses of the thyroglossal duct. Surg Gynecol Obstet 1928; 46:109–112.
29. Maddalozzo J, Venkatesan TK, Gupta P. Complications associated with the Sistrunk procedure. Laryngoscope 2001; 111:119–123.
30. Hancock BJ, St-Vil D, Luks FI, et al. Complications of lymphangiomas in children. J Ped Surg 1992; 27:220–226.
31. Kennedy TL. Cystic hygroma-lymphangioma: A rare and still unclear entity. Laryngoscope 1989; 99:1–10.
32. Chait D, Yonkers AJ, Beddoe GM. Management of cystic hygromas. Surg Gynecol Obstet 1974; 139:55–58.
33. Carr MM, Poje CP, Kingston L, et al. Complications in pediatric tracheostomies. Laryngoscope 2001; 111:1925–1928.
34. Rocha EP, Dias MD, Szajmbok FEK, et al. Tracheostomy in children: There is a place for acceptable risk. J Trauma Injury Inf Crit Care 2000; 49:483–486.
35. Dubrey SP, Garap JP. Pediatric tracheostomy: An analysis of 40 cases. J Laryngol Otology 1999; 113:645–651.
36. Donnelly MJ, Lacey PD, Maguire AJ. A twenty-year (1971–1990) review of tracheostomies in a major pediatric hospital. Int J Ped Otorhinolaryngol 1996; 35:1–9.
37. Halfpenny W, McGurk M. Analysis of tracheostomy-associated morbidity after operations for head and neck cancer. Br J Oral Maxillofac Surg 2000; 38:509–512.
38. Kenna MA, Reily JS, Stool SE. Tracheostomy in the preterm infant. Ann Oto Rhino Laryngol 1987; 96:68–71.
39. Matilla MAK, Suutarinen T, Sulamaa M. Prolonged endotracheal intubation or tracheostomy in infants and children. J Pediatr Surg 1969; 4:674–682.
40. Supance JS, Railly JS, Doyle WJ, et al. Acquired subglottic stenosis following prolonged endotracheal intubation. Arch Otolaryngol 1982; 108:727–731.
41. Bingol-Kolojlu M, Tanyel FC, Senocakv ME, et al. Surgical treatment of differentiated thyroid carcinoma in children. Eur J Pediatr Surg 2000; 10:347–352.
42. Steinmuller T, Klupp J, Wenking S, et al. Complications associated with different thyroid surgical approaches to differentiated thyroid carcinoma. Langenbeck's Arch Surg 1999; 384:50–53.
43. Herranz-Gonzalez J, Gavilan J, Matinez-Vidal J, et al. Complications following thyroid surgery. Arch Otolaryngol Head Neck Surg 1991; 117:516–518.
44. LaQuaglia MP, Corbally MT, Heller G, et al. Recurrence and morbidity in differentiated thyroid carcinoma in children. Surgery 1988; 104:1149–1156.
45. LaQuaglia MP, Corbally MY, Heller G, et al. Recurrence and morbidity in differentiated thyroid carcinoma in children. Surgery 1988; 104:1149–1156.
46. Harness JK, Thompson NW, McLeod MK, et al. Differentiated thyroid cancer in children and adolescents. World J Surg 1992; 16:547–554.
47. Stojadinovic A, Shaha AR, Orlikoff RF, et al. Prospective functional voice assessment in patients undergoing thyroid surgery. Ann Surg 2002; 236:823–832.
48. Bergenfelz A, Lindblom P, Tibblin S, et al. Unilateral versus bilateral neck exploration for primary hyperparathyroidism. Ann Surg 2002; 236:543–551.
49. Anderberg B, Gillquist J, Larsson L, et al. Complications to subtotal parathyroidectomy. Acta Chir Scand 1981; 147:109–113.

Thyroglossal Duct Cyst Excision

Expert: Richard G. Azizkhan, M.D.

QUESTIONS

1. **Is it necessary to perform a thyroid scan preoperatively?**
   It has not been my practice to routinely perform a thyroid scan preoperatively in patients who have a suspected thyroglossal duct cyst. However, it is common for ectopic thyroid tissue to exist within a thyroglossal duct remnant and is reported to be somewhere between 20% and 45% of the cases. I also do not obtain the thyroid function studies preoperatively unless there is a concern about hypo- or hyperthyroidism. If there is a significant amount of thyroid tissue removed at the time of operation, a postoperative radionuclide scan should be obtained to ensure that there is sufficient residual thyroid tissue remaining in the child's neck.

2. **How should the child with an infected thyroglossal duct cyst be managed?**
   Owing to the communication with the base of the tongue and the foramen cecum, the thyroglossal duct cyst commonly becomes infected and patients may report infection as the first manifestation. An area of tenderness and mild erythema overlying a thyroglossal duct cyst may be managed with oral antibiotics. However, if there is an obvious abscess with fluctuance, draining the thyroglossal duct cyst abscess may allow for a more rapid resolution of the infection.

3. **What technical steps should be performed to prevent recurrence?**
   A thyroglossal duct cyst is treated by complete excision of the thyroglossal duct tract and cyst up to the base of the tongue and should include the central portion of the hyoid bone. This procedure has been called the Sistrunk procedure after the surgeon who described and popularized this approach. Using the Sistrunk technique has reduced the incidence of recurrence to <5% from a recurrence rate of at least 25% to 30% for cystectomy alone. Complete surgical excision during an active infection is inadvisable because of the difficulty of the operation when infection is present and the risk of injury to surrounding structures which results in a higher incidence of recurrence.

4. **What technical steps should be performed if a thyroglossal duct cyst is recurrent?**
   Recurrence rate following primary resection of the previously uninfected thyroglossal duct cyst is now less than 5% and recurrence generally is observed within a year after the initial procedure. Recurrence has been attributed to incomplete excision of part of the cyst or its tract, but also can be caused by distortion of tissues due to significant inflammation or inadequate resection of the hyoid bone or the central stalk leading to the foramen cecum. Recurrence has also been described as a result of multiple tracts or rupture of the cyst at the time of excision. The procedure to resect the recurrence is performed through the same cervical incision. The surgeon is obliged to make sure that there's been an adequate resection of the central portion of the hyoid bone and follow the tract up to the foramen cecum. On occasion of the difficult dissection, the surgeon can place his/her left index and third finger through the mouth of the patient palpating the back of the tongue and at the same time palpating with the right hand through the incision to determine where the endpoint of the dissection from the neck should be. Unfortunately, even with a relatively wide secondary operation, recurrence rates after the secondary procedure can be as high as 25% to 30%.

5. **What unusual complications have you encountered following excision of a thyroglossal duct cyst?**
   In addition to recurrence, infection and localized hematomas are more of the common complications. Among the most unusual complications that have been seen is the presence of papillary adenocarcinoma in thyroglossal duct specimens. In adults, this occurs in up to 10% of the patients undergoing a Sistrunk procedure, although this has not yet been

reported in childhood. This observation lends further support to the rationale for early and complete excision of thyroglossal duct remnants.

An extremely rare complication that has been reported when the surgeon has misidentified the laryngocricoid complex for the hyoid bone and an injury has occurred to the airway. This has occurred in the face of distorted anatomy from a significant inflammatory process. This points out that the surgeon must be well familiar with the anatomy and experienced in doing this procedure. Finally, a rare complication in the thyroglossal duct cyst when the duct tissues are examined is that there is a significant amount of thyroid tissue associated with this. Occasionally, there is insufficient remaining thyroid tissue in the patient and a postoperative radionuclide scan would identify this problem and lead to appropriate thyroid replacement treatment.

6. **Is a specific margin of hyoid bone helpful in minimizing recurrence?**
During the surgical procedure, the hyoid bone is transected on either side of the duct leaving an approximately 0.5 to 0.75 cm margin on either side. Using this approach, I have not had any recurrences following thyroglossal duct excision.

7. **Is postoperative drainage no longer routinely indicated?**
The primary reason for postoperative drains being placed was the risk of significant wound hemorrhage within a closed space resulting in airway compression. Using meticulous hemostatic surgical technique has clearly reduced the need for routine drainage and it has not been part of my practice. However, in the days where bipolar cautery or unipolar cautery was not used, hemorrhage was a significant risk and these patients had drains placed to create a conduit to prevent airway compression by a large hematoma. I also believe leaving a drain in place increases the risk of postoperative infection.

9 | Complications of Pediatric Thoracic Surgery

Robert E. Kelly, Jr., M.D. and M. Ann Kuhn, M.D.

CARDIOPULMONARY COMPLICATIONS OF THORACIC SURGERY

Cardiopulmonary complications of thoracic surgery in children mirror those in adults in many ways. As in adults, preoperative efforts can prevent complications of surgery. Atelectasis should be discouraged. Smoking in teenage patients should be stopped prior to elective surgery. Asthmatic children should have their disease controlled as well as possible. The numerous medications available for chronic lung disease should be utilized under the direction of a pulmonary specialist to optimize lung function before operation. Intraoperatively, adequate inflation of the lungs by positive pressure ventilation should be assured by looking at the lung at time of closure or completion of thoracoscopy. After operation, pain relief is critical to allowing full opening of the lung. While some degree of atelectasis is a normal postoperative finding, it responds well to incentive spirometry, flutter valve, and other measures for pulmonary toilet. How frequently atelectasis leads to pneumonia is unclear, but not often. Family members can encourage the patient with these measures, and this helps them to realistically feel they are contributing to recovery.

Postoperative pneumonia in children occurs in several settings. Aspiration following regurgitation of gastric contents with general anesthesia occurs slightly more frequently in children (1 per 1200–2600 anesthetics) than in adults (1,2). Nonemergency operations should be performed with the patient fasted. In a large series of children undergoing general anesthesia at the Mayo clinic (63,180 anesthetics), pulmonary aspiration was noted in 24 patients (1:2632 anesthetics). Of those 24 children, 15 never developed pulmonary problems. No child died of sequelae of pulmonary aspiration (1). The bacteriology of the pneumonia is not predicted by the organisms cultured from the upper airway (3); of 91 heart surgery patients who underwent preoperative nasopharyngeal cultures, the risk of postoperative airway infection was the same (10%) whether or not the patient was colonized with pathogenic bacteria.

One pulmonologist noted, "An understanding of the epidemiology and bacteriology of pneumonia in childhood is frustrated by the difficulties in making an etiological diagnosis in young children" (4). Nosocomial pneumonia following cardiac surgery in children is better characterized in recent literature than pneumonia after the noncardiac thoracic surgery performed by pediatric surgeons. In a recent report of 311 cardiac surgical infants treated between 1999 and 2002, 21% developed nosocomial pneumonia. A total of 79 pathogenic microbial strains were identified. Gram-negative bacilli predominated, causing 86% of cases of pneumonia; fungi caused 7%, and the remainder were gram-positive cocci (7%) (5) (Table 1). In this series, there was only one case of infection with methicillin-resistant *Staphylococcus aureus*, and the susceptibility of extended-spectrum beta lactamase producing organisms to imipenem was 100%. With increasing antibiotic resistance recently reported in most centers, local susceptibility patterns must be followed.

In a study of adult patients undergoing pulmonary lobectomy, the species cultured from the cut end of the bronchus differed from those in the sputum (6), and were related significantly to postlobectomy pneumonia significantly. Pneumonia developed in 9% of patients postoperation; this low frequency may explain the dearth of reports on occurrence of this entity in children, who do not require pulmonary lobectomy frequently. It may be wise to obtain cultures from the cut end of the bronchus at time of pulmonary lobectomy to guide antibiotic therapy.

Nosocomial pneumonia also complicates care of patients with multiple trauma (7), and postoperative cancer patients (8). In adult cancer patients, piperacillin/tazobactam and amikacin or clindamycin, aztreonam, and amikacin were found to be equally efficacious and satisfactory choices in a prospective randomized study.

Table 1 Causes of Nosocomial Pneumonia in
Infants after Cardiac Surgery

Microbial strains	Isolates, No. (%)
GBN	68 (86.1)
A. baumannii	11 (13.9)
Other Acinetobacter	6 (7.6)
P. aeruginosa	10 (12.7)
Other Psudomonas	6 (7.6)
K. pneumoniae	7 (8.9)
F. meningosepticum	7 (8.9)
E. coli	6 (7.6)
Enterobacter cloacae	3 (3.8)
Other enterobacter	7 (8.9)
X. maltophilia	5 (6.2)
Gram-positive cocci	5 (6.3)
S. aureus	2 (2.5)
S. epidermidis	2 (2.5)
Other Staphylococcus	1 (1.3)
Fungi	6 (7.6)
C. albicans	5 (6.3)
Yeast	1 (1.3)
Total	79 (100)

Source: From Ref. 5.

Respiratory distress syndrome (RDS) arises in children from the same pathophysiologic processes as in adults. Pulmonary edema occurring as a result of oncotic and hydrostatic pressure differences leads to fluid in the alveolar spaces. Extensive literature on the topic is available to the reader for review of the pathophysiology and management of this condition. From the point of view of the surgeon, the differences rather than the similarities between the adult and the pediatric situation are important. Postobstructive pulmonary edema occurs in children usually after laryngospasm upon awakening from anesthesia. It often clears spontaneously following supportive measures. True RDS complicates the surgical care of children less frequently than adults. RDS in children is often complicated by infection of the edematous lung, and may require prolonged ventilatory support and tracheostomy. Management remains controversial. Despite years of efforts, no clear winner in the disputes over fluid administration and ventilatory management strategies has emerged. Efforts to minimize the toxicity of oxygen administration and barotrauma produced by the ventilator have included the use of pressure ventilation even in larger children. Pulmonary artery catheters, placed for more precise measurement of right heart pressures and left atrial pressure, and mixed venous oxygen saturation measurement have fallen out of favor, but may have application in a recalcitrant case.

Arrhythmias may complicate thoracic surgery in children. In a recent study of children with cardiac problems, the incidence was 15% (9). The occurrence is greatest in children with structural heart disease, and higher in cardiac than noncardiac surgery. Pectus excavatum patients may have associated arrhythmias, including bundle branch block and Wolf–Parkinson–White syndrome (10). Careful preoperative evaluation of thoracic surgical patients with an EKG or echocardiogram should be done as indicated. Unexpected arrhythmic arrest has complicated repair of chest wall deformities (11). Intraoperative attention to electrolyte abnormalities and EKG monitoring of high-risk patients should permit treatment for arrhythmias to proceed promptly. Management of arrhythmias has its own extensive literature, which cannot be briefly summarized.

COMPLICATIONS OF CHEST INCISIONS

Choosing the ideal incision for a thoracic operation involves a calculation of the best surgical exposure for the particular problem as well as the risks of that approach. The choice of chest incision in children is made difficult by the divergent information available on the complications

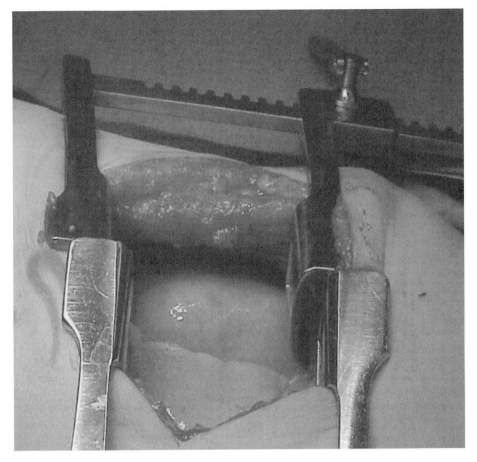

Figure 1 Posterolateral thoracotomy.

of any chest incision. Prior to the wide availability of thoracoscopic operations (video-assisted thoracic surgery, or VATS), the most widely used approach for a variety of problems was the posterolateral thoracotomy. In fact, it was used for so many types of procedures that it was called a standard thoracotomy by many surgeons. The long intercostal opening it provides gives good exposure of the esophagus, pulmonary hilus and parenchyma, descending aorta, and to a lesser extent the anterior mediastinum. However, the wide opening between the ribs (Fig. 1), commonly in the fourth or fifth interspace, is also associated with short- and long-term complications.

Posterolateral thoracotomy complications noted in a recent series of 49 children (12) were: scoliosis, 31%; elevation of the shoulder 61%; winged scapula 77%; asymmetry of the thoracic wall due to atrophy of the serratus anterior, 14%; deformity of the thoracic cage 18%, and asymmetry of the nipples 63%. While this frequency of problems seems high, prospective studies are lacking. Others have reported that shoulder asymmetry and electromyographic evidence of injury to nerves of the serratus and latissimus dorsi muscles occurred more frequently in children operated on in infancy (up to one year old) than in older children. A greater incidence of denervation problems was noted with more cephalad incisions. Most of the abnormalities were not functionally significant, but caused the authors to recommend that incisions should be as low as possible, and should be performed after the first year of life if possible (13). Anterolateral thoracotomy also leads to problems: a significant incidence of breast and pectoral maldevelopment has been reported after anterolateral thoracotomy (14).

For these reasons, several authors recommend techniques sparing the serratus anterior and latissimus dorsi. An excellent depiction of the technique is given by Horowitz (15). Muscle atrophy has been documented by CT scan following posterolateral thoracotomy as opposed to muscle sparing approaches (16). However, data showing that muscle-sparing thoracotomy

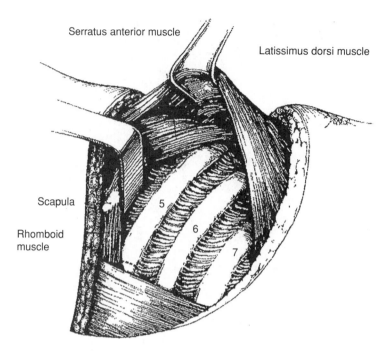

Figure 2 Muscle sparing thoractomy.

avoids problems are hard to find. Two studies showed no difference in complications, length of stay, and other difficulties when muscle sparing thoracotomy and posterolateral thoracotomy were compared (17,18). Some improvement in spirometry was seen in their (adult) patients. (Fig. 2)

Scoliosis (>10°) has followed repair of esophageal atresia (13% of 232 patients in one series (19), and in 50% of a different 18 patient report (20), aortic coarctation (22% of 160 cases) (21) via lateral thoracotomy. Importantly, most of the reports show modest degrees of scoliosis. The fraction of patients with a Cobb angle greater than 20° Was lower. In Chetcuti's report, only three of 30 patients with esophageal atresia and subsequent scoliosis were >20°. Durning's series showed that five of the nine patients had curves greater than 20°. So while the number of patients with "scoliosis" sounds impressive, a very small fraction needed treatment, and an even smaller number needed operation to correct scoliosis. Scoliosis of 20° to 30° is usually treated with bracing, and operative treatment is reserved for scoliosis of 40° to 50° or greater (19,20).

Median sternotomy in childhood has been followed by scoliosis in 34% of 128 patients followed to skeletal maturity (22). In 68 patients who underwent thoracotomy followed by sternotomy in childhood who were followed by the Nemours Clinic for a mean of 14.9 years, 26% developed scoliosis and 21% developed kyphosis (23). Patients with a cyanotic cardiac condition had a fourfold incidence of scoliosis. In patients with scoliosis, the mean kyphosis was 38°. In the Nemours data, the risk of developing scoliosis in children with congenital heart disease was more than 10 times that of idiopathic scoliosis.

Median sternotomy is sometimes complicated by mediastinitis or sternal wound infections. The incidence over a 9-year period ending in 2003 at the Children's Hospital of Philadelphia was 1.4% (24); the incidence of bloodstream infections in the same period was 6.3% in a randomly selected sample of the same group of patients (25). Wound infection incidence has been reported to be higher at other centers (26). Adult patients' incidence seems similar: those treated at University Hospital, Uppsala, Sweden during the period from 1980 through 1995 reported an incidence of 1.7% in 13,285 patients (27). At CHOP, the most frequent organisms found were *S. aureus* (46%), coagulase-negative staphylococcus (17%), and *Pseudomonas aeruginosa* (17%). For many years, surgical irrigation and debridement with wound coverage by omental flaps (28) have been used. Recently, vacuum-assisted closure devices have also been employed (29).

Thoracoscopy or VATS operations should minimize the incidence of the neurologic and chest wall complications which confound surgeons obliged to use a posterolateral thoracotomy. However, the approach is not without difficulties. Preparations should be made for rapid thoracotomy in case of unexpected massive hemorrhage, as has been done for years with mediastinoscopy. Reported series suggest a low likelihood of this problem; but published literature may underreport. Only the most expert surgeons publish, and there is every disincentive to report complications. While diminished pain after VATS when compared to posterolateral thoracotomy seems widely acknowledged, there is literature to suggest that there is no difference in post-thoracotomy pain and pain after VATS in adults (30). Wound infection does occur after VATS (31). Subcutaneous air is a frequent but usually benign and self-limited finding after thoracoscopy, especially if CO_2 insufflation is used.

Neurologic complications after open thoracotomy include paraplegia. The incidence of paraplegia after thoracotomy at one major center was 0.08% over a 40-year period (32). The mechanism in nonaortic surgery patients has been suggested to be the response to bleeding at the posterior end of the incision. Cautery and migration of topical oxidized cellulose resulting in mass effect within the spinal canal have been implicated. Experienced thoracic surgeons emphasize the hazards of bleeding at the costo-vertebral junction area, and avoid excessive retraction; it may be necessary to divide the rib posteriorly rather than tear the costo-vertebral angle. If bleeding occurs despite these efforts, minimal use of topical cellulose and avoidance of intercostals ligation are recommended (13).

COMPLICATIONS OF PULMONARY RESECTION

Pneumothorax or prolonged air leak from a thoracostomy tube following thoracic surgery may be a result of air leaking from the chest drainage device, air entering the chest along the chest tube as it passes through the chest wall, or leak from the lung, congenital pulmonary or bronchial lesion, bronchus, or esophagus. Troubleshooting the cause of air leaks begins with a check of connections beginning at the source of the suction and continuing up to the chest wall. Tape covering tube connections or the chest wall may obscure the cause of an air leak. Chest radiography can demonstrate malposition of the chest tube (33). Pulmonary sources of air leak include unrecognized bullous disease (34) as well as poorly sealed lung at a site of parenchymal transaction (Fig. 3). Unrecognized bullous disease may often be successfully managed by thoracoscopic stapling of the affected tissue (35,36). Parenchymal leak often resolves by continuing drainage of the air by a well-positioned (not intraparenchymal) chest tube.

Air leak from a bronchial stump leak is more troublesome. This complication is sufficiently infrequent in children that an incidence is hard to obtain. Often associated with debility, poor nutrition, infection, or malignancy, reoperation on a high-risk patient may occasionally be avoided by clever approaches. Recently, Tsunezuka reported video-assisted contralateral treatment for bronchial stump diastasis after left pneumonectomy. He exposed the left main bronchus extrapleurally with a right video-assisted thoracic surgical approach in the face of right and left pyothorax, thus avoiding a median sternotomy and potential sternal infection (37). Shimizu reported postoperative bronchial stump fistula occlusion by metallic coils and fibrin glue via a tracheostomy (38). More standard approaches employ repeat thoracotomy, thoracoscopy, and suture closure buttressed with pericardium or pleura.

COMPLICATIONS OF BRONCHIAL RESECTION

Pulmonary lobectomy by sleeve resection of the bronchus is infrequently indicated in children (Fig. 4). Large series of adults often include a few pediatric cases. One of the few pediatric series was reported in 1994 from the Massachusetts General Hospital (39). Of 12 patients treated over a 12-year period, 10 had malignancies; six required carinal resection and reconstruction, three main-stem bronchial resection, and three sleeve resection. Atelectasis was a persistent problem postoperative in three patients. With complete follow-up a mean of 64 months after operation, there was one death, no recurrences of tumor, and preservation of pulmonary function. While there is an extensive literature on this topic in adult patients (for example, a recent review of 1565 tracheobronchoplastic operations in Japan gives detailed subset analysis) (40), it is not

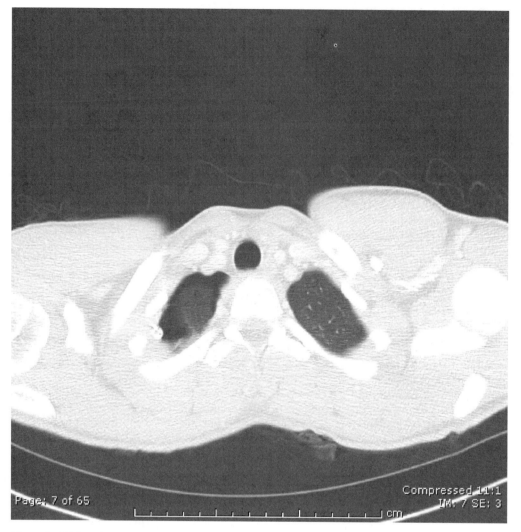

Figure 3 Right apical pulmonary blebs.

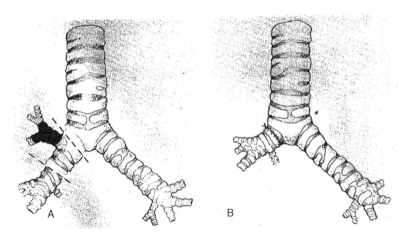

Figure 4 Sleeve resection.

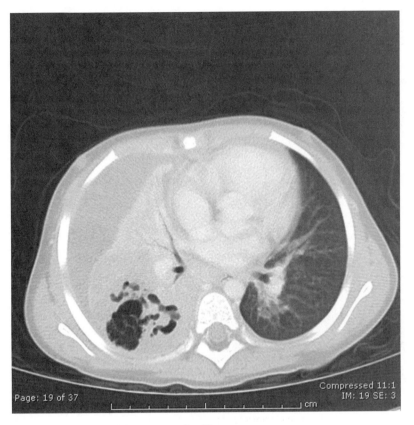

Figure 5   Right necrotizing pneumonia with empyema.

clear that the significant complication rates noted in adults can be generalized to children (41). Nevertheless, resection of the trachea or bronchi remains a significant undertaking which should be managed thoughtfully.

COMPLICATIONS INVOLVING THE PLEURAL SPACE

When nosocomial, pneumonia is accompanied by effusion or empyema, there is consensus in the surgical community that drainage by thoracostomy tube and/or thoracoscopy with decortication hasten recovery (42–45). CT scanning is very useful in determining the amount of fluid and the state of the pulmonary tissue, and should be strongly considered in evaluation of patients with pneumonia and effusion.

Even though the vast majority of surgeons advocate thoracoscopy for decortication of empyema, open thoracotomy is still an option. Recently (in 2003), a series of 44 children treated by open thoracotomy over a 10-year period was reported in the United Kingdom. In those patients, there was no mortality, minimal morbidity, short hospital stay, and rapid resolution of symptoms (46).

There are times when CT-guided radiologic drainage of a pulmonary abscess or open resection of necrotic, or infected pulmonary tissue is appropriate (47) (Fig. 5). Immunocompromised patients, including those with chronic granulomatous disease, may not respond to antibiotic therapy. Hardy organisms such as *Aspergillus fumigatis* may require resection in this setting (48). Though seldom necessary, pneumonectomy for bronchiectasis, aspergillosis, and/or tuberculosis has been reported in children to allow resolution of the underlying disease (49).

Pleural effusion following thoracotomy is more commonly an expected outcome of the operation rather than a complication, and is usually managed adequately by placing chest drains at the time of surgery. Reaccumulation after drain removal might indicate premature removal, but might also signal development of pneumonia with effusion, or hemorrhage (Fig. 6).

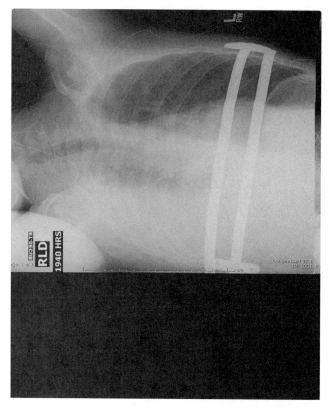

Figure 6 Lateral decubitus x-ray showing layering pleural effusion.

"Space problems," or intrapleural empty spaces not filled by lung, are not a frequent problem in general thoracic surgery in children. In adult practices, the lung fails to fill the intrathoracic cavity in about 11% to 29% of cases (50,51). In children, these spaces tend to resolve by slow expansion of the remaining lung or by accumulation of fluid. The use of a pleural tent intraoperatively has been advocated and has several features to recommend it. Pleural tents allow the lung to adhere to the pleural surface and help seal parenchymal air leaks. The space above the pleural tent fills with fluid and becomes fibrotic, which eliminates a space problem. Insufflation of air into the peritoneal cavity has been used to push the diaphragm cephalad and allow air leaks to seal. Phrenic nerve crush and thoracoplasty should be reserved for difficult situations (52).

Air collecting in the skull after thoracotomy is reported to be a well-recognized phenomenon, but a recent report cites only eight cases in the literature. A subarachnoid-space-to-pleural fistula can occur, and the occurrence of pneumocephalus must be considered when neurologic problems emerge after thoracotomy. It appears that if conservative treatment fails, surgical closure of the fistula via a thoracic or neurosurgical approach is indicated (53). Thoracoscopic sympathectomy is an operation which should be undertaken without insufflation of CO_2 to minimize the potential for gas accumulation in the central nervous system. This rare problem seems most frequent after that operation and others at the apex of the thorax. Meningitis and cerebritis with cerebral edema can follow. While the patients in the review article were aged 43 to 74 years, surgeons performing sympathectomy in older teenagers should be aware of the potential for this problem.

COMPLICATIONS OF MEDIASTINAL SURGERY

A variety of difficulties can complicate dissection of the mediastinum. In children, repair of congenital heart disease, while now well established, often involves complex rearrangement of the anatomy of a very disordered heart. Significant dissection is required, and it may be impossible to avoid damage to nearby structures like the lymphatic channels. Necessary cold cardioplegia solutions may adversely affect nerve function.

Chylothorax occurs after congenital heart surgery and other mediastinal operations. In a series of 5995 cardiac operations reported in Hong Kong, a prevalence of just under 1% was noted to occur at a median of 9 days postoperation (54). A series from Toronto shows an incidence of about 4% in 1257 operations (55). Both series report an increased incidence after Fontan procedures. The median duration of drainage was the same at 15 days. The great majority (about 90%) responded to treatment with dietary modification and/or octreotide. Surgical ligation of the thoracic duct was reported to decrease, but not eliminate drainage in the Toronto series. Both centers began octreotide drainage only after failure of dietary modification, which resolved about 60% (Hong Kong) or 80% (Toronto). A large series from Taiwan confirms the efficacy of medical treatment, and reports similar difficulties with chylothorax whether cardiac operations were performed by median sternotomy or lateral thoracotomy (56). Recent reviews in the critical care medicine literature note that there is no consensus about the optimal route of administration, dose, duration of therapy, or strategy for discontinuation of therapy; one calls for randomized controlled studies of the efficacy of octreotide (57,58). Thoracic duct ligation has been successfully performed thoracoscopically (59).

Dressler's syndrome, or postoperative pericarditis, has been reported to follow cardiac and noncardiac thoracic surgical procedures (60,61). First reported in 1956 after myocardial infarction, the process called "postpericardiotomy syndrome" need not follow opening of the pericardium (62,63). The cause is unclear but is likely an immunologic phenomenon (64). Clinical presentation is postoperative fever, anterior chest pain, and malaise, often accompanied by a pericardial friction rub. Diagnosis is by echocardiogram. Treatment is initially by nonsteroidal anti-inflammatory drugs, especially indomethacin. Steroids may be employed in refractory cases, and rarely drainage of the pericardial space by catheter or pericardial window may be necessary. Usually a self-limited condition, tamponade is rare, even following cardiac surgery (65).

Diaphragmatic paralysis after cardiac surgery can result from phrenic nerve injury by dissection, clamp, electrocautery, or ice used for cardioplegia (Fig. 7).

Phrenic nerve injury is a serious complication. Its frequency was reported to be 1.5% of 1656 cardiac surgical procedures over a 10-year period at one center (66) and 4.9% of 3071 children operated over 11 years elsewhere (67). Half of the patients in the first series required plication of the diaphragm, and all of the second series, mostly because of failure to wean from artificial ventilation. Video-assisted plication can be performed (68); open operation can be either by thoracic or abdominal incision (69).

COMPLICATIONS OF CHEST WALL RECONSTRUCTION

Operation for repair of chest wall abnormalities in pediatric surgery most frequently involves repair of pectus excavatum or carinatum. Published reports concerning sternal cleft, chest wall reconstruction following massive resection for tumor, and other uncommon problems do not provide sufficient information to offer other than general suggestions (70,71). Several authors report that complications of surgical treatment of pectus carinatum are infrequent, and complications few (72). Recently, pectus carinatum has been successfully managed by application of an external brace (73,74). Brace treatment appears to be almost eliminating the need for operation to treat pectus carinatum.

Repair of pectus excavatum is currently performed by two types of operation. The older technique, variously referred to as the open, Ravitch, or Welch repair, involves resection of all or part of the cartilages which join the ends of the ribs to the sternum. The Nuss operation places a metal bar beneath the sternum to push it anteriorly, but does not resect the cartilages. Because the two operations are fundamentally different, their complications will be treate separately.

General comments regarding avoiding complications with either operation for pectus excavatum include management by a team approach. Families often have many questions, which are the same for most families. Having advanced practice nurses and office staff familiar with these concerns is advantageous. Prior to operation, review of preoperative studies with

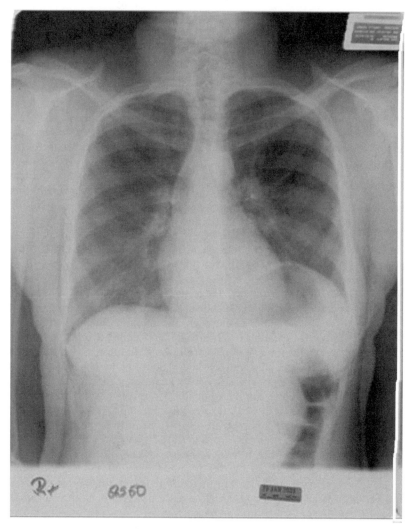

Figure 7 Left diaphragm elevation in phrenic nerve injury.

the family assures them of the anatomy and physiology of their child's condition, and that the surgeon has carefully considered the case. The preoperative discussion with a pectus excavatum patient and family generally takes the surgeon 45 to 60 minutes. Asking about metal allergy can prevent insertion of a nickel-containing stainless steel bar into a sensitive patient instead of nonreactive titanium. Surprisingly, most families who come to our institution indicate that no doctor has reviewed their CT scan, pulmonary function tests, or echocardiogram with them. Checking the CT scan with the family also allows the surgeon to look for a heart "hiding behind" the pectus depression or other potentially troublesome anatomic findings. Preoperative, intraoperative, and postoperative photographs of the patient are important if concerns arise later about the adequacy of treatment. While no one has defined the number of cases needed to pass the "learning curve," the operation does require the surgeon to be educated about the technique. It seems wise to look for proctoring or mentoring for at least the first 25 cases. While the "time out" process should identify whether all necessary support bars, tunneling equipment, and so forth are present, the surgeon should assure that he personally has the correct size bar, dissector, and so forth before the anesthetic is given. After the operation, frequent visits to the patient allow pain management concerns, questions about technique for mobilization out of bed, family anxiety, and other problems to be addressed as soon as they arise. It is a good idea for the surgeon to check a pectus patient twice daily, and in addition to having an advanced practice nurse visit the patient and family each day.

Table 2 Early (Perioperative) Complications

Complication N = 327	Number nuss patients w/complications within 30 days of surgery N = 284	Percent	Number open patients w/complications within 30 days of surgery N = 43	Percent	Total number patients w/complications within 30 days of surgery
Bar shift	7	2.46	0	0	7
Bar Reaction	1	0.35	0	0	1
Stabilizer Displacement	0	0	0	0	0
Wire Displacement	0	0	0	0	0
Wire Breakage	0	0	0	0	0
Pneumothorax >20	12	4.23	3	6.98	15
Hemothorax	0	0	0	0	0
Pericarditis	0	0	0	0	0
Pericardial Effusion with Tamponade	0	0	1	2.33	1
Homer's Syndrome	20	7.04	2	4.65	22
Wound Infection	5	1.77	1	2.33	6
Hematoma	2	0.70	0	0	2
Stitch Abscess	2	0.70	0	0	2
Stabilizer Breakage	0	0	0	0	0
Skin Rash	4	1.41	1	2.33	5
Pneumonia	0	0	1	2.33	1
Atelectasis	141	49.65	16	37.21	157
Pleural Effusion*	92	32.39	2	4.65	94

*$p < 0.001$ using a chi-square test.

COMPLICATIONS OF OPEN REPAIR OF PECTUS EXCAVATUM

The open operation has been performed since the early part of the 20th century, and in significant numbers for the last 60 years. Recently, a multicenter study of pectus excavatum made available prospective complication data on this procedure, which only recently were available by analysis of retrospective reports (75). Early complications of both the Nuss and open operations are listed in Table 2.

The complications unique to chest wall reconstruction for pectus excavatum or carinatum include recurrence and asphyxiating thoracic dystrophy. Asphyxiating thoracic dystrophy or acquired Jeune's syndrome are the names given to recurrence after repair in childhood followed by failure of chest wall growth (76). Recurrence rates following the open operation were reviewed and summarized by Ellis and colleagues in 1997 (77). Recurrence was reported in 2% of patients by Fonkalsrud, 2.4% by Shamberger, 5% by Haller et al. in a contemporary report, 6% by Sanger et al., 10% by Gilbert, 11.8% by Singh, 16% by Pena, and 20.5% by Willital and Meier if no internal supporting bar was used, but only 8.9% if a bar was used (77). Following that report, Lacquet reported unsatisfactory results in 16% of patients (3,72). Ellis et al. believed that that recurrence was related to a limited procedure at the first operation. When they operated on recurrences of other surgeons, deformed cartilages, which appeared to be untouched were often seen. Despite this observation, recurrence happens for unclear reasons. Recurrence affects patients of the most expert surgeons at all centers reporting in the literature.

Marfan syndrome may predispose to recurrence after open repair, since two reports cite a higher recurrence in Marfan patients (78, 79). Eleven of 28 patients with Marfan syndrome and pectus excavatum recurred in a report from Johns Hopkins (78). Haller and colleagues recommended delay in repair until skeletal maturity had been achieved, and use of an Adkins strut at operation for stabilization.

Timing of recurrence is affected by the type of repair. After open repair, recurrence is reported most frequently in the first 2 years following operation, and at the age of the pubertal growth spurt (79). After the Nuss operation, in which stainless steel bars are used to push the sternum to the normal anatomic position, recurrence in the first 6 months is almost always due to shift in the position of the support bars. The bars are secured to the chest wall with suture, if they move, the patient generally has significant pain. Recurrence is prevented by the metal bar while it is in place, and so for 2 to 3 years that the supporting bar is in place, recurrence is unlikely. If a supporting strut is employed to brace the sternum during open repair, the same logic applies. If the support bar is removed 6 weeks to 6 months following a Ravitch repair, recurrence can occur early after that operation. Early recurrence after open operation is thought by some surgeons to be due to inadequate removal of cartilages at the initial operation. Late recurrence at the pubertal growth spurt is noted after either repair (77). The patient or family notes the change in external appearance as the only symptom. Authorities agree that recurrence is associated often with periods of rapid growth at adolescence. Gilbert and Zwiren reported 60% of recurrences were after 12 years of age (80).

Migration of the supporting strut used for Ravitch repair has been reported, with the bar coming to rest in the myocardium, thoracic cavity, or peritoneal cavity, and with injury to the heart, lungs, or abdominal viscera (81–85). Bars (struts) should be removed when no longer required for sternal support, usually 6 weeks to 6 months postoperation.

Asphyxiating thoracic dystrophy was the name given in 1996 to a condition which was reported to follow early and extensive cartilage resection during operations to treat pectus excavatum (76). In children who underwent operation at less than 5 years of age, and whose cartilages were aggressively removed, the chest in later years failed to grow, and the thoracic cage was constricted to an inadequate size. Marked symptoms of exercise intolerance and shortness of breath with very mild exertion affected these patients. Subsequent reports have demonstrated replacement of the normally cartilaginous connection between the sternum and ribs with dense bone (86).

In explanation of the findings, Fonkalsrud notes, "When the deformed costal cartilages are removed with preservation of the perichondrial sheaths, the sheaths are often damaged, and the regenerated cartilage is often thin, irregular, and commonly rigid with varying amounts of bone and calcification ... If the regenerated cartilage is rigid, the chest essentially becomes a cylinder, with respiratory motions being largely dependent on diaphragmatic excursions, which limits the depth of lung expansion and requires more effort than normal respiration" (87). This problem remains very difficult to treat.

Cartilage resection must not be too extensive, or asphyxiating thoracic dystrophy may result. If it is inadequate, though, early recurrence is a risk. Most authors currently suggest freeing all deformed cartilages and their contralateral partners by a limited resection, but recommend leaving a few millimeters of cartilage on the rib and sternal ends. They hope that this technique will allow regrowth of the resected cartilage. Haller and associates, who first reported the problem, advise against operation in children younger than 4 years of age, and against removal of five or more pairs of cartilages (76).

REPAIR OF RECURRENT PECTUS EXCAVATUM BY THE OPEN OR RAVITCH OPERATION

Re-repair by the open operation has been well described by several writers. Recently, some have emphasized that only a small portion of the affected cartilages needs to be resected; earlier others have emphasized that all of the involved cartilages need to be treated to get a good result (77,87).

Open repair for recurrent pectus excavatum is performed under general endotracheal anesthesia (77). Because the pleura may be inadvertently opened, positive intrapulmonary pressure is an important safety measure to assure lung inflation. Thoracic epidural analgesia can be a useful adjunct in the hands of an anesthesiologist skilled in its use. A mixture of fentanyl and bupivacaine is very effective and can be continued as a means of postoperative analgesic. Appropriate anesthetic monitoring equipment includes pulse oximetry and end-tidal carbon dioxide monitoring to assure adequate gas exchange. Prophylactic antibiotics are appropriate; intravenous Ancef® (cefazolin) is a reasonable choice.

Either a transverse inframammary or a vertical midline incision is utilized and gives excellent exposure. Generally, the incision used for the initial repair is reopened. Skin flaps are elevated. The pectoralis major muscle is detached from its origin on the costal cartilages bilaterally, and the muscle is moved out of the way. Similarly the rectus abdominis muscles are detached. After inspection of the sternum and cartilages to determine which cartilages need to be

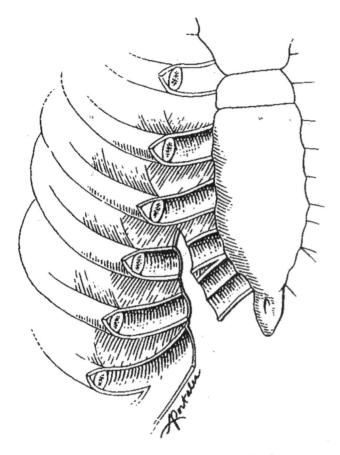

Figure 8   Costal cartilage resection in open operation for pectus excavatum.

divided, the perichondrial sheath is incised along the long axis of the cartilage. Costal cartilage can be freed from the perichondrial sheath with a Freer elevator or similar instrument. In a redo situation, there is often not a well-defined plane between the cartilage and the perichondrium (Fig. 8).

Some length of the cartilage must then be removed at each of the involved deformed cartilages. Most authors agree that only as much cartilage should be removed as is necessary to allow the ribs and sternum to come into good alignment. Since occurrence of asphyxiating thoracic dystrophy has complicated early and extensive operations by this procedure, removing as little cartilage as practical seems prudent. Some authors have proposed that only 3 to 8 mm of cartilage should be removed for a primary repair (87); but sometimes more must be removed to allow a twisted sternum with lengthy deformed cartilages to come into good alignment (77). Robicsek notes, ". . . the surgeon should not waste time in performing a meticulous 'classic' subperichondrial resection of the cartilages and ribs but should just leave enough perichondrium and periosteum behind to ensure the regeneration of the ribs. For the same reason, a segment of the most lateral portion of the cartilage should be left in continuity with the ribs" (88).

Sternal osteotomy may be needed to allow the sternum to come anteriorly. Fracturing the anterior table only with an osteotome is usually sufficient to allow twisting and fracturing the posterior table, allowing the deformed sternum to come into good position (Fig. 9). The process of sternal mobilization in a reoperative field may result in entering the pleural cavity, especially on the right. If so, a chest tube should be considered. Most surgeons place a stainless steel support behind the sternum, such as an Adkins strut or Lorenz bar. The support bar is secured to the soft tissues with suture or wire (Fig. 10). Occasionally, the support can be placed anterior to the sternum and held in place with sutures. In larger patients, more than one support bar may be necessary.

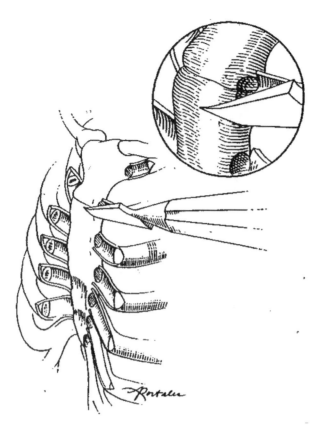

Figure 9 Wedge osteotomy.

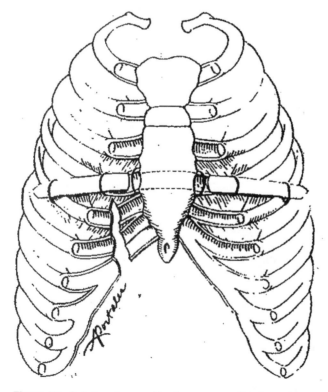

Figure 10 Substernal support bar in open operation for pectus excavatum.

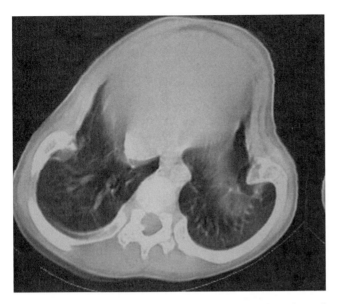

Figure 11   Asphyxiating thoracic dystrophy (acquired Jeune's syndrome).

The pectoralis major muscles are sutured together, and the rectus abdominis sutured to the inferior edge of the pectoralis muscles. Closed suction drains may be placed beneath the muscle layer. Skin closure may be with subcuticular suture.

Operation for treatment of acquired asphyxiating thoracic dystrophy or acquired Jeune's syndrome (Fig. 11) has been pioneered by Dr. Thomas R. Weber. A midline sternotomy is performed, and the pleura is widely opened bilaterally to allow the lung to herniate into the anterior mediastinum. This allows pulmonary compliance to improve immediately, with a marked increase in tidal volume with unchanged ventilatory pressures (89).

A subperiosteal lateral osteotomy of all ribs attached to the sternum bilaterally allows the sternal halves to be separated by 4 to 8 cm, increasing the mediastinal herniation of lung. Three straight bony rib segments of appropriate length are resected, generally from the lower ribs, and "wedged" and wired to hold the sternal halves apart permanently (Fig. 12).

After operation, all patients remain on a ventilator for 3 to 7 days. Because the heart is no longer covered entirely by bone, patients have been advised to wear a chest protector for sports after operation. Patients report tremendous subjective improvement in breathing, but pulmonary function studies do not show great improvement. Body image was a concern after operation in about 70% of patients (89). In selected patients, use of the vertically expandable titanium rib (VEPTER) may be necessary (Figs. 13 and 14, same patient as Figs. 11 and 13). This operation was pioneered by Campbell in San Antonio.

COMPLICATIONS FOLLOWING THE NUSS OPERATION

Complications of the Nuss operation have been documented in several reports from our institution and elsewhere. Early complications are given in Table 2. Late complications are listed in Table 3.

Metal allergy has recently been recognized. All patients should be asked about allergy to nickel or stainless steel, and whether they have had any rash with jewelry, wristwatches, belt buckles, and so forth. Any patient with a suspicious history should be referred to an allergist for testing. In the case of allergy to stainless steel, a titanium bar can be made to order at the factory. Because titanium must be highly polished to prevent tissue ingrowth to the bar, and because bending the bar scratches it, and because titanium is very stiff and hard to bend, the bar must be pre-configured (bent) at the factory. This is done by using computer-assisted design/computer-assisted manufacturing (CAD/CAM) technology to shape the bar to conform to the chest size and dimensions on CT scan (Table 4).

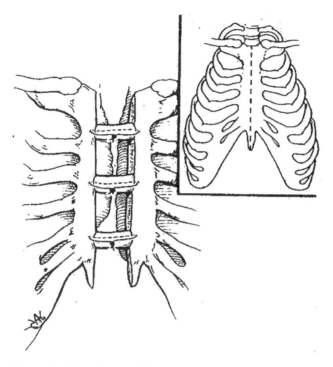

Figure 12 Rib grafts placed in sternal split to increase thoracic volume in acquired Jeune's syndrome.

The Nuss technique of repair of pectus excavatum has undergone several modifications since his initial description in 1997. Avoiding complications in primary repair of pectus excavatum can be aided by the following technical suggestions:

- Select the correct length of pectus bar. The bar should be 1 inch less than the distance from one anterior axillary line to the other.

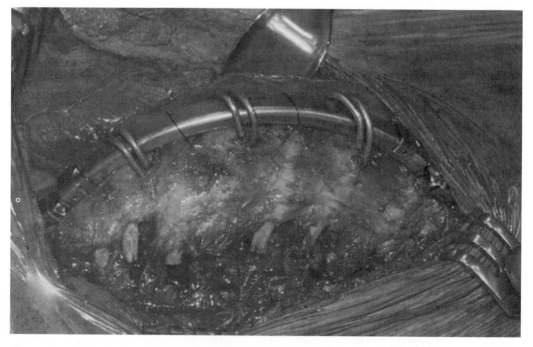

Figure 13 VEPTR device.

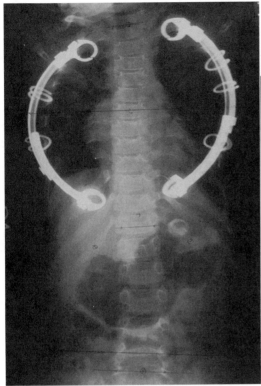
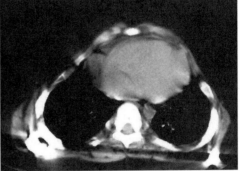

Figure 14   VEPTR device, same patient as Figure 11.

- Bend the bar to fit loosely on each side of the chest.
- When bending the bar, leave a 2 to 4 cm horizontal section in the middle of the bar to support the sternum.
- Thoracostomy entry and exit sites should be medial to the top of the pectus ridge. It the position where the bar enters the chest cavity from the subcutaneous space is lateral to the most anterior portion of the pectus depression's lateral margin, the weight will be borne entirely on the intercostal muscles, and they will tear under the load (Fig. 15).
- Usually the best position for the bar is directly under the deepest point of the pectus excavatum. In this position, it provides the most elevation of the sternum and is often in the most stable place—it is not resting on a sloped portion of the chest wall.
- Elevate the sternum with the introducer before inserting the bar. Especially in teenage and adult patients, anterior elevation with the introducer before passing the bar across prevents helical twisting of the bar as it is flipped over from the inverted position to its working location (Fig. 16).

Table 3   Late Complications of the Nuss
Operation, CHKD/EVMS 1996–2006

Bar displacements	55/900 (6.1%)
Requiring revision	28/55 (50.9%)
Overcorrection	22/900 (2.4%)
Bar allergy	22/900 (2.4%)
Wound/bar infection	8/900 (0.9%)
Recurrence	7/900 (0.8%)
Hemothorax (post-traumatic)	2/900 (0.2%)
Skin erosion	1/900 (0.1%)

Table 4 Metal Allergy, CHKD/EVMS

Metal allergy	22/900
Age	9–23 (average 14.7)
Males:Females	18:1
History of atopy	9 (56%)
Rash/erythema	10 (63%)
Pleural effusion	5 (32%)
Granuloma	1 (6%)
Preoperative screening identified	3 (15%)
Bar removal required for skin breakdown	3 (15%)
Bar replacement required	2 (10%)

- Apply one stabilizer per bar. Application of two stabilizers can lead to a wasp-waist phenomenon as the stabilizer prevents radial growth of the chest. With a single stabilizer, the bar can slip around the chest cage with growth by relative movement of the nonstabilized end toward the stabilized end.
- Use a figure of eight metal wire to attach the stabilizer to the bar. This prevents the stabilizer from sliding off the end of the bar with motion.

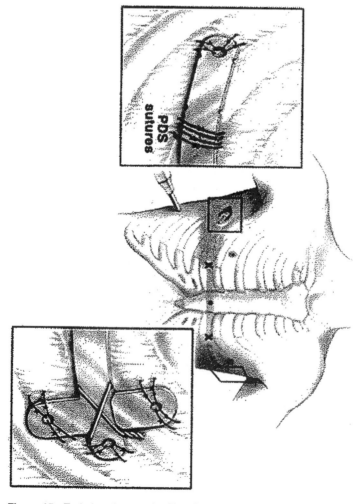

Figure 15 Technique for securing Nuss bar.

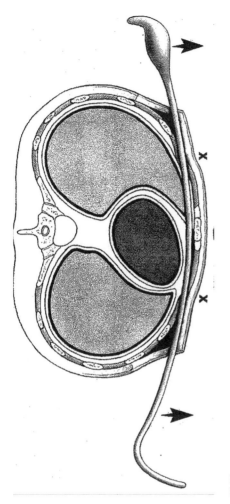

Figure 16 Lifting sternum anteriorly to loosen costal cartilages before bar placement.

- The most important factor in preventing displacement of the bar has been placement of double thickness heavy PDS sutures around the bar and underlying ribs with a laparoscopic fascial closure device under thoracoscopic guidance. Two or three of these should be placed as medially as possible via the lateral thoracic incisions around the bar and underlying rib(s).
- The patients in whom two bars are clearly necessary, consider placing the cephalad bar first. After passage of the introducer at the site of the anterior bar, the sternum is often dramatically elevated off the heart, and passage of the introducer through the lower bar location is facilitated and visualization made much easier. Leave the upper introducer in, or place the upper bar and then dissect the lower tract.
- If thoracoscopic visualization of the tract is difficult, consider:

  - Use of a 30° thoracoscope, which when rotated often gives excellent visualization;
  - Adding insufflation of 5 to 6 mm Hg pressure with CO_2 (we do this routinely) and using fingers to prevent the introduced CO_2 from escaping at the entry and exit sites of the dissector;
  - Passage of the thoracoscope anterior to the dissector through the same opening used to put the introducer in the chest;
  - Moving the thoracoscope from a location 1 to 2 interspaces inferior to the bar insertion site to 1 to 2 interspaces superior;
  - Elevating the sternum via a short incision below the xiphoid, allowing a bone hook or tenaculum to give upward traction to the sternum;
  - Passing a finger behind the sternum to guide the dissector via the same incision;

 – Moving the thoracoscope and dissection from the patient's right to the patient's left; and
 – Placing another thoracoscopic port to allow dissection of the mediastinal fat which often makes visualization more difficult.

After operation, antibiotics are continued intravenously until discharge from the hospital. When mobilizing patients after the operation, torsion, and flexion of the chest are minimized in the early postoperative period. Sports and athletic activities are prohibited for 6 to 8 weeks postoperatively, and while the bar is in place we ask that patients not do boxing, wrestling, hockey, football, or sports where the patient travels through space at high speed and the chest may come to rest suddenly against a fixed object, such as motocross or skiing. The bar or bars are removed after about 2 or more years.

During bar removal, the following technical considerations may help to avoid complications:

 – Complete division of the fibrous sheath which encases the bar posteriorly is helpful in getting the stabilizer off
 – Any bony ingrowth from the chest wall to the bar can be removed with rongeurs or an osteotome.
 – After division of the fibrous attachments, establish that the bar is free to move in its tunnel by placing a bone hook through the end of the bar, and move the bar with small amplitude movements along the course of the curve of the bar. If the bar moves easily for 2 cm, it should come out with minimal resistance.
 – Once the bar is free in its tunnel, slide one end of the bar posteriorly while leaving a Kocher clamp in the hole at the other end of the bar to prevent the opposite end of the bar from going into the chest. Use the Malti bender to straighten out the bar on the end which protrudes more. Then, pull the opposite side out and straighten it (Figs. 17–21). Once both ends of the bar are straight, it comes out with little resistance with traction along the long axis of the bar applied with a bone hook. The assistant may hold the chest stable with his hands to the sides of the patient as traction is applied.

Recurrence rates after the Nuss repair are less well established, since the operation only came into general use in 1997. Recurrence rates will not be deemed reliable by the surgical community until a large cohort of children can be evaluated. Early bar shift and recurrence after removal of the bars should be differentiated for the Nuss procedure. In 900 patients with pectus excavatum treated at Children's Hospital of The King's Daughters/Eastern Virginia Medical

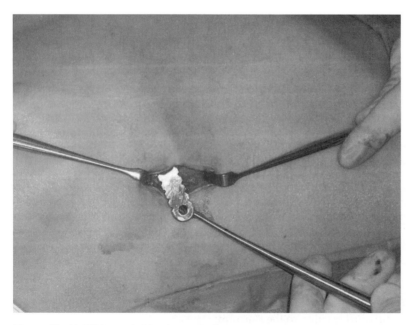

Figure 17 Mobilizing end of bar for removal.

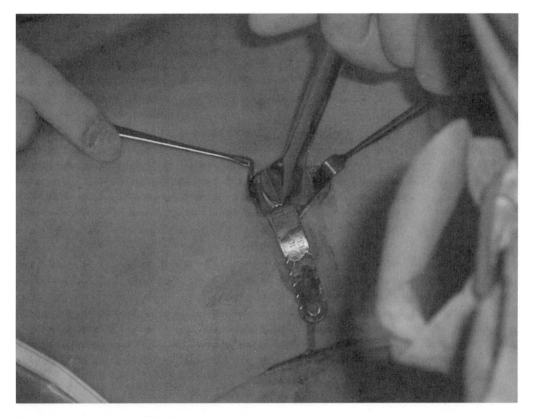

Figure 18 Applying anvil of Malti bender.

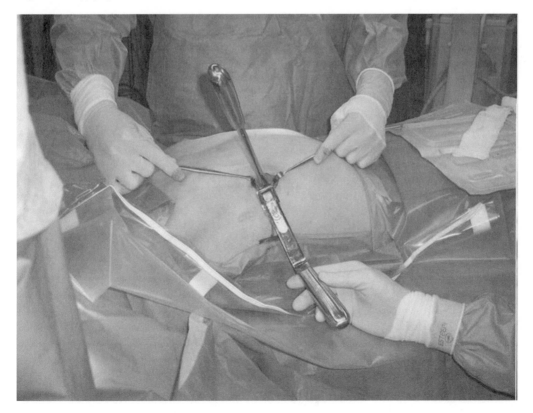

Figure 19 Both bending anvils of Malti bender in place.

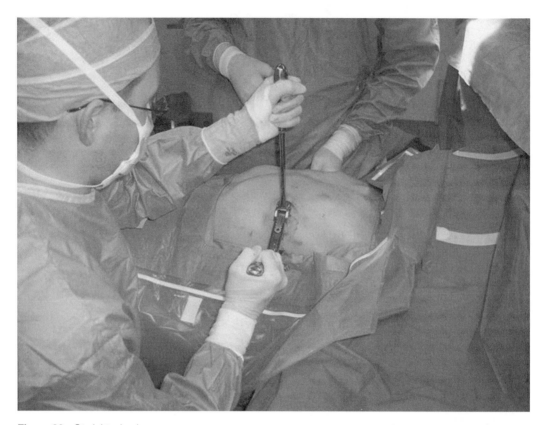

Figure 20 Straightening bar.

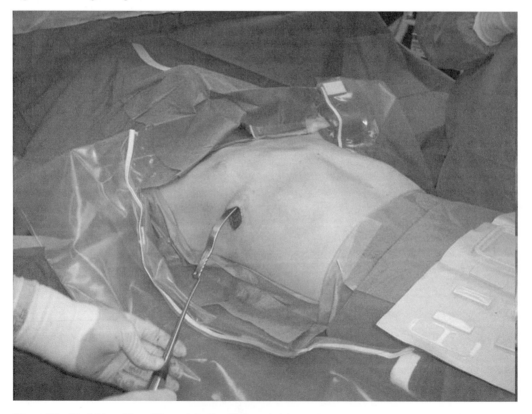

Figure 21 Straightened bar slides out easily with bone hook.

School (CHKD/EVMS), bar shift has occurred about 13% of the time in the first 100 patients. With current methods of securing the bar it is about 0.5% (1/245 patients). Park recorded bar displacement in 2.4% of 335 patients (90). Early bar shift is often related to some unexpected event such as being tackled by uninformed friends or a violent twisting motion. Late recurrence has occurred in 0.8% (7/900) of our patients with follow-up.

REPAIR OF RECURRENT PECTUS EXCAVATUM BY THE NUSS OPERATION

Minimally invasive repair (Nuss procedure) redo operation is accomplished with similar anesthetic and perioperative considerations as the primary repair: general endotracheal anesthesia, epidural analgesia supplement, full anesthetic monitoring, perioperative antibiotics, and bladder catheterization (91). As in first-time operations, allergy to nickel or other metal components of the pectus bar should be sought by application of a skin patch test (92).

Repair is performed through small bilateral midaxillary transverse incisions, subcutaneous tunneling, and intrathoracic placement of a stainless steel or titanium bar. The surgical technique is similar to the technique described for primary repairs with the addition of thoracoscopic lysis of adhesions as required to gain adequate visualization.

The width of the chest is measured in the operating room prior to surgery and the correct length steel bar is selected and bent to conform to the curvature of the anterior chest wall. A small transverse incision 2 or 3 cm long is made in each lateral chest wall between the anterior and posterior axillary lines. Subcutaneous tunnels are raised.

A site for entering the chest medial to the pectus ridge is selected. In a redo patient, it is crucial that the substantial pressure the bar exerts on the chest wall to oppose the pressure of the sternum is borne by the ribs, not the intercostal muscles. If the site of entry into the thorax is too lateral, no rib surface is available for load-bearing, and the intercostal muscles will tear since they cannot support that load.

A long clamp is used to enter the right hemithorax at this spot under direct visualization through a thoracoscope, with attention to be sure the clamp does not injure the adjacent (possibly adherent) lung. The long introducer is passed through this tunnel, posterior to the sternum and anterior to the heart, to emerge through the contralateral intercostal space. An umbilical tape is tied to the end of the introducer, and the umbilical tape is then pulled back through the tract. Once the umbilical tape is across the tract, the introducer is removed and the umbilical tape is transferred to the steel bar. It may be useful in a redo situation to pull a 24 French chest tube through the tract before the bar, and use it to guide the bar through the tract. Using the umbilical tape for traction, the steel bar is pulled through the tract with the convexity facing posteriorly, then the umbilical tape is removed. Once the bar is in position, it is rotated using the bar flipper so that the convexity faces anteriorly, thereby raising the sternum and chest wall into normal position. One end of the bar is secured to a lateral stabilizer using steel wire, and each stabilizer is secured to the musculature of the chest wall with absorbable suture. The bar should be secured to the ribs with a heavy absorbable suture such as PDS under direct vision with an endo-catch device. Before closing the incisions, positive end-expiratory pressure is added to prevent pleural air trapping, then each wound is closed in layers.

There are other several factors to consider for redo operations. In patients with an early recurrence, for example in the first two weeks after operation, the bar has usually flipped from its initial and desired position to one in which the sternum is not pushed anteriorly as much as desired. When this situation is recognized, it is important to put the bar or bars back where they belong. A group in Norway reported erosion of the arch of the aorta from a bar which had flipped to a position putting pressure on the aortic wall (93). Generally repositioning can be done through the initial incisions, even when bar displacement occurs more than a month postoperation (90–92,94). Thoracoscopy can be considered as needed. On-table radiography confirms the correct position of the bars.

It can be difficult at times to tell whether the bar has shifted in the first few days after operation. After repair a cross-table lateral chest X-ray taken in the recovery room can help with making decisions regarding the need to reoperate. Obtaining a chest radiograph on the operating table is wise in redo patients, since the potential for unrecognized residual air collections (pneumothorax) is greater.

Usually redo operations are in older patients. Two bars should be considered to support the sternum, rather than a single bar. One should have a low threshold to use two bars. The chest is often more rigid in redo operations, and two bars distribute the pressure over a broader area and bear less force on each bar. This may give a better result.

If two bars will be used, it may be better to put in the upper bar first. The deepest part of the depression is usually at the lower sternum or xiphoid process, where the lower bar will be placed. Cephalad to the deepest spot, it may be easier to tunnel between the pericardium and sternum.

After passing the first dissector, it should be left in place to support the sternum anteriorly before tunneling with a second dissector at the inferior bar's site. This greatly improves visualization for tunneling at the deeper part of the chest depression.

After the dissector is passed through successfully, the stiff chest of a redo patient should be slowly but firmly pulled toward the operating room ceiling by pressure from the surgeon and assistant. If this is not done, the bar may be twisted into a slightly helical shape when it is flipped over by resistance from the chest wall. We have had one sternal fracture on a redo patient, and the elevation of the sternum should be done gently but firmly.

A sternal saw should be in the room, and the team prepared to use it. We have had one patient suffer an arrhythmia leading to full cardiac arrest as the dissector was passed across the mediastinum. In his very rigid chest, pressure from the dissector may have produced bradycardia and then arrest. Sternotomy and open defibrillation were needed for resuscitation. We have had only one such event in almost 800 Nuss operations at our facility. However, a second patient developed profound bradycardia, treated medically, which apparently arose from a similar response to external pressure on the heart.

If the patient has numerous intrapleural adhesions, which can occur in considerable amount even after Ravitch repair, one should have a low threshold to leave a chest tube in place, since small air leaks may result from the dissection. In reoperative patients, the bars should be especially well secured to the ribs with heavy PDS sutures taken doubled back so two strands go around each rib. Thoracic epidural catheters are even more useful in redo patients because significant postoperative pain is to be anticipated (95). Miller et al. (96) have confirmed our findings that redo correction can be done safely with minimal blood loss and short operating time in patients who have undergone prior unsatisfactory open repair of pectus excavatum.

In conclusion, the variety of complications which occur in pediatric thoracic surgery prevents any simple formulation for preventing any problem. Careful attention to preoperative preparation, adherence to technical details during operation, and vigilant support of the patient's cardiorespiratory work after surgery minimize complications. Technologic improvements in equipment which allow operations to be done through minimal incisions also benefit patients in our time, especially when compared to children of only a few years ago.

ACKNOWLEDGMENTS

The authors thank Drs. Thomas Weber and Dick Ellis and their publishers for permission to use illustrations. We thank Mrs. Trisha Arnel for her help in preparing this manuscript.

REFERENCES

1. Warner MA, Warner ME, Warner DA, et al. Perioperative pulmonary aspiration in infants and children. Anesthesiology 1999; 90(1):66–71.
2. Janda M, Scheeren TW, Noldge-Schomburg GF. Management of pulmonary aspiration. Best Pract Res Clin Anaesthelsiol 2006; 20(3):409–427.
3. Gardlund Tan B, Rimeika D, Wedelin B, et al. Preoperative bacterial colonization of the upper airways does not predict postoperative airway infection in children. Acta Paediatr 1998; 87(4):375–377.
4. Heath PT. Epidemiology and bacteriology of bacterial pneumonias. Paediatr Respir Rev 2000; 1(1):4–7.
5. Tan, L, Sun X, Zhu X, et al. Epidemiology of nosocomial pneumonia in infants after cardiac surgery. Chest 2004; 125:410–417.

6. Lin CS, Hsu WH, Wu YC, et al. Effectiveness of short-term antibiotic prophylaxis on postoperative recovery course after pulmonary lobectomies. J Chin Med Assoc 2004; 67(6):275–280.

7. Cullen ML. Pulmonary and respiratory complications of pediatric trauma. Respir Care Clin N Am 2001; 7(1):59–77.

8. Raad I, Hachem R, Hannah, H, et al. Treatment of nosocomial postoperative pneumonia in cancer patients: A prospective randomized study. Ann Surg Oncol 2001; 8(2):179–186.

9. Delaney JW, Moltedo JM, Dziura JD, et al. Early postoperative arrhythmias alter pediatric cardiac surgery. J Thorac Cardiovasc Surg 2006; 131(6):1296–1300.

10. Coln E, Carrasco J, Coln D. Demonstrating relief of cardiac compression with the Nuss minimally invasive repair of pectus excavatum. J Pediatr Surg 2006; 41(4):683–686.

11. Zoeller GK, Zallen GS, Glick PL. Cardiopulmonary resuscitation in patients with a Nuss bar—A case report and review of the literature. J Pediatr Surg 2005; 40(11):1788–1791.

12. Bal S, Eishershari H, Celiker R, et al. Thoracic sequels after thoracotomies in children with congenital cardiac disease. Cardiol Young 2003; 13(3):264–267.

13. Emmel M, Ulbach P, Herse B, et al. Neurogenic lesions after posterolateral thoracotomy in young children. Thorac Cardiovasc Surg 1996; 44:86–91.

14. Cherup L, Siewers R, Futrell J. Breast and pectoral muscle maldevelopment after anterolateral and posterolateral thoracotomies in children. Ann Thorac Surg 1986; 41:492–497.

15. Horowitz MD, Ancalmo N, Ochsner JL. Thoracotomy through the auscultatory triangle. Ann Thorac Surg 1989; 47:780–781.

16. Frola C, Serrano J, Cantoni S, et al. CT findings of atrophy of chest wall muscle after thoracotomy: Relationship between muscles involved and type of surgery. Am J Roentgenol 1995; 164:599–601.

17. Lemmer J, Gomez M, Symreng T, et al. Limited lateral thoracotomy. Arch Surg 1990; 125:873–877.

18. Ponn R, Ferneini A, D'Agostino R, et al. Comparison of late pulmonary function after posterolateral and muscle-sparing thoracotomy. Ann Thorac Surg 1992; 53:675–679.

19. Chetcuti P, Myers NA, Phelan PD, et al. Chest wall deformity in patients with repaired esophageal atresia. J Pediatr Surg 1989; 24(3):244–247.

20. Durning RP, Scoles PV, Fox OD. Scoliosis after thoracotomy in tracheoesophageal fistula patients. A follow-up study. J Bone Joint Surg Am 1980; 62(7):1156–1159.

21. Van Biezen FC, Bakx PA, De Velleneuve VH, et al. Scoliosis in children after thoracotomy for aortic coarctation. J Bone Joint Surg Am 1993; 75(4):514–518.

22. Ruiz-Iban MA, Burgos J, Aguado HJ, et al. Scoliosis after median sternotomy in children with congenital heart disease. Spine 2005; 30(8):214–218.

23. Herrara-Soto JA, Vander Have KL, Barry-Lane P, et al. Spinal deformity after combined thoracotomy and sternotomy for congenital heart disease. J Pediatr Orthop 2006; 26(2):211–215.

24. Long CB, Shah SS, Lautenbach E, et al. Postoperative mediastinitis in children: Epidemiology, microbiology and risk factors for gram-negative pathogens. Pediatr Infect Dis J 2005; 24(4):315–319.

25. Shah SS, Kagen J, Lautenbach E, et al. Bloodstream infections after median sternotomy at a children's hospital. J Thorac Cardiovasc Surg 2007; 133(2):435–440.

26. Mehta PA, Cunningham CK, Collela CB, et al. Risk factors for sternal wound and other infections in pediatric cardiac surgery patients. Pediatr Infect Dis J 2000; 19(10):1000–1004.

27. Stahle E, Tammelin A, Bergstrom R, et al. Sternal wound complications-incidence, microbiology and risk factors. Eur J Cardiothorac Surg 1997; 11(6):1146–1153.

28. Weinzweig N, Yetman R. Transposition of the greater omentum for recalcitrant median sternotomy wound infections. Ann Plast Surg 1995; 34(5):471–477.

29. Agarwal JP, Ogilvie M, Wu LC, et al. Vacuum-assisted closure for sternal wounds: A first-line therapeutic management approach. Plast Reconstr Surg 2005; 116(4):1035–1040.

30. Furrer M, Rechstiener R, Eigenmann C, et al. Thoracotomy and thoracoscopy: Postoperative pulmonary function, pain, and chest wall complaints. Eur J Cardiothrac Surg 1997; 12:82–87.

31. Kaiser L, Bavaria J. Complications of thoracoscopy. Ann Thorac Surg 1993; 56:796–798.

32. Shapira OM, Shanian DM. Postpneumonectomy pulmonary edema. Ann Thorac Surg 1993; 45:190–195.

33. Baldt MM, Bankier AA, Germann PS, et al. Complications after emergency tube thoracostomy: Assessment with CT. Radiology 1995; 195(2):539–543.

34. Gervaix A, Beghetti M, Rimensberger P, et al. Bullous emphysema after Legionella pneumonia in a two-year-old child. Pediatr Infect Dis J 2000; 19(1):86–87.

35. Luh SP, Tsai TP, Chou MC, et al. Video-assisted thoracic surgery for spontaneous pneumothorax: Outcome of 189 cases. Int Surg 2004; 89(4):185–189.

36. Ellman BR, Ferrante JW, Tiedemann RN. Thoracoscopy for spontaneous pneumothorax 2.10 version with bleb stapling and pleurectomy. Am Surg 1995; 61(2):102–105.

37. Tsunezuka Y, Sato H, Kodama T. Video-assisted contralateral treatment for bronchial stump diastasis after left pneumonectomy. Chest 2000; 117(3):884–886.

38. Shimizu J, Takizawa M, Yachi T, et al. Postoperative bronchial stump fistula responding well to occlusion with metallic coils and fibrin glue via a tracheostomy: A case report. Ann Thorac Cardiovasc Surg 2005; 11(2):104–108.

39. Gaissert HA, Mathisen DJ, Grillo HC, et al. Trachobronchial sleeve resection in children and adolescents. J Pediatr Surg 1994; 29(2):192–197.

40. Maeda M, Nakamoto K, Ohta M, et al. Statistical survey of tracheobronchoplasty in Japan. J Thorac Cardiovasc Surg 1989; 97(3):402–414.

41. Al-Qahtani AR, Di Lorenzo M, Yazbeck S. Endobronchial tumors in children: institutional experience and literature review. J Pediatr Surg 2003; 38(5):733–736.

42. Chen LE, Langer JC, Dillon PA, et al. Management of late-stage parapneumonic empyema. J Pediatr Surg 2002; 37(3):371–374.

43. Ozcelik C, Ulku R, Onat S, et al. Management of postpneumonic empyemas in children. Eur J Cardiothorac Surg 2004; 25(6):1072–1078.

44. Kim BY, Oh BS, Jang WC, et al. Video-assisted thoracoscopic decortication for management of postpneumonic pleural empyema. Am J Surg 2004; 188(3):321–324.

45. Rowe S, Cheadle WG. Complications of nosocomial pneumonia in the surgical patient. Am J Surg 2000; 179(2 A Suppl):63 S–68S.

46. Alexiou C, Goyal A, Firmin RK, et al. Is open thoracotomy still a good treatment option for the management of empyema in children? Ann Thorac Surg 2003; 76(6):1854–1858.

47. Tseng YL, Wu MH, Lin MY, et al. Surgery for lung abscess in immunocompetent and immunocompromised children. J Pediatr Surg 2001; 36(3):470–473.

48. Kim YT, Kang MC, Sung SW, et al. Good long-term outcomes after surgical treatment of simple and complex pulmonary aspergilloma. Ann Thorac Surg 2005; 79(1):294–298.

49. Eren S, Eren MN, Balci AE. Pneumonectomy in children for destroyed lung and the long-term consequences. J Thorac Cardiovasc Surg 2003; 126(2):574–581.

50. Shields TW, Lees WMM, Fox RT, et al. Persistent pleural space following resection for pulmonary tuberculosis. J Thorac Cardiovasc Surg 1959; 38:523–536.

51. Barker WL, Langston HT, Naffah P. Postresectional thoracic spaces. Ann Thorac Surg 1966; 2: 299.

52. Burke SJ, Faber LP. Complications of pulmonary resection. In: Little AG, ed. Complications in Cardiothoracic Surgery. New York: Blackwell, 1994:67–91.

53. Malca SA, Roche PH, Touta A, et al. Pneumocephalus after thoracotomy. Surg Neurol 1995; 43(4):398–401.

54. Chan SY, Lau W, Wong WH, et al. Chylothorax in children after congenital heart surgery. Ann Thorac Surg 2006; 82(5):1650–1656.

55. Chan EH, Russel JL, Williams WG, et al. Postoperative chylothorax after cardiothoracic surgery in children. Ann Thorac Surg 2005; 80(5):1864–1870.

56. Wu, JM, Yao CT, Kan CD, et al. Postoperative chylothorax: Differences between patients who received median sternotomy or lateral thoracotomy for congenital heart disease. J Card Surg 2006; 21(3):249–253.

57. Helin RD, Angeles ST, Bhat R. Octreotide therapy for chylothorax in infants and children: A brief review. Pediatr Crit Care Med 2006; 7(6):576–579.

58. Kalomenidis I. Octreotide and chylothorax. Curr Opin Pulm Med 2006; 12(4):264–267.

59. Achildi O, Smith BP, Grewal H. Thoracoscopic ligation of the thoracic duct in a child with spontaneous chylothorax. J Laparoendosc Adv Surg Tech A 2006; 16(5):546–549.

60. Mott AR, Fraser CD Jr, Kusnoor AV, et al. The effect of short-term prophylactic methylprednisolone on the incidence and severity of postpericardiotomy syndrome in children undergoing cardiac surgery with cardiopulmonary bypass. J Am Coll Cardiol 2001; 37:1700–1706.

61. Nuss D, Croitoru DP, Kelly RE Jr, et al. Review and discussion of the complications of minimally invasive pectus excavatum repair. Eur J Pediatr Surg 2002; 12(4):230–234.

62. Dressler W. A post-myocardial infarction syndrome: Preliminary report of complication resembling idiopathic, recurrent, benign pericarditis. JAMA 1956; 160:1379–1384.

63. Velander M, Grip L, Mogenson L, et al. The postcardiac injury syndrome following percutaneous transluminal coronary angioplasty. Clin Cardiol 1993; 16:353–354.

64. Maisch B, Berg PA, Kochesiek K. Clinical significance of immunopathological findings in patients with postpericardiotomy syndrome. 1. Relevance of antibody pattern. Clin Exp Immunol 1979; 38:189–196.

65. Merrill W, Donahoo JS, Brawley RK, et al. Late cardiac tamponade: A potentially lethal complication of open-heart surgery. J Thorac Cardiovasc Surg 1976; 72:929–932.

66. Tonz M, von Segesser LK, Mihaljevic T, et al. Clinical implications of phrenic nerve injury after pediatric cardiac surgery. J Pediatr Surg 1996; 31(9):1265–1267.

67. Akay TH, Ozkan S, Gultekin B, et al. Diaphragmatic paralysis after cardiac surgery in children: incidence, prognosis and surgical management. Pediatr Surg Int 2006; 22(4):341–346.
68. Hines MH. Video-assisted diaphragm plication in children. Ann Thorac Surg 2003; 76(1):234–236.
69. Langer JC, Filler RM, Coles J, et al. Plication of the diaphragm for infants and young children with phrenic nerve palsy. J Pediatr Surg 1988; 23(8):749–751.
70. Cohen M, Ramasastry SS. Reconstruction of complex chest wall defects. Am J Surg 1996; 172(1): 35–40.
71. Richardson JD, Miller FB, Carrillo EH, et al. Complex thoracic injuries. Surg Clin North Am 1996; 76(4):725–748.
72. Lacquet LK, Morshuis WJ, Folgering HT. Long-term results after correction of anterior chest wall deformities. J Cardiovasc Surg 1998; 39:683–688.
73. Frey AS, Garcia VF, Brown RL, et al. Nonoperative management of pectus carinatum. J Pediatr Surg 2006; 41:40–45.
74. Egan JC, DuBois JJ, Morphy M, et al. Compressive orthotics in the treatment of asymmetric pectus carinatum: A preliminary report with an objective radiographic marker. J Pediatr Surg 2000; 35:1183–1186.
75. Kelly RE, Shamberger RC, Mellins R, et al. Prospective multicenter study of surgical correction of pectus excavatum: Design, perioperative complications, pain, and baseline pulmonary function facilitated by internet-based data collection. J Am Coll Surg 2007; 205:205–216.
76. Haller JA. Severe chest wall constriction from growth retardation after extensive and too early (<4 years) pectus excavatum repair: An alert. Ann Thorac Surg 1995; 60:1857–1864.
77. Ellis DG, Snyder CL, Mann CM. The 'redo' chest wall deformity correction. J Pediatr Surg 1997; 32(9):1267–1271.
78. Arn PH, Scherer LR, Haller JA Jr, et al. Outcome of pectus excavatum in patients with Marfan syndrome and in the general population. J Pediatr 1989; 115:954–958.
79. Willital GH, Meier H. Cause of funnel chest recurrences—operative treatment and long-term results. Prog Pediatr Surg 1997; 10:253–256.
80. Gilbert JC, Zwiren GT. Repair of pectus excavatum using a substernal metal strut within a Marlex envelope. South Med J 1989; 82:1240–1244.
81. Onursal E, Toker A, Bostanci K, et al. A complication of pectus excavatum operation: Endomyocardial steel strut. Ann Thorac Surg 1999; 68(3):1082–1083.
82. Dalrymple-Hay MJ, Calver A, Lea RE, et al. Migration of pectus excavatum correction bar into the left ventricle. Eur J Cardiothorac Surg 1997; 12(3):507–509.
83. Pircova A, Sekarski-Hunkeler N, Jeanrenaud X, et al. Cardiac perforation after surgical repair of pectus excavatum. J Pediatr Surg 1995; 30(10):1506–1508.
84. Kanegaonkar RG, Dussek JE. Removal of migrating pectus bars by video-assisted thoracoscopy. Eur J Cardiothorac Surg 2001; 19(5):713–715.
85. Elami A, Lieberman Y. Hemopericardium: A late complication after repair of pectus excavatum. J Cardiovasc Surg 1991; 32(4):539–540.
86. Pretorium ES, Haller JA, Fishman EK. Spiral CT with 3D reconstruction in children requiring reoperation for failure of chest wall growth after pectus excavatum surgery. Preliminary observations. Clin Imaging 1998; 22:108–116.
87. Fonkalsrud EW. Open repair of pectus excavatum with minimal cartilage resection. Ann Surg 2004; 240:231–235.
88. Robicsek F. Surgical treatment of pectus excavatum. Chest Surg Clin N Am 2000; 10:277–296.
89. Weber TR. Further experience with the operative management of asphyxiating thoracic dystrophy after pectus repair. J Pediatr Surg 2005; 40:173–175.
90. Park HJ, Lee SY, Lee CS. Complications associated with the Nuss procedure: Analysis of risk factors and suggested measure for prevention of complications. J Pediatr Surg 2004; 39:391–395.
91. Croitoru DP, Kelly RE Jr, Goretsky MJ, et al. The minimally invasive Nuss technique for recurrent or failed pectus excavatum repair in 50 patients. J Pediatr Surg 2005; 40:181–186.
92. Rushing GD, Goretsky MJ, Gustin T, et al. When it's not an infection: Metal allergy after the Nuss procedure for repair of pectus excavatum. J Pediatr Surg 2007; 42:93–97.
93. Hoel TN, Rein KA, Svennevig JL. A life-threatening complication of the Nuss procedure for pectus excavatum. Ann Thorac Surg 2006; 81:370–372.
94. Huang PM, Wu ET, Tseng YT, et al. Modified Nuss operation for pectus excavatum: Design for decreasing cardiopulmonary complications. Thorac Cardiovasc Surg 2006; 54:134–137.
95. Futagawa K, Suwa I, Okuda T, et al. Anesthetic management for the minimally invasive Nuss procedure in 21 patients with pectus excavatum. J Anesth 2006; 20:48–50.
96. Miller KA, Ostlie DJ, Wade K, et al. Minimally invasive bar repair for "redo" correction of pectus excavatum. J Pediatr Surg 2002; 37(7):1090–1092.

Nuss Procedure for Pectus Excavatum

Expert: Donald Nuss, M.B., Ch.B.

QUESTIONS

1. **What steps do you take to prevent cardiac injury during bar placement?**
   Before surgery, I review the CT scan to check the relationship between the heart and the sternum. If there is significant sternal torsion, then there may be a change in the normal relationship between the heart and the sternum, which may lead to cardiac perforation. It is, therefore, important to know where the heart is situated in relationship to the twisted sternum.

   Second, thoracoscopy is extremely important in preventing cardiac injury. I usually insert the thoracoscope on the right side, while other surgeons prefer the left side and some do bilateral thoracoscopy. In patients with a very severe pectus excavatum, I create the first tunnel one or two intercostal spaces superior to the deepest point of the pectus excavatum and then leave that introducer in place to keep the sternum elevated while I tunnel under the deepest point of the depression.

   The sternum may also be elevated by using the suction cup described by Schier et al., by placing anterior traction on either a suture through the anterior plate of the sternum, or a towel clip on the xiphisternum.

2. **In what situations do you use two bars?**
   Patients always look better on the operating table than they do when standing up because the supine position on the operating table obliterates the normal thoracic kyphosis. I will, therefore, add a second bar whenever I am not completely satisfied with the correction obtained with only one bar. I tell my residents "I have never regretted placing two bars, but I have frequently regretted placing only one bar". Patients who have Marfan's syndrome should receive two bars as the sternum may be too soft to be supported by only one bar, and postpubertal patients usually require two bars to diffuse the pressure over a wider area.

3. **How do you like to stabilize the bar?**
   I place a rectangular stabilizer with wire fixation suture on the patients left side, and on the right I place multiple "0" PDS sutures around the bar and underlying ribs. These sutures are placed through the right lateral thoracic skin incision under thoracoscopic control using a laparoscopic "endo-close" needle. I may also place sutures on the left side if I can get the thoracoscope through the substernal tunnel. Ideally, I like to place the bar under the deepest point of the depression as it is most stable in that position. A second bar helps to distribute the pressure over a wider area thereby minimizing the risk of displacement.

4. **Do you routinely place a chest tube?**
   No, the only patients who routinely receive a chest tube are "Re-do" patients who have had lysis of pulmonary adhesions. Primary repair patients almost never require a chest tube. The pneumothorax created with CO_2 for thoracoscopy is evacuated at the end of the procedure by using a water seal system with positive pressure ventilation to evacuate all the carbon dioxide. When there are no more air bubbles escaping from the water seal system, and the lungs are in full inspiration, the trocar is pulled and the incision is closed. If, however, air bubbles continue to escape from the water seal system for a prolonged period of time, then the system is checked for air leaks and if none are found, then a chest tube is inserted. Chest Xrays are taken immediately postoperatively, on day 1 and on day 3 to check for pneumothorax and bar displacement.

5. **How do you manage bar displacement?**
   If the bar is displaced more than 20° While the patient is still in the hospital, I take him back to the operating room and reposition the bar even if there is no recurrence. If the bar gets displaced after the patient has been discharged, it will be repositioned if he has a recurrence. If the patient returns for a check up at a later time and the bar

is mildly displaced, but the patient is asymptomatic and the repair remains in excellent condition then I will continue with observation and obtain another X-ray in a month. If the displacement progresses, then the bar will need to be repositioned.

6. **How do you manage an exposed bar in the early postoperative period?**

    This is preventable problem which I have not seen since I first started using the minimally invasive procedure and the bar we were using then was too soft—as the center caved in, the lateral portion would flare out. To prevent this from occurring, it is important to have the correct length bar and to bend the bar so that it does not protrude under the skin. When closing the incisions over the bar, all fascial layers need to be re-approximated over the bar. Prevention of infection is also important to prevent the incision from disrupting. If the bar does become exposed then the cause needs to be elucidated and treated—the bar may need more molding, infection needs to be treated and one needs to check for allergy.

7. **How do you manage the patient with a large seroma surrounding the endof the bar?**

    The seroma may be due to mechanical factors (bar movement causing tissue irritation, and hemorrhage), infection or allergy. I would aspirate fluid for culture and sensitivity and draw blood for a white count, ESR, and CRP. If all studies are negative then it is most likely due to tissue irritation and the patient needs to discontinue sports for 2 weeks, take anti-inflammatory pain medications and possibly antibiotics to prevent the seroma/hematoma from becoming infected. If aspiration shows pus and positive bacterial cultures are obtained, then one would treat it appropriately with antibiotics and drainage. I would start with IV antibiotics and then switch to oral antibiotics as appropriate until the ESR and CRP are back to normal which may take 1 to 2 months. If the seroma is due to allergy then there will be negative cultures, an elevated eosinophil count, elevated ESR, and CRP. In that case, I would test for nickel allergy and if that is positive I would treat with low dose prednisone until ESR and CRP are back to normal values which might also take 1 to 2 months.

8. **When do you remove the bar?**

    I generally remove the bar 3 years after insertion. Postpubertal patients are no longer growing so there is no urgency to remove the bar and some patients have kept their bar for as long as $4^{1}/_{2}$ years with no problems. If the patient grows more than 8 in ($\pm$16 cm) after bar insertion or becomes symptomatic after 2 years then I would remove the bar before 3 years. I encourage all patients to continue with their deep breathing exercises and aerobic sports.

9. **After bar removal what technical factors can be offered to the patient dissatisfied with the cosmetic result?**

    This depends on the severity of the recurrence. Patients who have a significant recurrence and wish to have it corrected may undergo repair. We have performed 81 re-do operations of which 45 were previous closed cases (four done at our institution) and 35 previous open cases (all done elsewhere). Thoracoscopy is essential in these patients since they all tend to have adhesions that may need to be lysed. Our results in these cases are only slightly less satisfactory than in the primary cases. If the patients' dissatisfaction is due to minimal irregularity of the anterior chest wall, and not severe enough to warrant surgery, then we prescribe a breathing, posture, aerobic exercise, and weight training program.

10. **What athletic activity restrictions are imposed while the bar is in place?**

    For the first 6 weeks after pectus repair all sports are prohibited although the patients may return to school after 2 weeks. Six weeks after the surgery they may slowly resume sports and by 8 weeks we encourage all our patients to participate in aerobic activities including swimming, basketball, soccer, dancing, etc. We do not permit heavy contact sports such as boxing, American football, ice hockey, or sports in which there is a high probability of chest injuries. We have had several patient involved in major car accidents without sustaining bar displacement. We have patients who have excelled in sports after pectus repair including basketball, swimming, water polo, diving, track, and athletics.

11. How do you diagnose and treat bar allergy?

If the patient gives a preoperative history of metallic allergy (cannot wear jewelry, watch or clothes with metal buttons) then the patient receives a titanium bar. If the patient or family gives a history of metal allergy or the patient suffers from atopy, eczema, or asthma, then he should be tested for nickel or cobalt allergy. He should probably receive a titanium bar even if he tests negative because these patients may not be positive at the time of the test but may become positive later. If the patient develops an allergy while the bar is in place as evidenced by persistent pleural or pericardial effusion, erythema over the anterior chest, sterile wound drainage, malaise and persistent pain, then he should be tested with a TRUE skin test and have a CBC, ESR, and CRP checked. If the tests are positive then the patient should be treated with prednisone until the ESR and CRP return to normal levels. This may take 1 to 2 months. The other alternative is to remove the steel bar in insert a titanium bar.

12. How to manage the patient with persistent pain?

Most patients no longer require pain medication after 1 to 3 weeks depending on age. A few patients (1–2%) complain of persistent pain. The causes may be chronic infection, allergy, bar displacement, bar too tight, bar too long, stabilizer displaced or fractured, sternal or rib erosion, or drug dependence. A chest X-ray, white blood count, ESR, CRP, and TRUE skin test are usually able to elucidate the correct diagnosis. Treatment will be directed at correcting the underlying problem. If the pain persists despite testing and treatment, then switching from a steel bar to a titanium bar may be helpful.

10 | Complications of Extracorporeal Membrane Oxygenation

Kimberly W. McCrudden, M.D. and Ronald B. Hirschl, M.D.

INTRODUCTION

Infants and children with severe, acute, reversible cardiac, and respiratory failure face significant mortality. Failure to respond to conventional medical and pharmaceutical treatment leaves these patients with little recourse. These patients are candidates for extracorporeal life support (ECLS) or extracorporeal membrane oxygenation (ECMO). This invasive intervention is not a cure or a therapy, but a mechanism to provide cardiorespiratory support while the underlying pathophysiologic processes resolve with time, medical management, or surgical intercession. ECLS spares the body from the harmful effects of hypoxia, acidosis, barotrauma, and end-organ hypoperfusion as it struggles to recover. However, management of severely ill neonates and children with ECMO is associated with many complications, some of which have significant long-term consequences for the patient. The goal of this chapter is to review the techniques of ECMO cannulation in infants and children with attention to preventing known surgical complications, discuss the short-term mechanical and patient-related complications of ECMO, and examine the long-term outcomes of ECLS in the neonatal and pediatric populations.

PERTINENT ANATOMY

Neonatal ECMO is usually performed through an open neck cutdown. Just under the skin is the platysma muscle, which spreads out like a sheet in the subcutaneous tissue and is pierced by small cutaneous nerves. The anterior triangle of the neck is bounded laterally by the medial border of the sternocleidomastoid muscle (SCM), which has two heads running from the top of the sternum and medial clavicle to insert on the mastoid process. This important triangle is defined superiorly by the angle of the mandible and medially by the sternohyoid muscle. The anterior triangle can be further divided into a submandibular, carotid, and muscular triangles. The carotid triangle lies in the inferior-most portion of the anterior triangle and is medial to the SCM, lateral to the sternohyoid, and inferior to the omohyoid.

Dissection lateral to the SCM will expose the external jugular vein, which is often available for cutdown insertion of indwelling catheters in infants. The carotid sheath runs medial to the SCM in the superior portion of the anterior triangle and then courses underneath the inferior portion of the SCM and omohyoid. It lies medial and posterior to the internal jugular vein. Within the carotid sheath, the common carotid artery lies medial and posterior to the vein and has no major branches. It bifurcates at about the level of the hyoid bone where the external carotid artery gives off the thyroid arteries. The internal jugular vein, located lateral to the carotid, often gives off a small branch medially (like the middle thyroid vein) which must be ligated during cannulation. The vagus nerve generally runs posterior and lateral to the common carotid artery in the carotid sheath.

Other structures to be aware of during a neck dissection for ECMO include the superior and inferior roots of the ansa cervicalis, which run over the inferior carotid sheath. The omohyoid muscle crosses the bottom of the carotid triangle and must be occasionally divided to provide adequate exposure to the vessels. Overzealous dissection posteriorly behind the carotid sheath might lead to damage of the phrenic nerve (which runs over the scalenus anterior) and the sympathetic trunk or even cause bleeding from the ascending cervical arteries.

Cannulation in larger children is often performed using a modified Seldinger technique and a two-cannula drainage system utilizing the femoral vein. Review of the vascular anatomy below the inguinal ligament finds the common femoral vein located medial to the femoral artery. The femoral nerve lies lateral to the artery, and the lymphatic channels run medial to the vein.

Palpation of the femoral artery pulse aids in accurate percutaneous access to the femoral vein. Open infrainguinal dissection just below the inguinal ligament will expose several branches of the greater saphenous vein (superficial epigastric, external pudendal, and superficial circumflex iliac vein) and their accompanying arteries in the superficial space. The deeper femoral sheath has three compartments: lateral containing the artery, middle holding the vein, and medial (also known as the femoral canal) carrying lymphatics. The proximal portion of the femoral canal is bounded medially by the lacunar ligament, anteriorly by the inguinal ligament, posteriorly by the pectinius muscle, and laterally by the femoral vein.

OPERATIVE DETAILS

Neonatal Cannulation

Neonatal ECMO is performed through an open neck cutdown technique. This is usually performed in the neonatal intensive care unit using intravenous sedation and neuromuscular blockade. Adequate paralysis is essential to prevent air embolization during insertion of the venous cannula. The patient is placed supine on the bed with the head facing toward the center of the room to allow for space to cannulate. A shoulder roll is placed transversely and the head is turned to the left. After ensuring that the endotracheal tube is not kinked, the entire neck, chest, and right face are prepped and draped in a sterile fashion.

A 2 to 3 cm transverse cervical incision is made approximately one finger's breadth above the medial portion of the clavicle. The platysma and subcutaneous tissues are divided with electrocautery to expose the underlying SCM. Blunt dissection between the sternal and clavicular heads of this muscle will expose the underlying carotid sheath. Occasionally, complete exposure of the sheath will require division of the omohyoid tendon, which lies superiorly. One or two self-retraining retractors are then placed to maintain exposure. Generous but controlled use of electrocautery may prevent later oozing from the surgical incision following heparinization.

The carotid sheath is then carefully opened and the common carotid artery, internal jugular vein, and vagus nerve are identified. Dissection begins with the vein, which is followed proximally and distally. Often, a branch is noted on the medial aspect of the vein, which should be ligated. Excessive dissection of the vein must be avoided as it often leads to severe venospasm, which makes insertion of large venous cannulas more difficult. Two 2–0 silk sutures should then be placed proximally and distally around the vein. A similar dissection is performed proximally and distally on the artery, and 2–0 silk ties are placed around the vessel. Even if only veno-venous bypass is planned, it is wise to dissect out both vessels, which requires little additional operative time and can greatly facilitate conversion to veno-arterial (VA) bypass, if needed. A small vessel loop is placed around the common carotid artery and the two ends either tied or clipped together. This identifying loop can be easily removed after successful veno-venous (VV) bypass is established or at the time of decannulation.

Following isolation of the vessels, intravenous heparin (100 U/kg) is administered. While the heparin is circulating, papaverine is instilled into the wound to aid venous dilation and the cannulas are selected and prepared. For VA bypass, the arterial cannula is selected (usually 8–10 French) and marked with a 2–0 silk ligature at approximately 2.5 cm from the tip. This provides a rough estimate of the location required for the cannula to lie at the junction of the brachiocephalic trunk and the aorta in most infants. The venous cannula is chosen (usually 12–14 French) and similarly marked with a 2–0 silk suture at a point that approximates the distance from the venotomy site to the right atrium (6 cm from the tip) (1).

After the heparin has been circulated for a minimum of 3 minutes, the common carotid artery is ligated distally and proximal control is obtained using an angled ductus clamp.

It is advisable to leave long tails on the proximal silk ligatures as these provide excellent traction that facilitates cannula placement. A transverse arteriotomy is made using an 11 blade near the distal ligature. Full-thickness 6–0 prolene stay sutures are then placed along the proximal edge of the arterial wall. These stay sutures are essential as they both prevent subintimal dissection and assist in placement of the arterial cannula. The cannula is inserted up to the 2.5 cm mark and secured in place using two 2–0 silk sutures tied over a small piece of silastic vessel loop (sometimes referred to as the "bumper"). Use of silastic bumpers is important in protecting the vessel wall from necrosis secondary to the tight ligatures and from injury during decannulation. The cannula is allowed to fill with blood, then quickly clamped using a tubing

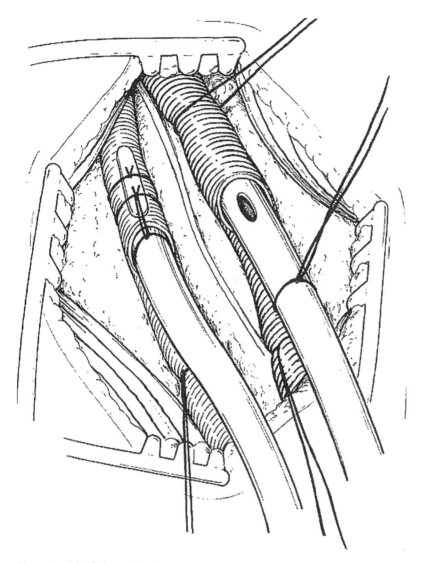

Figure 1   ECMO Cannulation.

clamp. Following arterial cannulation, the vein is ligated cephalad and traction applied to the caudal silk ligature to provide venous control. A transverse venotomy is then performed using the 11 blade and the venous cannula with obturator is inserted up to the 6 cm mark (Fig. 1). The cannula obturator is removed, filling the cannula with blood before clamping. This will occasionally require gentle pressure applied over the liver to enhance venous return. The venous cannula is then secured in place using two 2–0 silk sutures over a silastic bumper. Additional cannula security is provided by tying the ends of the silk ties marking the cannulas to the most distal ligature around the vessel. It is essential that the cannulas be well secured prior to initiating bypass to avoid accidental decannulation.

At this point, preparations are made to initiate bypass. Short segments of adaptor tubing are placed onto both cannulas. The cannulas and adaptive tubing are then filled with heparinized saline and examined for air bubbles. All bubbles, especially those in the arterial cannula, must be removed prior to initiation of flow. The adaptive tubing is then connected to the bypass circuit using sterile technique under a continuous flow of heparinized saline. Security of the cannulas must be maintained by the surgical team at all times during this connection process. Prior to wound closure, bypass flow should be gradually increased to full support to ensure that the cannula size and position support the infant. In addition, a chest radiograph should be performed to roughly confirm appropriate cannula placement.

After cannula placement and function have been assessed, the wound is irrigated and hemostasis assured. The skin is closed using a running monofilament suture and dressed with gauze. The exposed segments of each cannula are placed behind the ear, and then secured at several sites of the skin by using interrupted 2–0 silk sutures. When securing a double-lumen VV cannula in place, the reinfusion port (red port) must be oriented anteriorly to minimize recirculation. Once the final position of both the baby and the bypass pump is chosen, the cannulas must be secured to the bed.

Pediatric Cannulation

Children less than 10 kg have very small femoral vessels that are not generally suitable for bypass access. Open neck cutdown technique is preferred in this group, allowing access for VV bypass using a double-lumen cannula or standard VA bypass using the common carotid. However, children more than 10 kg have larger vessels, allowing a two-cannula venous technique to be utilized. If the vessel size permits, it is best to drain blood from the femoral vein and reinfuse it into the internal jugular vein. This technique results in higher overall arterial saturation despite lower total flow by minimizing recirculation (2). The femoral cannulas used should reach the lower inferior vena cava, a large vessel that does not collapse.

The cannula placement for veno-venous bypass in larger children is usually performed percutaneously over a wire using a modified Seldinger technique. Alternatively, some have described a semiopen technique in which the vessels are exposed via an open dissection, and then the needle and catheter are placed through the skin approximately 2 cm away from the incision. The needle and catheter are placed in the vessel under direct visualization; the needle is removed, a guidewire advanced through the catheter, and the catheter is withdrawn. A Teflon obturator is placed over the wire and into the appropriate location (right atrium or inferior vena cava) and the skin exit site enlarged with an 11 blade. Systemic heparinization is performed as described above and allowed for 3 minutes of circulation. The cannula and obturator are advanced over the wire into the vein under direct visualization. Since the vein was dilated to the exact catheter size and the venous system is in low pressure, hemostasis using the percutaneous technique is usually adequate without the placement of ligatures. Placement of a ligature around the cannula in the semiopen technique may in fact kink thin-walled cannulas and is therefore not recommended. Of note, it is very important that the cannula chosen for venous drainage have several side holes in addition to the end hole to maximize flow and prevent circuit shutdown should the end of the cannula become obstructed.

Cardiac Cannulation

Pediatric patients of any size with cardiac failure can be cannulated through the neck using the common carotid artery and internal jugular vein. The technique used is the same as described for neonatal cannulation. If children with cardiac failure are placed on ECMO through the neck, reinfusion through common carotid cannulas may increase cardiac afterload by increasing aortic pressure. This can prevent a failing left ventricle from ejecting blood, leading to left atrial distention and subsequent pulmonary edema. Left atrial overload should be managed by either a balloon atrial septostomy or direct cannulation of the left atrium with a drain connected to the venous side of the bypass circuit. For children placed on ECMO in the operating room after cardiac surgery, cannulation is most often performed through the chest, utilizing cannulas that had been placed for cardiopulmonary bypass. These cannulation sites often include a right atrial cannula or bicaval cannulas for venous drainage and infuse catheters into the proximal aorta.

SHORT-TERM COMPLICATIONS

Operative Complications

Many complications can be encountered in cannulation for ECMO. The most common problem is difficulty in threading the venous cannula. This may be secondary to size mismatch between the cannula and the vein, severe venospasm, mediastinal shift from congenital diaphragmatic hernia, or aberrant anatomy such as a left-sided superior vena cava. In addition, aggressive positioning may lead to obstruction of the vein by the clavicle or first rib. This can be addressed by careful repositioning of the head and neck.

Difficulties in venous cannulation or misguided venotomy may lead to complete division of the jugular vein. In this case, the first step to recovery is obtaining vascular control of the caudad portion of the vein with a small vascular clamp or placement of sutures into the exposed vein. Careful introduction of a guidewire can then aid cannula placement. On occasion, the caudad portion of the divided vein will invert into the mediastinum. Immediate control of bleeding is obtained by direct pressure. Attempts should then be made to retrieve the vein with vascular forceps. If this is unsuccessful and no other suitable vascular access is available for cannulation, median sternotomy is necessary to recover the vein. A thoracic approach to venous cannulation is then undertaken via the right atrium.

If there is no venous return after an uneventful cannulation and adequate volume resuscitation, all cannulas and the entire circuit tubing should be examined for kinks. Chest radiograph and transthoracic echocardiogram can be used to detect catheter malposition and direct appropriate repositioning or replacement. If the lack of flow is accompanied by significant hemodynamic instability, an intrathoracic perforation should be suspected and a median sternotomy performed, followed by vascular repair and open thoracic cannulation.

With respect to the arterial cannula, subintimal placement may lead to dissection of the common carotid artery and possible extension to a lethal aortic dissection. Alternatively, subendothelial cannula placement may lead to left ventricular disruption or perforation. This is best prevented by the placement of small prolene stay sutures after performing the anterior arteriotomy. Variations in arterial catheter position may cause significant problems. As mentioned above, cannula placement in the ascending aorta increases afterload and may cause left ventricular failure. Improper cannula position across the aortic valve leads to aortic valve insufficiency. Inadvertent selective cannulation of the right subclavian artery directs the entire flow of oxygenated blood into the right upper extremity while leaving the rest of the body in a state of hypoxia. Lastly, placement of the arterial cannula in the descending aorta leads to considerable compromise of coronary and cerebral blood flow.

Mechanical Complications

Thrombosis

The most common mechanical complication of ECMO remains clot formation in various portions of the bypass circuit. According to the recent Extracorporeal Life Support Organization (ELSO) registry data, thrombosis in the circuit accounts for 53% of the mechanical complications in neonatal respiratory failure cases and 28% in pediatric respiratory failure cases. While small clots are nearly ubiquitous and generally not dangerous to the patient, larger clots can lead to oxygenator failure, consumptive coagulopathy, and systemic embolization. Systemic heparinization, carefully monitored by serial measurements of the activated clotting time (ACT), minimizes clot formation but cannot prevent all thrombosis. Newer heparin-coated systems have been trialed in some centres with mixed results. Most studies have demonstrated that minimal clotting can be achieved with lower systemic heparin doses when heparin-coated circuits are used, but it remains unclear if this translates to any clinical benefit (3).

Oxygenator Failure

Oxygenator failure represents the second most common mechanical complication of ECMO. Although it represents only 5.9% of mechanical complications in neonatal respiratory failure, this percentage increases to 13.4% and 18.9% in pediatric and adult respiratory cases, respectively (4). This may reflect the longer time that neonatal and pediatric patients spend on ECMO when compared to adults. Oxygenator failure may be manifested as increased premembrane pressures in the setting of stable postmembrane pressures, deterioration in gas exchange, or unexplained platelet consumption. A failing membrane should be replaced immediately after deterioration in function is detected.

Air Embolism

Air embolism remains a dangerous and potentially fatal mechanical complication of extracorporeal support. There are several ways in which air emboli may develop. When the partial pressure of oxygen in blood is very high, oxygen can be forced out of solution by operating the circuit in an environment with low ambient pressure or by accidentally striking the membrane. It is therefore advisable to keep the postmembrane PO_2 less than 600 mmHg. Operating the pump in the setting of venous occlusion (caused by a tubing kink or an inappropriate clamp) generates significant negative pressure and subsequent cavitation. Massive venous airlock can occur when the venous cannula is dislodged to the point where the sideholes are outside the vessel. This situation requires immediate cessation of ECMO support followed by either removal of the air or replacement of the entire circuit. Lastly, a small tear in the membrane of the oxygenator may lead to a sizable air embolus. The tear allows blood to leak into the gas path of the oxygenator, where a clot may form that obstructs the outlet of gas. As the pressure in the gas portion of the oxygenator exceeds the blood phase pressure, a large bolus of air crosses the membrane into the blood path. This air embolus often exceeds the air trapping capacity of the heat exchanger and can lead to severe air embolization. This circumstance is managed by immediate clamping of all patient cannulas and opening of the bridge to allow recirculation. If air embolus is thought to have entered the patient, the head should immediately be lowered, relative to the rest of the body to direct circulating air pockets away from the cerebral circulation. Air emboli entering the coronary vasculature may cause acute cardiac decompensation requiring inotropic support.

Tubing Rupture
Tubing rupture is no longer a major problem in extracorporeal support since polyvinyl chloride tubing has been replaced by Supertygon raceway tubing (Norton Performance Plastics, Inc, Akron, OH, U.S.A.). It now occurs in only 1% of neonatal and 3.9% of pediatric patients. However, the raceway should be walked every 10 to 14 days in circuits using $1/4$-inch tubing, and every 4 to 6 days in circuits for older children using 3/8-inch tubing. All tubing clamps should be carefully applied, taking care not to squeeze the tubing in the proximal aspect of the clamp. Use of penetrating towel clamps should be avoided in all cases.

Other Mechanical Problems
Mechanical complications involving other components of the extracorporeal circuit are less common. Heat exchanger failure leads to significant hypothermia in neonates. Although pump failure is rare, the pump will cut out in situations of impaired venous return. This may occur secondary to hypovolemia, kinks in the cannula or tubing, improper venous cannula position, inadequate cannula size in relation to desired flow, inadequate bed height, pneumothorax, or cardiac tamponade.

Patient Complications
The incidence of patient complications in extracorporeal support is almost twice that of mechanical events. These adverse occurrences manifest in almost every organ system and present a significant challenge in management. Patient complications include bleeding, cerebral infarction, intracranial hemorrhage, renal insufficiency, hypertension, electrolyte disturbances, cardiac dysfunction, arrhythmias, gastrointestinal bleeding, and infection.

Cannulation Site Bleeding
Of the aforementioned complications, bleeding remains not only the most common but also the most potentially devastating problem. The need for systemic heparinization to prevent circuit thrombosis must be balanced against the risk of hemorrhage. Bleeding from the neck incision following open cannulation can often be managed with the use of topical hemostatic agents. Continued oozing is most often from a small vessel and can be controlled using a combination of direct pressure with a finger, decreasing the ACT, and maintaining the platelet count above 125,000 until the bleeding has stopped. Higher volume blood loss (>10 cc/hr in a neonate) is suggestive of a more serious vascular injury or cannula displacement and warrants reexploration of the wound. Cannulation site bleeding is most recently reported at 6.4% in neonatal respiratory cases. This increases to approximately 8.5% in children less than 1 year placed on ECMO for cardiac indications, 11.4% in pediatric respiratory ECMO cases, and 13.4% in older cardiac ECMO children (4).

Postoperative Bleeding
Performing procedures on ECMO creates an additional challenge in managing blood loss. It is currently recommended that the ACT be lowered and the platelet count be greater than 100,000 prior to any surgical procedure. It may also be helpful to transfuse platelets and fresh frozen plasma (FFP) (10 cc/kg) at the start of the operation. Dissection should be performed

slowly with liberal use of electrocautery. All identifiable vessels should be ligated rather than coagulated and topical hemostatic agents used liberally. Hemostasis should be assured prior to closure of fascia or skin. Postoperatively, the platelet count should be closely monitored and kept over 100,000. In addition, many centres use a 100 mg/kg bolus of 6-aminocaproic acid followed by a continuous infusion of 25– to 30 mg/kg/hr for 24 to 48 hours postoperatively. The data supporting the use of Amicar are limited, but suggest that the drug is safe for use in neonates and children and that it may decrease the rate of postoperative bleeding following cannulation. In 1993, Wilson et al. reported that administration of a bolus of Amicar (100 mg/kg) at the time of cannulation followed by a continuous infusion at 30 mg/kg/hr until the termination of ECMO decreased both the rate of intracranial hemorrhage and cannulation site bleeding in neonates (5). A more recent review of ECMO patients on Amicar out of the same institution suggested a significant reduction in surgical site bleeding (particularly in cardiac patients), but no alteration in the rate of intracranial hemorrhage (6). However, a prospective, randomized multicenter trial using a similar protocol (100 mg/kg bolus, followed by 25 mg/kg/hr for 72 hours) found no difference in either the incidence of significant intracranial hemorrhage or hemorrhagic complications (7).

Despite adherence to the above guidelines, bleeding from surgical sites remains a significant problem, especially in older children and cardiac patients. Surgical site hemorrhage is documented in 6.2% of neonatal respiratory cases and 15.2% of pediatric respiratory cases. In postoperative cardiac ECMO patients, this bleeding rate averages around 32% in children less than 16 years of age. Recently, recombinant coagulation factor VIIa has been reported to be effective in preventing reexploration in children on ECMO with uncontrolled postoperative bleeding following cardiac surgery (8). Recombinant factor VIIa has been shown to decrease chest tube output and reduce the need for blood products in postoperative pediatric cardiac surgery patients but has been associated with major thrombotic complications including ECMO circuit thrombosis and arterial line thrombosis leading to limb ischemia (9). In addition, novel anticoagulation strategies are being tried, such as continuous antithrombin infusion in combination with intermittent heparinization (10).

Hemorrhage

In addition to bleeding from the cannulation sites and surgical incisions, there are several other potential sites of spontaneous hemorrhage in the child on ECMO. These include intracranial, intra-abdominal, gastrointestinal, intrathoracic, and retroperitoneal bleeding. Gastrointestinal hemorrhage is reported in 1.7% to –4.2% of neonatal and pediatric patients on ECMO (4). Clinical manifestations of acute hemorrhage include persistent tachycardia or intermittent bradycardia, low hemoglobin, hypotension, peripheral cyanosis, decreased urine output, or an unexplained rise in the PaO_2 on venoarterial ECMO (11). Any acute changes in neurologic status such as seizures or dilated pupils must be treated as an intracranial hemorrhage until proven otherwise. Appropriate work-up for unexplained blood loss includes intracranial ultrasound, head CT, abdominal imaging, chest X-ray, and echocardiogram to rule out tamponade.

Cardiopulmonary Complications

Systemic hypertension is a common and potentially serious complication of ECMO, and it has been associated with a higher rate of intracranial hemorrhage (12). This may be managed by a variety of agents, including hydralazine, nitroglycerine, captopril, and isradipine. Studies utilizing an aggressive medical management regimen in neonates requiring ECMO demonstrated a decreased incidence of clinically significant intracranial hemorrhage from 50% to 9% (12).

Deterioration in myocardial function is seen in approximately 7% of neonates following initiation of ECLS (13–15). This "myocardial stun" is defined by decreased left ventricular shortening following initiation of bypass and return of normal function after 48 hours of ECMO. It is most often encountered in patients with severe hypoxia, cardiac arrest, and significant epinephrine pressor support requirements prior to going on ECMO. In addition, many of the infants and children placed on ECMO require inotropic support during their bypass run. Over 60% of all infants and children placed on ECLS for cardiac failure of postcardiotomy support still require inotropes to maintain adequate blood pressure (4).

Intrathoracic Complications

Intrathoracic complications such as pericardial tamponade, tension pneumothorax, and tension hemothorax occasionally develop in children on ECMO. These often present as a narrowed pulse pressure, decreased peripheral perfusion, increased PaO_2, and decreased mixed venous oxygen saturation. As venous return is impaired, the relative contribution of native cardiac output and pulmonary blood flow is decreased and peripheral perfusion is maintained by flow from the ECMO circuit. However, decreased venous return soon leads to decreased achievable ECMO flow and progressive deterioration. Any patient on ECMO with the aforementioned hemodynamic changes should be immediately be evaluated with a chest X-ray and echocardiogram. Cardiac tamponade with blood, serous fluid, or air is seen in 0.5% of neonatal respiratory cases and 1.7% of pediatric respiratory cases. However, this complication is much more common in infants and children undergoing ECMO for cardiac support, where tamponade is seen in 4.9% to 6% of children less than 16 years of age (4). The reverse is true for pneumothorax, which requires treatment in 6.1% of neonates and 12.9% of children on ECMO for respiratory failure, but in only 2.7% to 3.5% of children placed on ECMO for cardiac support. This may be related to the fact that postoperative cardiac cases often have multiple intrathoracic chest tubes placed in the operating room.

Neurologic Complications

Intracranial hemorrhage (ICH) remains a significant and devastating problem for infants and children requiring ECLS. Radiographically detected ICH is seen in 6.1% of neonatal respiratory and 4.9% of pediatric respiratory ECMO cases; this number increases to 10.3% of neonatal cardiac cases (4). It is the most common cause of death in infants managed with ECLS (16). Factors contributing to ICH in the critically ill neonatal population include hypoxia and hypercapnea secondary to respiratory failure, acidosis, hypotension and subsequent tissue ischemia, sepsis with subsequent thrombocytopenia and coagulopathy, birth trauma, and infusion of hypertonic solutions. Hypoxia alone can injure the endothelial cells lining the cerebral capillaries, predisposing them to disruption, and subsequent bleeding. Infants placed on ECMO are exposed to additional risk factors, including ligation of cerebral blood supply and venous drainage, systemic heparinization, refractory thrombocytopenia, and systemic hypertension (17). Ligation of the common carotid artery and internal jugular vein during cannulation for VA ECMO results in simultaneous decrease of regional cerebral blood flow and increase in cerebral venous pressure and thereby encouraging ICH (18). Initiation of ECLS in the setting of hypoxia results in the augmentation of cerebral blood flow and loss of cerebral autoregulation (19). Additional insult occurs when decreased $PaCO_2$ following successful initiation of ECMO results in further decrease in cerebral blood flow (20). All these factors play a role in predisposing critically ill infants placed on ECMO to ICH. Some studies have demonstrated that administration of bolus of Amicar around the time of cannulation, followed by a continuous infusion over the next 72 hours, decreases the incidence of ICH in high-risk neonates being placed on ECMO (5). However, other published data have found that Amicar administration does not change the rate of ICH in these infants (6,7).

Premature infants are at the highest risk for developing ICH on ECMO, and postconceptual age has been shown to be the best predictor of ECLS-related ICH in infants less than 37 weeks of gestational age. In a retrospective cohort study of premature infants treated with ECMO over a recent 8-year period, Hardart et al. (2004) reported that 26% of patients less than or equal to 32 weeks of postconceptional age developed ICH versus only 6% of patients with a postconceptual age greater than 38 weeks (21).

Given the frequent occurrence and significant morbidity and mortality associated with ICH in neonatal and pediatric ECMO, it is imperative to identify intracranial bleeding as soon as possible. It is recommended that infants on ECMO have cranial ultrasounds at least every other day while on ECMO, and immediately in the setting of seizures or neurologic deterioration.

In addition to ICH, intracranial infarction and seizures are other neurologic complications associated with ECMO in children. Intracranial infarction, documented by ultrasound or CT, is seen in 8.3% of neonatal respiratory and 3.4% of pediatric respiratory cases. Seizures, clinically documented or electroencephalographically detected, have been reported in 9.1% of neonatal respiratory and 4.7% of pediatric respiratory ECMO cases (4). The presence of seizures is clinically important as up to 50% of newborns with electroencephalographic seizures during ECMO either died or were found to be developmentally handicapped at 1 to 2 years of age (22).

Patients on VV ECMO have a lower rate of major neurologic complications when compared to children placed on VA ECMO. The incidence of seizures (6% versus 13%) and infarction (9% versus 14%) are less in children placed on VV ECMO when compared to VA ECMO (23,24). Lastly, clinical brain death in children on ECMO is seen in 1% of neonatal respiratory patients and 5.8% of pediatric respiratory patients. The rate of clinical brain death in infants and children on ECMO for cardiac causes ranges from 1.2% in newborns up to 30 days of age to as high as 8.8% in children aged 1 to 16 years (4).

Hematologic Complications

Thrombocytopenia is a common and expected problem in patients on ECLS, especially in those with severe hypoxia prior to initiation of support. Exposure to the ECMO circuit leads to platelet activation, adhesion, and aggregation. Reduction in the circulating platelet count occurs as platelet aggregates are preferentially sequestered in the lung, liver, and spleen (25). Thrombocytopenia results from decreased production, dilution, and sequestration or removal to extravascular sites. The acquired platelet dysfunction is not reversed by transfusion, and the survival rate of transfused platelets is reduced while the child remains on ECMO (26). Thrombocytopenia may persist for several days following discontinuation of ECLS, so platelet counts should be closely monitored during this period (25).

Heparin-associated thrombocytopenia (HIT) is a rare but challenging problem in managing patients on ECMO, as unfractionated heparin is the anticoagulant of choice in most extracorporeal support. HIT is an immune-mediated adverse reaction to heparin that paradoxically increases the risk of thrombosis. Susceptible patients form an IgG antibody to the heparin-platelet factor 4 complex causing platelet activation, aggregation, and eventual destruction. The most common clinical manifestation of HIT is venous thrombosis, which is seen in 30% to 70% of patients and includes deep vein thrombosis, pulmonary embolus, adrenal vein thrombosis, and cerebral sinus thrombosis. Arterial thrombi, known as "white clots," are seen in 15% to 30% of patients with HIT and are present most dramatically as stroke, myocardial infarction, or limb-threatening ischemia. Patients with HIT may also exhibit disseminated intravascular coagulation, acute reactions to heparin infusions, and skin lesions at injection sites. Recent reports suggest that argatroban, a synthetic direct thrombin inhibitor, may be safely used in patients on ECMO that develop HIT (27,28). Earlier reports also document the success of recombinant hirudin in these difficult situations. Argatroban reversibly binds to both free and clot-associated active thrombin sites and inhibits thrombin-catalyzed reactions including fibrin formation, activation of coagulation factors, and platelet aggregation. In our institution, argatroban is the drug of choice in ECMO patients with heparin-associated sensitivities or HIT. It may be initiated as a bolus of 0.1 mg/kg, then treatment administered as a continuous infusion with an initial dose range of 0.2 to 0.5 mcg/kg/min. Efficacy and appropriateness of dosing is monitored via serial ACTs, PTT, and argatroban levels.

Hemolysis, defined as a serum hemoglobin >50 mg/dL, occurs in 8.6% to 11.6% of infants and children on ECMO. Red cell breakdown is sometimes secondary to mechanical trauma related to the circuit, especially when using a centrifugal pump. Hemolysis is increased when clot forms within the circuit or oxygenator as erythrocytes adhere to and lyse on fibrin strands. A rise in the serum free hemoglobin is often accompanied by a rise in the fibrin split products and a decrease in fibrinogen, and change of the ECMO circuit is followed by normalization of all these levels (29). A new silicone, hollow fiber membrane lung has been demonstrated to have improved gas exchange, less hemolysis, and lower blood flow resistance when compared to conventional silicone, coil-type oxygenators (30). Eventual use of this novel membrane may decrease the rate of hemolysis in prolonged ECMO support.

Renal Insufficiency

Renal insufficiency develops in many children requiring ECMO and appears to be more common in the pediatric population. Oliguria is common in the first 48 hours of ECMO and is often secondary to extensive fluid shifts, variable renal blood supply, and mild acute tubular necrosis. Elevated creatinine (>1.5) occurs in 9.1% of neonatal respiratory ECMO cases, but at least 13.5% of infants on ECMO for respiratory failure require either dialysis, hemofiltration, or continuous arteriovenous hemodialysis (CAVHD) (4). Indications for renal replacement therapy are hypervolemia, hyperkalemia, acidosis, and azotemia. Continuous hemofiltration on ECMO, described by Sell et al. in 1987, involves placement of a small apparatus in-line to the

Table 1   Outcomes in Neonatal and Pediatric ECMO

	Total patients	Survived ECLS	Survived to D/C or transfer
Neonatal			
Respiratory	20,993	17,889 (85%)	16,005 (76%)
Cardiac	2898	1684 (58%)	1095 (38%)
ECPR	274	176 (64%)	109 (40%)
Pediatric			
Respiratory	3390	2173 (64%)	1895 (56%)
Cardiac	3658	2199 (60%)	1624 (44%)
ECPR	523	263 (50%)	200 (31%)

Source: Adapted from Ref. 40.

ECMO circuit and allows removal of excess plasma water and dissolved solutes while retaining intravascular proteins and cellular components (12). In children placed on ECMO for respiratory failure, elevated creatinine is seen in 14.7% of cases, and over 17% of the cohorts require renal replacement therapy. These numbers are fairly similar to the documented renal insufficiency in cardiac children on ECMO. Initial evaluation of the ECMO patient with oliguria unresponsive to diuretics should include a renal ultrasound to exclude anatomic abnormalities.

Infection

Critically ill infants and children on ECMO are at risk for infectious complications, especially given the severity of their illness and exposure of blood in the circuit to multiple infusions of medication and parenteral nutrition. Culture-proven infection is reported in 6.3% of neonatal respiratory ECMO cases. However, this percentage increases to 20.1% in pediatric respiratory ECMO patients and from 8.2% to 12.7% in cardiac ECMO patients (4). All ECMO patients should be placed on prophylactic antibiotic coverage against gram-positive organisms, and frequent surveillance cultures obtained to look for occult sepsis. ECMO patients with sepsis appear to have a higher rate of complications such as seizure, gastrointestinal hemorrhage, and renal dysfunction (31).

LONG-TERM OUTCOMES

Survival

Among neonates on ECMO for respiratory failure, overall success in weaning off extracorporeal support was 85%, while survival to discharge or transfer was 76% (Table 1) (4). Table 1 summarizes the survival of all neonatal and pediatric ECMO outcomes as published by the ELSO Registry. Infants with congenital diaphragmatic hernias requiring ECMO support continue to have the lowest survival (52%), likely secondary to severe pulmonary hypoplasia associated with the defect (Table 2). Table 2 summarizes the five most common neonatal respiratory diagnoses and their respective outcomes. Pediatric respiratory ECMO patients have an overall survival to transfer or discharge of 56% (Table 1), with the highest survival in patients with aspiration pneumonia (67%) and viral pneumonia (64%). Table 3 outlines survival in patients with pediatric respiratory failure requiring ECMO. In neonates requiring ECMO for cardiac support, 58% of the patients are successfully weaned and decannulated, but only 38% survive to discharge or transfer. Survival to discharge in pediatric cardiac ECMO patients is only somewhat better at 44%.

Table 2   Neonatal Respiratory ECMO Outcomes

	Total runs	Survival (%)
Meconium aspiration	7044	94
Congenital diaphragmatic hernia	5105	52
PPHN	3342	78
Sepsis	2482	75
RDS	1425	84

Source: Adapted from Ref. 40.

Table 3 Pediatric Respiratory ECMO Outcomes

	Total runs	Survival (%)
Viral pneumonia	829	63
Acute respiratory failure (non-ARDS)	658	48
Bacterial pneumonia	376	56
ARDS (not postoperative or trauma)	325	53
Aspiration pneumonia	177	67

Source: Adapted from Ref. 40.

The Collaborative UK ECMO Trial, the results of which were published in 1996, recruited 185 infants with severe respiratory failure meeting entry criteria (including gestational age > 35 weeks, weight > 2 kg, and age < 28 days) were randomized to conventional treatment or transfer to one of five ECMO centres for extracorporeal support. The principal outcome was death or disability at one year of age. Survival was 68% in the ECMO-allocated group versus 41% in the conventional group with no significant difference in disability, demonstrating ECMO to be the preferred management of children meeting the inclusion and exclusion criteria of the study (32).

Neurologic Outcomes

Neurologic injury occurring either before or during ECMO is a major concern in neonatal and pediatric critical care. Hypoxia and ischemia are frequently present even before the initiation of extracorporeal support, putting these infants and children at particular risk for a poor neurodevelopmental outcome. However, neurologic disability extends to critically ill infants managed with conventional ventilation as well as those requiring ECMO. In 1995, a study out of Case Western Reserve University prospectively evaluated 26 critically ill neonates managed with conventional treatment and 48 neonates treated with ECMO during a 1-year period (33). Survival was 69% in the conventional group and 90% in the ECMO group. With respect to long-term outcomes, 24% of the 17 survivors in the conventional group had neurodevelopmental impairment, compared to 25% of the 38 ECMO survivors at 8 to 20 months of age.

In the initial reports from the UK Collaborative ECMO Group, two infants of the 99 survivors (one child from each group) available for follow-up were severely disabled. The incidence of any neurodevelopmental impairment at 1 year of age was 28% among survivors in both groups (34). Seven-year follow-up from the UK trial demonstrated that 76% of the 89 children available for follow-up had a cognitive level within the normal range (35). Specific patterns of learning disability included global cognitive loss, poor spatial skills, and difficulty with reading comprehension and visual and verbal memory. In terms of neuromotor development, 39% of the ECMO children and 50% of the conventionally treated children were classified as having an impairment of neuromotor development, defined as abnormal signs on neurologic examination but normal function scores on the Movement Assessment Battery for Children.

A more recent study compared two groups of 5-year-old children—76 treated with ECMO versus 20 who were "near-miss" ECMO candidates managed with conventional treatment at the same institution (36). Rates of severe mental handicap (full-scale IQ < 70) were similar at 11% in the "near-miss" group and 12% among ECMO survivors. Both groups appeared at moderate risk for school failure with rates of 37% to 38%. Rates of parent-reported child behavior problems were also similar and fairly high in both groups (35% ECMO versus 24% "near-miss"). This retrospective study reveals that the risk of cognitive disability and social or adaptive difficulties are high in both ECMO survivors and "near-miss" candidates, suggesting both groups are at risk for school failure and will require close follow-up.

Other Late Sequelae

With respect to respiratory outcomes, the aforementioned study out of Case Western Reserve demonstrated that infants in the conventionally treated group had significantly more chronic lung disease, longer duration of oxygen therapy, more chronic reactive airway disease, and more rehospitalizations than the infants treated with ECMO (33). One-year follow-up from the UK Collaborative Trial revealed that one child from each arm of the study was still in the hospital, and five children still required supplementary oxygen (approximately 5% of each group). Seven-year follow-up from the UK trial revealed a higher respiratory morbidity and increased risk of behavioral problems among children treated in the conventional arm. In the conventionally treated children, 32% reported intermittent attacks of wheezing in the 12 months prior to examination and 42% regularly required an inhaler while in the ECMO group only 11% reported wheezing and 25% required an inhaler. The most commonly described behavioral abnormality was hyperactivity, and total deviance score was higher in the conventionally treated group (38%) versus the ECMO group (18%) (35). Bilateral high-tone sensineural hearing loss has been identified in 3% to 21% of patients treated with neonatal ECMO (37). This appears to correlate with duration of ventilation, degree of alkalosis in conventionally managed infants, and low $PaCO_2$ prior to ECMO support.

Congenital Diaphragmatic Hernia

Although more than two-thirds of neonatal respiratory ECMO patients survive, the poorest survival in this group is seen in infants with congenital diaphragmatic hernias. The average survival to discharge or transfer in these extremely ill neonates is documented at 52% (4). Review of the long-term outcome following ECMO for congenital diaphragmatic hernia in the United Kingdom, Davis et al. reported a 63% success in weaning from ECMO, a 58% survival in hospital discharge, but only a 37% survival at 1 year of age or more (38). This retrospective review of 73 neonates found "pre-ECMO" predictors of long-term survival including higher birth weight, higher 5-minute Apgar score, and postnatal diagnosis of the diaphragmatic hernia. Morbidity in survivors is significant, with 48% suffering from respiratory symptoms, 59% displaying gastrointestinal problems, and 19% exhibiting severe neurodevelopmental problems. A recent study aimed at determining if the data collected by the ELSO registry can be used to predict infants with congenital diaphragmatic hernia had difficulty reliably predicting infants at high risk for death (>90%) (39). However, this study did reveal that nonsurvivors were more likely to be of younger gestational age, have lower birth weights, have an earlier age at cannulation, and to be prenatally diagnosed.

SUMMARY

ECLS is a high-risk but life-saving intervention available to infants and children with acute respiratory and cardiac failure. Attention to detail during cannulation can reduce the risk of catheter-site bleeding. Careful optimization of preoperative coagulation parameters and use of Amicar and other agents may reduce the rate of postoperative hemorrhage when surgery is required in patients on ECMO. Long-term follow-up of neonatal ECMO survivors reveal that over 75% have normal cognitive function, suggesting that the documented reduction in mortality when compared to conventional therapy does not occur at the expense of severe disability among survivors. ECMO will likely continue to be an effective resource for management of critically ill children until that time when advances in clinical management obviate the need for its existence.

REFERENCES

1. Pranikoff T, Hirschl RB. Neonatal extracorporeal membrane oxygenation. In: Carter DC, Russell RCG, eds. Rob and Smith's Operative Surgery. 6th ed. London, England: Butterworth-Heinemann, 2005.
2. Pranikoff T, Hirschl RB, Remenapp R, et al. Venovenous extracorporeal life support via percutaneous cannulation in 94 patients. Chest 1999; 115:818–822.
3. Wand D, Alpard SK, Savage C, Yamani HN, Deyo DJ, Nemser S, Zwischenberger JB. Short term performance evaluation of a perfluorocopolymer coated gas exchanger for arteriovenous CO_2 removal. ASAIO J 2003; 49(6):673–677.
4. ELSO Data Registry Report: International Summary. Ann Arbor, MI, January 2007.
5. Wilson JM, Bower LK, Fackler JC, et al. Aminocaproic acid decreases the incidence of intracranial hemorrhage and other hemorrhagic complications of ECMO. J Pediatr Surg 1993: 28(4):536–540.
6. Downard CD, Betit P, Chang RW, et al. Impact of AMICAR on hemorrhagic complications of ECMO: A ten-year review. J Pediatr Surg 2003; 38(8):1212–1216.

7. Horowitz JR, Cofer BR, Warner BW, et al. A multicenter trial of 6-aminocaproid acid (Amicar) in the prevention of bleeding in infants on ECMO. J Pediatr Surg 1998; 33(11):1610–1613.

8. Dominguez TE, Mitchell M, Friess SH, et al. Use of recombinant factor VIIa for refractory hemorrhage during extracorporeal membrane oxygenation. Pediatr Crit Care Med 2005; 6(3):348–351.

9. Agarwal HS, Bennett JE, Churchwell KB, et al. Recombinant factor seven therapy for post-operative bleeding in neonatal and pediatric cardiac surgery. Ann Thoracic Surg 2007; 84(1):161–168.

10. Agati S, Cicarello G, Salvo D, et al. Use of a novel anticoagulation strategy during ECMO in a pediatric population: Single-center experience. ASAIO J 2006; 52(5):513–516.

11. DeBerry BB, Lynch J, Chung DH, et al. Emergencies during ECLS and their management. In: Von Meurs KV, Lally KP, Peek G, Zwischenberger, eds. ECMO Extracorporeal Cardiopulmonary Support in Critical Care. 3rd ed. Extracoporeal Life Support Organization, Ann Arbor, 2005:133–156.

12. Sell LL, Cullen ML, Whittlesey GC, et al. Experience with renal failure during extracorporeal membrane oxygenation: Treatment with continuous hemofiltration. J Pediatir Surg 1987; 22(7):600–602.

13. Hirschl RB, Heiss KF, Bartlett RH. Severe myocardial dysfunction during extracorporeal membrane oxygenation. J Pediatr Surg 1992; 27:48–53.

14. Hirschl RB, Bartlett RH. Extracorporeal life support for cardiopulmonary failure. In: Grosfeld JL, O'Neill JA, Fonkalsrud EW, Coran AG, eds. Pediatric Surgery. 6th ed. Philadelphia, PA: Mosby 2006:134–145.

15. Martin GR, Short BL, Abbott C, et al. Cardiac stun in infants undergoing extracorporeal membrane oxygenation. J Thorac Cardiovasc Surg 1991;101:607–611.

16. Jarjour IT, Ahdab-Barmada M. Cerebrovascular lesions in infants and children dying after extracorporeal membrane oxygenation. Pediatr Neurol 1994; 10:13–19.

17. Hardart GE, Fickler JC. Predictors of intracranial hemorrhage during neonatal extracorporeal membrane oxygenation. Pediatrics 1999; 143:156–159.

18. Schumacher RE, Barks JD, Johnston MV, et al. Right-sided brain lesions in infants following extracorporeal membrane oxygenation. Pediatrics 1988; 82(2):155–161.

19. Short BL, Walker LK, Traystman RJ. Impaired cerebral autoregulation in the newborn lamb during recovery from severe, prolonged hypoxia, combined with carotid artery and jugular vein ligation. Crit Care Med 1994; 22:1262–1268.

20. Walker LK, Short BL, Traystman RJ. Impairment of cerebral autoregulation during venovenous extracorporeal membrane oxygenation in the newborn lamb. Crit Care Med 1996; 24(12):2001–2006.

21. Hardart GE, Hardart MK, Arnold JH. Intracranial hemorrhage in premature neonates treated with extracorporeal membrane oxygenation correlates with conceptional age. J Pediatr 2004; 145:184–189.

22. Campbell LR, Bunyapen C, Gangarosa ME, et al. Significance of seizures associated with extracorporeal membrane oxygenation. J Pediatr 1991; 119(5):789–782.

23. Upp JR Jr, Bush PE, Zwischenberger JB. Complications of neonatal extracorporeal membrane oxygenation. Perfusion 1994; 9:241–256.

24. Zwischenberger JB, Nguyen TT, Upp JR, et al. Complications of neonatal extracorporeal membrane oxygenation: Collective experience from the Extracorporeal Life Support Organization. J Thorac Cardiovasc Surg 1994; 107:838–848.

25. Anderson HL III, Cilley RE, Zwischenberger, et al. Thrombocytopenia in neonates after extracorporeal membrane oxygenation. ASAIO Trans 1986; 32:534–537.

26. Robinson TM, Kickler TS, Walker LK, et al. Effect of extracorporeal membrane oxygenation on platelets in newborns. Crit Care Med 1993; 21:1029–1034.

27. Scott LK, Grier LR, Conrad SA. Hepain-induced thrombocytopenia in a pediatric patient receiving extracorporeal support and treated with argatroban. Pediatr Crit Care Med 2006; 7(3):355–357.

28. Young G, Yonekawa KE, Nakagawa P, et al. Argatroban as an alternative to heparin in extracorporeal membrane oxygenation. Perfusion 2004; 19(5):283–288.

29. Steinhorn RH, Isham-Schopf B, Smith C, et al. Hemolysis during long-term extracorporeal membrane oxygenation. J Pediatr 1989; 115(4):625–630.

30. Motomura T, Maeda T, Kawahito S, et al. Development of silicone rubber hollow fiber membrane oxygenator for ECMO. Artif Organs 2003; 27(11):1050–1053.

31. Douglass BH, Keenan AL, Purohit DM. Bacterial and fungal infection in neonates undergoing venoarterial extracorporeal membrane oxygenation: An analysis of the registry data of the extracorporeal life support organization. Artif Organs 1996; 20:202–208.

32. UK Collaborative ECMO Group. UK collaborative randomized trial of neonatal extracorporeal membrane oxygenation. Lancet 1996; 348:75–82.

33. Walsh-Sukys MC, Bauer RE, Cornell DJ, et al. Severe respiratory failure in neonates: Mortality and morbidity rates and neurodevelopmental outcome. J Pediatr 1994; 125(1):104–110.

34. UK Collaborative ECMO Group. UK collaborative randomized trial of neonatal extracorporeal membrane oxygenation: Follow-up to age 7 years. Pediatrics 1998; 101:E1–10.

35. McNally H, Bennett CC, Elbourne D, et al. United Kingdom collaborative randomized trial of neonatal extracorporeal membrane oxygenation: follow-up age 7 years. Pediatrics 2006; 117:E845–E854.

36. Rais-Bahrami K, Wagner AE, Coffman C, et al. Neurodevelopmental outcome in ECMO vs near-miss ECMO patients at 5 years of age. Clin Pediatr 2000; 39(3):145–152.
37. Cheyng PY, Robertson CM. Sensineural hearing loss in survivors of neonatal extracorporeal membrane oxygenation. Pediatr Rehabil 1997; 1:127–130.
38. Davis PJ, Firmin RK, Manktelow B, et al. Long-term outcomes following extracorporeal membrane oxygenation for congenital diaphragmatic hernia: The UK experience. J Pediatr 2004; 144(3):309–315.
39. Heiss KF, Clark RH. Prediction of mortality in neonates with congenital diaphragmatic hernia treated with extracorporeal membrane oxygenation. Crit Care Med 1995; 23(11):1915–1919.
40. ECLS Registry Report, International Summary, January, 2007.

ECMO Cannulation

Expert: Kevin P. Lally, M.D., M.S.

QUESTIONS

1. **What incision do you perform for access to the neck?**
   A short transverse incision just above the clavicle.

2. **How do you choose what size cannula to use?**
   A combination of experience and the Red Book in older patients. If using the Biomedicus in the newborn, I don't try to push too hard on size since the 12 French works very well. Veno-venous ECMO is much easier in the neonate if you can get the 15 French cannula in, but I avoid try to push too hard.

3. **How do you secure the cannulas?**
   Several 2–0 silk sutures.

4. **What steps to do take to reduce operative site bleeding?**
   Cautery and flood the field with cryoprecipitate and thrombin. Re-exploration of the site has become a very uncommon event.

5. **What criteria do you use to explore the neck for bleeding after cannulation?**
   As mentioned, this is very unusual anymore. Traditionally, I would use an output of >10 cc/hr in a newborn.

6. **What do you do if the vein tears during cannulation?**
   Grab the edges with fine hemostats for traction and use a smaller cannula.

7. **How do you check cannula position?**
   Chest radiograph with the wound still open.

8. **How do you manage a clot in the arterial cannula?**
   Use a Fogarty catheter. Again, an uncommon occurrence, but they can be declotted this way.

9. **How do you manage a clot in the venous cannula?**
   Same as with the arterial cannula.

10. **How do you avoid dissection of the arterial intima during passage of the cannula?**
    I use two 5–0 prolene sutures places at the 2 and 10 o'clock positions to facilitate cannula insertion.

11. **When do you give heparin and how much?**
    I give 100 units per kilogram once the vessels have been isolated. I give less if there is a pre-existing coagulopathy and rapidly check ACT levels.

12. **Empirically, how far in should the venous and arterial cannulas be placed?**
    Venous around 7 cm in the newborn. Arterial 3–4 with recheck on CXR.

13. **How would you select a patient for VV versus VA ECMO?**
    We try veno-venous ECMO in almost every circumstance. Some children fall in a cannula size range where veno-arterial ECMO is the only option. Occasionally, if we are effectively doing ECPR, we'll go to veno-arterial ECMO right away.

11 | Complications of Fetal Surgery

Oluyinka O. Olutoye, M.B.Ch.B, Ph.D.

INTRODUCTION

Fetal surgical procedures are increasing in number and frequency. A quantitative analysis of complication rates of fetal treatments is not possible with these relatively new treatment modalities. Outcomes of fetal surgeries are highly dependent on the expertise of the practitioner, and our overall degree of expertise is increasing as these treatments become more available. In addition, the techniques are constantly improving and the rates of complications are changing in kind. This summary is a compilation of cumulative experience in the field, anecdotes, discussions with colleagues, and a review of the literature.

In-depth details of the indications and operative techniques in fetal surgery are beyond the scope of this text, but are covered in other texts on the subject (1). In fetal surgery (or more appropriately, maternal-fetal surgery), two patients undergo surgery simultaneously. Thus, complications can occur with the mother and/or fetus(es). Fetal procedures can be broadly classified by their mode of access to the fetus: 1) Percutaneous image-guided therapy—where access to the fetus or placenta is obtained via needles or instruments guided typically by ultrasound. The instruments used are small and inflict minimal injury to the mother. However, due to the limitations with imaging, inadvertent injuries to the mother or fetus are possible. 2) Fetoscopic or fetendo approaches—where endoscopic techniques are used to guide therapy. A small endoscope (fetoscope <2 mm outer diameter) with a working port for therapy and manipulation is used to view the fetus or placenta through a 3-mm sheath. This approach is utilized frequently for selective laser photocoagulation of placental vessels in twin–twin transfusion syndrome, for fetal diagnostic procedures and for fetal endoscopic balloon tracheal occlusion for some cases of severe congenital diaphragmatic hernia. About 10 to 12 French trocars are used to gain access through the uterus and direct visualization of the fetus is a benefit. These trocars can be inserted percutaneously with image guidance, following a laparotomy or by a laparoscopic-assisted percutaneous approach. (3) Open hysterotomy approaches—where the fetus is accessed via a direct hysterotomy incision. Following a maternal laparotomy, the uterus is opened and direct access to the fetus obtained. Gross visualization of the fetus is achieved and extirpation of large tumors (lung masses and sacrococcygeal teratomas, (SCT)) or performance of delicate complex surgical procedures (repair of myelomeningocele) can be performed with this degree of access. Clearly, the impact to the mother is most significant in this approach. The hysterotomy can be performed at midgestation following which the pregnancy is allowed to continue, or it may be performed at the time of delivery when intrapartum treatment of the fetus is the objective. The latter is termed the EXIT (ex-utero intrapartum treatment) procedure.

These three different approaches to the fetus carry their own unique sets of risks and complications. Certain complications are possible with all types of approaches, but the approaches are associated with different degrees of risk. Contemporary variations in the techniques have also affected the morbidity related to these approaches. For example, the complication rate with fetal endoscopic procedures was high in the early experience prior to 2003 (2), but has since drastically declined as more endoscopic procedures are now being performed with fewer smaller trocars than the earlier surgeries (3). As published literature typically lags behind, current practice in rapidly advancing fields like fetal surgery, the complication rates cited in earlier publications may no longer be applicable as they may not reflect more recent modifications in technique.

In this chapter, the complications are divided into maternal and fetal complications, although in reality one complication may lead to the other. Unfortunately, there is limited outcome and long-term follow-up data that specifically address the complications of maternal fetal surgery. Where available, these have been incorporated in this text. When applicable, corollaries have been drawn from related surgical procedures, e.g., classical cesarean sections.

MATERNAL COMPLICATIONS

While there are no published reports of maternal deaths from maternal-fetal surgery (2), there are one or two anecdotal reports of procedure-related deaths in mothers following percutaneous image-guided procedures. To my knowledge, there has been no maternal death following open fetal surgery reported to date. Complications are significantly less following percutaneous approaches than with open hysterotomy (2). Refinement of the endoscopic technique (from multiple large ports to a single small port) has reduced the complication rates, but limits the types of procedures that can be performed with this approach.

Mirror Syndrome

The complications related to fetal surgery may be due to the procedure itself or complications related to the disease. In severe cases of fetal hydrops, the mother can manifest signs and symptoms that mimic or mirror the fetus's state. A severe preeclamptic state with hypertension, proteinuria, elevated liver enzymes, thrombocytopenia, ankle and pedal edema, or even generalized fluid retention. This condition, in which the mother's symptoms mirror the fetal state is referred to as the "Mirror Syndrome" (4). The exact mechanism of the mirror syndrome is unknown. However, it is thought that small molecules, present in the fetoplacental unit, cross the placenta and mediate this response in the mother. Mirror syndrome resolves with evacuation of the fetoplacental unit. Thus, fetal surgery is contraindicated in mothers who already have signs of mirror syndrome; rather the fetus should be delivered for the mother's well-being. Occasionally, the mirror syndrome may manifest after fetal surgery. Resolution of the fetal hydrops may start being apparent within a few days of the fetal surgical correction. As the hydrops resolves, the propensity to develop mirror syndrome also reduces. As the maternal health and well-being are paramount in every fetal procedure, if mirror syndrome becomes apparent and progressive after fetal surgery, the fetus should be delivered to allow the mother to recover.

Pulmonary Edema

Following open fetal surgery, pulmonary edema may be noted in the mother (2,5). This manifests as increased oxygen requirement and pulmonary infiltrates in the pregnant patient and some require endotracheal intubation. In the earlier experience with open fetal surgery, the incidence of pulmonary edema was as high as 29% (2). The pulmonary edema is neither associated with increased central venous pressure (6) nor with increased serum oncotic pressure. While the precise etiology is unclear, pulmonary edema following fetal surgery is thought to be due to increased vascular permeability (6), and was more common in the era when intravenous nitroglycerin was commonly used for tocolysis. In recent times, with judicious fluid restriction during surgery, and avoidance of intravenous nitroglycerin for tocolysis, the incidence of nonhydrostatic pulmonary edema following fetal surgery appears to have declined. However, hydrostatic pulmonary edema may occur as fetal hydrops resolves, as seen in some cases of large SCT with hydrops (7). Those mothers, who may already have excessive total body water, need to be aggressively diuresed to prevent this complication.

Injury to Maternal Viscera

In every fetal surgical procedure, there is the risk of injury to adjacent viscera. The risks differ with percutaneous and open approaches. With open fetal surgical procedures, a laparotomy incision (typically a Pfanenstiel or lower abdominal midline procedure) is made to gain access to the uterus. The risk of bladder injury is similar to that for a cesarean section. Typically, the intestines are reflected cephalad by the gravid uterus, thus injury to the intestines can be easily avoided as pregnancy progresses. Visceral injury may occur more with percutaneous procedures. However, the risk of these complications can be reduced by judicious use of the ultrasound during image-guided access to the uterus.

Bleeding

Maternal bleeding requiring blood transfusion can occur in as high as 12.6% of patients undergoing open fetal surgery cases (2). The frequency is much less with the minimal access techniques having a much lower risk of maternal bleeding. Maternal bleeding is a particular risk in any fetal surgery because of the very vascular nature of the gravid uterus. The uterine sinusoids are engorged, especially adjacent to the placenta. Some of these venous lakes can be seen grossly on the serosal surface of the uterus (during open fetal surgery) or by ultrasound (during image-guided approaches). With percutaneous needle approaches, there is no option to hold pressure on the bleeding sites. Fortunately, the muscular uterus closes on the tract of these needles and controls the hemorrhage.

Recent experience with laparoscopic-guided uterine access for posterior approach to an anteriorly placed placenta suggests that the amount of bleeding from needle or trocar sites is underestimated. The bleeding risk is greater when the uterus is relaxed. Halogenated anesthetic agents or other tocolytics can cause effective uterine relaxation. The inability of the uterine muscles to contract around the entry sites increases the risk of bleeding. This is readily seen in cases when needle decompression of a relaxed uterus for amnioreduction is performed prior to an open hysterotomy. Therefore for needle-guided or fetoscopic procedures that require a general anesthetic, care should be taken to minimize the degree of uterine relaxation to reduce blood loss.

Blood loss during open fetal surgery can be excessive if proper technique is not utilized. Full thickness hemostatic sutures are placed prior to incising the uterus with the electrocautery. The incision is then extended by the application of the uterine stapler. An absorbable lactomer stapler (U.S. Surgical Corp, Norwalk, Connecticut, U.S.A.) is useful for approximating the fetal membranes to the myometrium and also creates a hemostatic incision on the uterus. Large venous lakes seen on the serosal surface are avoided as much as possible. Bleeding from the lateral edges of the incision is common and the surgeon should be prepared for this. Carefully placed sutures or clamps at these corners can arrest the bleeding and allow for a bloodless operating field (Fig. 1).

Another major bleeding risk in the mother can occur following the EXIT procedure (8,9). The EXIT procedure is performed at the time of delivery for a variety of fetal indications. The most common indication is for airway access in fetuses with large neck or oral lesions.

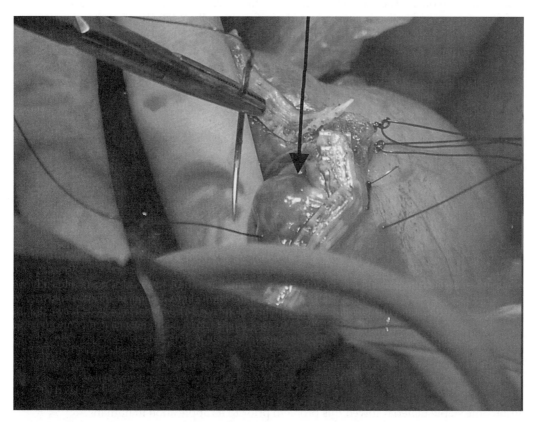

Figure 1 Extra-amniotic hematoma (*black arrow*) at the cut edge of the uterus following an open hysterotomy. Additional full-thickness sutures are being placed to control the bleeding.

To maintain uteroplacental circulation during the procedure, the uterus is kept relaxed until a secure fetal airway is achieved. The umbilical cord is then cut and the fetus delivered. Once uteroplacental flow is no longer required, the uterus is made to contract prior to delivering the placenta. If the placenta is delivered prematurely, profuse bleeding from the placental bed may occur due to the failure of the uterine muscles to contract the uterine sinusoids. Reversal of anesthesia and administration of pharmacologic agents to evoke uterine contraction are usually effective. Effective communication between the anesthesiologists, surgeons, and obstetricians is crucial to coordinate the timing of uterine relaxation and reversal during the EXIT procedure. Other local strategies for vascular control include inflation of an intrauterine balloon or direct compression of the uterine vessels. If uterine atony persists and bleeding is uncontrollable, a hysterectomy may have to be performed as a life-saving measure. Thus, informed consent for an EXIT procedure should include discussions about the possibility of a hysterectomy for bleeding. Fortunately, this is a very rare complication.

Uterine Rupture and Dehiscence

The risk of uterine rupture following fetal intervention is highest with open hysterotomy. Theoretically, every site of uterine access is a potential weak point. The needle-based interventions have little or no risk of rupture associated with them. The fetoscopic or trocar-based interventions use trocars that can vary in size from 3 to 5 mm in diameter. The larger ports create larger injury to the uterus. When multiple trocars are used or multiple insertions are attempted, the injury is multiplied. EXIT procedures are performed at term and the incision is usually located in the lower uterine segment. Thus, the risk of uterine rupture following an EXIT procedure should be no greater than the risk following a routine cesarean section, although a slightly larger incision may be required for delivery of fetuses with large neck masses. The greatest risk of uterine rupture occurs following open hysterotomy for fetal surgery. The incisions for fetal surgical procedures are not usually in the lower uterine segment. The uterine incision site is selected based on placental location and access to the specific portion of the fetus to be operated upon. These incisions could be on the body or fundus of the uterus (Fig. 2). A classical cesarean section incision is associated with a higher risk of uterine rupture, 4% to 9% (10) than the low-segment cesarean section incision 0.18% to 1.2% (11,12). Classical cesarean sections are performed at the end of pregnancy after which the uterus contracts and has time to heal. The uterine incision from fetal surgery is typically created between 19 and 28 weeks of gestation. This is a time when the gravid uterus continues to distend. As the uterus starts healing, the growth of the fetus stretches the wound even further. In addition, the uterine incision following fetal surgery is closed with the absorbable lactomer staples left *in situ* to ensure the fetal membranes remain approximated to the myometrium. The incision is therefore further separated by the thickness of these staples. Given these factors, one can postulate that the risk of uterine rupture of the fetal surgical hysterotomy incision should even be greater than that of classical cesarean section scar. However, due to meticulous surgical technique, the incidence of uterine rupture following fetal surgery in the major centers is 6% (13) and is comparable to that of classical cesarean section (4–9%) (10). Uterine dehiscence has a higher incidence of 12% (13) following open fetal surgery compared to 6% to 9% (14,15) following a classical or 0% to 3.5% (12,14,16) after low segment cesarean section (LSCS). These uterine dehiscences are typically asymptomatic and noted as "windows" in the uterus at the time of repeat surgery. Fortunately, uterine dehiscence is not associated with the same maternal morbidity and mortality as uterine rupture (15). The risk of uterine rupture is greatest at the time of labor. Hence, all women who undergo hysterotomy for open fetal surgery are committed to having an LSCS delivery of that pregnancy and all subsequent pregnancies. The deliveries should be performed prior to the onset of labor, when possible. These women are also encouraged to defer subsequent pregnancies for about 2 years following the open fetal surgery to allow for adequate healing of the uterine scar.

Fertility Risk

Fetal surgery can potentially impact the fertility of the woman. In the earlier animal experience with nonhuman primates, titanium staples left on the healing uterine incisions acted like intrauterine contraceptive devices and prevented subsequent conception (1). The use of absorbable staple material solved this problem prior to its application in humans.

Rarely, following a fetal procedure, uterine bleeding can be so severe that an unplanned cesarean hysterectomy may be necessary (13). Many women who desire to have children after

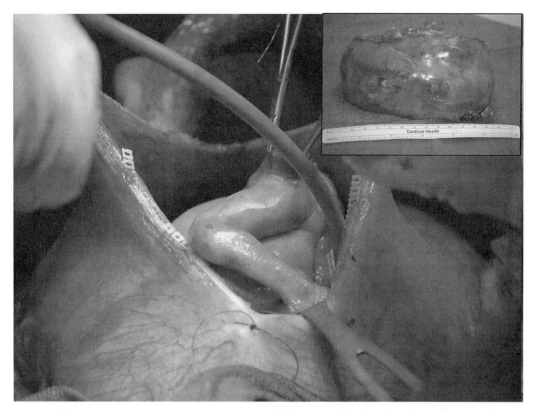

Figure 2 A very large hysterotomy is at times required for large fetal masses. In this case, a 10-cm hysterotomy was performed for resection of a large fetal sacrococcygeal teratoma (*inset*). These large incisions involving the body and fundus are at greater risk of dehiscence and rupture.

fetal surgery have gone on to have them (13,17). Following a fetal procedure, many maternal patients have opted not to have other children for a variety of reasons. The role of emotional stress and the psychosocial impact of a prior ill fetus on these decisions are unclear and poorly studied. When pregnancy does occur, there is the risk of abnormal placentation related to the uterine scar (18). These women are therefore at risk of placenta accreta or percreta that may place them at risk for severe bleeding and uterine rupture. A detailed assessment of the placenta in subsequent pregnancies is therefore essential in these women.

COMPLICATIONS RELATED TO THE FETO-PLACENTAL UNIT

Chorioamnionitis
Infection of the product of conception is always a possibility following fetal intervention. The incidence of chorioamnionitis following fetal surgery is as high as 8.9% (2,19). The incidence is higher following open surgery than with percutaneous or endoscopic techniques. Sterile technique is essential to avoid this complication. Repeated instrumentation and prolonged procedures increase the risk. Cultures of the amniotic fluid are obtained at the conclusion of the fetal procedure as a screening tool. Following open hysterotomy, antibiotic is instilled into the amniotic fluid at the time of uterine closure.

Placental Abruption
Placental abruption can complicate any fetal intervention. It is a distressing cause of bleeding that usually results in fetal demise and substantial maternal bleeding. A placental abruption rate of 8.9% has been reported after open hysterotomy (2). Following endoscopic or percutaneous procedures, the incidence may range from 0% to 10.7% (2,19). Prompt recognition of this

complication and delivery of the fetus may result in fetal salvage and limitation of maternal hemorrhage.

Membrane Separation

Chorioamnion separation can occur with any form of fetal access. During open fetal surgery, the uterine stapler is employed to prevent membrane separation. Yet the incidence of chorioamniotic membrane separation following open hysterotomy is 20% to 34% (2,20). A water-tight hysterotomy closure is also essential to prevent leakage of amniotic fluid from the incision. Controlling the membranes during percutaneous uterine access is more challenging. The membranes may be tented and pulled away from the myometrium as the trocar is inserted, thus endoscopic procedures have a higher incidence of membrane separation (64%) (2) compared to open hysterotomy. A sharp trocar readily pierces the membranes without tenting it, but may also leave a gaping hole in the amnion and chorion. Separation of the amnion and chorion releases prostaglandins that induce labor. Patients with chorioamniotic membrane separation after fetal surgery also have a higher incidence of premature rupture of membranes, preterm labor, and chorioamnionitis (21).

Premature Rupture of Membranes

Premature rupture of membranes (PROM) is a major concern following any instrumentation of the gravid uterus. There is a very small risk of PROM with needle amniocentesis 0.8% to 3.3% (22–24). The risk increases with the size of the trocar or incision and the number of attempts or sites (22). The fetal membranes heal poorly. Incidence of PROM can be as high as 52% (2) after fetal surgical procedures. Every puncture site is a potential leak site. Initial endoscopic procedures using several trocars had a higher incidence of PROM (44%) (2) compared to the newer single trocar techniques used for laser ablation or bipolar cord coagulation (17–38%) (19,25) and fetoscopic tracheal occlusion (35%) (3). Development of strategies to treat premature rupture of membranes remains an area of active interest in obstetric research (26–29). Some groups are attempting to close the membrane defect with gelfoam plugs to seal the hole and prevent membrane separation (30).

Preterm Labor and Premature Delivery

Preterm labor and delivery remains the Achilles heel of all fetal intervention. Differences in the documentation of preterm labor preclude adequate comparison between studies. The preterm delivery may be due to the underlying fetal condition, secondary to uterine stimulation, or both. Uterine stimulation appears to be less of a problem the smaller the instrument or incision. Hence the risk of premature delivery increases from needle amniocentesis on one end to open hysterotomy on the other extreme. Bigger incisions/trocars or multiple trocars, or multiple attempts all predispose to preterm labor. Incidence of preterm labor leading to delivery ranges from 12.9% for the percutaneous approaches to 32.9% for open hysterotomy (2). Following laser or bipolar cord coagulation in discordant monochorionic twins, Lewi et al. (25) reported a preterm delivery rate prior to 37 weeks of 62%, but only 21% were delivered before 32 weeks. Ilagan et al. (19) reported a 25% preterm labor rate following bipolar cord coagulation in twins.

Tocolytics to manage preterm labor is the key to successful fetal therapy. Indomethacin is an effective tocolytic but can cause premature constriction of the fetal ductus arteriosus. Thus, these fetuses need to be monitored closely with serial echocardiography and the treatment discontinued if ductal constriction is observed. Treatment with indomethacin is typically limited to 48 to 72 hours. Magnesium sulfate has withstood the test of time as an effective tocolytic agent. It is administered as an intravenous bolus and continued as an infusion. Serum magnesium levels are monitored and frequent neurological examination and tendon reflexes are monitored to assess toxicity. Treatment with high dose magnesium sulfate is frequently accompanied by nausea, vomiting, blurred vision, and malaise. Magnesium sulfate is useful as an adjunct to indomethacin to suppress uterine contractions in the first few days following maternal-fetal surgery or subsequently as rescue therapy when other agents have failed. When contractions have been suppressed for about 24 to 48 hours, patients who underwent needle or trocar access procedures typically do not require further tocolysis. However, following open hysterotomy, maintenance tocolysis may be required for several weeks and often for the remainder of the pregnancy. Agents used for maintenance therapy include calcium channel blockers (nifedipine) administered orally, and beta-adrenergic agonists (terbutaline) administered as a continuous subcutaneous infusion.

If the preterm labor cannot be effectively controlled, preterm delivery may be inevitable. Following needle or trocar access therapies, a vaginal delivery may be an option provided there are no obstetric contraindications. Following open fetal surgery, given the risk of uterine rupture, a cesarean section delivery is required. Depending on the time interval between the open hysterotomy and the need for preterm delivery and the location of the hysterotomy, that incision may be opened again to deliver the fetus if feasible. If the lower uterine segment has had time to develop over the course of the pregnancy, a standard lower segment cesarean section is the preferred mode of delivery. The typical issues related to premature neonates are relevant. These may be confounded by the underlying fetal condition that required intervention (fetal hydrops, intrauterine growth retardation, etc.) if not fully resolved by the time of preterm delivery.

Fetal Bradycardia

Acute drop in fetal heart rate during fetal surgery is not uncommon. This is readily identified with continuous fetal echocardiography (31,32). The most common cause is compression of the umbilical cord. Ensuring adequate uterine volume and repositioning the umbilical cord usually solves the problem. Fetal bradycardia can also occur during fetal thoracotomy for a large intrathoracic space-occupying lesion. These large chest masses compress the mediastinum and limit blood return to the heart resulting in heart failure and nonimmune hydrops. When the fetal thoracotomy is performed and the large mass exteriorized, the cardiac tamponade-like physiology is relieved acutely. This results in a marked reduction in systemic vascular resistance and hypotension, bradycardia and may lead to fetal demise. Hemodynamic instability during resection of a large intrathoracic mass can be ameliorated by volume-loading the fetus prior to performing the thoracotomy. In addition, the mass should be extruded gradually, allowing the fetus to equilibrate as monitored by continuous fetal echocardiography. The echocardiogram is also useful to assess the volume needs of the fetus prior to, during and after resection of the intrathoracic mass (31,32).

PROCEDURE-RELATED COMPLICATIONS

In addition to the complications that are related to the mode of access, some complications are specific to certain interventions and surgical procedures.

Collateral Damage from Radiofrequency Ablation

Radiofrequency ablation (RFA) is useful for the fulguration of tumors. There has been extensive experience with its use in adults but disappointing experiences so far when used for fetal tumors. RFA is commonly used for fetal conditions that are expected to result in the demise of the fetus. It is commonly used in the selective termination of the acardiac twin in twin-reversed arterial perfusion (TRAP) (33) sequence where the RFA needle is deployed at the umbilical cord insertion or even within the torso of the fetus to occlude the vessels and cause fetal demise. The advantage of RFA over bipolar cord coagulation is that the RFA can be administered via a percutaneous, transuterine needle puncture without the need for a trocar. When used for selective fetal termination (in TRAP or other indications), RFA has been quite effective and associated with few complications (34,35). The risk of bleeding, uterine irritation, premature rupture of membranes, and preterm labor are only slightly higher than that associated with amniocentesis as the needle is slightly bigger (14 gauge versus 20 gauge). The success of RFA in treating adult tumors and its use in fetal cord occlusion has resulted in its being utilized for occlusion of large feeding vessels in fetal SCT. Large SCTs in the fetus can result in high output cardiac failure as the fetal heart struggles to perfuse the rapidly growing mass which may contain arteriovenous connections. In this rare setting, fetal heart failure and hydrops occur and are invariably fatal (36–39). Changes in umbilical venous Doppler waveform can predict impending doom in these fetuses (40). However, fetuses with such large SCTs may benefit from fetal intervention. The goal in these cases is to limit the blood flow through the major vascular communications in the tumor. Successful attempts with open fetal surgery and debulking of the mass have been reported (7,41,42). RFA was conceived as a potential minimally invasive mode of achieving the same goal. However, reports to date have been dismal (43). Fetal bleeding and damage to surrounding structures, requiring extensive reconstructive surgery are reported (43). The fetal tissue has a very high water and electrolyte content that can easily disperse the energy beyond the intended target. While RFA is a useful treatment modality in other settings, its efficacy in fetal treatment will require further investigation: the unique fluid-filled intrauterine environment, the differing aqueous characteristics of fetal and adult tissues are complications that render research on adult patients irrelevant to the fetal setting.

Bleeding and Chest Wall Deformity Following Shunt Placement

Percutaneous insertion of thoracoamniotic shunts is performed for cases of fetal hydrothorax or large cystic lung lesions with hydrops (44). These shunts are placed through trocars percutaneously inserted through the fetal intercostal spaces. The shunts are deployed with a coil inside the thorax and another coil in the amniotic cavity. The unidirectional shunt thus allows fluid to flow from the thoracic cavity into the amniotic fluid. Any transthoracic procedure is at risk for injury to the intercostal neurovascular bundle. Bleeding from the intercostal vessels can worsen the intrathoracic fluid accumulation and also lead to hemorrhagic shock and death. Proper technique of accessing the intercostal space above the rib cannot be overemphasized. This is not trivial in a fetus whose intercostal space may only be a few millimeters in width. Intercostal vessel bleeding in the fetus can be seen as streaming from the puncture site on ultrasound and can be fatal. When thoracoamniotic shunts are placed in fetuses less than 21 weeks gestation, rib fractures and chest wall deformity have been noted postnatally (45). These risks should be weighed when these thoracic interventions are considered.

Shunt Dislodgement, Migration, and Cord Entanglement

Thoracoamniotic shunts or vesicoamniotic shunts (placed for lower urinary tract obstruction) can become dislodged (44,46). As the fetus grows, the shunts may become dislodged from their original location or migrate inwards into the thoracic or abdominal cavity. The shunt dislodgement rate is about 30% to 50% (46). At times, the shunts get clogged with vernix and become nonfunctional. There have been several cases where the fetus is seen on ultrasound holding on to the end of a shunt. How many cases of dislodgement are due to fetal actions is unknown. The greatest concern is the risk of cord entanglement, where the umbilical cord gets caught up in the coils of the shunt. This is more common with the vesicoamniotic shunts due to the proximity of these shunts to the umbilical cord insertion. The tangled cord can become compressed and/or occluded and lead to fetal demise. Some successful shunt procedures have resulted in untimely death of the fetus from cord entanglement. Keeping the external coils of the shunt as flat against the fetal body as possible may help reduce the risk of umbilical cord entanglement.

In conclusion, maternal-fetal surgery has a unique set of risks and complications. The actual incidence and prevalence of these complications are not well known because the surgeries are so new and methodology is rapidly changing. Surgeons involved in the care of these patients should be cognizant of the possible complications and measures to avoid and treat these complications. As more of these cases are performed and long-term outcomes reported, a better understanding of the relative risks and complication rates will be possible. A registry of complex fetal cases recording outcomes and complications would be helpful in this regard.

REFERENCES

1. Harrison MR, Golbus MS, Filly RA, eds. The Unborn Patient. 2nd ed. Philadelphia, PA: WB Saunders Company, 1990.
2. Golombeck K, Ball RH, Lee H, et al. Maternal morbidity after maternal-fetal surgery. Am J Obstet Gynecol 2006; 194(3):834–839.
3. Deprest J, Jani J, Gratacos E, et al. Fetal intervention for congenital diaphragmatic hernia: the European experience. Semin Perinatol 2005; 29(2):94–103.
4. Adzick NS. Management of fetal lung lesions. Clin Perinatol 2003; 30(3):481–492.
5. DiFederico EM, Burlingame JM, Kilpatrick SJ, et al. Pulmonary edema in obstetric patients is rapidly resolved except in the presence of infection or of nitroglycerin tocolysis after open fetal surgery. Am J Obstet Gynecol 1998; 179(4):925–933.

6. DiFederico EM, Harrison M, Matthay MA. Pulmonary edema in a woman following fetal surgery. Chest 1996; 109(4):1114–1117.

7. Hedrick HL, Flake AW, Crombleholme TM, et al. Sacrococcygeal teratoma: Prenatal assessment, fetal intervention, and outcome. J Pediatr Surg 2004; 39(3):430–438.

8. Noah MM, Norton ME, Sandberg P, et al. Short-term maternal outcomes that are associated with the EXIT procedure, as compared with cesarean delivery. Am J Obstet Gynecol 2002; 186(4):773–777.

9. Hirose S, Farmer DL, Lee H, et al. The ex utero intrapartum treatment procedure: looking back at the EXIT. J Pediatr Surg 2004; 39(3):375–380; discussion 375–380.

10. The American College of Obstetricians and Gynecologists. Vaginal birth after previous cesarean delivery. In: 2004 Compendium of Selected Publications. Washington, DC: The College, 2004. Practice Bulletin Number 5.

11. Ofir K, Sheiner E, Levy A, et al. Uterine rupture: risk factors and pregnancy outcome. Am J Obstet Gynecol. 2003; 189(4):1042–1046.

12. Durnwald C, Mercer B. Uterine rupture, perioperative and perinatal morbidity after single-layer and double-layer closure at cesarean delivery. Am J Obstet Gynecol 2003; 189(4):925–929.

13. Wilson RD, Johnson MP, Flake AW, et al. Reproductive outcomes after pregnancy complicated by maternal-fetal surgery. Am J Obstet Gynecol 2004; 191(4):1430–1436.

14. Halperin ME, Moore DC, Hannah WJ. Classical versus low-segment transverse incision for preterm caesarean section: Maternal complications and outcome of subsequent pregnancies. Br J Obstet Gynaecol 1988; 95(10):990–996.

15. Chauhan SP, Magann EF, Wiggs CD, et al. Pregnancy after classic cesarean delivery. Obstet Gynecol 2002; 100(5 Pt 1):946–950.

16. Durnwald CP, Rouse DJ, Leveno KJ, et al. The Maternal-Fetal Medicine Units Cesarean Registry: safety and efficacy of a trial of labor in preterm pregnancy after a prior cesarean delivery. Am J Obstet Gynecol 2006; 195(4):1119–1126.

17. Farrell JA, Albanese CT, Jennings RW, et al. Maternal fertility is not affected by fetal surgery. Fetal Diagn Ther 1999; 14(3):190–192.

18. Silver RM, Landon MB, Rouse DJ, et al. Maternal morbidity associated with multiple repeat cesarean deliveries. Obstet Gynecol 2006; 107(6):1226–1232.

19. Ilagan JG, Wilson RD, Bebbington M, et al. Pregnancy outcomes following bipolar umbilical cord cauterization for selective termination in complicated monochorionic multiple gestations. Fetal Diagn Ther 2008; 23(2):153–158.

20. Wilson RD, Johnson MP, Crombleholme TM, et al. Chorioamniotic membrane separation following open fetal surgery: pregnancy outcome. Fetal Diagn Ther. 2003; 18(5):314–320.

21. Sydorak RM, Hirose S, Sandberg PL, et al. Chorioamniotic membrane separation following fetal surgery. J Perinatol 2002; 22(5):407–410.

22. Nassar AH, Martin D, González-Quintero VH, et al. Genetic amniocentesis complications: is the incidence overrated? Gynecol Obstet Invest 2004; 58(2):100–104.

23. Centini G, Rosignoli L, Kenanidis A, et al. A report of early (13 + 0 to 14 + 6 weeks) and mid-trimester amniocenteses: 10 years' experience. J Matern Fetal Neonatal Med 2003; 14(2):113–117.

24. Brumfield CG, Lin S, Conner W, et al. Pregnancy outcome following genetic amniocentesis at 11–14 versus 16–19 weeks' gestation. Obstet Gynecol 1996; 88(1):114–118.

25. Lewi L, Gratacos E, Ortibus E, et al. Pregnancy and infant outcome of 80 consecutive cord coagulations in complicated monochorionic multiple pregnancies. Am J Obstet Gynecol 2006; 194(3):782–789.

26. Cortes RA, Wagner AJ, Lee H, et al. Pre-emptive placement of a presealant for amniotic access. Am J Obstet Gynecol 2005; 193(3 Pt 2):1197–1203.

27. Young BK, Roman AS, MacKenzie AP, et al. The closure of iatrogenic membrane defects after amniocentesis and endoscopic intrauterine procedures. Fetal Diagn Ther 2004; 19(3):296–300.

28. Mallik AS, Fichter MA, Rieder S, et al. Fetoscopic closure of punctured fetal membranes with acellular human amnion plugs in a rabbit model. Obstet Gynecol 2007; 110(5):1121–1129.

29. Ochsenbein-Kölble N, Jani J, Lewi L, et al. Enhancing sealing of fetal membrane defects using tissue engineered native amniotic scaffolds in the rabbit model. Am J Obstet Gynecol 2007; 196(3):263.e1–263.e7.

30. Luks FI, Deprest JA, Peers KH, et al. Gelatin sponge plug to seal fetoscopy port sites: technique in ovine and primate models. Am J Obstet Gynecol 1999; 181(4):995–996.

31. Keswani SG, Crombleholme TM, Rychik J, et al. Impact of continuous intraoperative monitoring on outcomes in open fetal surgery. Fetal Diagn Ther 2005; 20(4):316–320.

32. Rychik J, Tian Z, Cohen MS, et al. Acute cardiovascular effects of fetal surgery in the human. Circulation 2004; 110(12):1549–1556.

33. Hirose M, Murata A, Kita N, et al. Successful intrauterine treatment with radiofrequency ablation in a case of acardiac twin pregnancy complicated with a hydropic pump twin. Ultrasound Obstet Gynecol 2004; 23(5):509–512.

34. Tsao K, Feldstein VA, Albanese CT, et al. Selective reduction of acardiac twin by radiofrequency ablation. Am J Obstet Gynecol 2002; 187(3):635–640.

35. Livingston JC, Lim FY, Polzin W, et al. Intrafetal radiofrequency ablation for twin reversed arterial perfusion (TRAP): a single-center experience. Am J Obstet Gynecol 2007; 197(4):399.e1–399.3.

36. Hirose S, Farmer DL. Fetal surgery for sacrococcygeal teratoma. Clin Perinatol 2003; 30(3):493–506.

37. Langer JC, Harrison MR, Schmidt KG, et al. Fetal hydrops and death from sacrococcygeal teratoma: rationale for fetal surgery. Am J Obstet Gynecol 1989; 160(5 Pt 1):1145–1150.

38. Flake AW, Harrison MR, Adzick NS, et al. Fetal sacrococcygeal teratoma. J Pediatr Surg 1986; 21(7):563–566.

39. Bond SJ, Harrison MR, Schmidt KG, et al. Death due to high-output cardiac failure in fetal sacrococcygeal teratoma. J Pediatr Surg 1990; 25(12):1287–1291.

40. Olutoye OO, Johnson MP, Coleman BG, et al. Abnormal umbilical cord Doppler sonograms may predict impending demise in fetuses with sacrococcygeal teratoma. A report of two cases. Fetal Diagn Ther 2004; 19(1):35–9.

41. Adzick NS, Crombleholme TM, Morgan MA, et al. A rapidly growing fetal teratoma. Lancet 1997; 349(9051):538.

42. Graf JL, Albanese CT, Jennings RW, et al. Successful fetal sacrococcygeal teratoma resection in a hydropic fetus. J Pediatr Surg 2000; 35(10):1489–1491.

43. Paek BW, Jennings RW, Harrison MR, et al. Radiofrequency ablation of human fetal sacrococcygeal teratoma. Am J Obstet Gynecol 2001; 184(3):503–507.

44. Wilson RD, Baxter JK, Johnson MP, et al. Thoracoamniotic shunts: fetal treatment of pleural effusions and congenital cystic adenomatoid malformations. Fetal Diagn Ther 2004; 19(5):413–420.

45. Merchant AM, Peranteau W, Wilson RD, et al. Postnatal chest wall deformities after fetal thoracoamniotic shunting for congenital cystic adenomatoid malformation. Fetal Diagn Ther 2007; 22(6):435–439.

46. Wilson RD, Johnson MP. Prenatal ultrasound guided percutaneous shunts for obstructive uropathy and thoracic disease. Semin Pediatr Surg 2003; 12(3):182–189.

12 | Complications of Herniorrhaphy

Sara K. Rasmussen, M.D., Ph.D. and Jeffrey H. Haynes, M.D.

INTRODUCTION

Herniorrhaphy represents the most common procedure performed in pediatric surgical practice and the vast majority of such repairs are inguinal, umbilical, and epigastric. The incidence of inguinal hernia is between 0.8% and 4% of live births and occurs secondary to the failure of the processus vaginalis to obliterate during the seventh gestational month. The patent processus thereby allows a spectrum of pathologies to manifest, including scrotal hernias, communicating hydroceles, and hydrocele of the cord. Similarly, failure of the umbilical ring to undergo spontaneous closure results in an umbilical hernia. The true incidence of this hernia is unknown due to the high rate of spontaneous closure, but predilection for the African-American race and the premature infant is well known. Epigastric hernias result from defects in the linea alba and while occurring in about 5% of children, the etiology is unknown.

Overall, complication rates of herniorrhaphy are low. Those reported include wound infection, recurrence, injury to the vas deferens or testicular vessels, hematoma, stitch abscess and more rarely, infarcted testis or ovary, necrotizing fasciitis and small bowel, or bladder injury. The most common complications reported in large series include wound infection, recurrence, and testicular atrophy.

In the following chapter, the complications of pediatric herniorrhaphy will be reviewed and their management outlined. Most of the discussion will center on inguinal, umbilical, and epigastric hernias; however, other congenital hernias will be briefly discussed. It is to be emphasized that proper patient selection, timing of operation and meticulous technique will be most effective in the avoidance of any particular complication.

HERNIORRHAPHY

Inguinal Hernia

Due to a high risk of incarceration in male infants (see "Complications" section) inguinal hernias should be scheduled for repair at the time of diagnosis. Some pediatric surgeons opt to delay herniorrhaphy in female infants until their corrected gestational age is on the order of 45 to 50 weeks to minimize the small risk of postoperative apnea and so that an outpatient setting may be used. However, this approach must be balanced against a small risk of incarceration of the ovary.

An incarcerated and then reduced hernia presents a special consideration in both timing and extent of operation. The reduced hernia should generally be repaired during that hospitalization. Delay of a day or more under observation to allow swelling to abate is at the surgeon's discretion. Similarly, the decision to explore the contralateral groin in an infant after reduction should be considered in light of the duration of incarceration, difficulty in reduction, probability of contralateral hernia, and findings at operation when repairing the affected side.

The operative technique has been well described and is based on the high ligation of the patent processus vaginalis at the internal ring. An incision is made over the external ring and dissection carried down through Scarpa's fascia to expose and mobilize the spermatic cord in males. In infants, it is not necessary to open the external ring. The cord should be gently skeletonized, teasing the anteromedially located hernia sac away from cremasteric muscle fibers, vas deferens, and vessels. It is important to perform this dissection in as atraumatic a fashion as possible. If the hernia sac is found to be devoid of contents at the level of the internal ring, it is twisted and then ligated. Use of absorbable suture may avoid a late presenting stitch abscess. It is unusual to have to repair the inguinal floor although large premature infant hernias as well as recurrent hernias may need this anatomy addressed via a Bassini or Cooper's ligament repair. Prosthetic mesh may rarely be used in cases of native tissue deficiency. Hemostasis of the cord is essential as is assuring its normal anatomic position along with the testicle at the beginning of the closure. Local anesthetic blocks are effective. A meticulous skin closure assuring epidermal to epidermal apposition along the entire course of the wound will give the best chance for precise healing without infection. Repair in females is similar while the hernia sac is separated from the round ligament and then ligated. Note should be made here to exclude the presence of a sliding hernia, more common in females. The overlying external oblique may then be closed at the external ring to buttress the repair.

While an open repair may be considered the gold standard, there is a growing body of literature advocating a laparoscopic approach for both diagnosis of a contralateral patent processus vaginalis (1) as well as primary herniorrhaphy. Laparoscopic diagnosis of a contralateral patent processus vaginalis which then prompts exploration and repair has been shown to be safe and effective. Unanswered is the question of whether a patent processus represents a consistent risk of developing a metachronous clinical hernia.

Primary laparoscopic inguinal herniorrhaphy has been reported in several large series (2–5). All approaches involve peritoneal cavity entrance and direct visualization of the internal ring. As such there is a minimal but reported risk of bowel and vascular injury during accession and manipulation which is not present during open herniorrhaphy. Laparoscopic repair of the internal ring has been reported both transperitoneally as well as percutaneously. Postoperative risks include wound infection, stitch abscess, and postoperative hydrocele which are roughly equivalent to an open approach. Recurrence rates, however, vary widely and have been reported as low as 0.73% in two of these series to as high as 4% to 5% in both percutaneous and transperitoneal approaches.

Umbilical Hernia

The umbilical ring may undergo progressive closure with hernia resolution until age 3 to 5 years. Generally accepted indications for repair prior to this include incarceration, pain, or a fascial defect larger than 2 cm. Repair of a defect based on size may be best deferred until 12 months of age or later when the child is ambulating to allow the abdominal wall sufficient time to strengthen, and may result in fewer recurrences.

Umbilical herniorrhaphy is usually performed through a curvilinear incision nestled at the base of the umbilicus. Dissection is then carried around the hernia sac, which is then disconnected from the overlying skin. It is not necessary to remove the entire sac from the under surface of the umbilicus as this does not result in postoperative seromas and may result in "button-holing" the overlying skin. The hernia sac is then resected at the level of strong fascia and the defect re-approximated. As in inguinal hernias, the use of absorbable suture in the fascial repair may result in fewer late stitch abscesses. Hemostasis is attained and a local anesthetic infiltration employed. The overlying umbilical skin is then inverted and tacked at its apex to the mid-portion of the fascial closure, resulting in an inward configuration to the umbilicus. A perfect skin closure is then achieved and the incision dressed in a sterile fashion. A compression dressing is employed for 48 hours in the hope that it will be effective in preventing postoperative hematoma and seroma formation.

Epigastric Hernia

Small defects in the linea alba, usually between the umbilicus and the xyphoid process, result in epigastric hernias. While the etiology is unknown, they are almost always asymptomatic. The diagnosis is made by either an intermittent or constant pea-sized swelling in this region which is a result of prolapsed preperitoneal fat. Epigastric hernias may occur more frequently in the presence of a diastasis recti, due to the thinned out central fascia.

Elective fascial repair through a small transverse incision with resection of any prolapsed fat is curative. Attention should be paid to marking the site preoperatively as many of these defects are impalpable under general anesthetic relaxation.

Spigelian Hernia

Spigelian hernias occur spontaneously through the semilunar line at the lateral border of the rectus abdominus muscle. They are quite rare in children, but when encountered, can have life-threatening consequences if not treated promptly. There are 34 case reports in the literature and most are diagnosed on physical examination and confirmed at exploration. Most commonly the defect size in the fascia is 1 to 3 cm, but has been reported to be as large as 7.5 cm. Repair involves closing the fascial defect using available endogenous tissues.

COMPLICATIONS

Incarceration

The natural history of inguinal hernias in children demonstrates a high rate of incarceration (6) and is estimated to be around 10% to 12% (6–8). More than 50% of children who presented in one study with incarcerated inguinal hernia had a prior episode of incarceration. These children were more likely to need emergency surgery and had a higher postoperative complication rate (10.4%). Delay in operative repair after reduction almost always results in the child returning with a second episode of incarceration. Therefore, the standard of care for children who present with incarcerated inguinal hernia is repair during the next elective opportunity. Incarcerated inguinal hernias that are irreducible of course warrant immediate operation. The risks associated with open repair intraoperatively are primarily damage to the cord contents, which can lead to vas deferens damage and testicular atrophy in males and ovarian infarction in females. One prospective study evaluated the effectiveness of longitudinally splitting the hernia sac versus high ligation with sac excision; although the study was small (798 patients), the splitting technique had comparable results compared to high ligation and perhaps less severe complications (9). The hernia sac is known to be fragile and during dissection the sac can be shredded which may result from or contribute to over-handling of the cord structures.

Recent advances in laparoscopic techniques suggest that laparoscopy can aid in the treatment of incarcerated inguinal hernia. The main advantage of laparoscopy in the setting of incarceration is the ability to reduce the hernia under direct vision. Additionally, the pneumoperitoneum that is established during the laparoscopy may assist in the reduction of the hernia by potentially enlarging the internal ring. Patients that have laparoscopy to reduce their inguinal hernia may then undergo repair at the same operation. A small study investigating laparoscopic reduction of incarcerated inguinal hernia showed no complications and a greatly reduced hospital stay for affected children (10).

Anesthetic Risk

Anesthesia for inguinal herniorrhaphy also deserves careful planning and consideration. Preterm infants have a high rate of respiratory complications including postoperative apnea. As mentioned previously, an extended period of observation may be best for infants undergoing herniorrhaphy via general anesthesia if their corrected gestational is under 45 to 50 weeks. Infants who present with incarcerated hernias while affected by bronchiolitis are of special concern. The standard of care mandates quick operative repair surgically yet the anesthetic standard of care is to delay operation until pulmonary pathology resolves. Cases have shown that operating in this situation under a general anesthetic can be done safely (11,12). Nevertheless, regional and local anesthesia has been used for herniorrhaphy in high-risk infants. This is usually safe, but perforation of the small bowel during regional nerve block has been reported (13).

Recurrence

The recurrence rate after open inguinal hernia repair in many series is 1.2% (14). One major factor that has been identified as a risk for recurrence is the effect of surgeon training. Two different studies have independently found that general surgeons who perform pediatric hernia repair have a higher rate of hernia recurrence than pediatric surgeons. In another study, however, this difference in recurrence was not seen in general surgeons who performed a high volume of pediatric inguinal hernia repairs (8). For now, most studies investigating laparoscopic inguinal hernia repair also report a higher recurrence rate of around 3% to 5%, although this risk seems to decrease as a function of surgeon experience.

Wound Infections

The rate of wound infection after inguinal hernia repair is quite low, 1.2% in a large single-surgeon series. This is the expected infection rate for clean surgical wounds. Interestingly, in one series that examined stitch abscess formation, of six patients with stitch abscess formation, two had wound complications (15). Another case report of postoperative umbilical fistula demonstrated that the patient had a history of wound infection requiring drainage (22). Simple abscesses should be drained and antibiotics used for surrounding cellulitis be drained. Necrotizing fasciitis has been reported after inguinal herniorrhaphy although fortunately it is quite rare. High fevers in the immediate postoperative period should prompt careful wound evaluation. If any concern exists, the wound should be opened and assessed. Cultures should be taken and the health of the fascia assessed. Debridement is necessary to achieve a healthy margin in confirmed cases.

Testicular Atrophy and Vas Injuries

Perhaps one of the most serious postoperative complications from inguinal hernia repair is that of testicular atrophy and/or direct injury to the vas deferens during the operation. The blood supply of the testis is very delicate, and damage to the vessels can lead to testicular atrophy. The rate of testicular atrophy in one large series was 0.3% (7). Laparoscopic Palomo varicocelectomy has been shown to reverse, or at least stabilize, testicular atrophy in patients who have had inguinal hernia repair, but this has not been widely applied (18). Similarly, if a patient has a cryptorchid or "trapped" testis after inguinal hernia repair and it is not corrected in a timely fashion, the testis will have impaired sperm production (16). The incidence of boys requiring postoperative orchiopexy for trapped testis was 0.5% in one study. Interestingly, of boys noted to have a trapped testis postoperatively, 50% had an episode of incarceration (7). Finally, the vas deferens must be handled in the least traumatic fashion possible to prevent subsequent fibrous obliteration of the lumen and in cases of bilateral manipulation, possible infertility. This postoperative complication is often not recognized for more than 20 years after the initial operation. Damage caused by over-handling the vas tend to cover large lengths of the vas, and as such, are more difficult to repair. Microsurgical repair of impaired vas deferens has been done, but the success rate, while significant, does not assure every patient of fertility (17). The need for a gentle dissection is well known and accordingly the rate of vas deferens injury is low, 0.06%.

Stitch Abscess

There are a few reports of postoperative stitch abscesses requiring reoperation to remove offending suture. Most often, these stitch abscesses are in children who have had ligation of the sac performed with silk suture, which has been shown to cause clinically significant infections when colonized with as little as 10 CFU of *Staphylococcus aureus* per stitch. The rate of stitch granuloma formation is approximately 0.6% (20). Patients with stitch abscess can present either in the more immediate postoperative period or relatively late after herniorrhaphy—from 5 months to 7 years. To treat this complication, re-operation with drainage of the abscess and most importantly removal of the foreign body is curative. In some cases, repair of sliding inguinal hernia with incomplete reduction of the sliding component may lead to stitch granuloma formation in the bladder. This may present as repeated urinary tract infections and may necessitate local exploration and in severe cases removal of the trapped portion of bladder. Children with stitch abscess involving the bladder may not present with fever or leukocytosis, but microscopic hematuria is usually present (15,19).

Bladder Injury

As introduced above, the urinary bladder is quite close to the inguinal canal in infants, making this structure vulnerable to injury during herniorrhaphy, especially as a sliding component. The lateral bladder wall can protrude into the canal, making careful dissection during difficult herniorrhaphy essential. If the bladder is suspected to comprise the medial wall of the floor, it may either be repaired with a purse string suture or its presence confirmed by placing a feeding tube and filling up the bladder to identify the bladder wall. In cases of suspected bladder injury postoperatively, cystoscopy and VCUG may aid diagnosis. Bladder injury must be suspected in a postoperative patient that has continuous drainage from his or her wound, repeated urinary tract infection or persistent hematuria. In one reported case, bladder injury during herniorrhaphy was so significant that reconstruction with sigmoid colon was required (21).

Umbilical Fistula

There are reported cases of acquired umbilical fistula after hernia repair in children. Most of the cases had an associated postoperative wound infection. It is hypothesized that inguinal wound infection in small children can easily travel to the umbilicus with the guidance of the remnant umbilical artery. Treatment of the condition requires drainage, antibiotics, and eventual fistulectomy (22).

Necrotizing Enterocolitis

Necrotizing enterocolitis is a rare complication after hernia repair; it has been reported in one series examining the risk of poor nutritional status in infants undergoing herniorrhaphy. Interestingly, the reported case of necrotizing enterocolitis was found in an infant with appropriate nutritional status (23).

UNEXPECTED FINDINGS AT OPERATION

There are reports of male pseudohermaphroditism discovered at the time of bilateral inguinal hernia repair in apparent females. This condition occurs when a genotypic (XY) male has incomplete masculinization or complete feminization of the external genitalia. Classically, the affected child is a phenotypic female who presents with bilateral hernias. At exploration, bilateral gonads are discovered leading to the suspected diagnosis. Appropriate handling of this finding includes biopsy of the gonads to confirm the diagnosis, repair of the hernias, vaginoscopy, genetic consultation, and parental counseling.

CONDITIONS REQUIRING SPECIAL CONSIDERATION

Bladder Exstrophy

One other condition that warrants discussion is herniorrhaphy in the patient with bladder exstrophy. These patients are thought to be predisposed to inguinal hernia formation because of the effect the widely splayed pubic bones have on the obliquity of the inguinal canal, poorly developed abdominal musculature, and perhaps yet unknown but proposed anatomical defect in the inguinal canal. The incidence of inguinal hernia is much higher in this population than in the general population (66% in one series). Additionally there is a much higher incidence of bilateral inguinal hernia (81.8% of bladder exstrophy patients in one series) and a much higher incidence of recurrence (8.3%). Consequently, contralateral exploration is recommended in all patients with bladder exstrophy who develop inguinal hernia (24). The incidence of incarcerated hernia in these patients is generally similar to the rate of incarceration in patients without bladder exstrophy.

Prematurity

Premature infants are more likely to have inguinal hernias, principally owing to the patent processus vaginalis which in general obliterates in the seventh month of intrauterine life. An additional factor may be the small shorter distance between the internal and external rings in the neonate, and their less oblique relationship when compared to internal and external ring location in full-term infants. Accordingly, bilateral exploration is widely accepted in cases of unilateral clinical hernia.

Ventriculo-Peritoneal Shunts

The presence of a ventriculo-peritoneal (VP) shunt is a generally accepted indication for bilateral groin exploration in cases of unilateral clinical hernia. A minimally patent processus vaginalis may manifest as a hernia at a later date when subjected chronically to an increased intraperitoneal fluid burden. Additionally, VP shunts are thought to increase the rate of hernia recurrence because of the increased intra-abdominal pressure against the internal ring. Patients with VP shunts in one series had a recurrence rate of 10%, a rate eight times higher than the general population.

SUMMARY

Herniorrhaphy remains one of the most common operations performed by the pediatric surgeon. Although inguinal hernias have been one of the most long-standing and most successfully treated conditions encountered by the pediatric surgeon, challenges remain. Complications, though fortunately rare, can have devastating consequences for the children unfortunate enough to experience them. An emphasis on patient selection and meticulous technique should avoid most of these problems. The pediatric surgeon may never know of some complications, namely male infertility, that may plague their patient long after he or she has retired. Therefore, the standard of a meticulous dissection and repair and newer techniques such as laparoscopy that protect the cord structures and ensure careful visualization will ensure optimal results with few complications.

REFERENCES

1. Miltenburg DM, Nuchtern JG, Jaksic T, et al. Laparoscopic evaluation of the pediatric inguinal hernia— A meta-analysis. J Pediatr Surg 1998; 33:874–879.
2. Takehara H, Yakabe S, Kameoka K. Laparoscopic percutaneous extraperitoneal closure for inguinal hernia in children: Clinical outcome of 972 repairs done in 3 pediatric surgical institutions. J Pediatr Surg 2006; 41:1999–2003.
3. Schier F. Laparoscopic hernia repair: An option in babies weighing 5 kg or less. Pediatr Surg Int 2006; 22:1033.
4. Ozgediz D, Roayaie K, Lee H, et al. Subcutaneous endoscopically assisted ligation (SEAL) of the internal ring for repair of inguinal hernias in children: Report of a new technique and early results. Surg Endosc 2007; 21:1327–1331.
5. Spurbeck, WW, Prasad R, Lobe TE. Two-year experience with minimally invasive herniorrhaphy in children. Surg Endosc 2005; 19(4):441–443.
6. Niedzielski J, Kr l R, Gawlowska A. Could incarceration of inguinal hernia in children be prevented? Med Sci Monit 2003; 9:CR16–CR18.
7. Ein SH, Njere I, Ein A. Six thousand three hundred sixty-one pediatric inguinal hernias: A 35-year review. J Pediatr Surg 2006; 41:980–986.
8. Borenstein SH, To T, Wajja A, et al. Effect of subspecialty training and volume on outcome after pediatric inguinal hernia repair. J Pediatr Surg 2005; 40:75–80.
9. Gahukamble DB, Khamage AS. Prospective randomized controlled study of excision versus distal splitting of hernial sac and processus vaginalis in the repair of inguinal hernias and communicating hydroceles. J Pediatr Surg 1995; 30:624–625.
10. Kaya M, Huckstedt T, Schier F. Laparoscopic approach to incarcerated inguinal hernia in children. J Pediatr Surg 2006; 41:567–569.
11. Cox RG: Repair of incarcerated inguinal hernia in an infant with acute viral bronchiolitis. Can J Anaesth 2004; 51:68–71.
12. Melo-Filho AA, de Fatima Assuncao Braga A, Calderoni DR, et al. Does bronchopulmonary dysplasia change the postoperative outcome of herniorrhaphy in premature babies? Paediatr Anaesth 2007; 17:431–437.
13. Amory C, Mariscal A, Guyot E, et al. Is ilioinguinal/iliohypogastric nerve block always totally safe in children? Paediatr Anaesth 2003; 13:164–166.
14. Perlstein J, Du Bois JJ. The role of laparoscopy in the management of suspected recurrent pediatric hernias. J Pediatr Surg 2000; 35:1205–1208.
15. Imamoglu M, Cay A, Sarihan H, et al. Paravesical abscess as an unusual late complication of inguinal hernia repair in children. J Urol 2004; 171:1268–1270.
16. Imthurn T, Hadziselimovic F, Herzog B. Impaired germ cells in secondary cryptorchid testis after herniotomy. J Urol 1995; 153:780–781.
17. Sheynkin YR, Hendin BN, Schlegel PN, et al. Microsurgical repair of iatrogenic injury to the vas deferens. J Urol 1998; 159:139–141.
18. Barqawi A, Furness P, III, Koyle M. Laparoscopic Palomo varicocelectomy in the adolescent is safe after previous ipsilateral inguinal surgery. BJU Int 2002; 89:269–272.
19. Calkins CM, St Peter SD, Balcom A, et al. Late abscess formation following indirect hernia repair utilizing silk suture. Pediatr Surg Int 2007; 23:349–352.
20. Nagar H. Stitch granulomas following inguinal herniotomy: A 10-year review. J Pediatr Surg 1993; 28:1505–1507.
21. Miyano G, Yamataka A, Okada Y, et al. Sigmoidocolocystoplasty for augmentation of iatrogenic small capacity bladder caused by direct injury to the bladder during inguinal hernia repair: Long-term follow-up. Pediatr Surg Int 2004; 20:61–64.

22. Okuyama H, Fukuzawa M, Nakai H, et al. Acquired umbilical fistula after repair of inguinal hernia: A case report. J Pediatr Surg 1998; 33:737–738.
23. Turkyilmaz Z, Sonmez K, Numanoglu V, et al. Postoperative necrotizing enterocolitis following incarcerated inguinal hernia repair: Report of a case. Surg Today 2001; 31:550–552.
24. Connolly JA, Peppas DS, Jeffs RD, et al. Prevalence and repair of inguinal hernias in children with bladder exstrophy. J Urol 1995; 154:1900–1901.

Repair of Inguinal Hernia

Expert: Frederick J. Rescorla, M.D.

QUESTIONS

1. **How should the hernia sac be managed if it is torn during the separation from the vas deferens and blood vessels?**
   Initially, I try to start the dissection several centimeters from the internal ring so that if this happens there is room to gain proximal control. Although relatively rare, it seems to happen most in the premature children. I place hemostats on the edges and work from the inside of the sac to separate it from the vas and vessels and gradually lift all of the hemostats and place a clamp around the entire sac.

2. **What should be done if the vas is divided during repair of an inguinal hernia?**
   In a young child, place a fine (5–0) Prolene suture through the two ends anticipating a later repair by a urologist experienced is vas repair.

3. **What steps can be performed to prevent injuries to the vas and blood vessels?**
   Approach the sac on the anterior surface, lift carefully and "brush" the vas and vessels off laterally. I do not pick up either the vas or the vessels with forceps.

4. **How should the premature infant with a hernia and an undescended testicle be managed?**
   If the hernia is large and symptomatic, repair with simultaneous orchiopexy. If not symptomatic, wait to see if the testes come down and repair later. Orchiopexy in the premature infant is very difficult.

5. **What approach should be taken to repair a recurrent hernia?**
   Inguinal if appears to be a definite inguinal recurrence. I would have a low threshold for laparoscopy especially if there is concern that it was a missed femoral hernia.

6. **What technical problems lead to recurrence of an indirect hernia?**
   Missed sac, torn sac with a portion not included in ligation and not a high enough ligation.

7. **If a child presents with a inguinal groin bulge and no indirect hernia is identified during the operation what repair should be done?**
   Look for direct and femoral hernias. I would consider putting a scope in to evaluate and sort out the anatomy.

8. **Do you twist the sac?**
   No

9. **Do you inspect the testicle?**
   Not routinely. If it incarcerated, I try to visualize.

10. **In a female hernia, what techniques do you make to check for a fallopian tube?**
    I always try to see the fallopian tube and ovary. I am not always successful but I do attempt to visualize these structures.

11. **Which patients should undergo a contralateral exploration?**
    Premature infants.

12. **In the multiply recurrent hernia, is a prosthetic repair indicated?**
    Sometimes. I would be prepared to place a mesh, but it would depend on operative findings. If there was tension, I would place mesh. If it was postpubertal, I would place mesh.

13. **Should silk sutures be avoided due to risks of late stitch abscesses?**
    No, I have never seen a stitch abscess from a high ligation which is the only place I utilize the silk suture.

Congenital Diaphragmatic Hernia

Expert: Charles J. Stolar, M.D.

QUESTIONS

1. **How do you decide when to operate to repair congenital diaphragmatic hernia (CDH)?**
   Surgery for CDH is *elective* not emergent. The preoperative resuscitation is infinitely more important than the surgery timing. Surgery is scheduled on an elective basis defined by resolution of pulmonary hypertension. Evidence that pulmonary hypertension has resolved is developed by echocardiography regarding the position of the interventricular septum, direction of shunting at the foramen ovale and ductal level, degree of tricuspid regurgitation, and acceleration times of the main pulmonary artery. Clinically resolution/stabilization of pulmonary vascular tone is evidenced by disappearance of the pre-/postductal oxygen saturation gradient. Also, the patient is able to be weaned from aggressive respiratory and pharmacologic support. At the time of surgery, supplemental oxygen requirements are minimal and no cardiotonic agents or pulmonary antihypertensives are needed. This usually takes 3 to 7 days. There are exceptions where after a much more extended period of attempted stabilization pulmonary hypertension is unabated. At this time, extracorporeal membrane oxygenation (ECMO) can be added to the preoperative resuscitation if indicated or an operation can be considered in an otherwise stable baby.

2. **How do you decide when to patch a defect?**
   A patch for the diaphragmatic defect is used if, after mobilization of the posterior leaflet, a nominally tension free primary closure cannot be achieved. A tension free closure must separate the chest and abdomen medially and laterally. When repairing a CDH while on ECMO, the threshold for using a patch is even lower so as to minimize dissection and potential bleeding surfaces.
   A patch is also used for the anterior abdominal wall if the loss of abdominal domain is severe and primary closure would cause a compartment syndrome. An abdominal wall patch is also used if repairing CDH on ECMO to minimize tissue trauma when closing and lower the threshold for re-exploration if there is postoperative bleeding on ECMO. Also, in this circumstance, a J-P drain is left in the abdomen to drain accumulating blood.

3. **How you decide where to put sutures if there is no posterior rim?**
   This can be challenging. Medially there is usually a small amount of diaphragm muscle available. If not, the adventia of the aorta and muscle wall of the esophagus can be "used" but this is not terribly secure. I favor, in this circumstance, rotating a flap of pericardium into the field and using this to anchor a patch medially. As the surgeon comes laterally, nonabsorbable sutures can be passed around/between/or through successive ribs. Anterior there is usually a bit of muscle tissue for the patch to be sewn to. I do not favor rotating a flap of abdominal wall muscle because (a) this bleeds when on ECMO (usually the case in this circumstance) and (b) it creates a troubling flank hernia. I also tell the family that if the baby survives the chances of recurrence are significant.

4. **How do you repair a recurrent defect?**

First the abdominal organs have to be returned to the abdomen . . . again. The possibility of dense adhesions to the lung/mediastinum should be anticipated by positioning and prepping the patient for thoracic exposure if exposure from re-exploration of the abdomen proves inadequate. If the recurrence is dehiscence of a primary muscle closure, a patch of gortex is sewn to fresh edges over the defect. If the recurrence is in the context of a previous gortex repair, the initial patch of gortex is augmented with a second patch and sewn in place rather than remove and replace the entire initial patch. Nonabsorbable sutures are used.

5. **Does visceral incarceration occur in the newborn with a CDH that has not been repaired?**

Yes, but it's very unusual. In my 26-year experience with about 500 CDH newborns, I have had experience with a single CDH infant whose stomach (cardia only) was incarcerated in a diaphragmatic defect. The defect was about 2 cm in diameter, medial and not the usual posterolateral defect. There were no other viscera in the chest. The neonatologists thought it was a tension pneumothorax and called us when gastric contents came from their chest tube!

6. **What are the most common complications following CDH repair and how can they be avoided?**

The most common complication is death (about 10%). This can be minimized by excellent attention to iatrogenic injury to the lungs and respiratory care strategies that minimize lung injury, baro trauma, and oxygen toxicity. What constitutes lung sparing care is a long discussion, but this "expert" thinks a significant portion of CDH deaths are iatrogenic and preventable.

Persistent pulmonary hypertension occurs in 3% to 7% of survivors. Generally, these patients do not survive long term. The best pharmacologic management is not yet determined but it may be that proactive management with agents such as prostacycline, sildenafil, and other investigational drugs will be of value.

Recurrent CDH has been discussed above.

Foregut dysmotility occurs in almost al CDH infants. It cannot be avoided but can be usually managed medically, not surgically.

7. **What unusual complications have you seen occur in the treatment of an infant with CDH?**

The spectrum of complications is limited only by your imagination!

8. **Do you patch a large defect with a synthetic or muscle flap?**

See #4. Prosthetic materials are used only.

9. **Do you place a chest tube postoperatively? Do you place it on suction?**

The *only* indication for a chest tube is the presence of active bleeding or and active air leak. When repairing a CDH on ECMO, because of the bleeding risk, it may be of value to place a chest tube prophylactic ally. The ipsilateral lung is hypoplastic, not ateletatic. It is smaller than the thorax and will not "expand" to fill it. In those unusual circumstances where a chest tube is indicated, there is no reason to put it on suction. A small amount of water seal is sufficient combined with fastidious attention to maintaining patency of the tube. Applying suction only distorts the lungs and makes the unstable pulmonary vascular tone worse. Don't do it!

10. **How do you approach an inability to close the abdominal wall fascia post CDH repair?**

See #2. The threshold for placing an abdominal wall patch is very low even in the non-ECMO patient. It is temporary and can be removed with delayed primary closure 1 to 2 weeks later in a much calmer environment. Dealing with an abdominal wall patch is a lot easier than dealing with a compartment syndrome or ventral hernia/ dehiscence.

11. Any special techniques for dealing with a right-sided CDH?

The chest should always be prepped into the field for a right-sided diaphragmatic hernia because of uncertainty regarding the liver. On occasion the liver is fused to the lung (hepatopulmonary fusion). This can be best appreciated from the chest and abdomen. It also cannot be corrected surgically. On occasion the hepatic veins enter the right atrium directly instead of the IVC. Also, on occasion there is azygous continuation of the inferior vena cava. If the chest and abdomen are going to be separated in these circumstances a patch will be needed and it may be helpful to see both the chest and the abdominal cavities simultaneously.

Repair of Abdominal Wall Defects

Expert: Michael D. Klein, M.D.

QUESTIONS

1. How do you decide between the use of a silo and primary closure?

More than half of the patients I operate on can be closed primarily. This is, in part, because I make a big effort to operate early, in the delivery room when possible. If I have a question about whether it will be too tight, I use skin flaps, and if that will be too tight, I then use a silastic prosthesis. When I use skin flaps, I recognize that there will be a diamond of white skin, but that this skin seldom dies. I do ask the anesthesiologist to tell me the ventilatory pressure they are using. If it is more than 24 as I begin a fascial closure, I will not continue. Certainly, a requirement for pressures over 30 bodes ill. I do occasionally measure intra-abdominal pressure when reducing a silo (either from the nasogastric [NG] tube or from the Foley catheter), but for some reason, I do not do this in the operating room. It would certainly be a reasonable thing to do. It is not only the tightness of the closure that is important. When treating a newborn with an omphalocele, it is possible to close with very little tension and still have a patient who develops a persistent metabolic acidosis due to kinking of the hepatic veins as the liver angulates when it is reduced.

2. How do you attach a silo to the fascia? Has the preformed silo obviated the need for fascial attachment?

The work of Bianchi, Jona (and I am sure many others) has demonstrated that the intestines will gradually return to the abdominal cavity without pressure being applied, at least in most cases. Thus, I think it is perfectly acceptable to place a Bentec bag (performed silo with spring wound base to hold it in the abdomen) without stitches. Different from what Dr. Schuster introduced us to years ago when he developed the plastic prosthesis concept, it is NOT necessary to apply pressure to reduce the contents. There is even a group in South America that uses a female condom as a less expensive Bentec bag with excellent results.

   There are still occasions when a preformed silo cannot be used, as when a stoma is being created at the same time and the ring within the abdomen would put too much pressure on or angulate the bowel going to the stoma. In this case, I use two sheets of 0.007 inch thick Dacron impregnated with silicone rubber. I sew one sheet to each side of the defect in a vertical manner using running 3–0 prolene. I put the shiny side down next to the bowel and evert the silo material and the fascia so that the bowel sees a very smooth surface. I then use the same suture material in a running fashion to close the prosthesis to the prosthesis trimming where possible.

3. What steps can be taken to minimize silo disruption?

As noted above, the first step is to not reduce the silo too vigorously. Dr. Schuster originally used an inner layer of polyethylene to prevent fluid loss and bowel adhesion to the mesh. He then used a Dacron mesh on top to provide the strength layer. Tissue would grow into the mesh and provide a very strong attachment so that it could be reduced slowly. His concept was that the pressure was providing impetus for the development of the abdominal cavity. When surgeons changed to using the silastic impregnated Dacron as one piece, tissue would not grow in and we learned that we needed to remove the prosthesis by two weeks or it would just separate from the abdominal wall. Several surgeons developed measurement techniques (via g.t., NG tube, or bladder) so that aggressive reduction could be done (sometimes more than once a day). I have found that in most cases the prosthesis can be removed and the abdomen closed by 1 week. This suggests that the abdominal wall is not growing, but we are squeezing the edema out of tissues, emptying the lumen of the bowel, and stretching the abdominal wall. Now we know that reduction will usually occur without exogenous force.

A second step to prevent silo disruption when one is sewed on, is to take bites of rectus muscle and not just the midline fascia. This is also true for the final closure. The avascular abdominal wall midline is easily disrupted.

4. Do you monitor intra-abdominal pressure? What technique do you use?
In fact, I rarely monitor intraabdominal pressure. When I do, I use a simple CVP water manometer connected to the Foley catheter.

5. What do you do if the silo separates from the fascia?
I treat the separated area with topical antibiotics and dressings until the OR is ready. I try to go to the OR in less than 24 hours. Usually, by the time separation has occurred, one can cover the defect with skin. I do not like to use a permanent fascial repair material such as Marlex mesh or Goretex, unless I can entirely cover it with skin. In my experience without skin coverage, infection and separation will occur. By that time, however, there will be a peel on the bowel and treatment with dressings will allow for epithelialization.

6. What do you do with a large defect that cannot be reduced?
While I have not tried this yet, I might very well use one of the body wall flap methods that have been described where one can leave the posterior fascia intact and swing the anterior fascia over the defect, perhaps even employing very lateral relaxing incisions. The back up plan for what to do when the prosthesis MUST come off for some reason and neither fascia nor skin will come together is to sew thick Alloderm to the fascia and try to bring skin over to cover the suture line. As I have noted, this is likely to extrude, but it will leave a thick capsule of granulation tissue that can be treated with any number of dressings until epithelialization and scar contracture have occurred. One can then wait another few months (TPN cholestasis allowing) and venture back into the abdomen.

7. What do you do if an atresia is identified during initial inspection of the gastroschisis? Are allografts useful?
If there is a significant peel, edema, and induration of the bowel, I put it back in the abdomen along with everything else and repair the abdomen with fascia, skin flaps, or a prosthesis. I have seen several patients who have had an "obvious atresia," just eat and go home without further intervention. If the atresia is real, I am happy to reoperate in 3 to 6 weeks when the abdominal wall is more normal and the bowel inflammation has reduced.

If the peel is minimal, and especially if the atresia is high and very dilated, I bring out the dilated proximal end as a stoma through normal abdominal wall. Thus, if a prosthesis is being used, this may need to be quite lateral.

If I see a testicle (or two), I just put it back in the abdomen. The few I have dealt with in this manner ended up in the scrotum without another operation.

8. What procedures would you recommend if the fascia cannot be approximated at the time of abdominal wall closure?
Skin coverage is my first choice, if it seems easy. If I do not think I will be able to get skin coverage, however, I will not dissect back to the vertebral spines and stretch and pull. I will just place a prosthesis. I like to save all the skin maneuvers for when the silo is removed.

13 | Complications of Intestinal and Vascular Access

Nicholas C. Saenz, M.D.

"Man cannot live by bread alone (1)."

Access for the administration of medicines as well as nutritional support is achieved using two main routes, the gastrointestinal tract and the bloodstream. Devices are required to access each of these systems and their placement is performed by those from many disciplines of medicine. Enteral and parenteral access in children is a particular challenge given the size of these patients as well as their dependence on others for the administration of care and the use of these devices. This care and use is often performed by parents and therefore these systems must be simple and straightforward. This chapter will explore the complications encountered in performing enteral and parenteral access procedures and attempt to list some of the pitfalls in order that these potentially life-threatening complications may be avoided.

INTESTINAL ACCESS

To determine the type of intestinal access warranted, many aspects of the patient must be considered. How long will the child need to be fed before oral feeds are possible? Is the child able to take any nutrition by mouth? Many central nervous system anomalies preclude the eventual ability to feed independently. Are the mouth and oropharynx patent and functional? Is the esophagus intact? Is there normal gastric capacity and is the stomach able to empty? Is there intestinal continuity? Is the peristaltic function of the small intestine normal? Is the colonic motility normal and is defecation possible? These questions help to determine the type of enteral access required, the duration of access, and therefore the complications encountered.

Nasoenteric Feedings

The duration of enteral feedings plays a major role in determining at which location the gastrointestinal tract is accessed. For short-term access, the nasoenteric route is the most common. While used more for aspiration of gastric contents, such as in the treatment of postoperative ileus, nasogastric "gavage" feeding route is very common in the neonatal nursery. Even these small-caliber tubes (which may be as smaller than spaghetti) are not without risk. Placement of a firmer tube guided too far posteriorly may result in perforation of the posterior oropharynx. This complication is well recognized in the very small premature infant (2). A high index of suspicion often leads to the establishment of this diagnosis. If any resistance is met during the placement of even the softest tube, either orally or nasally, repositioning must be done. Grasping the tube between the thumb and index finger for gentle placement assists in preventing excess force from being generated. Auscultation while instilling air through the tube may be misleading as a tube in the inferior mediastinum or pleural cavity may still sound as though it is in the correct position. Radiographic confirmation is often warranted, especially if placement has been difficult or if a perforation is suspected. Administration of a small amount of water-soluble contrast will confirm the placement and rule out any violation of esophageal mucosal integrity.

Immediate recognition of perforation is vital and a high index of suspicion should be present if placement was difficult. Prompt removal of the tube is necessary. Pneumomediastinum or pneumothorax may be demonstrated by plain radiography. Contrast study of the esophagus is useful, but may not always demonstrate a very small injury. Rigid esophagoscopy is a very useful technique. Continuous insufflation with 0.5 to 1.0L/min of air through the rigid telescope during endoscopy helps to show the details of the wall of the esophagus.

If the hypopharngeal or esophageal injury is minor, simple avoidance of oral or nasogastric feeds is done for 2 to 3 days, at which point clear liquids may be started. Broad-spectrum antibiotics are added. If the injury is severe, operative drainage of either the neck or mediastinum may be necessary, with placement of a gastrostomy for distal feedings. Repeat radiological study may be warranted prior to reintroduction of feeds.

Misplacement of the nasoenteric tube is a common problem. The correct position of the tube must always be documented prior to the institution of enteral feeds. Simple instillation of air during auscultation is most common. The most devastating location for misplacement is the tracheobronchial tree. If uncertainty exists, radiographic confirmation must be obtained. Passage of the tube through the pylorus has been thought to reduce the risk of aspiration. There is a lack of conclusive data to support the placement of all nasoenteric feeding tubes in a postpyloric position.

Epistaxis and sinusitis are also complications of nasoenteric tube feedings. Nasoenteric feedings have been shown to increase the risk of nosocomial sinusitis (3). A syndrome described as the "nasogastric tube syndrome" has been described. This sudden bilateral vocal cord paralysis is thought to result from paresis of the posterior cricoarytenoid muscles secondary to ulceration and infection over the posterior lamina of the cricoid. Prompt investigation with esophagoscopy should be performed if hoarseness or evolving stidor occurs (4).

Gastrostomy

Gastrostomy placement is a very common and useful procedure that is now performed by physicians from many different specialties. Interventional radiologists, gastroenterologists, and surgeons are all consulted for intestinal access. The type of tube placed and the method of placement depend on the clinical scenario encountered.

Percutaneous endoscopic gastrostromy (PEG) has gained favor for patients requiring only enteral access without any history of gastroesophageal reflux. Contraindications include situations in which the stomach may not be placed in adequate apposition to the abdominal wall. Previous abdominal operations, esophageal abnormalities precluding upper endoscopy, and bleeding disorders also preclude PEG placement.

There are a variety of complications related to PEG. Complications of placement are often related to the inappropriate choice of attempting to pursue PEG as the method of enteral access. Injury to the esophagus as the button is "pulled" is possible if the esophageal lumen is too small. Either this complication is immediately recognized and addressed or may present late as an esophageal leak with mediastinitis. If the injury is very small, a period of rest with intravenous antibiotics may suffice. If the injury is larger, effective drainage of the mediastinum with tube thoracostomy and broad-spectrum antibiotics is adequate therapy. If the injury is substantial, open thoracotomy, primary repair of the injury, and effective drainage may be warranted. Long-term sequelae of such a complication may include esophageal stricture necessitating repeated dilations.

Improper placement of the gastrostomy on the stomach may occur. Locations too close to the pylorus may result in the inability of the stomach to act as an adequate reservoir and result in dumping. During placement of the gastrostomy, one must be assured that the stomach is directly opposed to the abdominal wall in order for the intracath to be placed. If intestine (large or small) is interposed between the stomach and the abdominal wall, the intracath and therefore the gastrostomy may pass directly through the intestine resulting in leakage or fistula formation. Other problems of apposition to the abdominal wall may result in the stomach not sufficiently adhered to the abdominal wall which may result in tube feedings directly into the peritoneum.

Open surgical gastrostomy is still a common procedure, particularly in the pediatric population. Failure to thrive is a common diagnosis resulting from a wide range of clinical problems including feeding aversion, severe neurological impairment, or respiratory embarrassment during feedings secondary to congenital heart disease. Pediatric surgeons are frequently consulted for enteral access and it is important to determine the best approach to the stomach. When considering this, the patients overall status must be reviewed carefully. In the pediatric population, the patient's neurological status may be compromised and the ability to protect from gastroesophageal reflux and aspiration may be diminished. In this scenario, fundoplication in addition to gastrostomy is warranted. The debate of laparoscopic fundoplication versus open fundoplication is beyond the scope of this chapter.

Stamm gastrostomy remains a reliable modality for achieving enteral access and provides the parents a relatively easy tube to use and replace as necessary. As with most complications in surgery, complications of open gastrostomy may often be traced to the initial operation. Inadequate purse-string sutures, inadequate "dunking" of the gastrostomy site resulting in poor tract formation, and inadequate tacking of the stomach up to the abdominal wall, are all complications which may result in the leaking of feeds into the peritoneal cavity. These are all preventable complications. Two purse sting sutures may be used at the site on the greater curvature chosen. The first of these is placed in a four quadrant box fashion. This affixes the tube to the stomach. The second purse string suture is placed wide in a true "purse string" fashion. This is the key suture that creates the tract as described by Stamm. Once tied, these sutures may be left long and used to attach the stomach to the abdominal wall. Additional suture(s) are also used to attach the stomach to the abdominal wall as necessary. Inadequate suturing of the stomach to the abdominal wall may result in the stomach "falling" off of the abdominal wall. The tract will fail to form thus making it impossible to change tubes easily. Failure to place the tacking sutures close enough to the tube may result in the formation of a puddle of feeds just below the peritoneal surface in a pocket resulting in eventual leakage.

Stamm gastrostomy provides parents and caretakers an easy and reliable tube which may be changed at home. Tube dislodgement is a common problem. Should the tube become dislodged within the first month, parents are asked to return immediately for tube replacement by the surgeon. An attempt to replace the tube immediately is performed and saline is then run in under gravity. Usually if the tube becomes dislodged early after placement, confirmation by contrast study is warranted. If the tube has been out for a significant amount of time, the tract may close. Parents of our patients are given a red rubber catheter to place immediately upon recognition that the tube has become dislodged. They may also place the same tube directly back in and tape it down until the child may be seen. Finally, if the tract has completely closed, the patient is taken to the operating room and while under anesthesia, the tract is sequentially dilated with Hagar dilators until a satisfactory tube may be placed. We have abandoned the initial placement of a Malecot mushroom-tipped catheter. Our practice was to place this type of tube at the time of operation and change to a lower profile tube after the tract had matured. Our practice now is to place a Mic-Key (Kimberly Clark/Ballard Medical Products) as the initial tube and provide the parents additional tubes of the same size. Eventually most parents become comfortable changing the tubes themselves and are able to avoid an emergency room visit.

Once gastrostomy tubes are no longer needed, they may be removed. With Mic-Key buttons, this is easily accomplished in an office setting by simply deflating the ballooning and removing the button. Approximately 95% of these stoma sites will close spontaneously. This leaves the 5% in whom the stoma site becomes a persistent gastrocutaneous fistula. We will give the site up to two months to close spontaneously, even with the augmentation of closing with applications of silver nitrate. Should all nonoperative means be exhausted, formal closure of the gastrocutaneous fistula is performed. This may be done as an outpatient procedure. Successful treatment of a gastrocutaneous fistula requires dissection of the stomach off of the abdominal wall, formal closure of the gastrostomy in two layers, followed by a layered closure of the abdominal wall. Patients are allowed to take liquids initially and advance to a regular diet the following day.

Jejunostomy

As with gastrostomy tubes, jejunostomy tubes are also placed by those from many disciplines. Surgeons and radiologists are by far the most common physicians involved in placing these tubes. Jejunostomy tubes are used in patients where gastrostomy may be precluded or con-traindicated. These situations may include gastroparesis, gastric outlet obstruction, postoperative feeding, neurological dysfunction, and gastroesophageal reflux. It has been my practice to primarily use gastrostomy tubes over other methods of access for long-term enteral access. It is mainly due to the complications associated with jejunal tubes and the relative ease of the use of gastrostomy tubes that this approach has been adopted. Studies aimed at demonstrating the frequency and types of complications associated with jejunostomy have been well documented. Carucci and colleagues showed a 14% incidence of one or more complications associated with jejunostomy tubes. These included small bowel obstruction, bowel narrowing, extraluminal tracks or collections, extravasation, and jejunal hematoma. Mechanical problems were reported in 19% of patients and included coiling, kinking and knotting, malpositioning, retrograde flow, and occlusion.

Needle catheter tube complications have been reported at a lower rate. Myers reported a 16-year period with over 2000 catheters with an overall complication rate of 1.5%. Complications encountered were similar to those seen with an open technique (5,6).

The process of troubleshooting jejunostomy problems is more complicated than with gastrostomy. These issues usually require a visit to either a physician's office or the hospital for replacement of the tube, which may involve a radiology procedure, performed using fluoroscopy.

VASCULAR ACCESS

Achieving secure vascular access in neonates, infants, and children is challenging and may be gratifying or frustrating. Dealing with the complications of securing vascular access may only intensify the above. Almost every hospitalized pediatric patient will require some form of venous access, and many of these patients will require central venous access. This central venous access will be required either short term or long term. The complications associated with the placement of these catheters and implantable central venous access devices (CVADs) are numerous and may be divided into 1) complications of placement; 2) complications during the period of use; and 3) complications of removal. This section of this chapter focuses mainly on the use of silastic implantable catheters. These are divided into two groups, 1) tunneled catheters with a cuff (Hickman or Broviac) and 2) subcutaneous reservoirs placed into a surgically created subcutaneous pocket (portacath/mediport or Port). Due to the scope of this chapter, venous access using intraosseous and percutaneously placed, nontunneled catheters will not specifically be addressed. Additionally, complications of arterial access will not be discussed.

Complications of Placement

The recent use of percutaneous intravenous central catheters (PICCs) has obviated the need for surgical placement of central venous catheters in many neonatal settings and warrants brief mention. Complications of placement of PICC are twofold, one of which bears close resemblance to insertion of peripheral venous catheterization, which is hematoma formation. The other main complication of PICC is malpositioning of the catheter. This has even resulted in the classifications of PICC to be either deep PICC or high/arm PICC. High positioning of the catheter results in the inability to use higher dextrose solutions. Malpositioning of the catheter as determined by postprocedure radiographs is said to be as high as 13%. Additionally, these malpositioned catheters have a higher rate of complication (7).

Placement of CVAD in the pediatric population is a procedure that has also crossed over into many specialties. These include surgeons, intensivists, anesthesiologists, and interventional radiologists. Risk of complication during placement is a function of device type, vein chosen for insertion, method of insertion, and level of expertise of those performing the procedure. The most common access sites to the central venous system in the neonatal and pediatric population includes but are not limited to the facial vein, external and internal jugular veins, subclavian vein, saphenofemoral junction, and the common femoral vein. Other less common sites include the gonadal veins, intercostal veins, azygous and hemiazygous veins, and direct access to the right atrium. Those veins in and around the neck are best performed using a cut-down technique in a sterile operating environment under general anesthesia. Cut-down procedures on the facial, external, and internal jugular veins are required for placement of silastic catheters into the right heart. Injury to the vein being used may result in the need to ligate that vein and proceed to approach other nearby veins. A common example occurs with the inability to cannulate the facial vein or external jugular vein results in the need to access the internal jugular vein. Ligation of the internal jugular vein must be avoided at all costs and a purse string suture is recommended. Injury to nearby structures in the very small patient is among the pitfalls of such a procedure. In the instances in which the internal jugular vein is used, the carotid artery, vagus nerve, trachea, esophagus, and thyroid are all vulnerable structures within the field of dissection. If one "wanders off course" in the dissection, what may result is an injury to any of these structures. Injury to these structures may be avoided by proper illumination and magnification. Loupe magnification and high-intensity headlights are extremely useful when dissecting in the neck through a small incision.

Catheter malpositioning is rare when either the facial vein or the internal jugular vein is used; however, anatomic anomalies must be considered, especially in the pediatric cardiac patient. The rate of catheter tip malpositioning increases with the use of the external jugular vein. Inability to maneuver the catheter tip into the right atrium is higher when using the left external jugular vein because of a more tortuous course to the right heart. For this reason, when cut-down is performed it is recommended that the right neck be chosen when possible as a first choice.

Percutaneous approach using the subclavian in children has gained popularity and has been shown to be safe and effective (8). A large multi-institution study demonstrated a trend among pediatric surgeons to use the percutaneous (subclavian) approach as the patients became older (9). There were minimal approaches using the subclavian vein in those patients under the age of one; however, this approach is safe in even the neonatal population. Size cutoff for percutaneous approach is operator-dependent and should be based on the level of expertise and the frequency with which it is performed. Acute complications arising from the subclavian approach are many. These include arterial puncture, hemothorax, pneumothorax, chylothorax, hemopericardium, air embolism, phrenic nerve injury, brachial plexus injury, tracheal injury, cardiac arrhythmia, and catheter malposition.

Arterial puncture is frequent and may usually be treated easily. Immediate recognition, withdrawal of the needle (or wire, if it has been passed), and direct pressure on the site usually are sufficient maneuvers and often will allow that particular side to be used. When accessing the subclavian vein, confirmation of wire position by fluoroscopy is required. The presence of premature atrial contractions is an early clue to intracardiac placement of the wire. Demonstration of the wire in the right heart is necessary prior to dilation of the tract. When it is unclear as to the position of the wire, as may happen when anatomic anomalies are encountered, a small angiocath may be passed over the wire and the pressure may be transduced. This is sometimes helpful in babies with congenital heart disease in which low arterial oxygen saturations are seen. Finally, a small amount of intravenous contrast may be used to delineate the anatomy. Positioning of the wire within the subclavian vein must be demonstrated prior to dilation of the vessel. Dilation of the subclavian artery with eventual recognition that the catheter is an arterial position as opposed to a venous location may result in significant injury to the vessel requiring operative repair. The subclavian vessels are more difficult to tamponade with digital pressure and hemothorax may result from either arterial or venous lacerations.

Dilation of the tract must also be done carefully, especially with the stiff dilators found in most CVAD insertion kits. Dilation should be directly observed using fluoroscopy to insure avoidance of passing out of the vein. This may occur when the wire is kinked and the dilator "catches" the kink and bends the wire, allowing the tip to pass out of the vein. In a more catastrophic scenario, the dilator may be passed too far laterally and exit the lateral aspect of the superior vena cava or superior vena cava/right atrial junction and result in communication with the pericardium. The patient may then bleed out of the injury site into the pericardium resulting in hemopericardium. This complication can be avoided by watching the passage of the dilator under fluoroscopy and not letting it pass across the midline. In small infants, the caliber of the catheter is very small and may pass out of the venous defect, thereby providing tamponade to the defect. Because the course of the catheter may lie parallel to the superior vena cava/right atrial junction, this may be "missed" and fluids may be administered using the catheter resulting in cardiac tamponade.

Less serious but often most frustrating is the malpositioned catheter. Strict attention to the wire position, and the use of wires of sufficient length to reach the right atrium, assists in avoidance of malpositioning. One study has shown a higher incidence of passage of the catheter incorrectly into the jugular vein to have a fourfold increase in incidence when using the right subclavian versus the left (10). Two main reasons for use of the left subclavian over the right subclavian exist. The first is anatomic and the second is operator-dependent. The left subclavian vein passes into the innominate vein and then on to the superior vena cava/right atrial junction with a smoother, less angulated course when compared to the right. The right subclavian vein "turns" into the superior vena cava more sharply. In the event of the wire passing either into the jugular vein or into the contralateral subclavian, placement of a small angiocath over the wire without formal dilation of the vein allows for access to the subclavian to be maintained while the wire is manipulated under direct vision using fluoroscopy as it is passed into the right heart. The operator-dependent issues relate to whether the surgeon is right-hand dominant or left-hand dominant. For the more common right-hand dominant surgeon, access to the left subclavian vein allows a natural position standing on the patient's left side with the syringe in the operator's right hand. To orient the direction of the needle appropriately for approach to the right subclavian vein, the angle that the needle must be held in is less "natural" and the operator's wrist requires an unnatural position. Maximum comfort while performing these procedures is as important as exposure and lighting.

Brief mention of cardiac arrhythmias must be made in that passage of the wire into the right atrium may often result in harmless premature apical contractions. Premature ventricular contractions occur more frequently when the wire is passed through the tricuspid valve. These are usually not serious and resolve upon withdrawal of the wire. All patients must be monitored during placement. Communication between anesthesiologist and surgeon is crucial during these procedures. When passing the wire while observing the monitor, particular attention by the surgeon should be made listening to the monitor and the anesthesiologist. Additionally, the control of the wire should never be lost within the lumen of the needle or dilator. This will prevent loss of the wire into the central venous system and the need for removal by an interventional radiologist or cardiologist. After successful placement of the wire through the needle, the wire should not be "snapped" on to the drapes as this may fracture the wire and lead to it unraveling. Chylothorax, vagus nerve injury, and tracheal injury all result from errant passes with the needle and are avoidable. These complications usually occur due to passing the needle too deeply. Based on the size of pediatric patients, it is extremely rare that the entire needle be passed to access the vein, except in the morbidly obese patient.

The most frequently discussed complication of the subclavian approach is pneumothorax. This complication usually occurs with frequencies less than 5% and in a Children's Cancer Study Group (CCSG) study not a single pneumothorax was reported (11). A learning curve has clearly been demonstrated using this technique. Attention to technique with particular attention to the relatively medial position of the subclavian vein in the smaller patient may help to avoid the pitfall of arterial puncture. Orientation of the needle with respect to the patient is critical in avoiding the pleura. The needle must be kept parallel to the anterior chest wall avoiding angulation of the needle toward the spine. Avoidance of the pleural space may be enhanced by removing the patient from positive pressure ventilator support during advancement of the needle. Proper positioning with a vertical roll between the scapulae displacing the shoulders posteriorly helps to "expose" the vein. Patients should be adequately hydrated and placed into Trendelenberg position to avoid attempts at cannulation of a collapsed vein. On a practical (yet superstitious) note, when approaching the subclavian vein, the contralateral side of the chest and bilateral necks should be adequately prepped. This allows for those sites to be accessed should the initial approach be unsuccessful. It is the cavalier and inappropriately overconfident surgeon that prepares only one vein for insertion. There is no such thing as "just a Broviac."

Complications During the "Life" of the Line

As previously mentioned, nonthreatening arrhythmias are commonly encountered during placement of a CVAD. Should arrhythmias persist after catheter placement, tip position should be confirmed using plain radiography. Final tip position is still controversial. The advantage of a "high-lying" tip is the avoidance of arrhythmias and some feel that the incidence of clot in the right atrium is lower. A tip in a higher location, however, is more prone to lie against the wall of the vena cava and when attempts are made at aspiration, the catheter tip may aspirate the wall of the lumen and temporarily occlude the lumen precluding aspiration. Catheters in this position will still flow, however. A catheter with a "high" tip originating in the innominate vein is also more prone to migrate either out into the right subclavian or flip up into the right jugular vein. Because of the relatively low incidence of problems when the tip of the catheter is just into the atrium, it is the preferred placement.

One of Broviac's contributions to catheter design was the cuff that was molded around the catheter (12). This cuff is meant to provide a surface area for adherence into the tract within the chest wall. Dislodgment of this cuff so that it has moved distance enough to translate into tip movement may be significant. Additionally, if the cuff becomes visible, the catheter is technically contaminated and therefore replacement is warranted if the catheter is to remain. The new catheter may be brought out of the same exit site. When catheters are initially placed, sutures are used to anchor the line while the cuff becomes adherent into to the subcutaneous tissue. When these sutures eventually erode through the skin level, they are usually not removed from around the catheter as one errant swipe with the scissors or blade may result in a hole in the catheter resulting in repair or necessitating complete replacement.

Infectious complications of indwelling ports as well as external devices are a controversial topic. Literature citing either a difference in infection rates or no difference in infections rates between the two types of devices is available (13,14). Institutional biases and physician preference end up dictating the type of line used many institutions. Additionally, the care and maintenance of these devices vary from institution to institution. In general, a healthy suspicion of the line as the source in any patient's sepsis evaluation is warranted. This is regardless of placement technique, device type, anatomic location, or line management algorithm. Treatment with empiric antibiotics until culture information is available is begun followed by organism-specific treatment. Fungal isolates and coagulase-negative staphylococci usually warrant early removal, with subsequent replacement only after an adequate course of therapy has been administered.

Failure of a line to flow or aspirate warrants an algorithmic approach beginning with checking the position of the tip of the catheter on chest radiograph. If tip position is satisfactory, a dye study of the line under fluoroscopy is performed. This will identify whether a distal thrombus is present and whether attempt at lytic therapy is warranted versus line removal and replacement. Occlusion of the catheter with thrombus was performed with urokinase until its production was discontinued. Recombinant tissue plasminogen activator (t-PA) is now frequently used with great success in re-establishing patency of occluded lines. Newer forms of t-PA have become available which have been reported to increase thrombus penetration allowing fibrinolysis to occur throughout the thrombus (15,16).

Complications During Line Removal

Device removal is performed as frequently as device placement and therefore complications occur as well. Removal is performed because of infection, nonfunction or malpositioning of the tip, or termination of therapy. This procedure is performed in many different areas, ranging from the operating room under general anesthesia to the bedside in the intensive care unit. Most agree that since port removal requires formal closure of the pocket, this procedure is best performed in the operating room. Removal of an externalized catheter usually goes smoothly if enough soft-tissue dissection is performed to free the cuff from the chest wall. Some prefer to cut down directly on the cuff rather that to dissect it free using blunt dissection. Some insist on cuff removal at all costs while others are less stringent that the cuff need be removed. Difficulty with cuff removal may warrant cutting down to it rather that risk catheter fracture. Early recognition of possible "sticking sites" and proper surgical exposure of those sites will result in safe removal of an intact catheter rather than loss of the catheter into the central venous system, often all the way to the heart. If, however, this does occur, catheter fragment removal if may be performed using a percutaneous approach in the cardiac catheterization laboratory by the interventional cardiologist. It is best performed there, rather than in the radiology department, as arrhythmias may arise while the catheter is being removed.

In summary, the size of our patients, the number of patients undergoing multiple procedures, and the many hazards possible, require the adoption of mind-set that these procedures are never routine. It is when one has become "too comfortable" doing these procedures that the "line that would not end" usually occurs, reminding us of our humility.

REFERENCES

1. Deuteronomy 8: 2–3. The phrase "Man doth not live by bread only" is one of many from the Torah that Jesus quotes in the New Testament, though he changes "does" to "shall" and "only" to "alone" (Matthew 4: 4 and Luke 4: 4). Thus the familiar "man does not live by bread alone" is a hybrid of two versions.
2. Sapin E, Gumpert L, Bonnard A, et al. Iatrogenic pharyngoesophageal perforation in premature infants. Eur J Pediatr Surg 2000; 10:83–87.
3. Desmond P, Raman R, Idikula J. Effects of nasogastric tubes on the nose and maxillary sinus. Crit Care Med 1991; 19(4):509–511.

4. Sofferman RA, Haisch CE, Kirchner JA, et al. The nasogastric tube syndrome. Laryngoscope 1990; 100(9):962–968.
5. Myers JG, Page CP, Stewart RM, et al. Complications of needle catheter jejunostomy in 2,022 consecutive applications. Am J Surg 1995; 170:547–550.
6. Carucci LR, Levine MS, Rebesin SE, et al. Evaluation of patients with jejunostomy tubes: Imaging findings. Radiology 2002; 223(1):241–247.
7. Racadio JM, Doellman DA, Johnson ND, et al. Pediatric peripherally inserted central catheters: Complication rates related to catheter tip location. Pediatrics 2001; 107:E28.
8. Newman BM, Jewett TC Jr, Karp MC. Percutaneous central venous catheterization in children: First line of choice for venous access. J Pediatr Surg 1986; 21:685–688.
9. Wiener ES, McGuire P, Stolar CJ, et al. The CCSG prospective study of venous access devices: an analysis of insertions and causes for removal. J Pediatr Surg 1992; 27:155–163; discussion 163–164.
10. Unal AE, Bayar S, Arat M, et al. Malpositioning of Hickman catheters, left versus right sided attempts. Transfus Apheresis Sci 2003; 28:9–12.
11. Mirro J, Jr., Rao BN, Kumar M, et al. A comparison of placement techniques and complications of externalized catheters and implantable port use in children with cancer. J Pediatr Surg 1990; 25:120–124.
12. Broviac J, Cole B, Scribner B. A modified right atrial catheter for access to the venous system in marrow transplant recipients. Surg Gyn Obst 1979; 148:871–875.
13. LaQuaglia MP, Lucas, A, Thaler HT, et al. A prospective analysis of vascular access device-related infections in children. J Pediatr Surg 1992; 27:840–842.
14. Sariego J, Bootorabi B, Matsumoto T, et al. Major long-term complications in 1,422 permanent venous access devices. Am J Surg 1993; 165:249–251.
15. Noble S, McTavish D. Reteplase: a review of its pharmacological properties and clinical efficacy in the management of acute myocardial infarction. Drugs 1996; 52:589–605.
16. Terril KR, Lemons RS, Goldsby RE. Safety, does, and timing of reteplase in treating occluded central venous catheters in children with cancer. J Pediatr Hematolo Oncol 2003; 25:864–867.

Broviac and Mediport Placement

Expert: Charles E. Bagwell, M.D.

QUESTIONS

1. **What steps do you take intraoperatively to prevent infection?**
    Infectious and septic complications of central venous catheter placement are of grave concern; accordingly prevention of these complications is paramount. Preparation of both the patient and the surgical team must be meticulous with care to assure that responsible individuals do not "cut corners" on hand scrub or patient prep techniques, including draping to avoid hair exposure or "corners" at drape margins to become exposed. Those patients who are immunocompromised on the basis of weight loss, chronic illness, or neoplasm should receive preoperative and postoperative antibiotics, and others may be considered on a case by cases basis. In the course of catheter insertion, all attempts should be made to see that the catheter itself is not allowed to lie in on the patient's skin for lengthy periods of time to minimize the possibility of colonization from *Staphlococcus epidermis.*

2. **What approach do you take for catheter placement in a patient with thrombocytopenia?**
    Many patients with neoplasms, especially leukemias, may have platelet counts which require preoperative platelet transfusion. The platelet count should exceed 50,000 for any surgical approach and double that if a percutaneous technique is to be employed. If persistent thrombocytopenia is an issue and correction is difficult, access is preferable by a cut-down technique on a more superficial vein (such as the external jugular) to minimize hemorrhagic risks from percutaneous subclavian or internal jugular access approaches.

3. **What technical strategies do you apply to avoid the creation of a pneumothorax during subclavian puncture?**
    Most studies indicate a roughly 1% incidence of pneumothorax from subclavian puncture, although this is clearly dependent on operator experience. To minimize risk of pneumothorax, technique for percutaneous access of the subclavian vein should direct the needle at

a relatively parallel position to the skin below the clavicle and gently advance it to "walk under" the bone rather than orienting the needle at a more perpendicular angle relative to the skin surface. If possible, the patient should be breathing spontaneously to decrease the lung volume at the time of needle stick. As the process of venous access can be both frustrating and irritating for any operator, no more than three needle passes should be performed by any member of the surgical team; if the vein is not accessed by the third try, the procedure should be passed on to a more senior member of the team. Fluoroscopy used in the operating theater to check position of the guidewire and final central line tip placement should also include examination of both lung apices for pneumothorax. In addition, a film should also be obtained in the recovery room area, not only to document catheter tip position, but also to detect delayed pneumothorax. This allows placement of a chest tube before complications develop later in a less monitored setting.

4. **Where is the Dacron cuff located to help prevent Broviac catheter dislodgement?**
Selection of the appropriate catheter size and cuff configuration (one or two cuff types) should be a prime consideration by the surgical team prior to the operation itself. Central lines needed for a relatively limited time (i.e., for vascular access in the perioperative and immediate postoperative period) may be located with the Dacron cuff just outside the skin, sutured in place to prevent dislodgement but to allow easy removal at the bedside prior to discharge from hospital. Those catheters needed for a longer time for patients undergoing long-term chemotherapy or intravenous feedings (for short-gut or other conditions) should have the Dacron cuff well within the subcutaneous tissues, but close enough to the exit site that removal can be accomplished through the exit site without the need for multiple counter-incisions and lengthy periods of dissection.

5. **How soon can a Mediport catheter be accessed following placement in a patient with hemophilia?**
Most such ports can be used immediately after placement, since patients with hemophilia will have their factor-VIII levels optimized at the time of operation and for the immediate postoperative period of 24 to 48 hours. It is easier in most pediatric patients for access of the port to be accomplished in the operating theater once the port is appropriately positioned, the wound closed and the patient still asleep under an anesthetic. Once the patient's postoperative factor administrations are complete and discharge is imminent, the port can be flushed with heparin and the needle removed prior to discharge from hospital.

6. **What are the most common complications following Broviac placement?**
The most common complications of any central venous catheter placement are clearly related to catheter malfunction or malposition, although many of these are still salvage-able and can be used, as catheter tips may "flip up" into a subclavian position on one film yet return to central venous location on another. Catheters that are occluded can often be cleared with hemolytic preparations instilled through the catheter or port. Other common complications include catheter-related infections or dislodgement. Postopera-tive fevers or fevers in any patient with a central line or port in place should prompt surveillance cultures, both through the catheter and by peripheral venipuncture. If indi-cated, antibiotics should include vancomycin for coverage of MRSA and staph epidermis. Uncommon, though potentially serious complications, include pneumothorax (discussed above) and the rare, although potentially lethal complication of bleeding from hemoth-orax with catheter insertion. On a previous review of this subject (1), a number of such cases were documented by respondents to a survey on this topic, but the actual number is difficult to ascertain. This complication should be discussed preoperatively as part of the consent process with awareness of the family that such a complication may require urgent thoracotomy for control of bleeding, although the incidence of this occurring is extremely rare. It is clear that some such cases of venous injury with catheter insertion are related to a passage of a stiff dilator across the mediastinum, especially in younger, smaller pediatric patients. Accordingly, estimation of the length of dilator to be passed intravascularly should be made on the chest wall prior to insertion.

7. **What unusual complications have you seen following Broviac or Mediport placement?**
A host of somewhat uncommon complications have been reported from these catheters including reports from past years (1) of a large mural thrombus in a neonate patient requiring long-term hyperalimentation and a young trauma patient following exploration. Erosion through vessels or intrathoracic structures (including the heart) have been described, although these appear much more common with the stiffer polyethylene catheters previously used than the currently utilized soft silastic catheters.

8. **Do you secure the port to the fascia with absorbable or nonabsorbable suture?**
Ports should be secured to the fascia of the underlying pectoralis major to prevent flipping or twisting in the subcutaneous pocket as well as to make them repeatedly accessible by percutaneous puncture. There are cases where the central line catheter has been seen to "wind up" and the tip no longer be central in location if the port becomes twisted in its pocket. Fixation can best be accomplished with a nonabsorbable suture by tacking opposite sides of the port in at least two places.

9. **At what points in the operation do you use fluoroscopy?**
Fluoroscopy should be available in the operating theater at *anytime* during the procedure when it is deemed necessary or the patient's stability is in question. This may include attempts to needle access the vein, pass the catheter itself, or with passage of dilator and/or sheath or the catheter in its final location. The surgeon should have no hesitation to bring the fluoroscopic unit over the surgical field at anytime he or she feels additional information regarding the catheter guidewire or chest anatomy needs further assessment. Obviously, lead shielding of the operating surgical team is necessary—sometimes for protracted periods if the access procedure is unduly difficult. Development of an arrhythmia during passage of the guidewire usually is a result of venous cannulation and advancement into the heart and will respond to withdrawal of the guidewire under fluoroscopy. One should fluoroscope the patient routinely to document venous placement of the guidewire and, if the procedure is uneventful, for final placement of the central venous catheter, but have little hesitation to do so anytime during the procedure if questions arise.

10. **What is your approach to the patient with and indwelling central venous line and positive blood cultures? Does the organism affect your decision to remove the line versus attempted antibiotic sterilization?**
Most patients with infected Broviac catheters can have these cleared with appropriate antibiotics. One exception to this is a positive culture with Candida, in which case the line should be removed. The patient should be treated with antifungal antibiotics through a peripheral IV site and replacement of the central venous catheter postponed for five to seven days to allow clearing of the fungemia.

11. **What surgical approach should be undertaken in the event of intraoperative hypotension with suspected venous injury after placement of a subclavian line?**
In such cases immediate fluoroscopy should be obtained to look for evidence of tension pneumothorax, widened mediastinum or hemothorax, and locate the affected side relative to the site of surgical approach by percutaneous puncture. If pneumothorax or hemothorax is identified, chest tube placement should be expediently performed. If significant blood is obtained through the tube thoracostomy, urgent resuscitative maneuvers should be undertaken with prompt thoracotomy of the affected hemithorax-remembering that the site of venous perforation may occur in either chest cavity even if the subclavian access is initially attempted through the preferred left side. A surgical dictum that "if somethings wrong, somethings wrong" should always be kept in mind, rather than discount hypotension as due to other, nonsurgical causes. The same should be said for these patients in the postoperative period, whether in the recovery area or on the floor. Any evidence of vascular instability or respiratory compromise with a central line in place mandates assessment for potential line-related complications, including a chest x-ray to rule out the conditions described above.

12. **Is there a weight below which a percutaneous subclavian approach should not be attempted?**
As noted in earlier responses, the key risk of central venous access by percutaneous route in a small child is clearly vascular injury especially with a stiff dilator, which in a small child only allows minimum passage before potentially abutting the innominate vein or vena cava. Accordingly, I prefer to approach venous access in the child less than 2 years (or 12 kg) usually by a cut-down technique, although others are more comfortable with percutaneous access routes, even in small infants and neonates.

REFERENCE

1. Bagwell CE, Sonnino RE, Haynes JH. Potentially lethal complications of central venous catheter placement. J Pediatr Surg 2000; 35(5):709–713.

Intestinal Stoma Formation

Expert: Sigmund H. Ein, M.D.

QUESTIONS

1. **How should the bowel be attached to the fascia/muscle to prevent prolapse?**
I'm not sure that attaching the bowel to the fascia/muscle really prevents prolapse, so I never did it. I do have a concern that suturing the bowel to the fascia/muscle runs the risk of creating a side fistula in the stoma, which is as much trouble as a prolapse.

2. **What are the contributing factors leading to stomal prolapse?**
No one that I have ever spoken to really knows the correct answer. Why does it most often happen to the distal limb of a loop stoma producing a retrograde prolapse? That must be the greatest contributing factor. The next commonest cause for prolapse has to be too wide a fascial opening for the stoma.

3. **What technical steps help avoid stomal prolapse?**
I believe that snugging up the hole through which the bowel comes does help prevent prolapse somewhat. A good rule of thumb for the hole to be snug enough to minimize the risk of a prolapse (and yet not obstruct the stoma) is for the stoma to be plum-colored at its completion. For some strange reason most stomal prolapses are retrograde from the distal loop. I found out early in my career, that a loop stoma nearly always prolapsed the longer you left it in place, and an almost foolproof way to prevent that was to divide the two stomas and bring them both out separate openings in the abdominal wall. An excellent (and easier) alternative is to bring out the usual loop stoma, and after closing the fascia, divide the loop and tunnel the distal stoma an inch or so away from the proximal stoma, so that each stoma comes out a different skin (only) opening (above the fascia). One can minimize an ileostomy from prolapsing by suturing (from within the abdomen) the serosa of the stoma to the peritoneum, and also suturing the terminal ileal mesentery to the peritoneal undersurface of the abdominal wall.

4. **Does bringing the stoma through the wound result in more complications?**
Yes. That has been the teaching and it seems to be true. Unless there is some technical reason why a stoma cannot be placed somewhere else, it probably should not be brought out through the wound. I think it's a good idea to keep intestinal contents as far away from any wound as possible to avoid the risk of wound infection, dehiscence ± evisceration, and ventral hernia.

5. **What special considerations should be applied to stoma formation in premature infants?**
   When it comes to making any kind of a stoma in a premature infant or the like, I was always happy to just get a viable piece of bowel up to the abdominal wall without any kind of fixation except to the skin (a so-called poststoma). Most of these newborn or infant stomas are temporary (weeks/months), so that whatever prolapse does occur can be tolerated and managed for a short while.

6. **In a temporary sigmoid colostomy, do you favor the use of a loop or divided ostomy?**
   I don't think it makes any difference; it really depends upon how long it's going to be there. If it is short term, temporary, a loop is sufficient. If it is long term, a loop, divided and tunneled colostomy has less risk of prolapse, which is the commonest complication (see Questions 2 and 3).

14 | Complications of Esophageal Surgery

Michael G. Caty, M.D., Stanley T. Lau, M.D., and Mauricio A. Escobar, M.D.

INTRODUCTION

Surgical management of diseases of the esophagus can be challenging for the pediatric surgeon. Successful management of esophageal problems requires knowledge of cervical, thoracic, and abdominal anatomy. In addition, the surgeon must be aware of functional abnormalities of the esophagus and stomach. Knowledge of potential complications due to technical problems and associated anomalies will allow the pediatric surgeon to anticipate and avoid these problems. In the following chapter, complications related to the treatment of esophageal atresia (EA), gastroesophageal reflux disease (GERD), and esophageal replacement will be presented.

ESOPHAGEAL ATRESIA

Introduction

The repair of esophageal atresia has been described as "the epitome of modern surgery" (1). While the first recorded case of EA was in 1670 by Durston, Thomas Gibson documented the first classic description of a child with EA with distal fistula in 1697 (2). In 1936, Thomas Lanman performed the first primary extrapleural anastomosis of this anomaly, but the child lived only 3 hours (3). Leven and Ladd reported the first staged survivors in 1939 (4,5), and Cameron Haight performed the first successful primary anastomosis in 1941 (6). Haight's original technique involved an extrapleural dissection with fistula division and a two-layer "telescoping" end-to-end esophageal anastomosis.

Epidemiology

Esophageal atresia with varying types of tracheoesophageal fistula (TEF) affects approximately 1:2400 to 1:3000 neonates (6,7). Associated chromosomal abnormalities include trisomy 13 and 18 (8). The majority of infants with EA have at least one associated congenital malformation. Cardiovascular anomalies account for approximately 35% of associated defects in patients with EA (9), and the majority of deaths associated with EA (10–12). A right-sided aortic arch is found in 5% of neonates with EA (13), and its presence may dictate the need for a left-sided thoracotomy in the operative approach to the EA repair (13–15). Common gastrointestinal anomalies associated with EA include anorectal malformations, duodenal atresia, and intestinal malrotation (11). Interestingly, many malformations may be clustered in the neonate as the VACTERL-H association, which includes vertebral, anorectal, cardiac, renal, limb abnormalities, and occasionally congenital hydrocephalus (16,17).

Esophageal atresia may be associated with a variety of syndromes, including Down's syndrome (11) and CHARGE syndrome (coloboma, heart defects, choanal atresia, developmental/growth delay, and ear anomalies with or without deafness) (18). Tracheomalacia is a commonly associated anomaly in patients with EA. Tracheomalacia results from a decreased ratio of circumferential cartilaginous trachea to membranous trachea (19). Clinical manifestations of tracheomalacia are noted below. A variety of lethal tracheobronchial abnormalities have been reported in association with EA, including tracheal agenesis, laryngeal atresia, congenital tracheal stenosis, and pulmonary agenesis. Other associated tracheobronchial malformations include ectopic bronchi such as tracheal bronchus and trifurcated trachea and absent right upper lobe bronchus. The observation of a trifurcated trachea in patients with EA supports current theories of its embryology.

Embryology

The most commonly accepted theory of the pathogenesis of EA is abnormal embryogenesis of the laryngotracheoesophageal groove and septum formation. Abnormal septation allows for persistent communication between the trachea and esophagus (20). Recently, Gittes and colleagues have demonstrated foregut trifurcation in Adriamycin-induced EA in Sprague-Dawley rats (7,21,22). Two of the tracheal branches formed lungs, and the third formed the TEF and distal "esophagus." It is interesting to note the identification of trifurcated tracheas in infants with EA (19) and the association of tracheobronchial remnants with EA (23).

Classifications

There are five basic types of EA ± TEF. The Gross classification is the most widely recognized (24). In order of prevalence, they are an EA with a distal TEF (86% incidence, Gross type C), EA without TEF (7%, Gross type A), TEF without EA ("H" type) (4%, Gross type E), EA with proximal and distal TEF (2%, Gross type D), and EA with a proximal TEF (1%, Gross type B) (2). In addition to anatomic classification, several risk stratifications have been utilized. The Waterston criteria stratified neonates based on birth weight, presence of pneumonia, and associated congenital anomalies (25). Spitz (26) noted that the two factors with the greatest impact on survival were very low birth weight (<1500 g) and major congenital cardiac malformations. Survival was grouped as follows: group I (birth weight >1500 g), 96%; group II (<1500 g *or* major congenital heart disease), 60%; group III (<1500 g *and* major congenital heart disease), 18% (2).

Diagnosis

Esophageal atresia should be suspected in neonates presented with feeding intolerance, choking, and respiratory distress. Diagnosis of EA is accomplished by carefully passing an oropharyngeal sump catheter until resistance is met. The tip of the catheter is identified in the proximal pouch on chest roentgenogram. Progressive abdominal distension and refluxed gastric contents resulting from a distal TEF may worsen the infant's pulmonary status. A "pouchogram" may demonstrate the upper esophageal pouch by injecting a few millimeters of air; alternatively, less than 1 mL of diluted barium or nonionic, water-soluble contrast may be injected under fluoroscopic guidance. A gasless abdomen on x-ray suggests an isolated EA without TEF (11). Prenatal ultrasonography is rarely accurate in diagnosing EA (18). Findings suggestive of EA include a small or absent stomach bubble in the presence of polyhydramnios (2).

Preoperative Management and Complications

Decompression of the upper pouch with a functioning sump catheter helps avoid aspiration from pooled secretions. Care must be taken to avoid perforating the proximal pouch. Mechanical ventilation should be avoided to prevent abdominal distension that further compromises the infant's respiratory status. Broad-spectrum antibiotics are started. Signs of VACTERL are sought on the physical examination, and a "midline workup" is initiated including echocardiography, renal ultrasonography, skeletal survey of extremities and the spinal column, and spinal ultrasonography if an anorectal malformation is detected.

Neonates with EA and distal TEF with severe respiratory distress pose a significant challenge in airway management. They are also at increased risk of gastric perforation as the stomach is insufflated through the TEF. Gastric perforation used to be universally fatal; however, survival after gastrointestinal perforation from EA has now been reported in low-birth weight infants (27). Techniques described to control the TEF in the infant with respiratory compromise include needle decompression of the stomach en route to the operating room, temporary occlusion of the gastroesophageal junction (28), placement of a gastrostomy tube to water seal, cannulating the fistula with a Fogarty catheter placed bronchoscopically (28), transgastric fistula occlusion, passage of a cuffed endotracheal tube distal to the fistula, and high-frequency jet ventilation (2,29). Spitz advocates emergency transpleural ligation of the fistula as the procedure of choice (2).

Operative Therapy

Preoperative Bronchoscopy

The operative approach to EA depends on the type of anomaly present and the occurrence of associated anomalies. Preoperative bronchoscopy is advocated by some pediatric surgeons to determine the level of the fistula (30), and hence the risk of a long gap EA and the presence of a proximal fistula. However, a proximal fistula may also be found with careful dissection of the upper pouch and may be missed by bronchoscopy. Preoperative bronchoscopy is by no means the standard of care, and most pediatric surgeons do not perform it routinely (31).

Esophageal Atresia with Distal Tracheoesophageal Fistula

Esophageal atresia with distal TEF is the classic presentation encountered by the pediatric surgeon. Division of the TEF and primary esophagoesophagostomy is the procedure of choice. Careful coordination with the anesthesia team is critical for optimal operative outcome. The anesthesiologist provides minimal ventilator support by allowing the infant to breathe spontaneously. This minimizes gastric insufflation through the TEF. The anesthesiologist and surgeon work in conjunction to provide the best exposure of the proximal pouch by placing a dilator or sump drain into the proximal pouch to provide gentle tension during the dissection. The operative approach is through a right posterolateral thoracotomy, unless a right-sided aortic arch is preoperatively diagnosed. This dictates a left-sided thoracotomy. Most pediatric surgeons prefer an extrapleural approach to avoid the possible complication of an empyema, but in the era of modern antibiotics, a transpleural approach is acceptable. For the extrapleural approach, the chest wall is dissected off the pleura by cotton swabs and gauze sponge-sticks in a lateral direction.

The azygous vein is identified and typically ligated as the fistula is usually posterior to the azygous arch. Some advocate the preservation of the azygous vein to maintain the normal venous drainage of the mediastinum (32,33). Small reports show a decrease in postoperative pneumonitis (33) and anastomotic leak (32) when the azygous vein is maintained. Kosloske advocates the preservation of the azygous to construct a flap to reinforce the esophageal anastomosis to prevent stricture and recurrent fistula (34).

The TEF is circumferentially dissected and controlled at the level of the trachea. Traction by a vessel loop or umbilical tape effectively seals gas flow and allows the anesthesiologist to sedate and paralyze the patient for the remainder of the operation. The majority of the infants in respiratory distress stabilize after this maneuver (2). The fistula is divided, leaving a 1 to 2 mm remnant of fistula on the trachea to hold suture for the closure. The fistula is closed with interrupted 5-0 or 6-0 silk, Ethibond, polyglycolic acid, or polypropylene suture. Polydioxanone (PDS) may also be used, but it has not been rigorously studied for outcomes. The closure is tested by positive pressure ventilation under saline.

The proximal pouch is then mobilized circumferentially to the level of the thoracic inlet. Great care is taken to minimize handling of this delicate tissue to prevent subsequent anastomotic leak and stricture. The anesthesiologist facilitates the mobilization by placing gentle pressure on the dilator or sump catheter to provide exposure. Additionally, a fine traction stitch may be placed at the apex of the proximal pouch. The surgeon takes great care to identify a second, proximal fistula, avoid inadvertently entering a possibly redundant membranous trachea, and preserving vagal branches. Cautery is avoided during this dissection to facilitate these surgical principles. Dissection of the distal esophagus is avoided if possible. The blood supply to the distal pouch is segmental; division of these arteries significantly increases the risk of ischemia to the distal esophagus. However, mobilization of the distal pouch may be acceptable if it ensures adequate length to complete a primary esophageal anastomosis.

The anastomosis is then created. An esophagotomy is made at the apex of the proximal pouch to match the circumference of the distal fistula. A 5-0 or 6-0 suture is utilized. The choice of suture is controversial. Chittmittrapap showed an increased incidence of anastomotic stricture formation with the use of silk compared to polyglycolic acid and polypropylene suture (35). A single-layer interrupted anastomosis has a decreased incidence of anastomotic stricture compared to a double-layer anastomosis (36,37). Two corner stitches are placed, but not tied. The posterior row of sutures is then placed in an interrupted fashion taking great care to take full thickness bites incorporating mucosa. The knots are then tied on the inside. The sump drain is then advanced carefully via the nares through the anastomosis into the distal esophagus and stomach. Choanal atresia is not present if the tube passes through the nares. Passage through the distal esophagus assures the absence of an obstructing tracheobronchial remnant associated with EA (23,38). The anterior row is then placed, tying the knots on the outside. A chest tube is inserted away from the anastomosis through a separate incision. The thoracotomy is then closed.

Additional technical considerations include reinforcement of the anastomosis, positioning of the drainage tube, and maintaining a high degree of suspicion for a second TEF. Postoperative respiratory failure in patients with a missed second TEF has been reported in a patient that did have preoperative bronchoscopy (31). Persistent drainage from an extrapleural chest tube that eroded into the esophageal anastomosis has also been reported (39). Some pediatric surgeons argue against the use of routine postoperative extrapleural drains in uncomplicated cases (40,41). A variety of techniques have been described to reinforce the esophageal anastomosis including using an azygous flap and applying fibrin glue (42). The application of fibrin glue was shown to decrease anastomotic leaks, stenosis, and mortality in a randomized trial of 22 patients compared to 23 patients who did not have fibrin glue applied to the anastomosis (42). Topical fibroblast growth factor application in rats demonstrates increased anastomotic strength, in part due to angiogenesis (43).

Of historical interest is the end-to-side repair for EA. The fistula is simply ligated, and a wide, oblique end-to-side anastomosis is performed. This technique has its proponents; however, there is an increased risk of fistula recanalization and mortality directly attributable to the EA in patients undergoing this technique (12). The end-to-end repair is safer than the end-to-side.

Thoracoscopic repair of an EA with TEF is a viable alternative for the pediatric surgeon with advanced laparoscopic skills. The baby is placed in the 45° prone position to allow the lung to fall away from the posterior mediastinum. Three cannulas are used for access to the thoracic cavity. A fourth port may be used for lung retraction. Carbon dioxide insufflation is used to affect lung collapse. The fistula is ligated using a variety of techniques including a suture ligature or a clip placed on the fistula tract with fistula division distal to it. The anastomosis is performed with either 4-0 or 5-0 PDS, polyglactin (Vicryl), or silk. The esophageal anastomosis is performed using either extracorporeal knot-tying techniques or intracorporeal suturing (44).

The incidence of postoperative complications is similar to the open end-to-end technique including the leak rate, stricture rate, rate of fundoplication, rate of recurrent fistula formation, and revision of the anastomosis. Thoracoscopic repair requires a transpleural approach. The operation is difficult in babies less than 2 kg and in babies with significant lung disease, since it requires the ipsilateral lung to be compressed with the operative pneumothorax to achieve an adequate working space. The primary advantage lies in the potential for a reduction in the musculoskeletal sequelae that may develop following thoracotomy in the newborn, although current open operative techniques minimize these complications. Advocates of the thoracoscopic repair feel there is superior visualization of the anatomy within the thoracic cavity (44).

Isolated Esophageal Atresia and Esophageal Atresia with Proximal TEF
"H" type fistulas and EA with an upper pouch fistula are special considerations. The diagnosis is established by a modified prone esophagram as the nasogastric tube is carefully retracted under fluoroscopic guidance by a skilled pediatric radiologist. The TEF without EA may be approached through a cervical incision. Bronchoscopy should be performed to identify and potentially stent the fistula to facilitate its identification during the dissection. The proximal fistula in an EA infant with proximal TEF is divided in the same fashion described for the distal TEF.

Technical Complications of the Repair of EA
The most common complications occurring after EA repair are anastomotic leak and stenosis. EA presents a unique surgical challenge because an anatomic gap exists between the esophageal ends that must be repaired. Several anatomic and physiologic considerations exist because of this and affect the integrity of the esophageal anastomosis. The submucosa is the strongest layer of the esophageal wall with the highest suture-holding capacity. Anastomotic strength during the early postoperative period relies upon the preexisting mature collagen network in the esophagus. This facilitates suture apposition of the divided ends of the esophagus. Postoperatively, this polymerized collagen is degraded, and synthesis of immature collagen

occurs, resulting in low mechanical strength. The thin esophageal wall, longitudinal muscle fiber distribution, absence of the serosal layer, and segmental distal esophageal vascularization also contribute to delayed and/or impaired healing (43). In patients with EA, the distance between the esophageal ends, the tension across the suture line, and the extent of mobilization of the esophageal segments are additional factors that further impair anastomotic healing (43).

Anastomotic Leak

Anastomotic leak results from a small, friable lower segment, ischemia of the esophageal ends, excess anastomotic tension, myotomy, sepsis, poor suturing techniques, type of suture, excessive mobilization of the distal pouch, and increased gap length (42). The incidence is approximately 15%, but has been reported to be as high as 27% (10). Anastomotic leaks after repair of EA are often subclinical and detected only through a barium swallow. Most leaks are managed nonoperatively and seal on their own by 4 weeks (10). Approximately 5% of leaks require reoperation in the setting of uncontrolled sepsis with persistent fluid collection or hydropneumothorax. The esophageal anastomosis should be revised if the tissues are healthy enough to hold sutures. Various approaches include simple reanastomosis, pleural patch overlay, intercostal muscle flap buttresses, simple debridement, and pericardial flap interposition (45,46). Otherwise, a segmental esophagectomy with cervical esophagostomy should be performed. This necessitates esophageal replacement later in life. The mediastinum and thoracic cavity should be widely drained.

Anastomotic Stricture

Predisposing factors implicated in the pathogenesis of esophageal anastomotic stricture are the use of a two-layer anastomosis, increased gap length, anastomotic tension, type of suture, anastomotic leak, and gastroesophageal reflux disease (35,42). Children with an anastamotic stricture have feeding difficulties, and vomiting, or dysphagia as their major symptoms. They may have chronic microaspiration, resulting in chronic lung disease. In babies, the first symptom is often "slow feeding" and regurgitation with or without cyanotic episodes (37). Surgeons define stricture after EA repair differently, and up to 50% to 80% of patients may develop a stricture (10). Chittmittrapap defined patients with swallowing problems or recurrent episodes of respiratory infection or foreign body impaction (including food), and narrowing of the esophagus noted on contrast esophagography or esophagoscopy, as having a stricture (35). Figures 1A and 1B compares an normal postoperative esophagram with and esophagram showing an anastomotic stricture.

Initial treatment is with dilation by either bougienage (10,35,37) or balloon dilation (47). The majority of patients (>80%) respond to less than four dilations (35,37). Complications from dilation such as perforation are rare (47). Stricture resection is reserved for patients who fail to respond to dilations (require more than five dilations) (35,37). The earlier the onset of symptoms, the more dilations are required and the higher the likelihood of needing surgery (37). It is extremely important to delineate the role of GERD in stricture formation. Many times, strictures will respond to dilation once the reflux is controlled; conversely, strictures will recur if resected without addressing the GERD first. Mitomycin C has been used to moderate fibrosis formation at the anastomotic site and help prevent stenosis (48).

Missed and Recurrent TEF

Missed TEF should be considered in infants with persistent respiratory compromise postoperatively. Bronchoscopy or barium swallow (as noted in the discussion for isolated TEF) is used for diagnosis. The management of the missed fistula is as outlined above.

Recurrent TEF occurs in 10% to 15% of EA repairs (37,49), and typically occurs in the first year of life, but may occur up to 10 to 15 years after repair (37). Recurrence of a TEF is more likely to occur if there has been leak from the anastomosis and following an end-to-side anastomosis. Minimal mobilization of the lower esophageal segment helps prevent a recurrent TEF by minimizing ischemia (37). The majority of patients with a recurrent TEF have coughing and sputtering episodes with feeding, usually associated with cyanosis (37). Diagnosis is made by esophagography, esophagoscopy, and bronchoscopy as described above. Spontaneous closure of a recurrent fistula is unlikely and there is little merit in deferring reoperation.

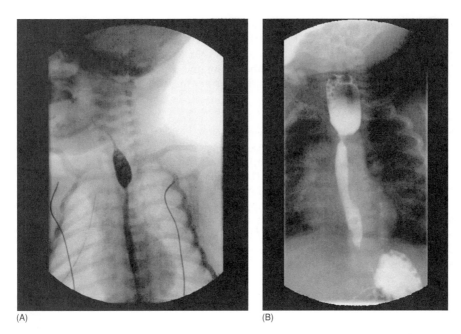

Figure 1   (A) Normal postoperative narrowing after repair of esophageal atresia. (B) Postoperative stricture following repair of esophageal atresia.

The fistula should be cannulated by bronchoscopy with a Fogarty catheter prior to repair. Thoracotomy with fistula ligation and division is the procedure of choice. Techniques described as above including pleural flap, pericardial flap, fibrin glue, and azygous vein flap interposed between the esophageal and tracheal suture lines have been used to prevent recurrence of the fistula, and must be used when repairing a recurrent TEF. Novel techniques such as laparoscopically harvested omental flap interposition between the suture lines have also been described (49).

Injury to the Vagus Nerve and Recurrent Laryngeal Nerve
The vagus nerve and its branches, including the recurrent laryngeal nerve, are intimately associated with the trachea and esophagus. These nerves may be damaged during dissection of the proximal esophageal pouch and distal esophagus. Injury to the vagus nerve and recurrent laryngeal nerve manifests as esophageal dysmotility and vocal cord paralysis, respectively. An incidence of 20% recurrent laryngeal nerve palsy has been reported in patients following EA repair (50). Interestingly, esophageal motor dysfunction is almost universal in patients with EA. Its role in the pathogenesis of GERD in patients with EA is becoming increasingly clear. It is unclear if vagal nerve and vagal nerve branch dysfunction after EA repair arises from injury to the nerves during dissection or if an underlying nerve abnormality exists preoperatively. It was initially thought that mobilization of the esophageal ends damaged branches of the vagal nerve, including the recurrent laryngeal nerve (51). Meticulous technique during dissection of the esophageal pouch is mandatory to preserve the vagal branches. However, it has been discovered in the Adriamycin-induced EA rats that the vagus and recurrent laryngeal nerves are absent and/or abnormal (52). Extrinsic and intrinsic innervation, including the vagus and laryngeal nerves, is abnormal in patients with EA with and without TEF (53). Injury to the recurrent laryngeal nerve certainly occurs, but recurrent laryngeal nerve dysfunction may be due to developmental abnormalities of the esophagus. Laryngoscopy should be performed to document vocal cord function at the time of the first operation.

Complications Related to Associated Conditions

Tracheomalacia
The differential diagnosis of respiratory symptoms following EA repair is anastomotic leak, recurrent TEF, GERD, and tracheomalacia. Tracheomalacia describes a generalized or localized

weakness of the trachea that allows the anterior and the posterior tracheal walls to collapse together during expiration or coughing. In addition, the flaccid trachea is easily compressed between the aorta anteriorly and the dilated esophagus posteriorly after EA repair. This situation can be exacerbated by esophageal distension during feeding. Presentation of tracheomalacia varies from a typical "brassy" or "barking" cough in mild cases, to life-threatening apneic spells or recurrent pneumonia in severe cases. Symptoms typically begin 2 months postoperatively (54,55). The incidence of severe tracheomalacia in patients with EA is 10% to 25% (55,56). Establishing the diagnosis includes studies to rule out leak, recurrent TEF, and GERD. Bronchoscopy with the child breathing spontaneously is diagnostic of severe tracheomalacia when the anteroposterior collapse of the tracheal lumen during coughing and expiration is more than 75%.

Mild to moderate tracheomalacia rarely requires operative repair. Aortopexy to the posterior surface of the sternum is the operative treatment of choice in patients with life-threatening anoxic spells (54,55,57). The approach is either via a left anterolateral thoracotomy (54,57), low transverse cervical incision (58), or thoracoscopically (59). The tissue plane between the vascular structures and the trachea should not be dissected to facilitate anterior displacement of the tracheal wall as the vessels are pulled forward (54). In patients with concomitant GERD and tracheomalacia, the tracheomalacia is treated first if the patient presents with dying spells or recurrent pneumonias (55). Filler et al. recommended that an airway stent be considered for children in whom aortopexy fails to relieve tracheal collapse (55). Failure of the stent necessitates tracheostomy.

Right-Sided Aortic Arch

The presence of a right-sided aortic arch occurs in 5% of cases with EA (13). A right-sided aortic arch may significantly complicate exposure and repair of the esophagus from the right side of the chest. Furthermore, a right aortic arch is frequently associated with congenital heart disease or a vascular ring that completely encircles the trachea and esophagus. When the aortic arch is on the right, the upper esophageal pouch lies on the left side of the aortic arch, and the distal TEF lies to the left of the descending aorta. Harrison et al. reported seven patients with right-sided aortic arch associated EA (13). Six were discovered at right thoracotomy. The authors encountered extreme difficulty completing the operation from a right thoracotomy, resulting in bilateral thoracotomy, staged repair of the EA and TEF, or esophageal replacement (13). One patient developed a postoperative aortoesophageal fistula and exsanguinated. Another patient developed left vocal cord paralysis, tracheobronchitis, subglottic narrowing, and tracheal stenosis requiring tracheostomy after primary esophageal repair through a left thoracotomy. It is important to determine the position of the aorta preoperatively. The gold standard for diagnosis is angiography; however, computed tomography (CT) angiography and magnetic resonance imaging has recently become a sensitive, less invasive, alternative (13–15,60). An umbilical artery line noted on x-ray may indicate the side of the aortic arch. Chest x-ray is not sensitive to diagnose a right-sided aortic arch (14). Echocardiography is operator dependent (13,15).

Tracheobronchial Remnants

Spitz was the first to demonstrate a congenital basis for distal esophageal stenosis associated with EA by showing the presence of tracheobronchial rests in an esophagectomy specimen (61). A de novo congenital esophageal stenosis may be encountered or one may present postoperatively after EA repair. Complications arising from tracheobronchial rests are signs and symptoms similar to those of postoperative anastomotic stenosis unrelated to tracheobronchial remnants. Gittes' model of EA with TEF formation readily explains the presence of tracheobronchial remnants in the distal esophageal pouch (7). A tracheobronchial rest, an esophageal membranous diaphragm, and segmental hypertrophy of the muscularis and diffuse fibrosis of the submucosa are different etiologies of congenital esophageal stenosis. Esophageal stenosis is typically diagnosed after EA with TEF repair, and infants present with symptoms of esophageal stricture. Bouginage or balloon dilation is recommended. If after three dilations symptoms and stricture persist, surgical resection of the stenotic segment with end-to-end anastomosis or esophageal replacement is the treatment of choice (23,38). Because the tracheobronchial remnants are limited to a short 1- to 2-cm length, a limited resection rather than a more extensive resection with esophageal substitution is all that is usually required (38). If the pediatric surgeon encounters an esophageal stenosis from tracheobronchial remnants during initial repair, the authors recommend the following approach. The anastomosis should be completed and a gastrostomy tube placed to preserve the native esophagus. The stenosis should be stented with a small nasogastric tube to ensure adequate drainage of saliva. The patient should then be allowed to grow, and after the anastomosis has healed, the stenosis may be evaluated with an esophageal swallow or CT scan. The patient should then undergo laparotomy if obstruction is present or persists. A Foley catheter may be placed through a gastrostomy, and passed proximally above the stenosis and the balloon inflated. The surgeon may then gently retract the esophagus into the abdomen, and the segment of esophagus with the tracheobronchial remnants may be resected. The specimen is sent for frozen section and the margins should be clear of any tracheobronchial rests. A primary anastomosis should then be completed in the abdomen. A postoperative esophagram should be performed 5 to 7 days postoperatively to check for an esophageal leak.

A leiomyoma at the site of EA repair has been reported (62). The patient presented with symptoms of persistent esophageal stricture.

Long-Term Complications

Pulmonary

It is obvious that the most common short-term postoperative complications following a thoracotomy will be pulmonary. Atelectasis and pneumonia are seen in up to 57% of patients who have undergone repair of EA (10). Aggressive pulmonary support is necessary to minimize these complications.

Late pulmonary function in patients with EA includes a variable incidence of restrictive and obstructive pulmonary disease, as well as airway hyperreactivity. In one study comparing a cohort of patients with EA and TEF to normal siblings, the incidence of respiratory symptoms was similar in both groups. However, pulmonary function tests were significantly abnormal compared to sibling controls. There was no difference in airway hyperreactivity. Pulmonary function abnormalities did not correlate with the presence or severity of current respiratory symptoms, with the presence of airway hyperreactivity, or with current gastrointestinal symptoms (63). There is an increased risk of aspiration in patients with EA and TEF. As discussed above, abnormal airway epithelium, excessive tracheal pliability, abnormal tracheal innervation, GERD, and abnormal esophageal motility all increase the risk of aspiration and subsequent risk of pneumonia. Respiratory problems tend to improve with age (64).

Gastroesophageal Reflux

Gastroesophageal reflux occurs in 30% to 82% of patients after EA and TEF repair; 30% of these patients require an antireflux operation (10,64–66). The bathing of the anastomotic line in stomach acid results in an increased incidence of stricture and leak. Feeding is affected and GERD contributes to aspiration as discussed above. Diagnosis is made by symptoms and pH probe. Tension on the anastomosis causing shortened intraabdominal esophageal length and blunting of the angle of His (65), intrinsic esophageal dysmotility (51), intrinsic innervation disorders (53), denervation from extensive esophageal pouch dissection, and gastric dysmotility (67) all contribute to the pathogenesis of GERD in EA.

Long-term consequences of GERD in these patients are manifold. It is important to note that the presence of pathologic changes of the esophagus, such as esophagitis and gastric metaplasia, do not always correlate with symptoms (68). Symptoms tend to decrease over time (66). Consequences of GERD in patients with a history of EA last well into adulthood (16), including respiratory symptoms (33%), dysphagia (52%), reflux esophagitis (58%), Barrett's esophagus (11%), and strictures (42%). In patients with a history of EA, men older than 35 years of age and individuals with episodes of reflux greater than three times per week have an increased risk of severe esophagitis and Barrett's esophagus (16). There have been two reported cases of esophageal squamous cell carcinoma in patients with EA, including one at the anastomosis (16). Long-term follow-up is mandatory to screen for these complications of GERD in EA.

The management of GERD is discussed elsewhere in this chapter. It is important to note that controversy surrounds the proper operative management of GERD in patients with EA. Nissen–Rossetti fundoplication has traditionally been considered the best option (69,70), but concerns for debilitating dysphagia and incidence of wrap disruption and recurrent GERD (33%) have challenged this notion (69). Some pediatric surgeons have begun to use partial wraps such as the Thal or Toupet procedure to ameliorate these problems. No clear improved outcome has been demonstrated using any of these procedures (69,70). Some surgeons modify their Nissen technique to create a shorter, floppier wrap (1.0 to 1.5 cm over a larger dilator) (70). In addition, some surgeons have used the Collis–Nissen fundoplication to gain intra-abdominal esophageal length (71).

Dysphagia

Dysphagia is a common symptom in individuals who have undergone surgical repair for EA, although in most patients this is mild and simply managed by drinking fluids with meals. The incidence of dysphagia appears to decrease slightly over time, with the majority of patients experiencing this during the first five postoperative years (40%). Most patients seem to grow accustomed to dysphagia and reflux symptoms, but these symptoms do persist well into adulthood (16,66). Impaired esophageal motility appears to be a major contributing factor to dysphagia (16). Gastric dysmotility has also been noted in patients with EA with dysphagia and dyspepsia (67). However, it is important to note that while gastric dysmotility documented by manometry and scintigraphy may persist to adulthood, they are not always responsible for symptoms. The much more common cause is GERD and esophageal dysmotility (67).

Long-Term Quality of Life

Swallowing function greatly affects the quality of life of children and adults with EA. Choking occurs in up to 30% of patients and contributes to dysphagia and esophageal foreign body obstruction including food boluses (66). Almost half of the children reviewed by Little et al. weighed less than the 25th percentile during the first 5 years; however, the children's weight and height steadily improved. By the time the children had reached 10 years of age, less than one-third of them continued to have weights or heights less than the 25th percentile (66). Most patients outgrow symptoms of choking, dysphagia, GERD, growth retardation, and respiratory problems after the first few years of life (>5 years old) (64,66,72), and enjoy a good quality of life and normal psychosocial functioning. The incidence of food entrapment requiring esophagoscopy or bouginage, which occurs in 38% of patient (72), lasts only a few years. Patients are able to train themselves to avoid certain foods or help themselves swallow appropriately. Importantly, patients do report feeling isolated when making the transition from childhood to adult medical services, suggesting that the pediatric surgeon should claim a larger role in preparing the adult physician to care for these patients (72). Table 1 shows the incidence of postoperative and long-term complications from long-term studies of the repair of EA.

Long Gap Atresia

In most instances, neonates who have EA and TEF have a short distance between the esophageal ends allowing for primary repair. Occasionally in infants with EA–TEF and usually in infants with isolated EA, the distance between the atretic esophageal ends limits the ability to easily complete a tension-free, end-to-end primary esophageal anastomosis. There is no precise agreed upon definition of the term "long gap EA." Various definitions include lengths between the esophageal ends ranging from 2 cm to 6 cm. The distance between vertebral bodies (>4) is also used. Regardless, long gap EA continues to be a therapeutic challenge for the pediatric surgeon. Maintaining the patient's native esophagus is a primary goal in the management of long gap EA.

In the case of isolated EA, most pediatric surgeons would proceed with the operative placement of a gastrostomy tube, a period of observation, and an attempted delayed primary repair. The proximal pouch is continuously suctioned to prevent microaspiration of pooled oral secretions. For isolated EA, it is important to exclude an upper pouch TEF. If at thoracotomy for EA and TEF, little or no intrathoracic esophagus is present and esophageal replacement is indicated, it is best to perform a gastrostomy tube and a cervical esophagostomy to avoid aspiration and allow the patient to go home before definitive repair (2).

During the initial procedure, the anastomosis may be attempted under tension. Good proximal and possibly distal mobilization of the esophageal segments may be necessary to facilitate this (73). Proximal esophageal circular Livaditis myotomy to lengthen the upper esophageal pouch and achieve a primary anastomosis in long gap EA can be used (74,75). A second or third proximal pouch myotomy may be performed via a cervical incision (76), and even a distal myotomy may be performed (77,78). Complications such as leak, impaction of food particles in the myotomy segment, pseudodiverticulum (79), and impaired esophageal motility (80) have been reported following the use of myotomies. A spiral upper pouch myotomy with oblique suture closure of the muscle layers may be used to prevent these complications (81,82).

Table 1 Complications of Repair of Esophageal Atresia

	Patients	Leak	Stricture	Recurrent TEF	GERD	Fundoplication	Tracheomalacia	Pulmonary[a]	Dysphagia[b]
McKinnon	64	21%	15%	5%	N/A	14%	N/A	N/A	N/A
Poenaru	111	12%	22%	9%[c]	21%[d]	N/A	5%	50%[e]	14.6%
Okada	141	26.5%	49.1%	7.2%	52%	20%	25.8%	57%	N/A
Schier	128	4%[g]	7%[g]	4%	46%	16%	13%[h]	80%	38%
Little[f]	69	N/A	N/A	N/A	48%	28%	4%[i]	29%	45%[j]
Koivusalo	128	8%	2%[g]	3%	19%	2%	6%[k]	32%	5%
Taylor	132	N/A	42%	N/A	63%	11%	N/A	33%	52%

a Pulmonary complications include postoperative atelectasis, pneumonia, empyema, and pneumothorax.
b Dysphagia includes difficulty swallowing and food impaction.
c Recurrent TEF occurred significantly more often when a side-to-side anastomosis was used compared to an end-to-end anastomosis.
d GERD occurred significantly more often when an end-to-end anastomosis was used compared to a side-to-side anastomosis.
e Pneumonia occurred significantly more often when a side-to-side anastomosis was used compared to an end-to-end anastomosis.
f Data presented from the first five years of follow-up.
g Required operation.
h Eight percent required aortopexy and 5% required tracheostomy.
i Did not require operation.
j Ten percent of patients suffered from choking.
k Required aortopexy.
Abbreviations: TEF, Tracheoesophageal fistula; GERD, Gastroesophageal reflux disease; N/A, Not analyzed.

An alternative approach is rows of short, horizontal, circumferential myotomies allowing the upper pouch to lengthen and narrow when stretched (83). An anterior flap may be constructed of the upper pouch, which can then be rolled into a tube for anastomosis (84). The stomach may be mobilized via an abdominal incision to achieve a primary esophageal anastomosis (85), or a Collis gastroplasty may be used to lengthen the distal end of the esophagus (86). Each of these maneuvers requires a fundoplication. Primary repair may be performed safely in the premature neonate. The presence of severe pulmonary disease is the critical factor that might necessitate a staged repair (87).

A delayed primary anastomosis may be performed. This may especially benefit high-risk premature infants (88). During the waiting period of 6 to 12 weeks, the gap between the two ends of the esophagus diminishes because of spontaneous growth, which makes primary repair more feasible (2). Bouginage of the proximal and/or distal esophageal ends (2,89), and magnetic bouginage may facilitate pouch growth (90). Transmediastinal silk or nylon thread bridging the gap between the two ends of the esophagus with and without silver olives has been used to allow directional grown and eventual fistulization between the two ends (91,92). A multi-stage mobilization of the proximal pouch is also described. This is accomplished as an end cervical esophagostomy and subsequent mobilization and translocation down the anterior chest wall subcutaneously. This is continued until sufficient length for a primary esophageal anastomosis is possible (93,94). Foker advocates the use of traction sutures placed at thoracotomy and externalized from the chest to stretch both the proximal and distal esophageal segments (95). Hydrostatic stretch techniques have also been described to stimulate growth of the distal esophageal pouch (96).

Infants may be prophylactically paralyzed and ventilated for an arbitrary period of 5 days postoperatively. The rationale for this is the prevention of disruptive forces at the anastomotic site by paralysis of the striated muscle in the proximal esophagus. Long gap atresia results in a loss of oral use in the neonate, and the baby is at risk for constant microaspiration because of bouginage to the proximal pouch. These infants experience the same complications as children with short gap atresias, but at somewhat higher rates (2,11,15). However, over time, these problems subside, even in children with long gap atresia (64,66,72).

SURGICAL TREATMENT OF GASTROESOPHAGEAL REFLUX

Background

Gastroesophageal reflux disease is a relatively common condition in children where gastric contents reflux into the esophagus. Symptoms may vary from occasional "spitting up" to persistent emesis. Pediatric GERD typically manifests within the first 6 weeks of life, and although approximately 60% of infants become asymptomatic by age 2, the remainder of the children, if left untreated, have persistent and significant symptoms until at least 4 years of age (97). Since the first description of the gastroesophageal reflux syndrome by Winkelstein (98), the management of this disorder has progressed significantly. Initial treatment consisted of positional therapy to alleviate symptoms (99). Until the 1990s, medical treatment was relatively ineffective. Surgical options were first introduced in the 1960s, and since then have been adapted and refined, and now antireflux procedures are one of the operations most frequently performed by pediatric surgeons.

Long-term outcomes of antireflux procedures in children are somewhat different than in adults, in large part due to the differences in the patient population. In pediatric centers, a large portion of patients are neurologically impaired, unlike most adult populations. And while nonsurgical management of GERD is the typical initial treatment in adults and normal children, neurologically impaired children almost always fail medical management, leaving surgery as the treatment of choice. Outcomes data have suggested a difference in the surgical outcomes between neurologically impaired children and normal children. Furthermore, there are a number of children with unique differences compared to adults, including those children with a repaired EA, a caustic esophageal injury, cystic fibrosis, congenital heart disease, and congenital diaphragmatic hernias.

In infants and children, the most frequent surgical operations that are used include the transabdominal and transthoracic fundoplications. The transabdominal fundoplications use either a circumferential (Nissen) or partial fundoplication. The partial fundoplications are either an anterior (Thal) or posterior (Toupet) fundoplication. Complications from these procedures include pulmonary difficulties as well as gastrointestinal problems. Such gastrointestinal dysfunction includes dysphagia, retching, gas bloat, dumping syndrome, diarrhea, and persistent or recurrent symptoms of gastrointestinal reflux. The long-term outcomes from these operations are a result of the unique aspects of a pediatric population.

Surgical Techniques

Nissen Fundoplication

A common antireflux operation performed in both adults and children is the Nissen fundoplication, which involves a loose, circumferential wrap of the gastric fundus around the intraabdominal esophagus. To accomplish this goal, the surgeon must fully mobilize the gastric fundus by dividing the short gastric vessels. A circumferential mobilization of the intraabdominal esophagus must also be performed. A 2- to 4-cm length of the gastric fundus is fashioned into a tension-free wrap around the intra-abdominal esophagus.

Partial Fundoplication

Partial fundoplications wrap around the intraabdominal esophagus up to approximately 270° rather than the complete 360° of the Nissen fundoplication. These partial fundoplications theoretically offer the functional benefits of an antireflux operation while decreasing the risk of obstructing the esophagus with too tight of a wrap.

Complications

As with all operations, complications can occur both intraoperatively and postoperatively. Intraoperative complications include pleural perforations, injury to the vagus nerve (particularly the posterior vagus nerve), esophageal perforations, and gastric perforations (100). Postoperative complications include wrap disruption, paraesophageal hernia, small bowel obstruction, dysphagia, retching, gas bloat, dumping syndrome, diarrhea, and persistent or recurrent symptoms of gastrointestinal reflux. Such symptoms might require a reoperation in up to 9% of patients (101–108).

Dysphagia

Some degree of immediate postoperative dysphagia is common, although it is typically mild and self-limited. Several authors have reported that up to 5.3% of children undergoing fundoplication have severe or persistent dysphagia postoperatively (100,102,103,107,108). The etiology of this dysphagia can be multifactorial, including a tight fundoplication, poor esophageal peristalsis, persistent or recurrent GERD, or a slipped or disrupted wrap. A tight fundoplication can often be treated with gentle endoscopic dilation, however slipped or disrupted wraps may need further surgical treatment.

Postoperative dysphagia results from esophageal obstruction that leads to difficulty in swallowing. While it is relatively common to have a small amount of mild dysphagia in the immediate postoperative period, this is usually self-limited and resolves within several weeks. One typically attributes this symptom to normal postoperative edema. However, dysphagia that persists beyond this time period is usually a result of a fundoplication that is wrapped too tightly around the distal esophagus. Some authors have suggested that division of the short gastric vessels reduces the risk of this complication (109). The risk of dysphagia can be minimized through the use of an intraoperative bougie to size the esophagus and to help ensure that a loose fundoplication is created. A rough estimate of the proper size of the bougie can be approximated by choosing a bougie that is the same diameter of the patient's thumb, or by using the child's weight as a guide. Ostlie et al. recommended a guide for choosing a bougie size (Table 2) (110).

Retching

Postoperative retching may occur in patients without recurrent reflux. In this case, the retching is a component of the emetic reflex, which is triggered by a variety of peripheral or central stimuli. Patients at risk for developing this complication primarily include those children who are neurologically impaired (111). Those with dietary intolerances and delayed gastric emptying may also be at a higher risk (112). The development of new-onset retching has been reported to

Table 2 Suggested Sizes for Bougie Placement during Fundoplication

Weight (kg)	Bougie size
2.0–4.0	20–24
4.0–5.5	24–28
5.5–7.0	28–32
7.0–8.5	32–34
8.5–10.0	34–36
10.0–15.0	36–40

occur in 1.25% to 25% of children undergoing fundoplication (102,106,112,113). The new-onset of retching might suggest a disrupted or herniated wrap, and requires appropriate evaluation with a barium study. Other nonsurgical causes of retching must also be considered, such as eosinophilic gastroenteritis or food allergies.

Gas Bloat Syndrome

Gas bloat syndrome describes an inability to belch and vomit, postprandial fullness, bloating, and abdominal pain. This complication occurs in 2% to 4% of children undergoing fundoplication (107,108,114). Symptoms of this syndrome are typically attributed to a tight wrap. Many surgeons advocate performing a shorter, looser wrap to avoid this complication. In those children with a gastrostomy tube, simply venting the tube will often relieve the symptoms.

Dumping Syndrome

Dumping syndrome has been reported to occur in up to 30% of children undergoing fundoplication (115). Early dumping is caused by a rapid entrance of hyperosmolar chime into the small intestines leading to a large rapid fluid shift into the intestinal lumen. This rapid change causes an increase in the amplitude and frequency of the peristaltic activity. Symptoms typically include sweating, palpitations, abdominal bloating and cramping, and diarrhea. Late dumping results from an overabundant insulin release causing reactive hypoglycemia. Symptoms include dizziness, confusion, headache, sweating, palpitations, and tremor.

Treatment of dumping syndrome is typically through dietary management, such as avoidance of simple carbohydrates and supplementation with complex carbohydrates. In resistant patients, drug therapy has been used to delay gastric emptying and inhibit insulin secretion.

Paraesophageal Hernia

In a retrospective review of 464 children undergoing an antireflux operation, Avansino et al. (116). reported a postoperative incidence of paraesophageal hernias in 4.5%. Of these 464 patients, 232 (50%) underwent a Nissen fundoplication, with 184 of these patients also receiving a simultaneous gastrostomy tube. Of the 464 patients 185 (40%) underwent a Thal fundoplication, 42 (9%) had a Boerema anterior gastropexy, and 5 (1%) had a Toupet fundoplication. Out of the 21 (4.5%) patients who had a postoperative paraesophageal hernia, 12 followed a Nissen fundoplication and 9 followed a Thal fundoplication. These authors performed a crural closure in all their patients, but additional esophageal plication sutures to the diaphragmatic crura were performed in 70% of those patients undergoing Nissen fundoplications. They reported a decreased incidence of postoperative paraesophageal hernia in these patients with additional plication sutures. However, two of these patients had an esophageal leak at these sites, requiring an emergent thoracotomy. After examining the preoperative symptoms, these authors suggested that the children at most risk for developing a postoperative paraesophageal hernia were those children with preoperative gagging or delayed gastric emptying.

Alrabeeah et al. performed a retrospective review of 89 patients who underwent a Nissen fundoplication at a single institution. These authors found that patients under 1 year of age as well as patients with significant neurologic dysfunction had a higher incidence of a postoperative paraesophageal hernia. These authors also noted an increased risk in those children who underwent a Nissen fundoplication without a crural repair compared to those who had a crural repair (21.9% versus 4%) (117). Still other authors have advocated both performing a crural repair as well as anchoring the wrap to the crural repair and to the diaphragm (118).

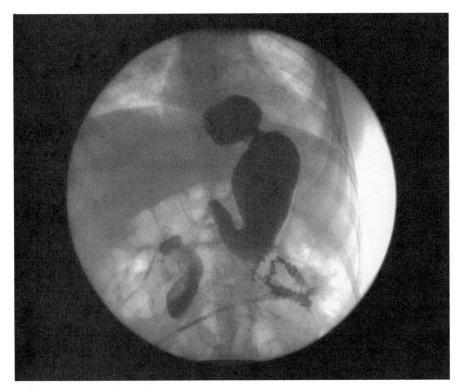

Figure 2 Slipped Nissen fundoplication.

Wrap Disruption and Wrap Slippage after a Nissen Fundoplication
In those patients who undergo a Nissen fundoplication, both a disruption of the wrap or a slippage of the wrap can lead to a postoperative failure and a recurrence of the reflux. With a wrap disruption, the fundoplication falls apart, essentially undoing the operation. A slipped wrap occurs when the fundoplication slips down over the fundus of the stomach, rather than around the esophagus. In these cases, a redo fundoplication is often necessary (Fig. 2).

The Laparoscopic Approach
Multiple studies have shown that the laparoscopic approach, whether with a partial or complete fundoplication, has a comparable complication rate to the open techniques. The failure rate after open Nissen fundoplication in children has been reported to range from 2% to 24% (119–121). In adults, the failure rate of open Nissen fundoplication has been reported from 9% to 30% (122). The laparoscopic failure rate in adults has been reported at a slightly better rate of 2% to 17% (121). Graziano et al. reported a failure rate of 8.7%, comparable to the adult literature (121). Further studies have reported success with performing redo laparoscopic fundoplications, particularly in those patients who initially underwent a laparoscopic operation.

Neurologically Impaired Children
Neurologically impaired children appear to have an increased risk of perioperative problems when undergoing an antireflux operation. Subramaniam and Dickson (108) performed a retrospective review of all children who underwent fundoplication during a period of 10 years at Booth Hall Children's Hospital in Manchester, England. They reported on 109 children, of whom 64.2% were neurologically impaired. During the first 5 years of the study, the preferred operation performed was the Boix-Ochoa procedure, in which an anterior wrap of fundus is anchored across the esophagus to the margins of the right crus and diaphragm. Fifty-three children underwent this procedure, and the remainder (56) underwent a Nissen fundoplication. Within the neurologically impaired group of children, 38 (54.2%) underwent a Nissen fundoplication and 32 (45.7%) underwent the Boix-Ochoa procedure. In the neurologically normal children, 18 (46.1%) underwent a Nissen fundoplication, and 21 (53.8%) underwent the Boix-

Table 3 Complications of Outcomes of Fundoplication in Neurologically Normal versus Neurologically Impaired Children

	Neurologically impaired (*n* = 70)		Neurologically normal (*n* = 39)	
	Boix-Ochoa	Nissen	Boix-Ochoa	Nissen
Total	32	38	21	18
Recurrence	14	2	6	0

Ochoa procedure. The rate of recurrent reflux is shown in Table 3. These authors concluded that the neurologically impaired group has a higher complication risk. Furthermore, they concluded that the Nissen fundoplication is more effective and has fewer complications compared to the Boix-Ochoa procedure.

Fonkalsrud et al. (103) performed a retrospective review of 7467 patients under 18 years of age who underwent antireflux operations for gastroesophageal reflux at seven participating hospitals. Fifty-six percent of their patients were neurologically normal and 44% were neurologically impaired. Sixty-four percent of patients underwent a Nissen, 34% had a Thal, and 1.5% had a Toupet. A laparoscopic fundoplication was performed in 2.6% of patients. A major complication occurred in 4.2% of neurologically normal patients and in 12.8% of neurologically impaired patients. The most frequent complications were wrap disruption leading to recurrent reflux (7.1%), respiratory complications (4.4%), gas bloat (3.6%), and intestinal obstruction (2.6%). Postoperative death occurred in 0.07% of neurologically normal patients and in 0.8% of neurologically normal patients. These authors reported no difference in the success or complications rates between the participating hospitals and no difference with respect to the type of antireflux operation that was performed. Neurologically impaired children, however, were four times more likely to have a complication than neurologically normal patients.

ESOPHAGEAL REPLACEMENT

Replacement of the esophagus is one of the most technically challenging procedures that the pediatric surgeon will perform. Performance of esophageal replacement must be preceded by the decision to abandon the native esophagus and to choose the replacement procedure. Although most pediatric surgeons choose one method of replacement as their mainstay, they must be knowledgeable of the other technical options. Anatomic variations such as a short colon may prompt the decision to use a gastric conduit while a poorly placed gastrostomy tube may require the abandonment of a reversed gastric tube. Complete necrosis of the conduit may also require the surgeon to utilize a secondary technique of esophageal replacement (Fig. 3).

Esophageal replacement is most frequently applied to pediatric patients with long gap EA or caustic ingestions. Public health measures in many countries, including the United States, have reduced the occurrence of caustic ingestions in children. However, the infrequent occurrence of intentional ingestion and farm accidents still result in caustic ingestions. Esophageal replacement for caustic ingestions is still a frequent problem in many countries. For example, Bassiouny performed 70 colon replacements of the esophagus during a 4-year period in Egyptian children who sustained caustic ingestions (123). The reduced incidence of caustic ingestion and options for esophageal lengthening reduce the frequency of the performance of esophageal replacement. The infrequent performance of these procedures places a greater responsibility for the surgeon to understand the complication profile for each type of esophageal replacement.

The ideal conduit between the stomach and the proximal esophagus or oropharynx should have aboral peristalsis and resistance to gastric acid. The ideal substitute for the esophagus must have appropriate length to bridge the distance between the stomach and proximal esophagus or pharynx. It should also have a reliable blood supply and relative ease of performance. The absence of the interposed segment from its native location should not result in problems for the patient. For example, use of the colon in a patient with short gut may result in refractory diarrhea. If all attempts to salvage the esophagus have failed, then an esophageal replacement is necessary.

The choices available for esophageal replacement include the colon, the stomach, and the jejunum. Each of the choices has specific advantages and disadvantages that the surgeon must consider. In addition, each of the procedures has their own complications that require recognition and management. Much of the introduction and development of the techniques of esophageal replacement has been due to adult surgeons treating esophageal cancer. While the basic procedures and categories of complications are similar between adults and children, the developmental issues and the length of time needed for conduit functioning make extrapolation from adult experiences to children difficult.

In the following section, colon and gastric replacement of the esophagus will be discussed. The focus of the discussion will be complication recognition, management, and avoidance.

Esophageal Replacement with Colon

The colon has been used to replace the esophagus for over 100 years and is the most frequently chosen form of esophageal bypass. Its use in adults preceded its application to children. Lund-blad used the colon to reconstruct the esophagus of a child with a corrosive injury in 1921 (124). In 1948, Sandblom was the first surgeon to use the colon as a replacement of the esophagus in a child with long gap EA (125).

The indications for colon replacement of the esophagus in children are long gap EA, caustic injury to the esophagus, and esophageal neoplasms such as extensive leiomyomatosis. Several situations make the choice of a colon conduit advisable. Children with microgastria or caustic gastric injury may not have the option of the stomach as a conduit. Children needing segmental lower esophageal replacement may be better served by retaining their gastric reservoir and using the colon as an interposition. In contrast, children needing the colon for future vaginal replacement or bladder augmentation should have a conduit created from the stomach. In addition, children who have previously undergone colon resection should have the remainder of their colon spared to prevent refractory diarrhea.

Anatomic Considerations

The surgeon performing replacement of the esophagus with the colon must have a thorough understanding of the vascular anatomy of the colon and the anatomic approaches that bridge the distance from the stomach to the cervical esophagus. The arterial blood supply of the colon is ideal for creation of a lengthy conduit because of the extensive collateral blood supply contained within the mesocolon. The proximal colon is supplied by the right colic artery and middle colic artery; both arteries are branches of the superior mesenteric artery (SMA). The colon distal to the middle of the transverse colon is supplied by the left colic artery; a branch of the inferior mesenteric artery (IMA). The ascending branch of the left colic artery connects with a descending branch of the middle colic artery to form the marginal artery of Drummond. The branches of the SMA supply the right and transverse colon and have greater variability than the arteries supplying the left colon. Sonnenland demonstrated that only 68% of autopsies showed standard arterial anatomy of the SMA, and the right colic artery was absent in 12.6% of autopsies (126). In contrast, the branches of the IMA were more often consistent. DeMeester analyzed colonic arterial anatomy by preoperative angiography and found that 92% of adults had an adequate ascending left colic artery. Further, 80% of patients had a single-trunked middle colic artery (127). The choice of colon segment is dependent upon the section with optimal collateralization. The transverse and left colon segments are used most often. The choice of either section of the colon may result in either an isoperistaltic or antiperistaltic segment. Although animal experiments suggest a difference in the emptying properties of the isoperistaltic versus the antiperistaltic colon, it is difficult to demonstrate clinically relevant differences in children (128).

The route of passage from the abdomen to the neck is a matter of surgeon preference. The choices include a transthoracic route, a transthoracic-retrohilar approach (Waterston), a subster-nal route, or a posterior mediastinal route. A potential advantage of the posterior mediastinal route is a reduction of dysphagia related to redundancy. A disadvantage of the procedure is the potential for recurrent laryngeal injury during the blunt esophagectomy (129). This injury may be obviated by the performance of a thoracotomy and open dissection of the esophageal remnant. Most pediatric surgeons prefer either the retrohilar transthoracic technique or the posterior mediastinal approach.

Principles of Colon Replacement of the Esophagus

The timing of the esophageal replacement requires good judgment, regardless of the conduit cho-sen. If a patient with long gap atresia does not have significant esophageal length for a primary esophogoesophostomy, most surgeons would perform a left-sided cervical esophagostomy. A minority of surgeons would leave the upper pouch intact and discharge the patient with upper pouch suctioning. My experience has been that families are uncomfortable with this approach, and the patients suffer from persistant, subclinical microaspiration. In addition, the inability to swallow extinguishes the desire and ability for oral feeding. The timing of esophageal replacement for caustic ingestion is also difficult. Refractory strictures are the most common indication for replacement. If the colon is the choice for esophageal replacement, a barium enema should be performed to demonstrate the length and position of the colon. Preoperative angiography and colonoscopy are not necessary in children. The patient should be admitted for a mechanical and antibiotic bowel prep. The choice of incision is determined by the intended operation. Patients undergoing a Waterston type replacement will undergo a left thoracoabdominal approach. Patients undergoing replacement of the esophagus through the bed of the esophagus (posterior mediastinal) may have a vertical midline abdominal incision. If a blunt esophagectomy is too difficult due to periesophageal inflammation, the incision can be curved over to either chest for completion of the esophagectomy. Upon entering the abdomen, the colon is inspected for its' arterial and venous anatomy. The patency of the right colic, middle colic, and left colic artery is confirmed. The presence of an adequate marginal artery is mandatory. After the segment has been chosen, inflow from the arteries should be interrupted by placing microvascular clamps on the marginal artery. This technique will assure that the graft can survive on its main arterial supply carried through the marginal artery. Test clamping the arteries can be done prior to the neck dissection or esophagectomy. The recurrent laryngeal nerve is at risk for injury during the takedown of the cervical esophagostomy. Injury can be minimized by confining the dissection to the wall of the esophagus. The cervical dissection is completed when an adequate passage through the thoracic inlet is established. When the surgeon is able to place two to three fingers through the thoracic inlet, constriction of the colon conduit is unlikely. Creating an adequate passage from the thorax minimizes the chance of venous obstruction and cervical leakage due to venous congestion. The lower anastamosis is performed first. Some surgeons believe that an anastamosis between the esophageal stump is preferable in the case of long gap EA. However, the size discrepancy between the colon and distal esophagus usually precludes this approach. On most occasions, it is better to suture the colon to the posterior aspect of the upper stomach to improve emptying. A small "collar" of stomach can be sewn around the anastamosis to prevent leakage. This should not be done circumferentially as this may obstruct the emptying of the colon conduit. Prior to the performance of the distal anastamosis, it is important to confirm that the conduit is not twisted as it is brought through its route to the neck. When the distal anastamosis is completed, the length of the conduit is checked, and if it is too long, it can be resected at the cervical end. The proximal anastamosis is usually completed in an end-to-end fashion with a single layer of absorbable suture. A soft drain is placed in the neck, and a feeding tube is placed in the stomach. The majority of surgeons perform a pyloroplasty. Intragastric feedings can be started within 48 to 72 hours. A contrast study of the conduit should be obtained prior to starting oral feeding. This is usually done 5 to 7 days after the operation.

Short-term Complications

Most short-term complications of colon replacement of the esophagus are either pulmonary or anastomatic leaks of the esophagocolonic anastamosis. Pulmonary complications result from exposures that are necessary during the operative dissection. Atelectasis is a common pulmonary complication that is the inevitable result of pulmonary compression during intrathoracic dissection. Pneumothorax results from either ipsilateral thoracotomy or pleural transgression when mediastinal dissection is necessary for native esophagectomy.

Cervical leaks most often result from vascular insufficiency. Rarely, a leak can result from blind insertion of a nasocolonic tube that perforates the anastamosis. Cervical leaks occur in 6.2% to 48.2% of reported series (Table 4). This range probably results from the absence of an accepted definition of an anastomotic leak. Some authors would only consider a clinically obvious leak as reportable while others would include a radiographically detected leak. Fortunately, most postoperative leaks of the esophagocolonic anastamosis heal spontaneously, and most do not result in a stricture. A leak will usually present with salivary secretions coming out of the cervical drain. Early discovery of a leak is achieved by a contrast study on the fifth to seventh postoperative day. If a leak is discovered, the child is not allowed oral feeding for 1 to 2 weeks, and a repeat contrast study is performed. If a stricture is noted, a gentle dilation under general anesthesia is performed.

Table 4 Complications of Colon Replacement of the Esophagus

Author	Patients	Mortality	Anastamotic leakage	Stricture	Redundancy	Graft failure
Ahmed	112	15 (13.3%)	54 (48.2%)	34 (30.3%)	N/A	9 (8%)
Bassiouny	100	3 (3%)	8 (8%)	6 (6%)	N/A	0
Mitchell	76	9 (11.8%)	23 (30.2%)	17 (22.3%)	N/A	8 (10.5%)
Rode	38	4 (10.5%)	8 (21%)	5 (13.1%)	N/A	3 (7.8%)
Ahmad	38	0	11 (29%)	10 (26.3%)	4 (11%)	7 (18%)
Stone	37	1 (2.7%)	12 (32.4%)	14 (37.8%)	N/A	0
Hendren	32	1 (3.1%)	2 (6.2%)	1 (3.1%)	4 (12.4%)	0
German	32	1 (3.1%)	9 (28.1%)	7 (21.8%)	N/A	1 (3.1%)

The key to minimizing the occurrence of anastamotic leaks and strictures is optimizing the blood supply to the most distal aspect of the colon. It is necessary to choose the conduit with a reliable blood supply, avoid torsion of the conduit, avoid narrowing the thoracic inlet, and minimize the length of the colon graft. Several authors have recommended strategies for improving the vascularity of the colon. Hadidi recommended ligation of the middle colic vessels at the time of gastrostomy for patients with long gap atresia and caustic ingestions. This strategy was pursued to increase the blood supply to the conduit through the marginal artery. Although no objective studies demonstrated increased blood flow in this report, only one out of 11 patients had a stricture of the esophagocolonic anastamosis, and no leaks occurred (130). Adult surgeons have suggested that arterial augmentation of the cervical part of the colon would improve circulation and diminish vascular insufficiency of the cervical anastamosis. This technique requires a microvascular anastamosis of the colic vessels at the terminus of the colon graft to cervical vessels. Using this technique, the rate of leakage (7%) was substantially lower in the "supercharge" group compared to the controls (54%). Disadvantages of this strategy are that the operation is prolonged for several hours, anticoagulation is required, and a microvascular surgeon must be available. Given the size differences of pediatric blood vessels, it is not certain that this strategy can be extrapolated to young children; however, it should be considered in the older child (131).

Strictures may occur at either the esophageal or gastric anastamosis. Strictures of the esophageal anastamosis usually result from the fibrosis that occurs following a leak that heals. Occasionally, a proximal stricture will occur in the absence of a leak. Early management should be dilations under general anesthesia. Refractory strictures may require resection of the anastamosis and a repeat esophageal to colon anastamosis.

Strictures at the gastric anastamosis are rare and may result from either subacute ischemia or acid reflux. A persistent stricture of the gastrocolonic anastamosis limits emptying of the conduit and results in food retention and the potential for aspiration. Most surgeons would not attempt dilation but would revise the anastamosis.

Long-term Complications
The ideal replacement for the esophagus should function long term as a conduit to the stomach. Large series demonstrate patient satisfaction with colon replacement of the esophagus. Kelly et al. reported on 22 patients with a follow-up of 12.8 years who had undergone colon replacement of the esophagus. Eighty-seven percent of the patients were eating a regular diet and had no upper intestinal symptoms (132). All of the 12 patients reported by Lindahl et al. had good outcomes with minimal symptoms (133).

Dysphagia following colon interposition may result from a proximal stricture (coloesophageal anastamosis), distal stricture (cologastric anastamosis), colonic redundancy, acid reflux, or alkaline reflux. A barium swallow will identify strictures and colonic redundancy. Strictures are discussed elsewhere (vida supra). Redundancy of the colon is thought to result from a combination of technical issues and differential growth of the colon. The colon is often longer than the marginal artery, and it is a natural inclination to leave the colon with some extra length. Unfortunately, this will predispose to redundancy and increases the amount of colon to perfuse. In Hendren's series of 32 patients, four had symptomatic redundancy. Several large series do not report redundancy as a complication, and others report it as an asymptomatic finding (134). When the patient is symptomatic and the barium esophagram demonstrates dilation

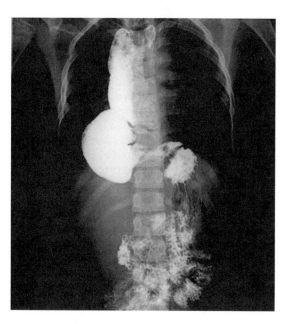

Figure 3   Redundant colon following a colon interposition graft.

and redundancy, the surgeon has several technical options. Several surgeons have reported a transthoracic "sleeve" resection of the colon, taking care to preserve the marginal artery on the mesenteric side of the colon. Other surgeons have performed a thoracoabdominal approach to resect the distal colon, resite the cologastric anastamosis, and taper the intrathoracic colon. We have successfully treated colonic redundancy by transhiatal mobilization and intrabdominal tapering coloplasty. One strategy to minimize the occurrence of redundancy is to perform the cologastric anastomosis last. Using this strategy, the colon can be pulled down onto the stomach and the redundant colon excised. It is not clear that the route of the colon influences redundancy as the colon has been observed to have symptomatic redundancy in all of the routes to the neck, including a case report of redundancy in a subcutaneous, presternal colon (135) (Fig. 3).

Intrinsic diseases of the colon occurring in the transplanted colon are extremely rare. No evidence exists for the occurrence of inflammatory bowel disease in the transposed colon. There are several case reports of adenocarcinoma of the colon esophagus, and one case report of synchronous adenomas in the native colon and colon esophagus (136–139). A juvenile polyp has been reported in the colon esophagus of an 11-year-old child (140). These reports suggest that any unexplained symptoms such as pain, hematochezia, or hematemesis in a patient with a colon esophagus may warrant endoscopic evaluation. Further, the colon esophagus should undergo surveillance endoscopy at the same time as it is warranted for the native colon. It is not uncommon for the patient who undergoes replacement of the esophagus with colon to have transient diarrhea postoperatively. This usually resolves with bulking agents and time.

A number of unusual and infrequent complications have been reported in patients undergoing replacement of the esophagus with colon. This includes formation of a colopericardial fistula, cardiac tamponade due to intrathoracic colonic volvulous, and peptic ulceration (141–143).

Gastric Transposition

The stomach has long been an esophageal substitute in adults undergoing esophageal resection for carcinoma. Application to esophageal replacement in children has been a recent event, with most of the experience concentrated in two centers (144,145). One advantage of using the stomach for esophageal replacement is that it requires only one anastamosis (esophagogastric) as opposed to the three anastamoses required for colon replacement of the esophagus. The blood supply to the stomach is reliable and easily managed during mobilization of the stomach. Conduit length is rarely an issue. Complication rates are comparable to colon replacement and gastric tube replacement.

Anatomic Considerations

The stomach is a hollow organ with a consistent size for use as a conduit to the proximal esophagus. One exception to this finding is the microgastria that can be associated with pure EA. The patient with microgastria should be considered for an alternative type of esophageal substitute. The blood supply to the stomach has rich submucosal collaterals that allow division of three of the four main blood vessels of the stomach with preservation of blood flow. The blood vessels contributing blood supply to the stomach are the right gastric artery, left gastric artery, right gastroepiploic artery, and left gastroepiploic artery. Mobilization of the stomach to the neck requires division of the left gastric artery. Occasionally, an aberrant left hepatic artery originates from the left hepatic artery. To avoid hepatic necrosis, this anatomic situation should be looked for, and the division of the left gastric artery should be done distal to the hepatic artery. Once the left gastric artery is divided, the stomach will depend upon the right gastroepiploic artery and its connection to the left gastroepiploic artery for its blood supply.

Surgical Procedure

Prior to the procedure, an upper gastrointestinal series should be performed to assess the size of the stomach. This information is usually ascertained at the time of gastrostomy tube placement. Patients with the potential for caustic gastric injury should undergo repeat upper endoscopy to ensure the viability of the proximal stomach. After mobilization of the stomach and proximal esophagus, esophagectomy is performed. Approximately half of the time this can be accomplished without a thoracotomy. Previous surgery on the esophagus and caustic injury are associated with the more frequent need to perform a thoracotomy to assist with esophagectomy. The most common route of passage for the stomach conduit is the posterior mediastinum. This minimizes, but does not eliminate the potential for respiratory compromise during gastric dilation. Alternatively, the stomach can be passed in a retrohilar, transthoracic approach. Due to the inevitable vagotomy during esophagectomy, a pyloroplasty is recommended. A jejunostomy tube is placed in younger patients who have not developed oral feeding habits. Patients are paralyzed and ventilated postoperatively for several days. This minimizes respiratory complications from the mediastinal dissection and relocation of the stomach. The stomach is decompressed by an indwelling nasogastric tube. A soft drain is placed adjacent to the esophagogastric anastomosis. On the seventh postoperative day, a water-soluble contrast study is performed to evaluate the proximal anastamosis, transgastric passage, and the state of the pyloroplasty. If the study does not show a leak, oral feedings are started.

Short-term Complications

Most of the significant intraoperative complications result from the mediastinal dissection to perform the esophagectomy. Different authors have reported tracheal perforation, hemorrhage, and death due to division of an aberrant subclavian artery. Most of the early deaths have resulted from respiratory complications in children with multiple previous thoracotomies. Patients with preexisting tracheomalacia may have airway collapse worsen with placement of the stomach within the posterior mediastium. Aortopexy may be required to alleviate this postoperative complication. In Spitz's series, 12% of patients developed anastamotic leakage. Twenty percent of his patients developed an anastomatic stricture (144). Coran reported that 36% of his patients who underwent gastric transposition developed an anastamotic leakage and 49% developed a stricture (145). In both of these series, leaks were self-limited and were treated with an extended period of avoidance of oral feeding. Strictures were treated with periodic dilation until swallowing was returned to normal. Children who undergo jejunostomy placement may develop mechanical complications of the jejunostomy. These complications include jejunostomy leakage, volvulous, and small bowel obstruction (Table 5).

Table 5 Complications of Gastric Transposition Replacement of the Esophagus

Author	Patients	Mortality (%)	Anastamotic leakage (%)	Stricture (%)
Spitz	173	5.2	12	19.6
Coran	41	0	36	49
Tannur	35	5.7	20	14.2

Long-term Complications
Transposition of the stomach into the mediastinum or thorax results in complete vagotomy of the stomach. The limited studies available demonstrate abnormal emptying of the transposed stomach. Adult studies have demonstrated improved emptying with the upright position. Spitz found that electric impedance tomography demonstrated abnormal emptying and retention of the gastric reservoir function (146). In Spitz' report of 173 patients undergoing gastric transposition, 30.6% were found to have significant swallowing problems. Half of these patients had prolonged swallowing problems. Severe delay of gastric emptying was evident in 8.7% of the patients. Abnormalities in gastric emptying and the intrathoracic position of the transposed stomach predispose to reflux. This reflux can either be acid reflux or nonacid reflux. Reflux induced injury to the vocal cords was noted by Casson et al. (147). The presence of unabated reflux into the proximal esophagus raises the concern for the development of Barrett's esophagus. Not enough long-term information is available to make recommendations regarding surveillance endoscopy.

Gastric Tube Replacement of the Esophagus
Tubularization of the greater curvature of the stomach creates a well-vascularized conduit that can bridge the gap between the attached stomach and the proximal esophagus. The abundant blood supply of the stomach permits this gastric reconstruction to function as a conduit. Tubularization of the stomach was successfully applied to adults by Heimlich in the 1960s (148). In 1968, Burrington and Stephens reported their experience in the management of EA with a gastric tube technique (149). The gastric tube technique was introduced at that time due to dissatisfaction with the pulmonary complications of total gastric transposition. Early attempts were accomplished in patients who needed an esophageal replacement but had anorectal malformations or failed colon conduits. Several studies have compared colon interposition with gastric tube outcomes and found comparable results (133,150).

Procedure
Creation of a gastric tube requires knowledge of the collateral blood supply of the stomach. The gastric tube relies upon blood flow from either the right or left gastroepiploic artery. The isoperistaltic tube derives its blood supply from the right gastroepiploic artery, and the antiperistaltic tube is supplied by the collaterals from the left gastroepiploic artery. When the stomach is approached intraoperatively, the omentum should be divided at a distance from the collateral blood supply that runs along the greater curvature. Splenectomy was performed in the past; however, most recent experiences do not recommend this component of the procedure. Surgeons have compelling arguments for either an isoperistaltic or antiperistaltic tube. The isoperistaltic tube is felt to have greater length by some surgeons. It is also believed to have less risk for kinking at the junction of the tube with the stomach when compared to the antiperistaltic tube. The antiperistaltic tube is felt to have less risk for compromise of the pylorus and ultimately gastric emptying. Long-term outcomes fail to demonstrate the advantage of either approach. After the orientation of the conduit is chosen, the stomach is divided along the axis of the greater curvature. This can either be done with a stapler or with a two-layer suture closure. All authors advocate using an intraluminal tube to standardize the size of the lumen of the conduit. The gastric tube can be brought to the neck through either the left thorax or the retrosternal space. Some authors perform the esophagogastric anastomasis in a delayed fashion. When this approach is taken, the surgeon must be aware of the cervical symptoms of reflux up the conduit. Some children report burning pain in the neck and others have developed skin changes while awaiting creation of the esophageal—gastric tube anastomasis. A gastrostomy tube is often placed in patients. If necessary, this can be placed through the posterior wall of the stomach due to the forward rotation of the body of the stomach. Prior placement of a gastrostomy tube is not a contraindication to gastric tube formation. If a gastric tube is contemplated, the gastrostomy should be placed either in the midbody of the stomach, or if permissible, on the lesser curvature. If a primary anastamosis is performed, a water-soluble contrast study is performed to assess the anatomy and rule out a leak. If the anastamosis is delayed, intragastric feedings can be started 5–7 days postoperatively. Patients with significant gastric tube reflux prior to closure of the proximal anastomosis may be fed with a transgastric jejunal feeding tube. Some surgeons place jejunostomy tubes at the time of gastric tube creation. A pyloroplasty is not necessary unless esophagectomy is performed concurrently owing to the

likely injury to the vagotomy. A few patients subsequently require pyloroplasty because of delayed gastric emptying.

Short-term Complications

Leakage of the anastamosis between the gastric tube and the proximal esophagus is common. Most surgeons perform the anastamosis in the neck, and the systemic impact of the leak is minimized. Ein et al. reported that 66% of the anastamoses leaked in his series of 36 patients (151). Schettini and Pinus reported a 63.3% rate of leakage in their series of 19 patients (152). Although delayed closure may minimize edema at the end of the gastric tube, it does not seem to reduce the rate of leakage when studies are compared. The long suture line and dependence upon collateral blood supply predispose to leakage. Unfortunately, no intraoperative evaluations are reliable at predicting vascular insufficiency. Vascular insufficiency also predisposes to anastomotic stricture. Ein et al. reported 41% of his patients developed a stricture and Schettini and Pinus reported a 42.1% stricture rate (151,152). In most studies, strictures responded to one or two dilations and only a small percentage required resection of the anastamosis. When the conduit is brought through the mediastinum or thorax, the long suture line may allow the formation of fistulas. Fistulas have been reported between the gastric tube and the pleura, bronchus, and heart (153–155). Several adults have been reported to have strangulation of the gastric tube by the azygous vein arch during passage of the gastric tube through the posterior mediastinum (156). In addition, several adults have been reported to have ST-T abnormalities that resulted from cardiac compression from a retrosternal gastric tube (157). These complications have not been reported in children.

Long-term Complications

The most important indicator of the success of replacement of the esophagus by any conduit is the ability to swallow and maintain normal nutrition and growth. All of the large series of gastric tube replacements indicate normal swallowing in the majority of their patients. Ein et al. reported that 29 of 32 patients followed for over a year had normal swallowing (151). Lindahl et al. reported that 7 of 10 patients followed long term had no swallowing symptoms (133). In all series, patients are noted to have minor symptoms with meat and bread that are alleviated with the consumption of liquids. A number of preoperative and mechanical factors influence swallowing. Children with long gap atresia who have not had oral intake prior to esophageal substitution have delayed onset of oral feeding and dysphagia. Children with proximal esophageal and pharyngeal burns from caustic materials also have impaired swallowing. Fortunately, most children adapt with time, and the majority regain swallowing function enough to discontinue intragastric or jejunal feeding. Several mechanical problems can result in difficulty swallowing. The most obvious cause is stricture. Approximately 40% of patients develop a stricture at the gastric tube—esophageal anastomosis. Most achieve normal size of the anastomosis with one or two dilations. It is unusual to have to perform a resection of the proximal esophagus to correct a recalcitrant stricture. Dysphagia associated with an anastamotic stricture should managed with dilations and possible resection. Strictures have also been noted in the distal gastric tube contained within the thorax or mediastinum (Fig. 4). This may also be dilated but caution must applied as perforation can result in mediastinal soilage and loss of the gastric tube. Anatomic obstruction of the tube has been noted at the junction with the stomach and the thoracic inlet. Several authors have reported reoperation for stenosis at the thoracic inlet. Surgical options have included widening of the Sibsons fascia in the thoracic inlet and division of the omohyoid muscle to enlarge the space. Kinking of the attachment of the gastric tube to the stomach may inhibit emptying. This has been treated by performing a side-to-side anastomosis of the distal gastric tube to the stomach (152) (Table 6).

Creation of a gastric tube allows unimpeded gastric reflux up the conduit. Reflux is present in all patients postoperatively, and is worsened in the supine position. In a series of 10 patients who had undergone gastric tube replacement, Anderson et al. found four patients with symptomatic nocturnal reflux, and an additional patient required a fundoplication of his gastric tube (150). Lindahl et al. reported one of ten patients with symptomatic reflux. This condition was controlled by elevating the head of the bed while sleeping (133). Pinus and Schettini reported 12 of 19 patients with reflux. They felt that only two patients had clinical manifestations of reflux, and that the main factors influencing reflux were a wider constructed gastric tube, gastric tube terminating near the pylorus, and a small gastric remnant (152). Due

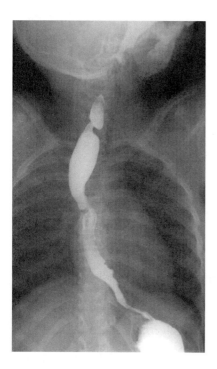

Figure 4 Postoperative stricture following a reversed gastric tube.

Table 6 Complications of Gastric Tube Replacement of the Esophagus

Author	Patients	Mortality	Anastamotic leakage	Stricture
Ein	36	3 (8.3%)	66%	41%
Burgnon	21	1 (4.7%)	2 (9.5%)	2 (9.5%)
Schettini	19	1 (5.2%)	63.3%	42.1%

to the fact that gastric mucosa lines the gastric tube, reflux damage to the conduit is unlikely. However, acid secretion in the tube can lead to bleeding and perforation of the tube due to ulcer formation. In addition, the proximity of acid and gastric mucosa to the cervical esophagus can result in the formation of Barrett's esophagus. Lindahl et al. found that 10 of 14 patients with gastric tubes had Barrett's type mucosa above the anastamosis (158). The presence of Barrett's esophagus in these studies suggests the need for routine endoscopy of the gastric tube and proximal esophagus. Another indication for surveillance endoscopy is the occurrence of gastric tube cancer. Although these cancers have only been reported in adults after esophagectomy, the length of time a child will have a gastric tube in place suggests the need for surveillance endoscopy to detect this rare but lethal cancer (159).

REFERENCES

1. Myers NA. Oesophageal atresia: The epitome of modern surgery. Ann R Coll Surg Engl 1974; 54:277–287.
2. Spitz L. Esophageal atresia: Past, present, and future. J Pediatr Surg 1996; 31:19–25.
3. Lanman T. Congenital atresia of the esophagus: a study of thirty-two cases. Arch Surg 1940; 41:1060–1083.
4. Leven N. Congenital atresia of the esophagus with tracheoesophageal fistula. J Thorac Cardiovasc Surg 1941; 10:648–657.
5. Ladd W. The surgical treatment of esophageal atresia and tracheoesophageal fistulas. N Engl J Med 1944; 230:625–637.
6. Haight C, Towsley H. Congenital atresia of the esophagus with tracheoesophageal fistula. Extrapleural ligation of fistula and end to end anastamosis of esophageal segments. Surg Gynecol Obstet 1943; 76:672–688.
7. Crisera CA, Connelly PR, Marmureanu AR, et al. Esophageal atresia with tracheoesophageal fistula: Suggested mechanism in faulty organogenesis. J Pediatr Surg 1999; 34:204–208.

8. Harris J, Kallen B, Robert E. Descriptive epidemiology of alimentary tract atresia. Teratology 1995; 52:15–29.

9. Morini F, Cozzi DA, Ilari M, et al. Pattern of cardiovascular anomalies associated with esophageal atresia: Support for a caudal pharyngeal arch neurocristopathy. Pediatr Res 2001; 50:565–568.

10. Okada A, Usui N, Inoue M, et al. Esophageal atresia in Osaka: A review of 39 years' experience. J Pediatr Surg 1997; 32:1570–1574.

11. Ein SH, Shandling B. Pure esophageal atresia: A 50-year review. J Pediatr Surg 1994; 29:1208–1211.

12. Poenaru D, Laberge JM, Neilson IR, et al. A more than 25-year experience with end-to-end versus end-to-side repair for esophageal atresia. J Pediatr Surg 1991; 26:472–476; discussion 6–7.

13. Harrison MR, Hanson BA, Mahour GH, et al. The significance of right aortic arch in repair of esophageal atresia and tracheoesophageal fistula. J Pediatr Surg 1977;12:861–869.

14. Berdon WE, Baker DH, Schullinger JN, et al. Plain film detection of right aortic arch in infants with esophageal atresia and tracheoesophageal fistula. J Pediatr Surg 1979; 14:436–437.

15. Canty TG, Jr., Boyle EM, Jr., Linden B, et al. Aortic arch anomalies associated with long gap esophageal atresia and tracheoesophageal fistula. J Pediatr Surg 1997; 32:1587–1591.

16. Taylor AC, Breen KJ, Auldist A, et al. Gastroesophageal reflux and related pathology in adults who were born with esophageal atresia: A long-term follow-up study. Clin Gastroenterol Hepatol 2007; 5:702–706.

17. Lomas FE, Dahlstrom JE, Ford JH. VACTERL with hydrocephalus: Family with X-linked VACTERL-H. Am J Med Genet 1998; 76:74–8.

18. Choudhry M, Boyd PA, Chamberlain PF, et al. Prenatal diagnosis of tracheo-oesophageal fistula and oesophageal atresia. Prenat Diagn 2007; 27:608–610.

19. Usui N, Kamata S, Ishikawa S, et al. Anomalies of the tracheobronchial tree in patients with esophageal atresia. J Pediatr Surg 1996; 31:258–262.

20. Rosenthal A. Congenital atresia of the esophagus with tracheoesophageal fistula: report of eight cases. Arch Pathol 1931; 12:756.

21. Crisera CA, Maldonado TS, Kadison AS, et al. Patterning of the "distal esophagus" in esophageal atresia with tracheo-esophageal fistula: Is thyroid transcription factor 1 a player? J Surg Res 2000; 92:245–249.

22. Crisera CA, Maldonado TS, Longaker MT, et al. Defective fibroblast growth factor signaling allows for nonbranching growth of the respiratory-derived fistula tract in esophageal atresia with tracheoesophageal fistula. J Pediatr Surg 2000; 35:1421–1425.

23. Yeung CK, Spitz L, Brereton RJ, et al. Congenital esophageal stenosis due to tracheobronchial remnants: A rare but important association with esophageal atresia. J Pediatr Surg 1992; 27:852–855.

24. Gross R. The Surgery of Infancy and Childhood. Philadelphia: WB Saunders, 1953.

25. Waterston DJ, Carter RE, Aberdeen E. Oesophageal atresia: Tracheo-oesophageal fistula. A study of survival in 218 infants. Lancet 1962; 1:819–822.

26. Spitz L, Kiely EM, Morecroft JA, et al. Oesophageal atresia: At-risk groups for the 1990s. J Pediatr Surg 1994; 29:723–725.

27. Holcomb GW III. Survival after gastrointestinal perforation from esophageal atresia and tracheoesophageal fistula. J Pediatr Surg 1993; 28:1532–1535.

28. Templeton JM Jr, Templeton JJ, Schnaufer L, et al. Management of esophageal atresia and tracheoesophageal fistula in the neonate with severe respiratory distress syndrome. J Pediatr Surg 1985; 20:394–397.

29. Domajnko B, Drugas GT, Pegoli W Jr. Temporary occlusion of the gastroesophageal junction: A modified technique for stabilization of the neonate with esophageal atresia and tracheoesophageal fistula requiring mechanical ventilation. Pediatr Surg Int 2007; 23:1127–1129.

30. McKinnon LJ, Kosloske AM. Prediction and prevention of anastomotic complications of esophageal atresia and tracheoesophageal fistula. J Pediatr Surg 1990; 25:778–781.

31. Hack H. Use of the esophageal Doppler machine to help guide the intraoperative management of two children with pheochromocytoma. Paediatr Anaesth 2006; 16:867–876.

32. Sharma S, Sinha SK, Rawat JD, et al. Azygos vein preservation in primary repair of esophageal atresia with tracheoesophageal fistula. Pediatr Surg Int 2007; 23:1215–1218.

33. Upadhyaya VD, Gangopadhyaya AN, Gopal SC, et al. Is ligation of azygos vein necessary in primary repair of tracheoesophageal fistula with esophageal atresia? Eur J Pediatr Surg 2007; 17:236–240.

34. Kosloske AM. Azygous flap technique for reinforcement of esophageal closure. J Pediatr Surg 1990; 25:793–794.

35. Chittmittrapap S, Spitz L, Kiely EM, et al. Anastomotic stricture following repair of esophageal atresia. J Pediatr Surg 1990; 25:508–511.

36. Spitz L, Kiely E, Brereton RJ, et al. Management of esophageal atresia. World J Surg 1993; 17:296–300.

37. Myers NA, Beasley SW, Auldist AW. Secondary esophageal surgery following repair of esophageal atresia with distal tracheoesophageal fistula. J Pediatr Surg 1990;25:773–777.

38. Neilson IR, Croitoru DP, Guttman FM, et al. Distal congenital esophageal stenosis associated with esophageal atresia. J Pediatr Surg 1991; 26:478–481; discussion 81–82.

39. Jardine LA, Kimble RM. An unusual cause of salivary leak post tracheoesophageal fistula repair. Pediatr Surg Int 2008; 24:443–445.

40. McCallion WA, Hannon RJ, Boston VE. Prophylactic extrapleural chest drainage following repair of esophageal atresia: Is it necessary? J Pediatr Surg 1992; 27:561.

41. Kay S, Shaw K. Revisiting the role of routine retropleural drainage after repair of esophageal atresia with distal tracheoesophageal fistula. J Pediatr Surg 1999; 34:1082–1085.

42. Upadhyaya VD, Gopal SC, Gangopadhyaya AN, et al. Role of fibrin glue as a sealant to esophageal anastomosis in cases of congenital esophageal atresia with tracheoesophageal fistula. World J Surg 2007; 31:2412–2415.

43. Fedakar-Senyucel M, Bingol-Kologlu M, Vargun R, et al. The effects of local and sustained release of fibroblast growth factor on wound healing in esophageal anastomoses. J Pediatr Surg 2008; 43:290–295.

44. Holcomb GW III, Rothenberg SS, Bax KM, et al. Thoracoscopic repair of esophageal atresia and tracheoesophageal fistula: A multi-institutional analysis. Ann Surg 2005; 242:422–428; discussion 8–30.

45. Chavin K, Field G, Chandler J, et al. Save the child's esophagus: Management of major disruption after repair of esophageal atresia. J Pediatr Surg 1996; 31:48–51; discussion 2.

46. Wheatley MJ, Coran AG. Pericardial flap interposition for the definitive management of recurrent tracheoesophageal fistula. J Pediatr Surg 1992; 27:1122–1125; discussion 5–6.

47. Ko HK, Shin JH, Song HY, et al. Balloon dilation of anastomotic strictures secondary to surgical repair of esophageal atresia in a pediatric population: Long-term results. J Vasc Interv Radiol 2006; 17:1327–1333.

48. Uhlen S, Fayoux P, Vachin F, et al. Mitomycin C: An alternative conservative treatment for refractory esophageal stricture in children? Endoscopy 2006;38:404–407.

49. Bonnard A, Paye-Jaouen A, Aizenfisz S, et al. Laparoscopically harvested omental flap for recurrent tracheoesophageal fistula in a newborn baby. J Thorac Cardiovasc Surg 2007; 134:1592–1593.

50. Bargy F, Manach Y, Helardot PG, et al. Risk of recurrent laryngeal nerve palsy in surgery of esophageal atresia. Chir Pediatr 1983; 24:130–132.

51. Kawahara H, Kubota A, Hasegawa T, et al. Lack of distal esophageal contractions is a key determinant of gastroesophageal reflux disease after repair of esophageal atresia. J Pediatr Surg 2007; 42:2017–2021.

52. Qi BQ, Merei J, Farmer P, et al. The vagus and recurrent laryngeal nerves in the rodent experimental model of esophageal atresia. J Pediatr Surg 1997; 32:1580–1586.

53. Pederiva F, Burgos E, Francica I, et al. Intrinsic esophageal innervation in esophageal atresia without fistula. Pediatr Surg Int 2008; 24:95–100.

54. Filler RM, Rossello PJ, Lebowitz RL. Life-threatening anoxic spells caused by tracheal compression after repair of esophageal atresia: Correction by surgery. J Pediatr Surg 1976; 11:739–748.

55. Filler RM, Messineo A, Vinograd I. Severe tracheomalacia associated with esophageal atresia: Results of surgical treatment. J Pediatr Surg 1992; 27:1136–1140; discussion 40–41.

56. Spitz L, Kiely E, Brereton RJ. Esophageal atresia: Five year experience with 148 cases. J Pediatr Surg 1987; 22:103–108.

57. Schwartz MZ, Filler RM. Tracheal compression as a cause of apnea following repair of tracheoesophageal fistula: Treatment by aortopexy. J Pediatr Surg 1980; 15:842–848.

58. Morabito A, MacKinnon E, Alizai N, et al. The anterior mediastinal approach for management of tracheomalacia. J Pediatr Surg 2000; 35:1456–1458.

59. Schaarschmidt K, Kolberg-Schwerdt A, Bunke K, et al. A technique for thoracoscopic aortopericardiosternopexy. Surg Endosc 2002; 16:1639.

60. Calcagni G, Gesualdo F, Brunelle F, et al. An unusual case of left aberrant innominate artery with right aortic arch: Evaluation with high-resolution CT. Pediatr Radiol 2008; 38:115–117.

61. Spitz L. Congenital esophageal stenosis distal to associated esophageal atresia. J Pediatr Surg 1973; 8:973–974.

62. Lee H, Morgan K, Abramowsky C, et al. Leiomyoma at the site of esophageal atresia repair. J Pediatr Surg 2001; 36:1832–1833.

63. Robertson DF, Mobaireek K, Davis GM, et al. Late pulmonary function following repair of tracheoesophageal fistula or esophageal atresia. Pediatr Pulmonol 1995; 20:21–26.

64. Koivusalo A, Pakarinen MP, Turunen P, et al. Health-related quality of life in adult patients with esophageal atresia—A questionnaire study. J Pediatr Surg 2005; 40:307–312.

65. Guo W, Fonkalsrud EW, Swaniker F, Kodner A. Relationship of esophageal anastomotic tension to the development of gastroesophageal reflux. J Pediatr Surg 1997; 32:1337–1340.

66. Little DC, Rescorla FJ, Grosfeld JL, et al. Long-term analysis of children with esophageal atresia and tracheoesophageal fistula. J Pediatr Surg 2003; 38:852–856.

67. Romeo C, Bonanno N, Baldari S, et al. Gastric motility disorders in patients operated on for esophageal atresia and tracheoesophageal fistula: Long-term evaluation. J Pediatr Surg 2000; 35:740–744.

68. Lindahl H, Rintala R, Sariola H. Chronic esophagitis and gastric metaplasia are frequent late complications of esophageal atresia. J Pediatr Surg 1993; 28:1178–1180.

69. Wheatley MJ, Coran AG, Wesley JR. Efficacy of the Nissen fundoplication in the management of gastroesophageal reflux following esophageal atresia repair. J Pediatr Surg 1993; 28:53–55.

70. Bergmeijer JH, Tibboel D, Hazebroek FW. Nissen fundoplication in the management of gastroesophageal reflux occurring after repair of esophageal atresia. J Pediatr Surg 2000; 35:573–576.

71. Kawahara H, Imura K, Yagi M, et al. Collis-Nissen procedure in patients with esophageal atresia: Long-term evaluation. World J Surg 2002; 26:1222–1227.

72. Schier F, Korn S, Michel E. Experiences of a parent support group with the long-term consequences of esophageal atresia. J Pediatr Surg 2001; 36:605–610.

73. Lessin MS, Wesselhoeft CW, Luks FI, et al. Primary repair of long-gap esophageal atresia by mobilization of the distal esophagus. Eur J Pediatr Surg 1999; 9:369–372.

74. Livaditis A. End-to-end anastomosis in esophageal atresia. A clinical and experimental study. Scand J Thorac Cardiovasc Surg 1969 :Suppl 2:7–20.

75. Livaditis A, Radberg L, Odensjo G. Esophageal end-to-end anastomosis. Reduction of anastomotic tension by circular myotomy. Scand J Thorac Cardiovasc Surg 1972; 6:206–214.

76. Coran AG. Ultra-long-gap esophageal atresia: How long is long? Ann Thorac Surg 1994; 57:528–529.

77. Giacomoni MA, Tresoldi M, Zamana C, et al. Circular myotomy of the distal esophageal stump for long gap esophageal atresia. J Pediatr Surg 2001; 36:855–857.

78. Lai JY, Sheu JC, Chang PY, et al. Experience with distal circular myotomy for long-gap esophageal atresia. J Pediatr Surg 1996; 31:1503–1508.

79. Slim MS. Circular myotomy of the esophagus: Clinical application in esophageal atresia. Ann Thorac Surg 1977; 23:62–66.

80. Orringer MB, Kirsh MM, Sloan H. Long-term esophageal function following repair of esophageal atresia. Ann Surg 1977; 186:436–443.

81. Kimura K, Nishijima E, Tsugawa C, et al. A new approach for the salvage of unsuccessful esophageal atresia repair: A spiral myotomy and delayed definitive operation. J Pediatr Surg 1987; 22:981–983.

82. Rossello PJ, Lebron H, Franco AA. The technique of myotomy in esophageal reconstruction: An experimental study. J Pediatr Surg 1980; 15:430–432.

83. Lindell-Iwan L. Modification of Livaditis' myotomy for long gap oesophageal atresia. Ann Chir Gynaecol 1990; 79:101–102.

84. Gough MH. Esophageal atresia—Use of an anterior flap in the difficult anastomosis. J Pediatr Surg 1980; 15:310–311.

85. Fernandez MS, Gutierrez C, Ibanez V, et al. Long-gap esophageal atresia: Reconstruction preserving all portions of the esophagus by Scharli's technique. Pediatr Surg Int 1998; 14:17–20.

86. Evans M. Application of Collis gastroplasty to the management of esophageal atresia. J Pediatr Surg 1995; 30:1232–1235.

87. Pohlson EC, Schaller RT, Tapper D. Improved survival with primary anastomosis in the low birth weight neonate with esophageal atresia and tracheoesophageal fistula. J Pediatr Surg 1988; 23:418–421.

88. Alexander F, Johanningman J, Martin LW. Staged repair improves outcome of high-risk premature infants with esophageal atresia and tracheoesophageal fistula. J Pediatr Surg 1993; 28:151–154.

89. Howard R, Myers N. Esophageal atresia: a technique for elongating the upper pouch. Surgery 1965; 58:725.

90. Hendren WH, Hale JR. Esophageal atresia treated by electromagnetic bougienage and subsequent repair. J Pediatr Surg 1976; 11:713–722.

91. Rehbein F, Schweder N. Reconstruction of the esophagus without colon transplantation in cases of atresia. J Pediatr Surg 1971; 6:746–752.

92. Shafer AD, David TE. Suture fistula as a means of connecting upper and lower segments in esophageal atresia. J Pediatr Surg 1974; 9:669–673.

93. Kimura K, Soper RT. Multistaged extrathoracic esophageal elongation for long gap esophageal atresia. J Pediatr Surg 1994; 29:566–568.

94. Kimura K, Nishijima E, Tsugawa C, et al. Multistaged extrathoracic esophageal elongation procedure for long gap esophageal atresia: Experience with 12 patients. J Pediatr Surg 2001; 36:1725–1727.

95. Foker JE, Linden BC, Boyle EM, Jr., et al. Development of a true primary repair for the full spectrum of esophageal atresia. Ann Surg 1997; 226:533–41; discussion 41–3.

96. Vogel AM, Yang EY, Fishman SJ. Hydrostatic stretch-induced growth facilitating primary anastomosis in long-gap esophageal atresia. J Pediatr Surg 2006; 41:1170–1172.

97. Boix-Ochoa J, Ashcraft KW. Gastroesophageal Reflux. In: Ashcraft KW, Holcomb GW, Murphy JP, eds. Pediatric Surgery. Philadelphia, PA: Elsevier Saunders, 2005:383–404.

98. Winkelstein A. Peptic esophagitis: A new clinical entity. JAMA 1935; 104:906–915.

99. Carre IJ. Postural treatment of children with a partial thoracic stomach ('hiatus hernia'). Arch Dis Child 1960; 35:569–580.

100. Esposito C, Montupet P, Amici G, et al. Complications of laparoscopic antireflux surgery in childhood. Surg Endosc 2000; 14:622–624.

101. Dalla Vecchia LK, Grosfeld JL, West KW, et al. Reoperation after Nissen fundoplication in children with gastroesophageal reflux: Experience with 130 patients. Ann Surg 1997; 226:315–321; discussion 21–23.

102. Esposito C, Van Der Zee DC, Settimi A, et al. Risks and benefits of surgical management of gastroesophageal reflux in neurologically impaired children. Surg Endosc 2003; 17:708–710.

103. Fonkalsrud EW, Ashcraft KW, Coran AG, et al. Surgical treatment of gastroesophageal reflux in children: A combined hospital study of 7467 patients. Pediatrics 1998; 101:419–422.

104. Fung KP, Seagram G, Pasieka J, et al. Investigation and outcome of 121 infants and children requiring Nissen fundoplication for the management of gastroesophageal reflux. Clin Invest Med 1990; 13:237–246.

105. Humphrey GM, Najmaldin AS. Laparoscopic Nissen fundoplication in disabled infants and children. J Pediatr Surg 1996; 31:596–599.

106. Rothenberg SS. Experience with 220 consecutive laparoscopic Nissen fundoplications in infants and children. J Pediatr Surg 1998; 33:274–278.

107. Steyaert H, Al Mohaidly M, Lembo MA, et al. Long-term outcome of laparoscopic Nissen and Toupet fundoplication in normal and neurologically impaired children. Surg Endosc 2003; 17:543–546.

108. Subramaniam R, Dickson AP. Long-term outcome of Boix-Ochoa and Nissen fundoplication in normal and neurologically impaired children. J Pediatr Surg 2000; 35:1214–1216.

109. Gotley DC, Smithers BM, Menzies B, et al. Laparoscopic Nissen fundoplication and postoperative dysphagia—Can it be predicted? Ann Acad Med Singapore 1996; 25:646–649.

110. Ostlie DJ, Miller KA, Holcomb GW III. Effective Nissen fundoplication length and bougie diameter size in young children undergoing laparoscopic Nissen fundoplication. J Pediatr Surg 2002; 37:1664–1666.

111. Richards CA, Milla PJ, Andrews PL, et al. Retching and vomiting in neurologically impaired children after fundoplication: Predictive preoperative factors. J Pediatr Surg 2001; 36:1401–1404.

112. Connor F. Gastrointestinal complications of fundoplication. Curr Gastroenterol Rep 2005; 7:219–226.

113. Bourne MC, Wheeldon C, MacKinlay GA, et al. Laparoscopic Nissen fundoplication in children: 2–5-year follow-up. Pediatr Surg Int 2003; 19:537–539.

114. Fonkalsrud EW. Nissen fundoplication for gastroesophageal reflux disease in infants and children. Semin Pediatr Surg 1998; 7:110–114.

115. Samuk I, Afriat R, Horne T, et al. Dumping syndrome following Nissen fundoplication, diagnosis, and treatment. J Pediatr Gastroenterol Nutr 1996; 23:235–240.

116. Avansino JR, Lorenz ML, Hendrickson M, et al. Characterization and management of paraesophageal hernias in children after antireflux operation. J Pediatr Surg 1999; 34:1610–1614.

117. Alrabeeah A, Giacomantonio M, Gillis DA. Paraesophageal hernia after Nissen fundoplication: A real complication in pediatric patients. J Pediatr Surg 1988; 23:766–768.

118. Tunell WP, Smith EI, Carson JA. Gastroesophageal reflux in childhood. The dilemma of surgical success. Ann Surg 1983; 197:560–565.

119. Caniano DA, Ginn-Pease ME, King DR. The failed antireflux procedure: Analysis of risk factors and morbidity. J Pediatr Surg 1990; 25:1022–1025; discussion 5–6.

120. Dedinsky GK, Vane DW, Black T, et al. Complications and reoperation after Nissen fundoplication in childhood. Am J Surg 1987; 153:177–183.

121. Graziano K, Teitelbaum DH, McLean K, et al. Recurrence after laparoscopic and open Nissen fundoplication: A comparison of the mechanisms of failure. Surg Endosc 2003; 17:704–707.

122. Hunter JG, Trus TL, Branum GD, et al. A physiologic approach to laparoscopic fundoplication for gastroesophageal reflux disease. Ann Surg 1996; 223:673–85; discussion 85–87.

123. Bassiouny IE, Bahnassy AF. Transhiatal esophagectomy and colonic interposition for caustic esophageal stricture. J Pediatr Surg 1992; 27:1091–1095; discussion 5–6.

124. Lundblad O. Ueber antethorakale oesophagoplastic. Acta Chir Scand 1921; 53:535–541.

125. Sandblom P. Treatment of congenital atresia of the oesophagus from a technical point of view. Acta Chir Scand 1948; 97:25–43.

126. Sonnenland J, Anson B, Beaton L. Surgical anatomy of the arterial supply to the colon from the superior mesenteric artery based on the study of 600 specimens. Surg Gynecol Obstet 1958; 106:385–398.

127. Peters JH, Kronson JW, Katz M, et al. Arterial anatomic considerations in colon interposition for esophageal replacement. Arch Surg 1995; 130:858–862; discussion 62–63.

128. Dreuw B, Fass J, Titkova S, et al. Colon interposition for esophageal replacement: Isoperistaltic or antiperistaltic? Experimental results. Ann Thorac Surg 2001; 71:303–308.

129. Freeman NV, Cass DT. Colon interposition: A modification of the Waterston technique using the normal esophageal route. J Pediatr Surg 1982; 17:17–21.

130. Hadidi AT. A technique to improve vascularity in colon replacement of the esophagus. Eur J Pediatr Surg 2006; 16:39–44.

131. Gorman JH III, Low DW, Guy T St, Gorman RC, Rosato EF. Extended left colon interposition for esophageal replacement using arterial augmentation. Ann Thorac Surg 2003; 76:933–935.

132. Kelly JP, Shackelford GD, Roper CL. Esophageal replacement with colon in children: Functional results and long-term growth. Ann Thorac Surg 1983; 36:634–643.

133. Lindahl H, Louhimo I, Virkola K. Colon interposition or gastric tube? Follow-up study of colon-esophagus and gastric tube-esophagus patients. J Pediatr Surg 1983; 18:58–63.

134. Hendren WH, Hendren WG. Colon interposition for esophagus in children. J Pediatr Surg 1985; 20:829–839.

135. Urschel JD. Late dysphagia after presternal colon interposition. Dysphagia 1996; 11:75–77.

136. Liau CT, Hsueh S, Yeow KM. Primary adenocarcinoma arising in esophageal colon interposition: Report of a case. Hepatogastroenterology 2004; 51:748–749.

137. Haerr RW, Higgins EM, Seymore CH, et al. Adenocarcinoma arising in a colonic interposition following resection of squamous cell esophageal cancer. Cancer 1987; 60:2304–2307.

138. Altorjay A, Kiss J, Voros A, et al. Malignant tumor developed in colon-esophagus. Hepatogastroenterology 1995; 42:797–799.

139. Kovacs BJ, Griffin RA, Chen YK. Synchronous adenomas in a colonic interposition graft and the native colon. Am J Gastroenterol 1997; 92:2303–2304.

140. Del Rosario MA, Croffie JM, Rescorla FJ, et al. Juvenile polyp in esophageal colon interposition. J Pediatr Surg 1998; 33:1418–1419.

141. Wetstein L, Ergin MA, Griepp RB. Colo-pericardial fistula: Complication of colonic interposition. Tex Heart Inst J 1982; 9:373–376.

142. Canivet JL, Piret S, Hick G, et al. Cardiac tamponade and pulmonary compression due to volvulus of oesophageal coloplasty. Acta Anaesthesiol Belg 2004; 55:125–127.

143. Holland RH. Peptic ulceration and perforation of a left colon bypass for esophageal carcinoma. J Thorac Cardiovasc Surg 1967; 53:733–734.

144. Spitz L, Kiely E, Pierro A. Gastric transposition in children—A 21-year experience. J Pediatr Surg 2004; 39:276–81; discussion –81.

145. Hirschl RB, Yardeni D, Oldham K, et al. Gastric transposition for esophageal replacement in children: Experience with 41 consecutive cases with special emphasis on esophageal atresia. Ann Surg 2002; 236:531–539; discussion 9–41.

146. Ravelli AM, Spitz L, Milla PJ. Gastric emptying in children with gastric transposition. J Pediatr Gastroenterol Nutr 1994; 19:403–409.

147. Koh P, Turnbull G, Attia E, et al. Functional assessment of the cervical esophagus after gastric transposition and cervical esophagogastrostomy. Eur J Cardiothorac Surg 2004; 25:480–485.

148. Heimlich HJ. Esophagoplasty with reversed gastric tube. Review of fifty–three cases. Am J Surg 1972; 123:80–92.

149. Burrington JD, Stephens CA. Esophageal replacement with a gastric tube in infants and children. J Pediatr Surg 1968; 3:24–52.

150. Anderson KD, Noblett H, Belsey R, et al. Long-term follow-up of children with colon and gastric tube interposition for esophageal atresia. Surgery 1992; 111:131–136.

151. Ein SH, Shandling B, Stephens CA. Twenty-one year experience with the pediatric gastric tube. J Pediatr Surg 1987; 22:77–81.

152. Schettini ST, Pinus J. Gastric-tube esophagoplasty in children. Pediatr Surg Int 1998; 14:144–150.

153. Nakagawa M, Seki M, Koike J, et al. Gastric tube-to-pleural fistula seventeen months after esophagectomy: Successful endoscopic treatment of an unusual complication. Jpn J Thorac Cardiovasc Surg 2005; 53:569–572.

154. Stringer DA, Pablot SM. Broncho-gastric tube fistula as a complication of esophageal replacement. J Can Assoc Radiol 1985; 36:61–62.

155. Schouten van der Velden AP, Ruers TJ, Bonenkamp JJ. A cardiogastric fistula after gastric tube interposition. A case report and review of literature. J Surg Oncol 2007; 95: 79–82.

156. Lin FC, Russell H, Ferguson MK. Strangulation of the reconstructive gastric tube by the azygos arch. Ann Thorac Surg 2006; 82:e8–e10.

157. Takato T, Ashida T, Sugiyama T, et al. Marked reversible ST-T abnormalities induced by cardiac compression from a retrosternal gastric tube used to reconstruct the esophagus after tumor resection. A case of a diabetic patient and mini-review of 7 reported patients. Int Heart J 2006; 47:475–482.

158. Lindahl H, Rintala R, Sariola H, et al. Cervical Barrett's esophagus: A common complication of gastric tube reconstruction. J Pediatr Surg 1990; 25:446–448.

159. Takeo H, Matsukuma S. Gastric tube cancer: Immunohistochemical study of 10 lesions in six patients. J Gastroenterol Hepatol 2007; 22:23–29.

Repair of Esophageal Atresia

Expert: Jay L. Grosfeld, M.D.

Esophageal atresia is one of the major congenital anomalies cared for by pediatric surgeons. The survival of these patients has improved significantly over the past three decades; however, management of the premature infants, cases of long gap atresia, and complications following repair still present a challenge to the physician.

QUESTIONS

1. **What steps should be taken to prevent a recurrent tracheoesophageal fistula?**

    We have attempted to reduce the risk of a recurrent tracheoesophageal fistula (TEF) in instances of Type C esophageal atresia in the following manner: In the majority of patients, the TEF is identified at the level where the azygos vein enters the superior vena cava. Once the mediastinal pleura is teased open the azygos vein is identified, ligated and divided, and the TEF becomes apparent A branch of the vagus nerve usually passes near the fistula. When dissecting the entry of the lower (distal) esophagus to the trachea, we usually leave a very tiny cuff of esophageal tissue on the tracheal side to avoid narrowing the trachea. We employ fine (5-0) monofilament or absorbable interrupted (PDS) sutures with the knots tied on the outside to repair the tracheal side. If the fistula is large, the suture line can be continuous. We check for an air-leak by placing the suture line under saline and asking the anesthesiologist to gently hyperinflate to check for air bubbles. When assured the tracheal closure is airtight, we cover the tracheal suture line with mediastinal pleura to interpose fresh tissue between this suture line and the subsequent esophageal anastomosis. It is imperative to observe for a second fistula from the proximal blind ending atretic segment which may occur in 2 to 3% of cases (Type D). One might suspect this by having difficulty mobilizing the proximal esophagus. Preoperative fiberoptic bronchoscopy may help identify instances of double fistula. This may aid in discerning between a true recurrence from a "missed" second fistula. By covering the tracheal suture line, our recurrence rate for primary repair cases has been in the 2% to 3% range. Others have employed fibrin glue, but we have no long-term data regarding the enduring effect of its application.

2. **How should a recurrent tracheoesophageal fistula be repaired?**

    A recurrent tracheoesophageal fistula usually presents with a clinical pattern of recurrent episodes of choking while eating and pulmonary infection. Identification of the recurrence can be accomplished by studies employing aqueous nonhypertonic contrast material or endoscopy. Repair of a recurrent tracheoesophageal fistula is challenging. Recent studies have shown that some recurrent fistulas will respond to endoscopic management using diathermy or electrocautery with a Bugbee electrode to de-epithelialize the fistula tract, followed by insertion of a sealing agent such as fibrin glue into the fistulous tract. This works best when the recurrent fistula is of small diameter with a long thin tract. In some instances, a second endoscopic application is necessary to achieve closure. The recent reported success rate has been as high as 85%. In cases unresponsive to endoscopic treatment, reoperative therapy is required. It has been our personal experience that reoperation has been required in a majority of patients.

    For recurrent H-type fistulas, a cervical approach to the fistula is usually possible. Identification of the exact location of the fistula is facilitated by inserting a small balloon catheter (Fogarty type) at endosocopy prior to making the incision. During the dissection, care should be taken not to injure the vagus or recurrent laryngeal nerve. The fistula is divided and the esophagus and tracheal walls are closed with interrupted 5-0 sutures of Vicryl or PDS monofilament suture. The suture lines are checked for leaks using saline injected in the cervical esophageal lumen by the anesthesiologist for the esophagus, and hyperinflation to check for an air-leak (seeing air bubbles) on the tracheal side following installation of saline in the wound over the tracheal closure site. The two suture lines are then separated by interposing a strap muscle flap in the neck (often the omohyoid muscle) to prevent another recurrence. Some have advocated applying fibrin glue over the suture lines before interposing the muscle flap. A soft drain is placed and brought out a stab wound separate from the neck incision. The esophageal suture line is checked with a contrast swallow at 5 to 6 days to assure an intact closure prior to resuming feedings.

Surgical management of a recurrent TEF following repair of a type C or D esophageal atresia has been successfully accomplished by open and thoracoscopic techniques. Preoperative endoscopic placement of a balloon catheter may again aid in locating the fistula. I have no personal experience performing this thoracoscopically. At thoracotomy, the fistula is identified and divided. The tracheal wall is closed with interrupted 5-0 monofilament suture. The esophageal side is similarly closed with interrupted 4-0 or 5-0 vicryl. The suture lines are checked for leaks as noted above. It is important to separate the two suture lines by interposing some type of "normal tissue." I would prefer to mobilize a flap of mediastinal pleura for this purpose. However, because of the previous surgery, the mediastinal pleura in the area may be inadequate to achieve this goal. A variety of tissues have been used to accomplish this, including the use of a pericardial flap, costal cartilage and an intercostal muscle flap, and a laparoscopically acquired omental pedicle flap brought up through the esophageal hiatus. This may be more difficult to accomplish during thoracoscopic repair, and biosynthetic mesh (Surgisis® Cook, Inc., Bloomington, Indiana, U.S.A.) has been employed as an alternative. Coating the two suture lines with fibrin glue prior to interposing tissue may have some advantages in reducing recurrence. We usually leave the endotracheal tube in place for 48 to 72 hours following the repair to allow the fistula site to seal. A contrast swallow is obtained at 5 to 6 days postoperatively to be sure the esophageal suture line is intact and then feedings are resumed.

3. **What technical steps are taken to prevent an anastomotic stricture?**
The incidence of anastomotic stricture following repair of esophageal atresia is variable and ranges from 15% to 30% according to the criteria employed to make this diagnosis. Because the size of the proximal and distal esophagus is discrepant, it is not uncommon for there to be a slight narrowing at the anastomosis. The baby may be entirely asymptomatic. Certainly severe constriction will be associated with symptoms and require dilatation.

A number of factors have been associated with an increased risk of stricture formation. These include; two layer anastomosis, devitalization of tissue (ischemia—particularly in the distal end), tension on the anastomosis (wider gap), use of braided silk suture for the repair, anastomotic leak, and gastroesophageal reflux disease where the anastomosis is constantly bathed with gastric acid.

The use of a two-layer anastomosis is more of historical interest and in general, most pediatric surgeons perform a full thickness one-layer anastomosis. It is important to mobilize the well-vascularized proximal atretic segment to acquire adequate length and reduce the tension on the anastomosis. This can be done by extending the dissection up into the thoracic inlet. The blood supply to the proximal pouch comes from the inferior thyroid artery. Ideally, it is best not to dissect and mobilize the distal segment of the esophagus extensively. Following the division of the TEF, the remaining blood supply to the mid-esophagus is from small direct branches from the aorta and dividing these may reduce the blood flow to the upper end of the distal esophagus resulting in ischemia. However, distal mobilization may occasionally be necessary in some cases to assure achieving an esophageal anastomosis, salvaging the native esophagus, and avoiding a replacement procedure. Although this may be associated with an increased risk of leak and stricture, these are complications that are often manageable.

Avoid using silk suture for the repair. Silk is a braided material and bacteria can reside in the interstices of the silk. Saliva bathes the anastomosis and bacterial flora can colonize in the braids. Although many surgeons prefer to place the knots of the sutures on the back wall of the anastomosis within the esophageal lumen, we believe this also can serve as a nidus for bacteria and choose to place all the knots on the outside. Pass a red rubber tube past the anastomosis to check for patency of the lower esophagus and avoid missing a distal cartilaginous remnant that may be present in 1% to 2% of cases. Not identifying this can result in obstruction. Insert the anterior row of anastomotic sutures over the tube to reduce the risk of excessive narrowing. Avoid an excessive number of sutures. Only use interrupted sutures to ensure adequate blood flow between stitches and allow growth. Make sure the suture line is watertight by having the anesthesiologist instill saline in a catheter in the lumen above the anastomosis. This may avoid missing an unrecognized unsealed area that may result in a leak. Postoperatively, maintain the baby in a head up, inclined position and institute reflux precautions including antacids to reduce the risk of gastric acid-induced stricture.

4. **If the patient develops an early stricture, what is your protocol for dilations?**
   The documentation of a postoperative stricture is usually achieved by obtaining a contrast study. The first contrast study is usually obtained 5 to 6 days after the procedure to simply document an intact suture line without a leak so that oral intake can be initiated. If there is no significant narrowing observed, then the child is followed expectantly and re-evaluated radiologically only if symptoms occur. If the first radiograph shows significant narrowing, a repeat study is done 2 weeks later. If significant narrowing is observed, the anastomosis is gently "sounded" by passing soft tapered Tucker rubber dilators starting at Fr # 10-12 size and continuing to Fr 22-24 or until some resistance is encountered. Alternatively, this can be done under anesthesia and fluoroscopy using a balloon dilator or a Maloney dilator. Savory dilators passed over a guide wire placed at esophagoscopy and monitored by fluoroscopy has also been effective. Reassessment is done at 1 month. If a narrowing persists, and the gastrostomy tube is still in place, a string can be passed from above and graduated Tucker dilators can be attached and guided through the narrowing on a weekly basis. Dilatation to a 32 to 34 Fr size usually denotes response of the stricture to the dilators. Persistence of the stricture may be due to gastroesophageal reflux and continued bathing of the stricture site by gastric acid, resulting in restricture. If reflux is not abated by conservative measures such as antacids, thickened feedings, and proton pump inhibitors, an antireflux procedure may be necessary to allow the stricture to successfully respond to dilatation. Most strictures resolve over time, however, rarely, resection and reanastomosis are required.

5. **What should be done when a right-sided aortic arch is encountered during the repair of esophageal atresia through the right chest?**
   The incidence of a right aortic arch in reports concerning babies with esophageal atresia ranges from 2.5% to 5.2%. Plain chest radiography and preoperative echocardiography are not always accurate in defining the location of the aorta. Right aortic arch is associated with an increased incidence of congenital heart anomalies and vascular rings. The right-sided aorta and latter anomalies often make the repair of esophageal atresia through the usual right thoracotomy approach more difficult. A higher complication rate has been observed in cases with a right aortic arch.

   If a right aortic arch is identified preoperatively, we usually employ a left thoracotomy to repair the esophageal defect. This allows better exposure of the esophagus without the aorta getting in the way. Further, if there is an associated vascular ring, the most frequent type is an aberrant left subclavian artery and left patent ductus arteriosus. The left thoracotomy allows easier access to divide the left patent ductus arteriosus.

   Although some success in identifying instances of right aortic arch in indeterminate cases has been achieved preoperatively with advanced imaging sources such as spiral computerized tomographic angiography and MR-angiography, not uncommonly, an unsuspected right aortic arch is encountered during the performance of a right thoracotomy to repair the esophageal atresia. Under these circumstances, surgical judgment must prevail. Although successful repair of the defect is possible, it is a more tedious procedure and is associated with a higher complication rate. If the dissection goes smoothly, a complete repair can be carried out. If the dissection and mobilization of the esophageal ends is difficult, the TEF can be ligated, the right chest wound closed, and a left thoracotomy performed to complete the procedure.

6. **What should be done if the ends of the esophagus cannot be approximated during the repair of esophageal atresia?**
   In some instances a longer gap exists between the two esophageal ends than anticipated and they cannot be brought together without excessive tension. There are a number of steps to consider in attempting to salvage the native esophagus and perform a primary anastomosis. First, one should ascertain that maximum mobilization of the well-

vascularized proximal atretic pouch has been achieved by making sure that the dissection is taken up through the thoracic inlet. One should be sure that distal mobilization of the proximal pouch is not restricted by an unrecognized proximal TEF. Although not ideal, mobilization of the distal esophagus can be done down to the level of the diaphragm. If the ends of the esophagus are still too far apart to achieve an anastomosis, performing a Livaditis extramucosal circular myotomy on the proximal pouch smooth muscle wall may be considered to attain an addition 1 to 2 cm in length. Rarely, this technical adjunct may be associated with ballooning of the myotomy site and impaired motility. Some surgeons have employed two proximal myotomies. An alternative technique is to use a spiral myotomy of the entire proximal pouch. Although some have also advocated myotomy of the distal esophageal segment, we have not employed this and believe it is risky. In our experience, in most Type C and D cases, these steps can successfully achieve a primary anastomosis.

Rarely, when significant tension still persists, we will seal both esophageal ends and tack them to chest wall for 5 to 7 days and re-explore the patient and be able to attain a delayed primary anastomosis. We have not externalized traction sutures on the closed ends of the esophagus as advocated by Foker.

In some type A cases, Kimura has employed spiral myotomies of the proximal pouch with staged mobilization of the proximal segment distally from the neck onto the chest wall fixed under tension to stretch the pouch over time and subsequently perform a primary anastomosis. We have attempted this twice and been successful once. Type A cases often have a very limited amount of distal esophagus (a nubbin) above the diaphragm and are a more complex group, of patients to manage and will be discussed further below.

7. **Do you favor daily bougienage preoperatively in long gap esophageal atresia? Is it safe for this to be done at home?**
Babies with Type A esophageal atresia without a TEF are a complex group of patients to deal with. These infants often have the longest gap between the two blind ends of the esophagus with the distal portion represented by a tiny nubbin above the diaphragm. They clinically present with excess salivation from a blind proximal pouch and have no air beneath the diaphragm on a plain abdominal radiograph. Rarely, these babies have a significant length of distal esophagus occasionally attached to the trachea by an occluded fibrous cord—that represents a TEF that spontaneously obliterated. This unusual subset of Type A infants are quite amenable to primary esophageal repair.

Typically, babies with Type A atresia are managed by gastrostomy feedings and watchful waiting to see if the proximal esophagus will grow and elongate spontaneously. In the past, daily proximal pouch bougienage was employed to stretch the cervical end of the blind esophagus. However, it has been subsequently shown that over time, babies simply observed achieved the same degree of lengthening. The infant requires care to prevent aspiration from overflow of excessive salivation from the blind proximal pouch. This care may be possible at home in the hands of intelligent parents. Careful assessment of the ability of the proposed caretakers to manage such a patient at home is critical. In some instances, this requires long-term hospitalization. Infants with extensive gaps between the ends of the atretic esophagus usually undergo attempts at trying to preserve the native esophagus as noted in the previous paragraphs. However, when the gap is greater than four vertebral lengths in a patient with almost no distal esophagus to speak of, it is unlikely that a primary anastomosis will be possible and an esophageal replacement procedure will be necessary using colon, stomach, or jejunum according to the surgeon's preference.

8. **How should the premature infant with pulmonary disease and esophageal atresia with distal fistula be managed?**
With all of the risk classifications that characterize esophageal atresia, severe prematurity and associated anomalies have an adverse effect on outcome, especially in babies that manifest hemodynamic instability and pulmonary disease. Staged repair has been advocated for the management of this subset of cases. The infants often require endotracheal intubation and mechanical ventilation. Because of the presence of a distal TEF, overinflation of the stomach is a risk factor associated with reflux of gastric acid and pneumonia.

A small Replogle tube is placed in the blind proximal esophageal pouch and attached to continuous suction to prevent excess collection of saliva and choking. The baby is placed on antibiotics. We would pay close attention to the positioning of the uncuffed endotracheal tube so that the beveled end is placed to hopefully occlude the fistula. A Stamm gastrostomy is performed to decompress the stomach and reduce the risk of reflux. In instances where the diameter of the fistula is large, significant loss of oxygenated inspired air may occur through the G-tube resulting in destauration and hypoxia. Placing the gastrostomy tube under water establishes a water seal and back pressure that may reduce loss of inspired air. Continued desaturation may require retrograde passage of a small balloon catheter through the gastrostomy site into the lower esophagus to prevent oxygen loss. Catheter displacement may occur once again placing the baby at risk of desaturation and hypoxic injury. This may require emergency thoracotomy and ligation of the TEF. This can be done thoracoscopically in older babies; however, the minimally invasive equipment may be difficult to employ in a tiny premature infant <1800 g. As the baby stabilizes, gastrostomy feedings can be safely started with the TEF ligated and allow the baby to grow. When the baby shows weight gain (>2500 g) and pulmonary improvement, a formal repair of the esophagus can be attempted During the waiting period, a systems workup looking for additional anomalies in other systems (cardiovascular, renal, central nervous system, and musculoskeletal), should be undertaken.

Gastric Transposition

Expert: Arnold G. Coran, M.D.

QUESTIONS

1. **How should the blood supply of the stomach be assessed to judge suitability for gastric transposition?**
   The blood supply for the gastric transposition is based on the right gastric artery and the right gastroepiploic arteries. To get adequate length on the stomach to bring it up to the neck, one must divide the short gastric vessels, the left gastroepiploic vessels, and the left gastric artery and vein. Because of the excellent submucosal blood supply of the stomach, the gastric conduit always maintains good blood supply in the fundic area which is anastomosed to the cervical esophagus in the neck. Even with previous surgery done on the stomach, such as one or more fundoplications even with a Collis extension, the blood supply always remains excellent.

2. **How can respiratory embarrassment from gastric dilation be avoided?**
   Although, in the earlier years, pediatric surgeons were concerned that a complete transposition of the stomach behind the trachea and left main stem bronchus could cause compression of these two structures, I have never seen this problem in 129 consecutive gastric transpositions. Only one patient in my series needed an aortopexy for severe respiratory distress; however, this patient had severe tracheomalacia which was probably the main cause for the need for an aortopexy. Even if gastric dilation occurs postoperatively, respiratory distress does not happen. I have never seen it in my own series. However, if it were to occur, I would place a nasogastric tube into the gastric transposition to decompress it.

3. **What route should the stomach take to get to the neck?**
   The best route for any esophageal replacement is through the posterior mediastinum in the bed of the original esophagus. I have been able to accomplish this in more than 95% of the cases. Occasionally, in a patient who has had multiple operations on the esophagus or in whom esophageal perforations secondary to dilations for esophageal strictures have occurred, the esophageal bed may be difficult to dissect. In these situations, I have brought the stomach behind the hilum of the left lung through a small left thoracotomy.

4. **How can anastamotic leaks and strictures in the neck be minimized?**
   All anastomotic leaks in the neck heal spontaneously. I have never had to operate upon a leak. The leak rate is about 20% to 25%, but the leaks always seal and do not create major

problems. The stricture rate is also about 25%; however, the percentage depends on how you define a stricture. I am very liberal in esophagoscoping my patients and routinely passing dilators at that time. The number of patients that need prolonged dilations is far less than 25%. Obviously, the way to minimize leaks and strictures is to maximize the blood supply in the area of the esophagogastric anastomosis by handling the tissues very gently and by doing the anastomosis under minimal tension. My own personal observation is that the correlation between what appears to be excellent blood supply or poor blood supply at the end of the stomach and the development of a leak or stricture is very poor. I have seen leaks and strictures when the blood supply appeared to be excellent and I have had cases where the blood supply appeared marginal and no leaks or strictures occurred.

5. **How do you manage the native esophagus?**
   I have always resected the esophagus in esophageal replacement surgery, whether I have used stomach, gastric tube or colon. I do this for two reasons: because the native esophagus is at risk of developing carcinoma in adult life and because, in lye strictures, mucoceles can form and cause compression on the trachea and left main stem bronchus.

6. **How would you manage necrosis of the gastric transposition?**
   I have never seen necrosis of the stomach in any of the cases I have done. If this were to occur, obviously, I would remove the stomach and use colon as an esophageal replacement.

Open Nissen Fundoplication

Expert: Dennis Lund, M.D.

QUESTIONS

1. **What steps can be taken to prevent slippage of the Nissen?**
   There is no question that the most common failure of a Nissen fundoplication is the slippage of the wrap up into the chest. This results from the development of a hiatus hernia postoperatively, and is most frequently seen in patients who stress their repair with seizures, gagging and retching, or spasticity. The technique of creation of the fundoplication wrap that I use is designed to try to prevent development of a "slipped Nissen."

   First, I always dissect out the entire hiatus and the esophagus well up into the mediastinum. The goal is to mobilize enough esophagus, so that at least 5 cm of esophagus is in the abdomen for the formation of the wrap. In my experience, when this mobilization is done thoroughly, I have virtually never had to resort to esophageal lengthening procedures, such as the Collis technique, and there is no tension on the wrap. Once this is done, with a Maloney or Tucker dilator in the esophagus, I close the hiatus using three nonabsorbable, braided sutures, such as Ethibond. The braided, nonabsorbable suture stimulates tissue response locally that leads to healing of the 2 two muscle edges, and I believe this material is less likely than monofilament to cut through the muscle. It is essential that these sutures be tied down securely but not so tightly that they cause ischemia of the muscle. In redo cases, where the integrity of the hiatus muscle tissue has already failed once, I use small Teflon pledgets on each side of the crura in order to keep the sutures from cutting through.

   After the hiatus has been secured, I suture the esophagus to the hiatus with 3 three or 4 four interrupted Prolene sutures. I push up on the hiatus as I place these sutures in order to add more length to the intra-abdominal esophagus. As the wrap is created, and I do this with 3 three rows of Prolene sutures for a Nissen wrap and 2 two rows for an open, Toupet wrap, the apical sutures of each row include stomach, esophagus, and hiatus in order to firmly anchor the wrap to the diaphragm. Finally, after the wrap is created, I suture the anterior portion of the wrap to the diaphragm with 2 two to 4 four Prolene sutures in order not only to pull the wrap forward in an effort to create some angulation, but also to further anchor the wrap in the abdomen. I also typically mark the gastroesophageal junction with 2 two titanium clips, so that this location can be visualized on a plain radiography.

2. **How should the left lateral segment of the liver be managed to improve exposure?**
Excellent exposure to the left upper quadrant is essential to for performing this procedure. The left triangular ligament is incised as far to the right as possible, and the left lateral segment of the liver is retracted to the right. This is best accomplished by bending it inferiorly and holding it gently in place with an atraumatic right angle retractor attached to either a Denis-Browne or Buchwalter self-retaining retractor ring. When incising the triangular ligament, one must be on the lookout for a phrenic vein, which may run in this region.

3. **How can postoperative small bowel obstruction be avoided or minimized?**
I absolutely minimize the handling of the small bowel in these cases. Occasionally, it is necessary to look at the location of the ligament of Treitz to exclude intestinal malrotation if there is any question of this on pre-operative studies. This should be done with the least possible bowel manipulation. The incision I use extends from the xyphoid to the umbilicus and this typically offers excellent exposure to the left upper quadrant. Using general anesthesia with good relaxation supplemented by an epidural catheter, there is rarely a need to pack the bowel away, which I try to avoid.

4. **How should a replaced left hepatic artery be managed?**
One must always be looking for an accessory left hepatic artery as the hiatus and the right crus of the diaphragm is dissected. There is virtually never any need to damage or divide one if it is present. Using the mobilization technique that is described with question #1 above, it should be possible to have an adequate length of esophagus (5 cm) in the abdomen above the GE junction in order to complete the wrap without interfering with an accessory left hepatic artery, which will remain below the wrap.

5. **What unusual complications have you seen after an open fundoplication?**
Fortunately, complications have been rare in patients in whom I have performed this operation. Prior to the liberal utilization of epidural catheters, the most common post-operative problem encountered was respiratory, especially in the neurologically impaired patients. This has become much more rare with the use of regional anesthesia for postoperative pain management.

Since the vast majority of children in whom I perform fundoplication have some neurological impairment, the most common gastrointestinal problem we encounter after surgery is delayed gastric emptying with gagging and retching. I do not routinely perform pyloroplasty in these children and I always take great care to visualize and preserve the vagi. If patient is undergoing a redo procedure, however, I will typically perform a Heinicke-Mickulicz pyloroplasty.

One unusual complication I have seen has led me to be quite wary of patients on high doses of anti-seizure medications. That is elevation of liver enzymes after retraction of the liver. In one extremely obese patient who was on very large doses of these medications, there was very severe liver injury simply from retraction of the liver. Therefore, in these patients, I am very careful to make a large enough incision, so that the liver retraction can be as gentle as possible.

I have also seen one case of gastric volvulus in a patient who had a Nissen fundoplication performed at an outside hospital and had her gastrostomy placed in the back wall of the stomach. This led to a twist of the stomach that eventually worked its way into a fully developed volvulus.

6. **Is it always necessary to mobilize the left lateral segment of the liver?**
Although I do not know that whether it is always necessary to mobilize the left lateral segment, I do always perform this maneuver. This allows the best view of the right crus of the diaphragm for proper placement of the sutures that close the hiatus.

7. **Do you always divide the short gastrics?**
Yes. Many have written and discussed doing a fundoplication without taking the short gastric vessels, but it seems to me that a goal of this operation is to obtain a wrap of adequate length that is tension-free. The short gastric vessels will always have the tendency to pull on the wrap if they are not divided.

8. **Do you place a primary button in open fundoplication?**
    I do not always place a gastrostomy if the child does not need it. Thus, if the patient has little or no neurological impairment and will be able to take adequate nutrition by mouth, a gastrostomy is not placed. If there is any question of nutrition or of the need to drain the stomach post-operatively, however, I will place a gastrostomy tube. Children with severe neurological impairment often swallow large amounts of air and need some degree of stomach venting from time to time, especially after an anti-reflux procedure. Since Because a gastrostomy tube vents are better than a button, in the immediate post-operative period, I use a gastrostomy tube rather than a primary button, usually a silicone gastostomy tube, sized 14F or 16 French. If the gastrostomy is going to remain long term for feeding, this is then changed in the clinic to a button at the first postoperative visit approximately 3 three weeks postoperatively.

Gastric Tube Replacement of the Esophagus

Expert: Kurt D. Newman, M.D.

QUESTIONS

1. **What steps can be taken to prevent leakage from the intrathoracic portion of the gastric tube?**
    The chief intervention to avoid suture line leakage is to oversew the long staple line and imbricate the staple line.

2. **How should gastroesophageal reflux after gastric tube replacement be treated?**
    The gastric tube should be constructed so that there is at least a 3-cm portion of intrabdominal neo-esophagus. Almost all patients will reflux so that maintenance on anti-reflux medications is routine. In the event of severe reflux, some surgeons have advocated a "half-Nissen" to decrease the regurgitation.

3. **What technical steps allow the straight passage of the tube into the thorax?**
    The orientation is almost always very straight, but care must be taken not to torque the neo-esophagus. When operating for pure atresia, the native esophageal stump should be removed to allow for a straight passage. The native bed of the esophagus is the preferred location for passage of the conduit.

4. **How does the surgeon decide upon performance of an antrally based gastric tube versus a reversed gastric tube?**
    This procedure is almost never done any more, since the gastric transposition has become popular.

5. **What are the most common complications from the performance of a gastric tube?**
    Approximately 50% of the reversed gastric tubes will leak at the esophageal anastamosis. This is usually self-limited and resolves, but in some cases leads to stricture. Virtually all of the patients with gastric tubes will have reflux.

6. **What unusual complications have you seen following performance of a gastric tube?**
    Gastric outlet obstruction from an improperly designed gastric tube narrowing the pylorus is a difficult problem to manage. Cyclic vomiting can occur and this is also a difficult problem to manage. Ulceration of the gastric tube with bleeding or perforation into the chest is a rare but reported complication.

7. **How have you performed the gastric tube if the original gastrostomy tube was not placed on the lesser curve?**
    Yes, although it makes the operation more difficult. If this is the situation, the gastrostomy can be oversewn and the gastric tube constructed.

15 | Complications of Surgery of the Stomach, Duodenum, and Small Intestine

Sani Z. Yamout, M.D., Michael G. Caty, M.D., and Philip L. Glick, M.D., M.B.A.

INTRODUCTION

Advances in neonatal and pediatric intensive care as well as refinements in the operative management of surgical diseases in children have greatly improved patient outcome in recent years. With improved outcome and longer survival, more information on long-term complications is becoming available. This chapter discusses complications related to the surgical diseases of the stomach and small bowel, as well as complications resulting from diagnostic and therapeutic interventions. As with other organ systems, knowledge of potential short- and long-term complications can help avoid or at least anticipate and ameliorate such complications. The following is a discussion of the complications related to pyloric stenosis, duodenal atresia, jejunoilieal atresia, malrotation, intussusception, necrotizing enterocolitis (NEC), and meconium ileus (MI).

PYLORIC STENOSIS

Pyloromyotomy for idiopathic hypertrophic pyloric stenosis (IHPS) is one of the more frequently performed nonelective operations on infants. Whether using an open or laparoscopic technique, the goal is to split the abnormal muscle fibers that are causing the obstruction without injuring the mucosal lining. Splitting the muscle fibers breaks the cycle of muscle spasm and opens the pyloric channel. As with many other procedures, several approaches to pyloromyotomy have been devised. In the traditional open approach, a transverse right upper quadrant incision is used to access the abdominal cavity. The pylorus is then delivered through the incision and a myotomy performed. A variant of the open technique is the transumbilical approach. In this approach, access to the peritoneal cavity is obtained through a supraumbilical skin incision, followed by a midline incision into the fascia through which the pylorus is delivered. The most recent advancement in pyloromyotomy is the laparoscopic approach, where laparoscopic instruments are used to perform the myotomy in an intracorporeal fashion. This approach has been shown equivalent to the open technique, with less discomfort and better cosmetic results (1).

Disease-Related Complications

Infants with IHPS usually present after days and sometimes weeks of emesis. This prolonged period of emesis from gastric outlet obstruction leads to fluid and electrolyte abnormalities, specifically dehydration and hypochloremic hypokalemic metabolic alkalosis. If left untreated, alkalosis predisposes patients to preoperative, intraoperative, and postoperative respiratory complications such as apnea, respiratory arrest, and cardiac arrhythmias (2). Blood tests easily identify electrolyte abnormalities which should be corrected by intravenous crystalloid solutions (potassium should be held until patients start voiding); however, the assessment of dehydration can be more challenging. Clues which help estimate the level of dehydration include the number of wet diapers, severity and duration of emesis, amount of tolerated oral intake, level of activity, condition of fontanelles, and vital signs. Steiner et al. noted that digital capillary filling time and skin turgor are some of the most reliable physical findings to reflect more than 5% dehydration. Digital capillary refill is normally less than 2 seconds when tested with the patient's hand at the level of the heart. Evaluation of skin turgor is more subjective. To assess skin turgor, the skin lateral to the umbilicus is pinched and the time for it to return to its original shape is noted. When skin turgor is normal, the skin rapidly returns to its original form (3). Children with severe dehydration and potassium depletion from a prolonged period of emesis may present with paradoxical aciduria. Normally, in an attempt to conserve sodium, the kidneys preferentially excrete potassium; however, in the setting of a potassium deficit, the kidneys begin to excrete hydrogen ions instead, which results in paradoxical aciduria (paradoxical because the patient usually has metabolic alkalosis because of loss of hydrogen ions due to emesis). A urine pH measurement can thus help estimate the extent of both dehydration and total body potassium deficit (4). It is important to realize that infantile hypertrophic pyloric stenosis is not a surgical emergency and ample time is available for fluid resuscitation and gradual correction of electrolyte abnormalities prior to general anesthesia and surgical repair.

Procedure-Related Complications

Pyloromyotomy for IHPS is a safe and effective procedure which results in a dramatic and rapid improvement in symptoms. Unfortunately, pyloromyotomy is not without complications. For a procedure to be successful, sufficient muscle fibers should be split without damaging the mucosal lining. Complications mainly occur when either insufficient abnormal muscle fibers are split (Torkelson's bands), resulting in persistent obstruction, or an overly aggressive myotomy results in mucosal injury. The overall complication rate of this procedure is reported to be 3%. However, this rate of perforation includes operations performed in low volume hospitals by general surgeons, and should probably be lower in specialized pediatric surgical center (5).

It is not unusual for emesis to persist for the first few days after a successful operation because of a transient dysfunction of gastric motility secondary to the prolonged period of obstruction that preceded the operation (6). The persistence of symptoms can be a source of frustration to both parents and physicians. In an attempt to manage the frequency and duration of transient postoperative emesis, some authors have advocated the use of specific feeding regimens that are based on advancing feedings slowly and in a controlled manner. Several studies have addressed the relationship between feeding regimens and postoperative emesis and have demonstrated variable results. Several studies have shown that infants do well and have a shorter hospital stay with rapid postoperative advancement of feeds (7, 8). In our institution, infants are started on formula feeds once they leave the recovery room and advanced in 30 mL increments at 3 hour intervals and then switched to ad libitum feeding prior to discharged (8). A more problematic cause for persistent postoperative emesis is an incomplete myotomy, where enough pyloric muscles are left intact that the obstruction is not relieved. Differentiating between transient postoperative emesis and emesis secondary to an incomplete myotomy can be challenging. An upper gastrointestinal (UGI) imaging study with oral contrast seems like the logical first step in evaluating a patient with a suspected persistent obstruction due to an inadequate myotomy. Unfortunately, an UGI study is not useful during the immediate postoperative period since it can remain abnormal for several weeks after a successful operation. If sufficient concern exists regarding the possibility of an incomplete myotomy, the only reliable method of evaluation is reexploration. Reexploration should be considered in infants who do not show signs of improvement after at least 1 week of supportive management (9).

Varying rates of an incomplete myotomy have been reported in different studies comparing the open and laparoscopic techniques. An incomplete myotomy can occur in either of the two approaches; however, the laparoscopic pyloromyotomy seems to be associated with a higher risk of incomplete myotomy when compared to the open approach (2.2% versus 0.0%) (10, 11). Once an incomplete myotomy is suspected, reexploration and a repeat myotomy should be performed through either an open or laparoscopic approach, based on surgeon preference (10).

Mucosal perforation, a potentially fatal complication of pyloromyotomy, results from accidental extension of the myotomy into the mucosal layer. Perforations are usually identified intraoperatively either by direct visualization of mucosa or leaking gastric content or during insufflation of the stomach at the end of the procedure. If a perforation is missed, patients can present with potentially life-threatening intraabdominal sepsis a few days postoperatively. The overall incidence of perforation is 2%, but varies with technique and surgeon experience (12). Yagmurlu et al. reported a significantly higher rate of perforation with open pyloromyotomy when compared to the laparoscopic approach (3.6% versus 0.4%). This was attributed to the magnification and better visualization associated with laparoscopy (10). If a mucosal perforation is identified, it is prudent to convert to an open approach. Management options include repairing the mucosal tear with interrupted fine absorbable sutures followed by placement of an omental patch or closing the myotomy and performing a new myotomy at a different site. The stomach should be decompressed by nasogastric suctioning while the repair heals, and a contrast study performed to document the absence of a leak prior to resuming feeds. Patients may also benefit from postoperative prophylactic antibiotics. Fortunately, if a perforation is recognized and repaired intraoperatively, the only consequence is an increased risk of wound infection and a longer hospital stay. On the other hand, if a perforation is missed, the consequences can be catastrophic (12).

Aggressive and repetitive manipulation of the duodenum may result in deserosalization or full thickness damage to the duodenal wall (10,13). This may be more common with the laparoscopic technique where the grasper stabilizing the duodenum is usually outside the field of vision while the myotomy is being performed. Adequate exposure of the duodenum is an important factor in minimizing the chance of injury. The duodenum must be gently but securely grasped with a bowel grasper, along its full circumference prior to any manipulation and inspected for damage at the end of the procedure. In an attempt to circumvent this potential complication, some surgeons grasp the stomach instead of the duodenum to stabilize the pylorus prior to the myotomy (14). The transumbilical approach may also predispose to deserosalizaion during attempts at delivering an enlarged pylorus through the umbilical incision (15).

Perioperative antibiotics are not routinely administered for a pyloromyotomy, since it is a clean operation. An uncomplicated pyloromyotomy, where the mucosal lining is not violated, should have a 3% or less rate of wound infection, similar to other clean operation (16). This correlates well with a 2% wound infection rate in open pyloromyotomies performed through a right upper quadrant incision. Ladd et al. noted that the rate of wound infection in patients undergoing a pyloromyotomy using a transumbilical approach was 7%, but dropped to 2.3% with the use of perioperative antibiotics. The authors attributed this increase in risk to the environment surrounding the umbilicus and tissue ischemia that results from traction exerted with this technique. They recommend the use of prophylactic antibiotics when using the transumbilical approach (17). Other risk factors for wound infection are a poorly epithelialized umbilical stump and mucosal perforation. In both these situation, the administration of perioperative antibiotics may decrease the chance of wound infection.

DUODENAL ATRESIA

Duodenal atresia (DA) is a condition where the duodenal lumen is partially or completely obstructed, resulting in proximal intestinal obstruction. It is the most common type of atresia in the gastrointestinal (GI) tract, occurring in 1 in 5,000 to 10,000 live births (18). During the early stages of duodenal development, rapidly proliferating endothelial cells transiently obliterate the intestinal lumen; this is later recanalized and the lumen reestablished. DA is believed to be a result of incomplete recanalization of the duodenum. The process of recanalization occurs during early stages of development, which may explain the high rate of anomalies associated with DA. DA can be divided into three types, based on the nature of interruption of the lumen. The most common type of atresia involves a membrane that partially or completely obstructs the duodenal lumen with no interruption of duodenal wall. This is referred to as Type 1 atresia and occurs in 90% of cases. Type 2 atresia, which occurs in 1% of cases, consists of a fibrous cord connecting two blind loops of duodenum with an intact mesentery. Type 3 atresia, which occurs in 7% of cases, represents two nonconnected blind loops with a V-shaped mesenteric defect (18).

Some of the signs of intestinal obstruction from DA may manifest prenatally, frequently as maternal polyhadramnios and a "double bubble" sign on ultrasound. Maternal polyhydramnios occurs in 75% of cases and predisposes to preterm labor and delivery of a premature infant. If maternal polyhydramnios is associated with signs of neonatal intestinal obstruction, but no "double bubble" is present one must always entertain the possibility of malrotation and midgut volvulus, and proceed to an upper gastrointestinal study to confirm the diagnosis. Up to 45% of infants with DA are born premature; these infants are at increased risk of perioperative complications and morbidity due to cardiac and respiratory problems associated with prematurity (29–21). DA is part of a set of abnormalities of various organ systems, where 50% of patients may have associated anomalies (22) (Table 1). This high rate of associated

Table 1 Anomalies Associated with Duodenal Atresia (22)

Type	Percentage (%)
Annular pancreas	37
Malrotation	32
Congenital heart disease	27
Esophageal atresia	8
Renal abnormalities	5
Imperforate anus	4
Anterior portal vein	3
Biliary atresia	1

anomalies is a main contributor to poor outcome. DA is not an immediately life-threatening condition, and time is available for a thorough search for associated anomalies prior to surgical intervention. Thirty percent of children with DA have Down's syndrome. Cardiac anomalies are present in 30% of patients with DA and are responsible for 50% of mortality (1818–2020). Other associated anomalies include esophageal atresia, renal anomalies and imperforate anus. Awareness and identification of such anomalies are vital in these children, since they can be a major cause of morbidity and mortality. A preoperative echocardiogram and renal ultrasound should be performed in all patients with DA. Esophageal atresia is evaluated by the passage of an orogastric tube into the stomach. Careful inspection of the anus identifies any anorectal anomalies.

Initial management of infants with DA consists of fluid resuscitation and gastric suctioning. Parenteral nutrition may be started if operative intervention is delayed while other anomalies, such as cardiac defects, are addressed. The aim of operative management is to resect an obstructing web if possible or bypass a complete obstruction. Intraoperatively, the GI tract should be evaluated for malrotation, which is known to be associated with duodenal obstruction. The duodenum should be adequately mobilized in order for it to be fully inspected; this also helps minimize tension on the anastomosis. The point of duodenal obstruction is usually located at the transition point between the dilated and decompressed segments of the duodenum. Once the obstruction point is localized, a duodenotomy is performed and the lumen inspected. In 5% of cases, a thin membrane is all that is obstructing the lumen and simple resection reestablishes continuity (18). More frequently, a duodenoduodenostomy or duodenojejunostomy is required to bypass the obstruction. The proximal duodenum is mobilized then brought down and anastomosed to the duodenum distal to the obstruction. Occasionally, when anastomosis to the duodenum is not possible, the proximal duodenum is anastomosed to the jejunum. Many of the complications associated with the management of DA are related to this anastomosis. Frequently, an annular pancreas is encountered intraoperatively. It is unclear if an annular pancreas, when present, is responsible for duodenal obstruction or is merely an associated anomaly. The management, however, does not change and the anastomosis in this case should be performed anterior to the abnormal pancreatic tissue which should not be violated to avoid pancreatitis or pancreatic leaks and fistulas.

A popular method of bypassing the point of obstruction is a diamond-shaped duodenoduodenostomy. For this anastomosis, a transverse duodenotomy is performed on the proximal dilated duodenum and then anastomosed to a longitudinal duodenotomy performed over the distal decompressed duodenum such that the corner of one incision is approximated to the midline of the other. This method of anastomosis is believed to result in a larger stoma than the traditional side-to-side anastomosis with subsequent earlier feeding and improved long-term patency (23, 24). A duodenojejunostomy can similarly be performed as either a diamond-shaped or side-to-side anastomosis. Historically, gastrostomy tubes were placed routinely because of the anticipated delay in anastomotic function. The advent of the diamond-shaped anastomosis, with the associated quicker return of bowel function, has made the routine placement of a gastrostomy tube unnecessary. In our institution, a gastrostomy tube is strongly considered in infants with Down's syndrome with associated cardiac disease which may require one or several operations. We also have a low threshold to place a gastrostomy tube in patients with Down's syndrome in general since they tend to progress slowly with feeding.

Intraoperative Complications

Duodenal dissection and anastomosis should be performed with great care, since proximal duodenal dilation distorts local anatomy. The ampulla of Vater is at risk for injury during dissection or construction of the anastomosis. Boyden et al. studied the location of the ampulla of Vater in patients with DA and noted that the ampulla is usually present in the immediate vicinity of the point of obstruction (25). This proximity places the ampulla at risk of injury during surgical repair (20). To minimize the risk to the ampulla, it should be identified by gently squeezing the gallbladder and observing bile flow before and after the anastomosis. When a thin membrane is the only source of obstruction, and a membrane excision is planned, the excision should be restricted to the lateral aspect of the membrane to avoid injuring the ampulla. A tapering duodenoplasty is sometimes required to improve postoperative bowel function. Studies have shown that tapering the duodenum prior to anastomosis is associated with an increased risk of injury to the ampulla. The disrupted anatomy of the dilated duodenum places the ampulla at higher risk of injury (26).

Persistent mechanical obstruction is another potential postoperative complication of DA repair. Obstruction may be a result of a missed second atresia or a windsock membrane. A second distal atresia is present in around 5% of patients. If such a lesion is not identified and corrected, patients will have a persistent obstruction that may jeopardize the proximal anastomosis. A preoperative contrast enema should be performed to identify any associated colonic atresia. Intraoperatively, saline should be injected into the bowel lumen and milked distally to check for concomitant small bowel atresias. Another source of persistent obstruction, present in 5% of patients, is a windsock membrane. A windsock membrane is an obstructing membrane that is stretched distally within the lumen of the duodenum. On external examination, the observed point of transition in caliber of the duodenum is actually distal to the origin of obstruction. If such a variant is not recognized, an anastomosis would be ineffective because of its location distal to the site of obstruction. Close inspection usually identifies a small area of constriction of the wall of the duodenum which marks the origin of the membrane and the actual point that needs to be bypassed (Fig. 1) (27). The presence of a windsock membrane is confirmed by passing an orogastric catheter into the lumen of the duodenum. If a windsock membrane is

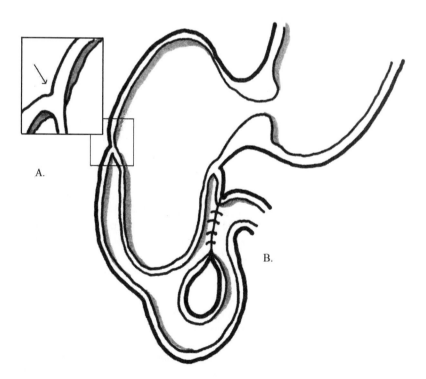

Figure 1 Windsock membrane. **(A)** Indentation in the wall of the duodenum marks the origin of the obstructing membrane. **(B)** An anastomosis performed distal to an unrecognized windsock membrane.

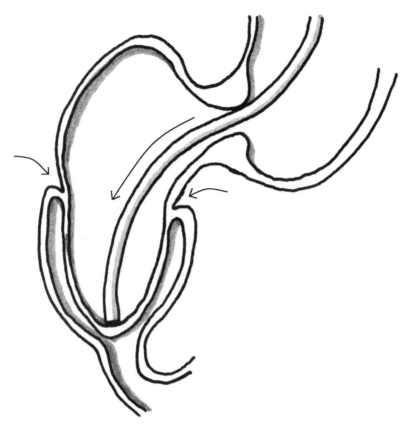

Figure 2   Windsock membrane identified by passing a tube into the duodenum.

present, pushing on the catheter results in tenting of the duodenal wall proximal to the transition point (Fig. 2).

Early Postoperative Complications

Delayed anastomotic function, with slow return of bowel function postoperatively, is one of the main complications associated with repair of duodenal atresia. Factors related to both the design of the anastomosis and intrinsic poor function of the proximal dilated duodenum may contribute to this problem. The original management of DA consisted of a side-to-side duodenojejunostomy. Patients frequently required gastrostomy tubes with transanastomotic feeding because of a delayed return of bowel function. Gastrostomy tubes are associated with their own set of complications, and exposed patients to further problems such as leaks, skin irritation, dislodgement, mechanical failure, gastroesophageal reflux, and persistent gastrocutaneous fistulae. Advent of the more physiologic duodenoduodenostomy, described by Weitzman et al. in the 1960s (28), and then the diamond-shaped anastomosis technique, described by Kimura in 1977, has greatly improved the results of this operation (24). The diamond-shaped duodenoduodenostomy results in quicker resumption of feeds and shorter hospital stay when compared to side-to-side duodenoduodenostomy and side-to-side deuodenojejunostomy (23). Because of the quicker return of intestinal function, gastrostomy tubes and trans-anastomotic feeding are no longer necessary (24).

Intrinsic dysfunction of the proximal dilated duodenum may also contribute to delayed anastomotic function. Dilated segments of intestine have been shown to be ineffective in bolus propulsion, regardless of the adequacy of peristaltic function. Even with normal peristalsis, the walls of a sufficiently dilated intestine cannot establish a pressure gradient within the lumen because they cannot coapt well (29). Studies have shown that an anastomosis functions sooner when the dilated intestinal segment proximal to it is resected or the size of the lumen reduced (20,30). The two main solutions to a dilated duodenum are a tapering duodenoplasty and duodenal plication (31). The tapering duodenoplasty involves the resection of part of the wall of a

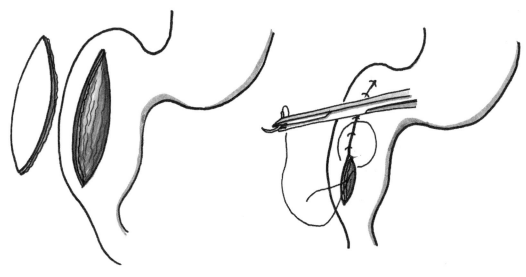

Figure 3   Sutured duodenoplasty.

dilated duodenum using either electrocautery followed by primary repair (Fig. 3) or using a GIA stapler (Fig. 4). A duodenal plication entails imbricating the redundant duodenal tissue, which avoids the long suture line associated with a duodenoplasty (Fig. 5) (32). Although reducing the caliber of the lumen has been shown to be beneficial in patients who present with postoperative functional obstruction from a dilated duodenum, the same cannot be said about the benefit of a prophylactic tapering procedure when a dilated duodenum is encountered during the initial operation (26). The extent of duodenal dilation observed at the initial operation has not been shown to predict outcome, and recommendations on prophylactic tapering procedures cannot be made based on intraoperative findings (18).

Late Complications

The importance of continued follow-up into adulthood has been reinforced by several recent long-term outcome studies that have reported a considerable rate of long-term complications after DA repair. Complications include late-onset duodenal dilation, blind loop syndrome, anastomotic stricture, gastroesophageal reflux disease (GERD), duodenogastric reflux, and small bowel obstruction. Escobar et al. reported a 12% rate of long-term postoperative complications (18).

Late-onset duodenal dilation is a condition that may result in a functional bowel obstruction despite early successful feeding. Progressive dilation of the duodenum after the anastomosis is constructed may result in a functional obstruction months to years postoperatively (33). Patients with a sufficiently dilated duodenum may experience failure to thrive, vomiting, abdominal pain, and blind loop syndrome (18,34). Along with causing a functional obstruction, the dilated stagnant duodenum may cause blind loop syndrome and malabsorption secondary to bacterial overgrowth. The functional obstruction is a result of poor propulsion of food through the dilated lumen. Late-onset functional obstruction secondary to a dilated duodenum occurs in 5% of patients. Earlier studies reported a 20% rate of duodenal dilation; however, those studies evaluated patients who had undergone a side-to-side anastomosis (21,30). Patients with a symptomatic dilated duodenum can be managed with either duodenoplasty or duodenal plication. Fortunately, the more prevalent use of the diamond-shaped anastomosis has decreased the rate of duodenal dilation, probably due to an improved anastomotic patency. Some reports suggest that tapering or plicating the duodenum during the initial operation may prevent this late complication; however, the exact amount of dilation that would benefit from a prophylactic tapering is unclear (33). Stagnation and bacterial overgrowth may also occur if the distal duodenotomy is not positioned close enough to the site of obstruction, leaving a segment of bowel which is not in continuity with flow. This condition is more common when a duodenojejunostomy is performed (24,33,35).

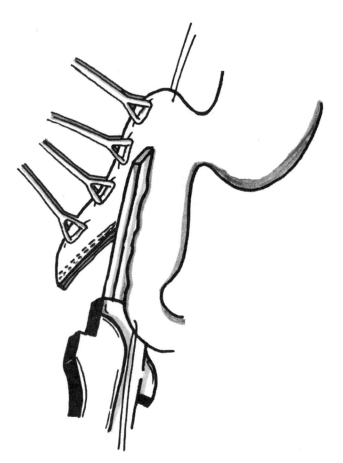

Figure 4 Stapled duodenoplasty.

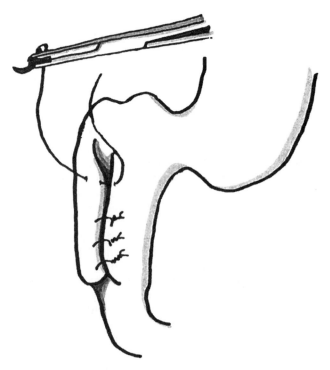

Figure 5 Duodenal plication.

Table 2   Survival of Patients with Duodenal Atresia (18)

Author/year	% Survival
Fonkalsrud et al. (22)	68
Nixon et al. (1970)	57
Grosfeld et al. (1985)	90
Escobar et al. (18)	91

Other long-term complications may be associated with DA repair. Anastomotic stenosis may be responsible for late-onset obstructive symptoms. The wide spread use of the diamond-shaped anastomosis has also made stenosis an uncommon problem (18,24). Gastroesophageal reflux requiring operative intervention occurs in 8% of patients after DA repair. A certain degree of functional obstruction distal to the stomach, secondary to poor intestinal motility, may account for this finding (36, 37). Duodenogastric reflux may also be present in some patients. Radiologic evidence of duodenogastric reflux can be seen in 30% of patients after DA repair (34). This may cause peptic ulceration and esophagitis from chronic exposure to alkaline biliary fluid. Duodenogastric reflux may be alleviated by prokinetic agents (35).

Mortality

Mortality in patients with DA is mainly a result of associated cardiac anomalies. Thirty percent of patients have cardiac anomalies; these anomalies are responsible for 50% of mortality (18–20). Advances in the diagnosis and management of pediatric cardiac disease, along with progress in neonatal cardiac surgery and critical care have resulted in a remarkable improvement in survival of patients born with DA. Patient survival has improved from 60% to over 90% in recent years (18,22) (Table 2).

JEJUNOILEAL ATRESIA

Jejunoileal atresia (JIA) is a condition where there is discontinuity in the lumen of the small bowel distal to the ligament of Treitz. The etiology is believed to be an ischemic insult to the intestines that occurs during the latter stages of fetal development. Conditions such as cystic fibrosis (CF), intrauterine volvulus, abdominal wall defects, or intussusception may coexist with JIA and are believed to be responsible for the ischemic insult (30). JIA can be divided into four types. Type 1 consists of a mucosal defect with intact mesentery. Type 2 defines a lesion where a fibrous cord connects two atretic bowel ends. Type 3a indicates two atretic ends with a V-shaped mesenteric defect. Type 3b refers to an apple peel lesion, where the distal piece of bowel is supplied by a single vessel. Type 4 denotes multiple atretic segments of bowel. Associated conditions in patients with JIA are not as frequent as they are with DA, and do not impact patient outcome to the same extent, except for coexisting atresias and should be evaluated for intraoperatively.

Disease-Related Complications

Short bowel syndrome (SBS) is a condition where not enough intestinal length is available for maintenance of a patient's nutritional needs. It is a quantitative and/or qualitative deficiency in bowel function that results in malnutrition, weight loss and diarrhea. The length and condition of residual intestinal segments, presence of an ileocecal valve, along with the operation performed are major determinants of outcome in terms of SBS. Patients with an apple peel deformity or multiple atresias are at highest risk for SBS, especially if the small intervening segments of intestine between points of atresia are resected. SBS, which occurs in 25% of patients with JIA, is a major cause of morbidity and mortality (19). Fortunately, when residual intestinal length is not sufficient to absorb nutrients and maintain growth, the intestine undergoes a series of changes referred to as adaptation, which may ultimately result in normal intestinal function. Adaptation is a process that involves morphologic and functional modifications of the residual intestine as it attempts to keep up with nutritional requirements. Exposure of the intestinal cells to nutrients plays a key role in adaptation. The method of administration as well as the composition of enteral feeds affects this process. Early, gradual and continuous feeding with formula containing complex nutrients and low in carbohydrates is advantageous since complex nutrients present more of a "work load" for the intestine and thus are more effective in promoting adaptation than simple nutrients. Enteral feeds should be hypoallergenic, low in carbohydrates, and high in fat content. Because of their abnormal mucosal barriers, infants with SBS are more prone to milk protein allergies. Subsequently, special formulas, designed to minimize milk protein allergy should be used while the intestinal barrier is still maturing. Similarly, carbohydrates should be limited in enteral feeds since they present a large osmotic load to the already compromised bowel of patients with SBS. Fats, particularly long-chain triglycerides, have the most trophic effect on intestinal cells and should be used as a main source of calories (38).

Operative intervention for SBS is usually reserved for patients who reach a plateau with bowel adaptation and continue to require total parenteral nutrition (TPN) to meet their nutritional needs and is usually not offered until at least a year has passed with nonoperative management. Several surgical options aimed at increasing transit time, intestinal length, or improving intestinal motility are available with variable success rates (39,40). Bowel transplantion is reserved for patients who fail all the above attempts at improving bowel function and continue to be dependant on hyperalimentation.

The advent of parenteral nutrition has made a marked contribution to the outcome of patients with SBS, allowing survival of patients with as little as 20 cm of residual bowel (9). Unfortunately, sepsis, and parenteral nutrition associated liver disease continue to be a significant cause of morbidity and mortality. Liver failure occurs in around 25% of patients with JIA receiving parenteral nutrition, most of whom are either too small for transplant or do not survive long enough to be transplanted. Parenteral nutrition associated liver disease is believed to be partly due to the inflammatory and hepatotoxic effects of the soybean-fat emulsion used as part of parenteral nutrition formula. A recent study by Gura et al. has shown promising results with the use of a fish-oil-based fat emulsion (Omegaven®). Parenteral nutrition dependant patients who were placed on the fish-oil-based emulsion were found to have signs of reversal of liver disease with no evidence of adverse effects. The benefit of a fish-oil-based fat emulsion is believed to be partly due to the anti-inflammatory effect of omega-3 fatty acid metabolites and the absence of some hepatotoxic substances found in soybean-based emulsions (41). Despite the promising potential of Omegaven, and because of the high morbidity and mortality associated with prolonged administration, weaning of parenteral nutrition is central in improving outcome in this patient population.

Associated conditions are less frequently encountered with jejunoileal atresia than duodenal atresia. When present, associated conditions are usually part of the pathophysiology of the ischemic insult that results in atresia. Coexisting conditions that may affect patient outcome and management include gastroschisis, CF, malrotation, and inherited thrombophilias. Small bowel atresia is present in 10% of patients with gastroschisis. Because of the thick peel enveloping the intestines of patients with gastroschisis, some atresias may not be recognized intraoperatively and are later identified during evaluation for a persistent postoperative obstruction. When an intestinal atresia is discovered during initial evaluation of gastroschisis several options for management are available. The atresia can be repaired primarily, observed, and repaired at a later date or fashioned into an ostomy. Primary repair may be considered when the intestines have minimal peel and primary closure of the abdomen is anticipated since an anastomosis between intestinal segments with a thick peel or in contact with a synthetic material is at increased risk of breakdown. If the atresia is not addressed at the time of gastroschisis reduction, delayed repair after a period of bowel decompression and parenteral nutrition is usually achievable since the peel softens with time (42). Stoma formation is generally restricted to cases where an intestinal perforation is present or the viability of bowel is in question. Ten percent of patients with JIA have associated CF (19). The surgical approach to this group of patient should include steps to evacuate the inspissated meconium, and aggressive postoperative respiratory and nutritional support while workup for CF is underway. Malrotation coexists with JIA in 10% of cases (43), and should be addressed when the condition of the intestines permits.

Inherited thrombophilias, such as the Factor V Leiden mutation, have recently been implicated in the etiology of intestinal atresia. Factor V Leiden is a form of factor V that is resistant to activated protein C, which normally regulates the coagulation cascade by inactivating factors V and XIII. Subsequently, patients with factor V Leiden have a tendency for vascular thrombosis, which is the postulated etiology behind small bowel atresia in newborns. Patients who are heterozygotes for the Leiden mutation have up to ten times the normal rate of thrombosis while those who are homozygotes have thrombosis episodes up to 100 times more frequently than the general population. Studies have identified a higher incidence of Factor V Leiden mutations in patients with intestinal atresia when compared to the general population (4% versus 18%) (44). These findings have helped shed light on the etiology of intestinal atresia, and have identified a patient population who may be at higher risk for complications of a hypercoagulable state.

Procedure-Related Complications

Many of the postoperative complications of JIA are related to the intestinal anastomosis, particularly in patients who have multiple atretic segments. Postoperative complications include adhesive bowel obstruction, functional anastomotic obstruction, and anastomotic leaks and strictures. With the less frequent use of stomas in these patients, complications of stomal prolapse and strictures are seldom encountered.

Adhesive bowel obstruction is a common complication to most intraabdominal operations and, as with other forms of adhesive bowel obstruction, most patients recover with nonoperative management (19). A more difficult condition to manage is persistent functional obstruction of the anastomosis. This is a situation where there is poor flow across an anastomosis despite it being of adequate caliber, and can occur if the proximal dilated intestine is not addressed prior to repair of the atresia. The walls of dilated loops of intestine are incapable of proper opposition; which may explain their poor ability to propel food. Resection of dilated bowel, in an attempt to circumvent this problem, is frequently not feasible due to the increased risk of SBS; this makes a tapering enteroplasty or intestinal plication more attractive options. A tapering enteroplasty or intestinal plication may help improve intestinal function without compromising bowel length, and should be considered when a patent anastomosis associated with dilated proximal intestinal loops fails to function. Another cause of persistent obstruction despite a successful anastomosis is a missed second atresia. Five percent of patients with JIA will have more than one atresia which, if missed, will cause persistent obstruction and may compromise the more proximal anastomosis. To avoid such a situation, one must perform a preoperative contrast enema to clear the colon. Intraoperatively, saline should be injected into the intestinal lumen and milked distally to help identify concomitant atresias. Other anastomotic complications, including leaks and stenosis occur in a small percentage of patients. In a study by Dalla Vecchia et al., the rate of anastomotic leak was 4% in patients treated for JIA (19).

Mortality

As with many of the other pediatric surgical diseases, advances in neonatal care and surgical technique have markedly improved survival. The major causes of mortality in patients with JIA are complications related to short gut syndrome and prolonged use of total parental TPN. Current long-term survival from JIA is 85%, with the vast majority of late mortality resulting from infectious complications of TPN (19). An interesting point to note is that the operative mortality for JIA is less than 1% as compared to a 4% operative mortality in DA. This lower early mortality is attributed to the less frequent association of JIA with other anomalies, specifically congenital heart disease.

MALROTATION

Embryology

The proper development of the intestinal tract depends on a series of precise steps that regulate rotation and fixation of the intestines. These steps result in a wide mesenteric base, which is central in preventing midgut volvulus. Intestinal rotation and fixation occurs during early fetal development. Around the fifth week of embryonic growth, the developing intestines exit the peritoneal cavity and begin a 270° counterclockwise rotation about the superior mesenteric artery (phase 1). The rotation is completed during the return of the intestines into the abdomen around the tenth week (phase 2). Once full rotation is accomplished, the mesentery is fixed to the posterior abdominal wall (phase 3). Proper intestinal fixation and stabilization depend on all three phases of this process being completed (45). Based on the timing of interruption of

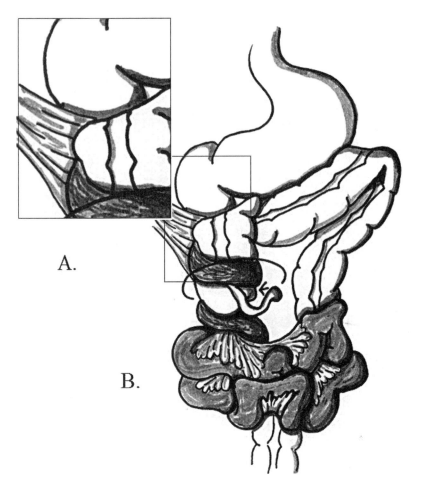

Figure 6 Malrotation. (**A**) Ladd's bands causing duodenal obstruction. (**B**) Midgut volvulus with small bowel mesentery twisted clockwise around the superior mesenteric artery.

progress, two main types of rotational anomalies are described. Nonrotation and incomplete rotation refer to conditions where phases 1 or 2 is interrupted, respectively.

Disease-Related Complications

Midgut volvulus, a condition where the small intestines twist around a narrow mesenteric pedicle, is the most dreaded complications of malrotation (Fig. 6). If not promptly treated, it can result in bowel ischemia, necrosis, and SBS. Fortunately, and because of increased awareness and more aggressive imaging, the rate of volvulus in patients with malrotation has dropped from 80% in the 1950 s to 30% in recent years (46). Midgut volvulus, one of the true emergencies in pediatric surgery, should be suspected in any child with bilious emesis. Malrotation with midgut volvulus must be operatively corrected as soon as it is diagnosed to minimize complications of intestinal necrosis. Since the volvulus usually occurs in a clockwise direction, counterclockwise rotation of the small bowel along its mesentery reverses the volvulus.

Patients with intestinal rotation anomalies may also have coexisting heterotaxia. Heterotaxia refers to any variant of organ position that lies between the normal situs solitus and situs inversus totalis (mirror image reversal of organs). Heterotaxia is an important contributor to patient outcome because of its association with asplenia or polysplenia, primary ciliary dyskinesia (Kartagener syndrome), and/or congenital heart disease (47). Asplenia and primary ciliary dyskinesia, when present, predispose patients to infectious complications related to an altered immune response to encapsulated organisms and respiratory complications, respectively. Additionally, some forms of heterotaxia are associated with congenital heart disease in up to 90% of cases. This association is not surprising considering the fact that proper cardiac development is dependant on correct right and left orientation. Because of the increased operative risk in patients with congenital heart disease, controversy exists regarding the need for operative intervention, particularly in asymptomatic patients with an incidentally found malrotation. Tashjian et al. recommend performing a Ladd's procedure on asymptomatic patients once their cardiac function is optimized. In their study, mortality was secondary to cardiac defects and not directly related to the operation (48). This seems to be the safest option given that the risk of volvulus in these patients is life long.

Procedure-Related Complications

Long-term complications occur in up to 50% of patients after a Ladd's procedure (49). Physicians caring for patients who have undergone a Ladd's procedure should be aware of these complications and their management. Knowledge of the potential operative complications of a Ladd's procedure is central to the management of patients with malrotation, particularly those who are asymptomatic or present with vague GI symptoms not clearly related to malrotation. Some of the long-term complications of malrotation and the Ladd's procedure are adhesive small bowel obstruction, persistent GI symptoms, and midgut volvulus (50, 51).

Adhesion formation is one of the goals of a Ladd's procedure, which entails performing multiple mesenteric incisions to release congenital adhesions and widen a narrow mesentery. These incisions result in numerous areas of raw surface which result in extensive adhesions. Although adhesions help fix the intestines and prevent volvulus, they also increase the risk of adhesive bowel obstruction. In a study by Murphy et al., 25% of patients who underwent a Ladd's procedure subsequently required admission for adhesive bowel obstruction; half of admitted patients required surgical intervention (49). It is important to keep in mind this high rate of adhesive small bowel obstruction when deciding on the management of asymptomatic patents with malrotation.

Persistence of GI symptoms after a Ladd's procedure is another problem surgeons and patients must be aware of. Infants who present with obstructive symptoms have delayed return of GI function after repair of malrotation. This delay is usually more severe in patients who have had midgut volvulus. Murphy et al. noted that 2% of patients with malrotation had chronic abdominal pain after a Ladd's procedure and 9% had persistent feeding difficulties (49). The problem of persistent GI symptoms is more significant in patients who are diagnosed with malrotation beyond the neonatal period who present with chronic abdominal pain, diarrhea, vomiting, and failure to thrive. Coombs et al. noted that 50% of their patients who presented after the first year of life with malrotation and chronic abdominal symptoms had persistence of symptoms after a Ladd's procedure. Persistent symptoms included recurrent pain, abdominal distension, pseudoobstruction, vomiting, and/or protein losing enteropathy. Motility studies were performed on some of the patients with persistent symptoms, and all were found to be abnormal. The authors concluded that symptoms of malrotation may have a functional as well as mechanical etiology (52).

An interesting group of patients are those with "atypical" malrotation on UGI studies. The normal position of the duodenojejunal junction, when seen on an UGI study, is to the left of midline rising to the level of the pylorus posteriorly. Atypical malrotation is diagnosed when the junction is abnormally located, but does not fit the criteria of classic malrotation. This usually consists of a duodenojejunal junction that is to the left of midline but lying lower than the level of the pylorus. Mehall et al. noted that this group of patients was at a higher risk for operative complications and persistence of symptoms; moreover, they were also less likely to present with midgut volvulus. Based on their findings, they raised the question of whether this group of patients should undergo a Ladd's procedure (53). Another problematic group of patients are those who present at an older age with an incidentally identified malrotation on radiologic studies performed for other indications. Unlike patients with symptomatic malrotation, the management of this group of patients is somewhat controversial. It is sensible to perform a Ladd's procedure on any patient with malrotation, unless there are associated comorbidities which place the patient at a high operative risk (54, 55). If nonoperative management is elected, close follow-up is mandatory.

Mortality from malrotation has been reported to be as high as 20%. In a study by Messineo et al., the mortality was 10% and mostly related to complications of midgut volvulus. Risk factors for mortality were the presence of necrotic bowel, associated anomalies and a younger age group (56). A high index of suspicion for malrotation and volvulus is critical in patients with bilious emesis since early diagnosis and operative intervention are central to improving patient outcome.

INTUSSUSCEPTION

Intussusception is one of the most commonly encountered abdominal emergencies in infants and children (57). Signs and symptoms may be nonspecific and a high index of suspicion is critical since a missed intussusception can result in a life-threatening intraabdominal catastrophe. Prompt recognition and reduction, prior to the onset of intestinal ischemia and gangrene, are the cornerstones of management and complication prevention. Advances in techniques of enema reduction have markedly improved the success and safety of nonoperative management (58).

Complications of Radiologic Diagnosis and Management

Prompt diagnosis and management are central to a good outcome in intussusception. Once the diagnosis of intussusception is entertained, an appropriate diagnostic radiologic study should be performed. Plain abdominal films may show evidence of intussusception such as identifying a soft tissue mass in the right side of the abdomen, but are not reliable in ruling out the diagnosis of intussusception. Traditionally, contrast enemas have been advocated as the "gold standard" for diagnosis. However, contrast enemas involve radiation exposure and do not evaluate the abdomen for other causes of abdominal pain. More recently, ultrasound has been shown to be up to 100% sensitive and specific in the diagnosis of intussusception, it involves no radiation exposure and can identify alternative causes of abdominal pain (59).

Air contrast enema reduction is considered the safest and most effective method (~90% success rate) of nonoperative management of intussusception. Since the first description of the use of a retrograde enema for the reduction of intussusception, many modifications have been made, which resulted in a safer and more successful procedure. In our institution, the air contrast enema is administered through a catheter placed into the child's rectum and secured with tape. The buttock cheeks are squeezed together as air is insufflated to no more than 120mmHg of pressure. The intussusception is then followed fluoroscopically until it completely reduces, as indicated by a rush of air into the ileum. Enema reduction is not attempted in patients with peritonitis, shock, or evidence of perforation on abdominal x-ray (60).

The main complications of enema reduction are bowel perforation and failure of reduction. These complications occur more frequently in younger children and those with a longer duration of symptoms. Other problems that may be encountered are incomplete reduction and recurrence of intussusception after successful reduction.

Bowel perforation is the most serious complication of enema reduction. Perforations occur in up to 3% of cases, and may involve either healthy or ischemic intestines (60, 61). The rate of bowel perforation has been shown to be higher in younger patients and those who have had a longer duration of symptoms. In one study of bowel perforation after enema reductions, patients who were younger than 6 months of age and those who had symptoms for more than two days were at a higher risk for perforation. Another risk factor for perforation is a high insufflation pressure. Limiting insufflation pressure to less than 120 mmHg may help prevent bowel injury, although perforations at pressures as low as 60 mmHg have been described. Unlike the amount of pressure used, the type of enema has not been shown to affect the rate of perforation. Pneumatic and hydrostatic pressure (barium or gastrograffin) enemas have been shown to have similar perforation rates; however, the morbidity of a perforation from a hydrostatic enema is higher. When perforations occur with barium, patients are more likely to require bowel resection and a longer hospital stay because barium, due to its higher viscosity, results in larger holes and markedly worse peritoneal soiling (61).

Intestinal perforation during enema reduction requires prompt surgical intervention. Surgical management of perforation depends on intraoperative findings. Once the intussusception is reduced intraoperatively, and depending on the extent of injury and condition of the intestines, the area of perforation may be repaired primarily or resected. Primary repair is more frequently possible with perforations from an air contrast enema, where the perforation is usually small with minimal spillage. Perforations secondary to barium more frequently result in larger tears (due its the higher viscosity) and worse spillage. Bowel resection with or without ostomy formation is a safer option in this scenario (61). Occasionally, when a perforation occurs during air enema administration, a tension penumoperitoneum may develop, resulting in hemodynamic and respiratory compromise. This is due to the increased intraabdominal pressure pushing up on the diaphragm and impeding venous return to the heart. An 18 guage needle should always be available to decompress the abdomen in the event of tension pneumoperitoneum (62).

Enemas fail to reduce intussusception in up to 20% of cases. The main risk factors related to failure of reduction are a younger age and longer duration of symptoms. Children younger than three months of age and those who have had symptoms for more than two days are at highest risk for failure of enema reduction (60,63). Enema reduction has a higher failure rate in patients with ileoileocolic intussusception. This form of intussusception, which appears as a fronded mass within a fluid-filled cecum on ultrasound, is associated with a 90% rate of failure of reduction and higher rate of bowel ischemia (64). Ultrasonographic findings of trapped fluid within the intussusception and the intussusceptum reaching the rectum are other conditions associated with less successful enema reduction (63,65). As long as the maximum pressure is not exceeded during enema administration and patients are stable, multiple attempts may be made to reduce an intussusception. If initial attempts only achieve partial reduction, waiting a few hours and repeating an air enema may lead to success. Improved perfusion and decreased edema of the intussusception after a partial reduction may account for success with repeat enemas (66).

An important criterion for confirming complete reduction of bowel is documenting reflux of gas into the small bowel. If gas does not reflux, the intussusception may have not been completely reduced or the patient may have an ileoileocolic intussusception. In this situation, an attempt can be repeated after a few hours. It is important to document the persistence of intussusception with sonography prior to repeated attempts, since spontaneous reduction may occur during the waiting period. Close observation between attempts is important to assure patient stability (66).

Five to ten percent of patients successfully reduced will have recurrence of their intus-susception (67, 68). The majority of recurrences will occur in the first few days after successful reduction. Daneman et al. noted that 50% of patients have the recurrence in the first 48 hours, with one-third having more than one recurrence. Patients with recurrence tend to present early, probably because of a higher index of suspicion, and quicker symptom recognition by parents. Once a recurrence is identified, usually by ultrasound, and if no contraindications are present, an air contrast enema should be attempted. Studies have shown that enemas have the same success rate with recurrent as with initial intussusception (68). No clear risk factors have been associated with recurrence of intussusception. Some surgeons recommend surgical resection of the intussusception that recurs because of concerns for a pathologic lead point. Daneman et al. noted only a slight increase in the presence of a lead point between initial and recurrent intussusception, 6% compared to 8%. None of the characteristics of the recurrence were asso-ciated with a higher risk of a pathologic lead point. Even though recurrence is associated with only a slight increase in risk, it is recommended that patients be evaluated for a pathologic lead point by either ultrasound, CT scan, or barium enema, particularly if they have had multiple recurrences (60).

Complications of Operative Intervention

Operative intervention is indicated in patients who demonstrate signs of perforation, those who fail attempts at enema reduction or are found to have evidence of a pathological lead point on contrast studies. Manual reduction with no further intervention is possible in up to 70% of cases (58). Resection with primary repair is indicated when manual reduction fails, the reduced segment of intestine is not viable or a pathologic lead point is identified. Caution should be used when palpating for pathologic lead points. Enlarged Peyer's patches can be confused for malignant growth; the former require no resection, the latter may. Occasionally, a small enterotomy is identified after reduction, which may safely be managed with primary repair (60). Temporary stoma formation is the safest option for patients who present with perforation and peritoneal soiling.

Complications of operative management include bowel injury from manipulating the intussusception, wound infection and dehiscence, recurrent intussusception, and adhesive small bowel obstruction (69). Improper handling of the intussusception may result in injury during manual reduction. The safest technique is to milk the intussusceptum free, and avoid pulling on the proximal bowel, which increases the risk of bowel injury and may lead to the need for bowel resection. Bowel resection in the unprepped patient increases the risk of postoperative complications such as wound infection, dehiscence, and abscess formation. Interestingly, recurrent intussusception after operative reduction has been reported to occur less frequently than after enema reduction. The 3% rate of recurrence after operative reduction is presumably due to postoperative adhesion formation (67).

NECROTIZING ENTEROCOLITIS

Necrotizing enterocolitis (NEC) is a condition involving an inflammatory process of the GI tract of newborns. It is the most common GI emergency seen in the neonatal intensive care unit (70). Patients at highest risk for NEC are preterm low birth weight infants who have received enteral feeds. The pathophysiology of NEC is believed to be related to the combination of ischemic changes to intestinal mucosa, bacterial colonization of the GI tract, and the presence of a substrate such a formula in the gut lumen (71). Once NEC is diagnosed, feeds are held; patients are started on broad spectrum antibiotics and followed up with serial abdominal plain films and exams. Approximately half of the patients with NEC will require surgical intervention because of evidence of intestinal perforation or persistent illness despite medical therapy (72).

Disease-Related Complications

Necrotizing enterocolitis may progress to intestinal gangrene and perforation in around 50% of patients. Intestinal perforation, which is evident by free air on abdominal plain films, is generally considered the only absolute indication for surgical intervention. The extent of intestinal injury in NEC ranges from segmental to massive intestinal involvement (NEC totalis). Intestinal failure and short bowel syndrome develop when residual intestinal function after resection or recovery from ischemia is insufficient to meet the nutritional demands of the infant. Short bowel syndrome is the most common long-term complication in patients who survive NEC and occurs in around 10% of these patients (70). Short bowel syndrome from necrotizing enterocolitis is one of the main causes for intestinal transplantation in infants (73). During operative exploration of patients with extensive intestinal involvement, the surgeon should attempt to preserve as much intestinal length as possible to avoid SBS. Deciding on the extent of bowel resection can be difficult. On one hand, there is a theoretical advantage to resecting ischemic segments of intestine to control the source of inflammation and abate the disease process. On the other hand, marginally viable bowel may recover if left behind, avoiding possible SBS. Several operative strategies have been devised to attempts to preserve as much intestinal length as possible. These will be discussed later in the section on procedure-related complications.

Intestinal stenosis is another entity that may complicate the course of NEC. Intestinal stenosis is a narrowing of the intestinal lumen due to either fibrosis (stricture) or edema and ulceration without fibrosis. Stenosis occurs when segments of intestine do not completely recover from the ischemic insult. The term stenosis, rather than stricture, emphasizes the concept that some of the radiologic findings of decreased lumen size are reversible and not necessarily due to permanent fibrosis (74). Schwartz et al. performed routine screening contrast enemas on patients after medical management of NEC and noted a 35% rate of stenosis. Intestinal stenosis was detected an average of 3 weeks after the episode of NEC and tended to occur in the left colon. Not all patients who were found to have stenosis were symptomatic; however, half of asymptomatic patients went on to develop signs and symptoms of obstruction within a month of discharge. The authors recommended frequent follow-up of asymptomatic patients with repeat enemas to follow the progression of the stenosis. When patients were symptomatic, they had either signs of intestinal obstruction or bloody bowel movements (75). Interestingly, Tonkin et al. noted that some patients with asymptomatic stenosis who were reevaluated with contrast enemas were found to have normal intestinal caliber, signifying resolution of the stenosis (74).

A few patients may have recurrent NEC despite initial successful medical or operative management. In 5% of cases, infants may have one or more recurrent episodes of NEC. In a study by Stringer et al., infants with recurrent NEC were noted to be either very low birth weight infants or have major associated cardiac anomalies. One patient had a superior mesenteric artery thrombosis and experienced four episodes of recurrent NEC. No relation to a particular feeding regimen or the method of management of the initial episode (medical or operative) was noted. Most of the patients with recurrent NEC were successfully treated medically, with a mortality of 12% as a consequence of parenteral nutrition associated liver failure (76).

Table 3 Complications of Operative Management of
NEC (70)

Complication	*n*	%
Sepsis	23	9
Stricture	23	9
Short gut	22	8.7
Wound infection	15	5.9
Stoma	12	4.7
Bowel obstruction	9	3.5
Renal failure	8	3.1
DIC	8	3.1
Intraabdominal abscess	6	2.3

Abbreviation: NEC, necrotizing enterocolitis; DIC, disseminated
intravascular coagulopathy.

Procedure-Related Complications

Patients treated for NEC are a heterogeneous group with variable degrees of illness and comorbidities; this makes comparing the outcomes of different modalities of therapy difficult. This is evident in several studies comparing laparotomy to peritoneal drainage in infants with NEC. These studies are confounded by the preferential treatment of smaller and sicker infants by peritoneal drainage and larger and less sick ones by laparotomy. The two different modalities offer theoretical advantages in terms of preservation of intestinal length. On one hand, peritoneal drainage avoids potentially unnecessary intestinal resection and gives marginally viable segments of intestine that might have otherwise been resected a chance to recover; on the other hand, laparotomy and intestinal resection may result in more rapid control of the disease process by eliminating the source of sepsis. The heterogeneity of the patient population and the multiple confounding factors related to the management of these patients makes data interpretation difficult.

Postoperative complications occur in 50% of patients treated for NEC. A study by Horwitz et al. showed a 63% rate of complications after peritoneal drainage and 44% after laparotomy (70). The rate of complications in that study was independent of the indication for operation, whether it was failure of medical therapy or perforation, and was higher in patients treated with drainage, probably because that group of patients tends to be sicker. Complications related to surgical intervention include postoperative sepsis, intestinal stricture formation, short bowel syndrome, wound infections, stoma complications, bowel obstruction, and intra-abdominal abscess formation (Table 3). Some of these complications may be related more to the extent of the disease process than the operation performed. For example, it is unclear if intestinal stenosis distal to a stoma is purely due to the natural progression of intestinal ischemia or if it is related to the diversion of enteric contents that may contribute to the maintenance of intestinal lumen caliber by their trophic properties and/or mechanical presence. The same applies for persistent postoperative sepsis, intra-abdominal abscess formation and short bowel syndrome.

In a study by Horwitz et al., postoperative sepsis occurred in 7% of patients who underwent laparotomy and 19% of patients who underwent peritoneal drainage. Sepsis was the main postoperative complication in both these two groups, and was more frequent in infants weighing less than 1000 g, presumably because of a more immature immune system (70). The significance of postoperative sepsis is that it is associated with a 30-day mortality of 50%. The presence and severity of preoperative sepsis were not addressed in that study, so it is unclear if the poor outcome was because the infants were initially sicker.

Intestinal strictures are a known complication of NEC, and result from ischemic changes to the affected intestinal segments. Some studies have shown that patients who undergo laparotomy with bowel resection have a lower incidence of intestinal stenosis than those treated with peritoneal drainage. Horwitz et al. noted that intestinal stenosis was twice as common in patients who underwent peritoneal drainage than those who underwent a laparotomy (15% versus 7%). This increased rate of stenosis is believed to be related to the fact that, with peritoneal drainage, the most affected segments of ischemic intestine are left behind, and those are more prone to stricture formation (70). Another theory behind the development of strictures in patients with NEC relates to the role of the absence of enteric contents in distal intestinal segments of patients treated with resection and stoma formation. O'Connor et al., in a study of patients after stoma formation, noted a 40% rate of intestinal strictures distal to the site of diversion. Intestinal content may play a role in decreasing the rate of stricture formation, both by a local trophic effect and through mechanical dilation of the intestinal lumen (77).

The objective of surgical management of NEC is to resect nonviable bowel and preserve as much salvageable intestinal length as possible. It is this balance that may mean the difference between insufficient bowel resection and SBS. Deciding on the extent of bowel resection depends on intraoperative judgment of intestinal viability and the procedure planned. Cikrit et al. reported on patient outcome after surgical management of NEC and noted a 38% rate of SBS; the majority of these patients underwent intestinal resection and enterostomy (78). Resection and primary anastomosis, despite its appeal and advantage of avoiding potential complications of stoma formation, may inherently promote excessive intestinal resection as the surgeon attempts to obtain clearly viable intestinal margins suitable for a safe anastomosis. As discussed earlier, procedures have been devised to help preserve as much intestinal length as possible, particularly in cases of massive intestinal involvement (NEC totalis). Procedures designed to preserve intestinal length include proximal diversion, the "clip and drop" technique, and "patch, drain, and wait" approach (79). When a diverting entersotomy is constructed proximal to the intestinal segments involved with NEC, the aim is to divert enteric content away from ischemic but potentially viable bowel while it recovers from its injury. The peritoneal cavity may be drained, but intestinal resection is avoided. Once the systemic inflammatory process is controlled, a second operation is performed, usually weeks to months later, and the ostomy is taken down and any stenotic or nonviable bowel is resected. Luzzato et al. reported a decrease in the length of diseased intestinal segments at reexploration when compared to the initial operation. Unfortunately, the patients are exposed to the risks associated with stoma construction, such as stricture formation, parastomal hernias, wound complications, the need for bowel resection, and anastomotic complications after reversal. The stoma also predisposes patients to complications of high ostomy output such as fluid and electrolyte abnormalities. Another operative strategy aimed at reducing the amount of bowel resected is the clip and drop back technique. With this procedure, only clearly nonviable intestinal segments are resected. Residual intervening segments are dropped back into the abdominal cavity. A second look operation is later performed and based on the viability of residual intestinal segments, they are either anastomosed or further resection performed and a third look operation planned. Still another technique aimed at the preservation of intestinal length is the "patch, drain, and wait" approach, where intestinal contents are evacuated through existing intestinal perforations which are then closed using either imbricating sutures or patched with adjacent segments of intestine. The basic principle behind this approach is avoiding bowel resection and enterostomies, thus minimizing the chance of SBS. Drains are placed into the peritoneal cavity and no further operative intervention performed for the next 14 days, while the patients receive antibiotics and TPN. Moore et al. reported their experience with 23 patients treated in this manner with excellent results (80).

Stoma formation is generally considered the safest approach to the patient who needs intestinal resection for NEC. The combination of unprepped bowel with questionable viability and a patient who is systemically ill makes the option of a stoma appealing. This offers the advantage of avoiding an anastomosis in suboptimal conditions within the peritoneal cavity between intestinal segments that may not have sufficient perfusion, which predisposes to complications such as strictures and anastomotic leaks. Patients are also frequently malnourished and a stoma allows time for optimization of nutritional status prior to formation of an anastomosis. Despite their appeal, enterostomies are not without complications. Potential problems include skin excoriation, strictures, parastomal hernias, prolapse or intussusception and high output resulting in fluid and electrolyte abnormalities, particularly in more proximally located enterostomies. Additionally, enterostomies divert luminal contents away from distal bowel, which may be associated with an increased rate of intestinal strictures because luminal contents may have a role in preventing stenosis by virtue of their nutritive and mechanical properties (77).

In selected patients with NEC, intestinal resection with primary anastomosis may be safely performed. The advantage to primary anastomosis is that it avoids the complications associated with enterostomies and the need for a second operation. Additionally, establishing intestinal continuity early may help decrease the rate of distal stricture formation and accelerate distal intestinal adaptation and thus help avoid SBS. The argument against primary anastomosis is that performing an anastomosis between segments of bowel with potentially compromised blood flow and in a suboptimal milieu may increase the risk of complications such as anastomotic leaks and strictures. In addition, and in an attempt to reach healthy intestinal segments suitable for anastomosis, surgeons may be forced to resect potentially viable bowel and increase the risk of SBS. Studies comparing resection and anastomosis to enterostomy formation report variable results (81–83). Unfortunately, selection bias in these retrospective studies where primary anastomosis might have been more readily performed in healthier patients with less extensive disease makes interpretation of the results difficult. If primary anastomosis chosen, distal irrigation of the bowel to washout residual stool is vital to help avoid anastomotic breakdown.

MECONIUM ILEUS

Meconium ileus is a condition where inspissated meconium results in obstruction of the intestines of neonates either directly by occluding the intestinal lumen or indirectly by causing atresia or segmental volvulus. The vast majority of the patients with MI have cystic fibrosis, which is why early detection is important to patient outcome. Prenatal ultrasound findings of dilated intestinal loops with increased echogenicity in fetuses after 15 weeks of gestation should raise the suspicion for MI and initiate parental CF screening to help with early detection (84). In the United States, with newborn screening programs, infants with MI can have their newborn screen results expedited, which can help make the diagnosis and initiate therapy early. Cystic fibrosis, through various mechanisms, results in the production of meconium of abnormal consistency, which is responsible for the spectrum of complications of MI. Meconium ileus is a unique example of a condition where complications and outcome are predominantly related to the underlying disease process. Approximately 50% of patients with MI present with what is referred to as simple MI, where the obstruction is due to the mechanical properties of the tenacious, intraluminal meconium, but otherwise intact GI tract. This group of patients can frequently be managed nonoperatively, with hydrostatic enemas. On the other hand, heavy meconium filled loops of bowel may twist on themselves causing gangrene, perforation, segmental volvulus, bowel atresia, giant meconium cyst, or meconium peritonitis. When an infant has any of the above conditions associated with MI, they are referred to as having complicated MI. The treatment of MI varies depending on the presentation. In simple MI, the goal is to evacuate the meconium from the intestinal lumen. This is done by irrigating the intestinal lumen using a retrograde enema or through an enterotomy. The management of complicated MI is always operative and varies from resection with anastomosis to resection with stoma formation (85).

Disease-Related Complications
The majority of morbidity and mortality of patients with MI is due to cystic fibrosis, which is almost universally present in this patient population. Subsequently, it is important to mention complications of CF that may directly affect surgical outcome.

Patients with CF produce thick respiratory secretions which are responsible for many of the pulmonary complications associated with this disease process. Pulmonary complications of CF may manifest at a very early stage as mucous plugging of the tracheobronchial tree of the neonate with inflammation and bacterial colonization developing over the first year of life. Aggressive perioperative pulmonary toilet (manual or using pneumatic drainage vests in children) and nebulizer treatment (particularly immediately preoperatively) with prompt weaning from any ventilator support are vital in improving outcome of patients with CF who require surgery (86). Studies have shown that surgery is relatively safe in patients with CF, especially with improvement of anesthesia and critical care. In a study by Saltzman et al. of 130 patients with CF who underwent surgery, the 5% rate of postoperative mortality was largely from progressive respiratory failure due to CF and not directly related to surgical intervention (87). Focal biliary cirrhosis, which occurs in around a third of patients with CF, is another contributor to morbidity. The pathogenesis is thought to be similar to that of lung disease and related to poor regulation of biliary ductal secretions, with resultant obstruction of biliary drainage by inspissated secretions and subsequent bile duct injury. Clinically, patients may have signs of portal hypertension, and less frequently, hepatocellular failure (88). In addition, in our experience, TPN associated cholestasis in patients with SBS from complicated MI is another contributor to morbidity and mortality in this patient population. The team approach to surgical patients with CF, with close involvement of pulmonary specialists, gastroenterologists, dieticians, and respiratory therapy, is critical in improving the outcome of this patient population.

Poor nutritional status is another problem associated with CF that influences surgical outcome by increasing the risk of postoperative complications. Patients with CF are at a higher risk for malnutrition because of an increase in metabolic requirements, exocrine pancreatic insufficiency, and bile stasis. A study by Lai et al. suggests that patients with CF with a history of MI are at an even higher risk of malnutrition than those with no previous history of MI (89).

A third of patients with CF experience intraabdominal complications of their disease (90). Distal intestinal obstruction syndrome (DIOS), formerly referred to as MI equivalent, is a condition where viscid intestinal contents cause a mechanical intestinal obstruction similar to MI. Patients are usually older children and present with abdominal pain and signs of intestinal obstruction. This condition is usually precipitated by poor patient compliance with their pancreatic enzyme supplementation. Most patients with DIOS respond to ployethylene glycol (Golytely®) administered orally or as an enema and do not usually require surgical intervention. Rectal prolapse and ileocolic intussusception are two other conditions that can be associated with CF. Children with rectal prolapse and those who present with ilieocolic intussusception at an older age should be evaluated for CF since both can be the initial presenting signs of this disease. Inguinal hernias can also be problematic in patients with CF. Many factors, including chronic cough and poor nutrition, play a role in the higher incidence and recurrence rate of inguinal hernias in patients with CF (87). Patients with CF are also at a higher risk of developing GERD. Because of nutritional considerations related to CF, gastrostomy tubes are frequently placed concomitantly with a Nissen procedure to help keep up with postoperative nutritional requirements. Advances in nutritional management, particularly the emphasis on maximizing enteral caloric intake, have made a notable impact on the outcome of patients with CF, which stresses the need for a thorough nutritional evaluation and aggressive nutritional optimization of this set of patients prior to any elective surgical procedures.

Fibrosing colonopathy (submucosal fibrosis of the colon) is a condition that occurs in patients with CF receiving high dose pancreatic enzyme supplementation. Patients present with colonic obstruction secondary to stricture formation due to submucosal fibrosis. Once the diagnosis is confirmed with contrast studies, the strictured segment of colon should be resected. Pancreatic enzyme doses should be limited to 2500 units per kilogram per meal to avoid injury to the colonic mucosa help prevent fibrosing colonopathy (91).

Complications of Diagnostic/Theraputic Enemas

Several alternative strategies have been proposed for the nonoperative management of MI, but hyperosomolar contrast enemas (Gastrografin) remain the mainstay for both the diagnosis and treatment of MI. Gastrografin enemas have been shown to be the most effective in relieving the obstruction. After administration of the enema, the hyperosmolar contrast material results in a fluid shift into the lumen of the bowel which subsequently helps soften and evacuate meconium. Unfortunately, this fluid shift may result in bowel distention and third space fluid loss; this places patients at risk for hypovolemic shock, mucosal and submucosal inflammation, intestinal perforation and ischemic enterocolitis (92). The most detrimental complication of enema administration is bowel perforation. Intestinal perforation, which has been reported to occur in around 5% of cases, may occur acutely during the procedure or several days later (90,93). Acute perforation is usually due to an increase in intraluminal pressure beyond the bursting pressure of the intestinal wall. Controlling the pressure at which an enema is administered and avoiding the use of a balloon tip catheter are the two main methods of decreasing the rate of perforation. Delayed perforation may be due to over distension of bowel and mucosal injury which later progresses to a transmural injury and perforation. Most enemas are administered at half strength to help avoid these complications and reduce fluid shifts into the intestinal lumen. Adequate fluid resuscitation, gentle enema administration and close supervision by a surgeon are important precautions that should be taken to assure the safety of this procedure (94). In simple MI, several contrast enemas, every 12 to 24 hours may be necessary to successfully evacuate the inspissated meconium and can be continued as long as progress is being made and the patient remains physiologically stable.

Complications of Operative Management

When repeated attempts at resolving the obstruction using enema irrigation fail, or patients present with complicated MI, operative intervention is necessary. The key operative goals are evacuation of meconium and resection of any nonviable bowel. In simple MI, meconium can be evacuated by irrigating the intestinal lumen through either an enterotomy or the base of the appendix after performing an appendectomy. Once accessible meconium is evacuated, Gastrograffin, 5% N-acetyl cysteine or normal saline is instilled into the bowel lumen and used to evacuate any residual meconium. Complicated MI requires resection of the segment of abnormal intestine with primary anastomosis or stoma formation. Adequate distal irrigation is crucial in cases where a primary anastomosis is performed to prevent distal obstruction that may jeopardize the anastomosis. Traditionally, stoma formation has been considered the most conservative way to manage infants who require unplanned intestinal resection. Several different types of stomas, such as the Santulli, Bishop-Koop, and double barrel enterostomies, have been devised to allow continued irrigation of the small bowel while allowing early feeding. Because of the inherent complications associated with an intestinal stoma, as well as the need for a second operation to reverse it, there has been a trend toward avoiding intestinal stomas in selected situations. The two circumstances where primary anastomosis may be considered a safe option are when volvulus or atresia is present, and there is no peritoneal soiling (95). Resection and primary anastomosis avoids potential complications of stoma formation such as stricture, fistula, prolapse, high volume output, and the need for a second operation for reversal. In a study by Weber et al., a third of newborns who underwent jejunostomy or ileostomy formation for various disease processes had complications related to the enterostomy within weeks of the operation. All of these patients required ostomy revision (96). The author attributed the high rate of complications to the use of marginally viable bowel while attempting to avoid excessive bowel resection and potential short gut syndrome.

If an enterostomy is placed too proximally in the small bowel, the length of intestine upstream of it may not be sufficient to absorb fluids and electrolytes adequately, which may result in a high output enterostomy. High output enterostomies can be particularly troublesome since they place the infants at risk of fluid and electrolyte imbalance, poor weight gain and metabolic acidosis from sodium and bicarbonate loss. These enterostomies should be reversed as soon as possible. Bower et al. studied the effect of sodium deficit on growth and noted that infants with enterostomies tended to have poor growth if the urine spot sodium was less than 10 mEq/L, even if their serum sodium levels were normal. They noted that when these infants were given supplementary enteral sodium until the urine sodium increased to more than 20 mEq/L, they grew satisfactorily. The mean ileostomy output that required supplementation in that study was 30 mL/kg/day (97).

There has been a significant improvement in operative mortality in patients treated for MI, where current mortality is around 5% (87). Overall one-year survival has increased from 50% to around 98%, in both simple and complicated MI (93,98). Much of this improvement in survival is due to advances in management of CF and the multidisciplinary approach to the disease. Despite progress in the management of this group of patients, patients with MI still fair worse in terms of their long-term nutritional status when compared to patients with CF but no MI, which is probably related to the nutritional insult suffered by these patients during the neonatal period (86).

REFERENCES

1. St Peter SD, Holcomb GW III, Calkins CM, et al. Open versus laparoscopic pyloromyotomy for pyloric stenosis: A prospective, randomized trial. Ann Surg 2006; 244 (3):363–370.
2. Naik-Mathuria B, Olutoye OO. Foregut abnormalities. Surg Clin North Am 2006; 86(2):261–284, viii.
3. Steiner MJ, DeWalt DA, Byerley JS. Is this child dehydrated? JAMA 2004; 291(22):2746–2754.
4. Rice HE, Caty MG, Glick PL. Fluid therapy for the pediatric surgical patient. Ped Clin North Am 1998; 45(4):719–727.
5. Safford SD, Pietrobon R, Safford KM, et al. A study of 11,003 patients with hypertrophic pyloric stenosis and the association between surgeon and hospital volume and outcomes. J Pediatr Surg 2005; 40(6):967–972; discussion 72–73.
6. Scharli AF, Leditschke JF. Gastric motility after pyloromyotomy in infants. A reappraisal of postoperative feeding. Surgery 1968; 64(6):1133–1137.

7. Adibe OO, Nichol PF, Lim FY, et al. Ad libitum feeds after laparoscopic pyloromyotomy: A retrospective comparison with a standardized feeding regimen in 227 infants. J Laparoendosc Adv Surg Tech 2007; 17(2):235–237.

8. Gollin G, Doslouglu H, Flummerfeldt P, et al. Rapid advancement of feedings after pyloromyotomy for pyloric stenosis. Clin Pediatr (Phila) 2000; 39(3):187–190.

9. Grosfeld JL, O'Neill JA, Jr., Fonkalsrud EW, et al. Pediatric Surgery. 6th ed. Philadelphia: Mosby Elsevier, 2006.

10. Yagmurlu A, Barnhart DC, Vernon A, et al. Comparison of the incidence of complications in open and laparoscopic pyloromyotomy: A concurrent single institution series. J Pediatr Surg 2004; 39(3):292–296; discussion-6.

11. Leclair MD, Plattner V, Mirallie E, et al. Laparoscopic pyloromyotomy for hypertrophic pyloric stenosis: A prospective, randomized controlled trial. J Pediatr Surg 2007; 42(4):692–698.

12. Stringer MD, Oldham KT, Mouriquand PD, et al. Pediatric Surgery and Urology: Long term outcomes. W. B. Saunders, 1998.

13. Levitt MA, Rothenberg SS, Tanotoco JG, et al. Complication avoidance in miniature access pyloromyotomy. Pediatr Endosurgery and Innovative Techniques 2003; 7(3):291–296.

14. Bufo AJ, Merry C, Shah R, et al. Laparoscopic pyloromyotomy: A safer technique. Pediatr Surg Int 1998; 13(4):240–242.

15. Fujimoto T, Lane GJ, Segawa O, et al. Laparoscopic extramucosal pyloromyotomy versus open pyloromyotomy for infantile hypertrophic pyloric stenosis: Which is better? J Pediatr Surg 1999; 34(2):370–372.

16. Duque-Estrada EO, Duarte MR, Rodrigues DM, et al. Wound infections in pediatric surgery: A study of 575 patients in a university hospital. Pediatr Surg Int 2003; 19(6):436–438.

17. Ladd AP, Nemeth SA, Kirincich AN, et al. Supraumbilical pyloromyotomy: A unique indication for antimicrobial prophylaxis. J Pediatr Surg 2005; 40(6):974–977; discussion 7.

18. Escobar MA, Ladd AP, Grosfeld JL, et al. Duodenal atresia and stenosis: Long-term follow-up over 30 years. J Pediatr Surg 2004; 39(6):867–871.

19. Dalla Vecchia LK, Grosfeld JL, West KW, et al. Intestinal atresia and stenosis: A 25-year experience with 277 cases. Arch Surg 1998; 133(5):490–496; discussion 6–7.

20. Grosfeld JL, Rescorla FJ. Duodenal atresia and stenosis: Reassessment of treatment and outcome based on antenatal diagnosis, pathologic variance, and long-term follow-up. World J Surg 1993; 17(3):301–309.

21. Spigland N, Yazbeck S. Complications associated with surgical treatment of congenital intrinsic duodenal obstruction. J Pediatr Surg 1990; 25(11):1127–1130.

22. Fonkalsrud EW, DeLorimier AA, Hays DM. Congenital atresia and stenosis of the duodenum. A review compiled from the members of the Surgical Section of the American Academy of Pediatrics. Pediatrics 1969; 43(1):79–83.

23. Weber TR, Lewis JE, Mooney D, et al. Duodenal atresia: A comparison of techniques of repair. J Pediatr Surg 1986; 21(12):1133–1136.

24. Kimura K, Mukohara N, Nishijima E, et al. Diamond-shaped anastomosis for duodenal atresia: An experience with 44 patients over 15 years. J Pediatr Surg 1990; 25(9):977–979.

25. Boyden EA, Cope JG, Bill AH, Jr. Anatomy and embryology of congenital intrinsic obstruction of the duodenum. Am J Surg 1967; 114(2):190–202.

26. Bowen J, Dickson A, Bruce J. Reconstruciton for duodenal atresia: Tapered or non-tapered duodenoplasty? Pediatr Surg Int 1996; 11:474–476.

27. Richardson WR, Martin LW. Pitfalls in the surgical management of the incomplete duodenal diaphragm. J Pediatr Surg 1969; 4(3):303–312.

28. Weitzman JJ, Brennan LP. An improved technique for the correction of congenital duodenal obstruction in the neonate. J Pediatr Surg 1974; 9(3):385–388.

29. de Lorimier AA, Norman DA, Goodling CA, et al. A model for the cinefluoroscopic and manometric study of chronic intestinal obstruction. J Pediatr Surg 1973; 8(5):785–791.

30. Nixon HH, Tawes R. Etiology and treatment of small intestinal atresia: Analysis of a series of 127 jejunoileal atresias and comparison with 62 duodenal atresias. Surgery 1971; 69(1):41–51.

31. Adzick NS, Harrison MR, deLorimier AA. Tapering duodenoplasty for megaduodenum associated with duodenal atresia. J Pediatr Surg 1986; 21(4):311–312.

32. de Lorimier AA, Harrison MR. Intestinal plication in the treatment of atresia. J Pediatr Surg 1983; 18(6):734–737.

33. Ein SH, Kim PC, Miller HA. The late nonfunctioning duodenal atresia repair—A second look. J Pediatr Surg 2000; 35(5):690–691.

34. Kokkonen ML, Kalima T, Jaaskelainen J, et al. Duodenal atresia: Late follow-up. J Pediatr Surg 1988; 23(3):216–220.

35. Rescorla FJ, Grosfeld JL. Duodenal atresia in infancy and childhood: Improved survival and long-term follow-up. Contemp Surg 1988; 33:22–28.

36. Takahashi A, Tomomasa T, Suzuki N, et al. The relationship between disturbed transit and dilated bowel, and manometric findings of dilated bowel in patients with duodenal atresia and stenosis. J Pediatr Surg 1997; 32(8):1157–1160.

37. Masumoto K, Suita S, Nada O, et al. Abnormalities of enteric neurons, intestinal pacemaker cells, and smooth muscle in human intestinal atresia. J Pediatr Surg 1999; 34(10):1463–1468.

38. Warner BW, Vanderhoof JA, Reyes JD. What's new in the management of short gut syndrome in children. J Am Coll Surg 2000; 190(6):725–736.

39. Glick PL, de Lorimier AA, Adzick NS, et al. Colon interposition: An adjuvant operation for short-gut syndrome. J Pediatr Surg 1984; 19(6):719–725.

40. Thompson JS, Langnas AN, Pinch LW, et al. Surgical approach to short-bowel syndrome. Experience in a population of 160 patients. Ann Surg 1995; 222(4):600–605; discussion 5–7.

41. Gura MK, Lee S, Valim C, et al. Safety and efficency of a fish-oil based fat emulsion in the treatment of parental nutrition associated liver disease. Pediatrics 2008; 121:c678–686.

42. Snyder CL, Miller KA, Sharp RJ, et al. Management of intestinal atresia in patients with gastroschisis. J Pediatr Surg 2001; 36(10):1542–1545.

43. DeLorimier AA, Fonkalsrud EW, Hays DM. Congenital atresia and stenosis of the jejunum and ileum. Surgery 1969; 65(5):819–827.

44. Johnson SM, Meyers RL. Inherited thrombophilia: A possible cause of in utero vascular thrombosis in children with intestinal atresia. J Pediatr Surg 2001; 36(8):1146–1149.

45. Snyder WH, Jr., Chaffin L. Embryology and pathology of the intestinal tract: Presentation of 40 cases of malrotation. Ann Surg 1954; 140(3):368–379.

46. Ford EG, Senac MO Jr, Srikanth MS, et al. Malrotation of the intestine in children. Ann Surg 1992; 215(2):172–178.

47. Brueckner M. Heterotaxia, congenital heart disease, and primary ciliary dyskinesia. Circulation 2007; 115(22):2793–2795.

48. Tashjian DB, Weeks B, Brueckner M, et al. Outcomes after a Ladd procedure for intestinal malrotation with heterotaxia. J Pediatr Surg 2007; 42(3):528–531.

49. Murphy FL, Sparnon AL. Long-term complications following intestinal malrotation and the Ladd's procedure: A 15 year review. Pediatr Surg Int 2006; 22(4):326–329.

50. Kirby CP, Freeman JK, Ford WD, et al. Malrotation with recurrent volvulus presenting with cholestasis, pruritus, and pancreatitis. Pediatr Surg Int 2000; 16(1–2):130–131.

51. Mazeh H, Kaliner E, Udassin R. Three recurrent episodes of malrotation in an infant. J Pediatr Surg 2007; 42(4):E1–E3.

52. Coombs RC, Buick RG, Gornall PG, et al. Intestinal malrotation: The role of small intestinal dysmotility in the cause of persistent symptoms. J Pediatr Surg 1991; 26(5):553–556.

53. Mehall JR, Chandler JC, Mehall RL, et al. Management of typical and atypical intestinal malrotation. J Pediatr Surg 2002; 37(8):1169–1172.

54. Malek MM, Burd RS. Surgical treatment of malrotation after infancy: A population-based study. J Pediatr Surg 2005; 40(1):285–289.

55. Burke MS, Glick PL. Gastrointestinal malrotation with volvulus in an adult. Am J Surg 2008; 4:501–503.

56. Messineo A, MacMillan JH, Palder SB, et al. Clinical factors affecting mortality in children with malrotation of the intestine. J Pediatr Surg 1992; 27(10):1343–1345.

57. West KW, Stephens B, Vane DW, et al. Intussusception: Current management in infants and children. Surgery 1987; 102(4):704–710.

58. Ein SH, Alton D, Palder SB, et al. Intussusception in the 1990 s: Has 25 years made a difference? Pediatr Surg Int 1997; 12(5–6):374–376.

59. del-Pozo G, Albillos JC, Tejedor D, et al. Intussusception in children: Current concepts in diagnosis and enema reduction. Radiographics 1999; 19(2):299–319.

60. Stein M, Alton DJ, Daneman A. Pneumatic reduction of intussusception: 5-year experience. Radiology 1992; 183(3):681–684.

61. Daneman A, Alton DJ, Ein S, et al. Perforation during attempted intussusception reduction in children—A comparison of perforation with barium and air. Pediatr Radiol 1995; 25(2):81–88.

62. Sohoni A, Wang NE, Dannenberg B. Tension pneumoperitoneum after intussusception pneumoreduction. Pediatr Emerg Care 2007; 23(8):563–564.

63. Applegate KE. Clinically suspected intussusception in children: Evidence-based review and self-assessment module. Am J Roentgenol 2005; 185(3 Suppl):S175–S183.

64. Peh WC, Khong PL, Lam C, et al. Ileoileocolic intussusception in children: Diagnosis and significance. Br J Radiol 1997; 70(837):891–896.

65. Britton I, Wilkinson AG. Ultrasound features of intussusception predicting outcome of air enema. Pediatr Radiol 1999; 29(9):705–710.

66. Connolly B, Alton DJ, Ein SH, et al. Partially reduced intussusception: When are repeated delayed reduction attempts appropriate? Pediatr Radiol 1995; 25(2):104–107.

67. Ein SH. Recurrent intussusception in children. J Pediatr Surg 1975; 10(5):751–755.

68. Daneman A, Alton DJ, Lobo E, et al. Patterns of recurrence of intussusception in children: A 17-year review. Pediatr Radiol 1998; 28(12):913–919.

69. Bruce J, Huh YS, Cooney DR, et al. Intussusception: Evolution of current management. J Pediatr Gastroenterol Nutr 1987; 6(5):663–674.

70. Horwitz JR, Lally KP, Cheu HW, et al. Complications after surgical intervention for necrotizing enterocolitis: A multicenter review. J Pediatr Surg 1995; 30(7):994–998; discussion 8–9.

71. Kosloske AM. Necrotizing enterocolitis in the neonate. Surg Gynecol Obstet 1979; 148(2):259–269.

72. Moss RL, Dimmitt RA, Barnhart DC, et al. Laparotomy versus peritoneal drainage for necrotizing enterocolitis and perforation. N Engl J Med 2006; 354(21):2225–2234.

73. Kato T, Mittal N, Nishida S, et al. The role of intestinal transplantation in the management of babies with extensive gut resections. J Pediatr Surg 2003; 38(2):145–149.

74. Tonkin IL, Bjelland JC, Hunter TB, et al. Spontaneous resolution of colonic strictures caused by necrotizing enterocolitis: Therapeutic implications. Am J Roentgenol 1978; 130(6):1077–1081.

75. Schwartz MZ, Richardson CJ, Hayden CK, et al. Intestinal stenosis following successful medical management of necrotizing enterocolitis. J Pediatr Surg 1980; 15(6):890–899.

76. Stringer MD, Brereton RJ, Drake DP, et al. Recurrent necrotizing enterocolitis. J Pediatr Surg 1993; 28(8):979–981.

77. O'Connor A, Sawin RS. High morbidity of enterostomy and its closure in premature infants with necrotizing enterocolitis. Arch Surg 1998; 133(8):875–880.

78. Cikrit D, West KW, Schreiner R, et al. Long-term follow-up after surgical management of necrotizing enterocolitis: Sixty-three cases. J Pediatr Surg 1986; 21(6):533–535.

79. Petty JK, Ziegler MM. Operative strategies for necrotizing enterocolitis: The prevention and treatment of short-bowel syndrome. Semin Pediatr Surg 2005; 14(3):191–198.

80. Moore TC. Successful use of the "patch, drain, and wait" laparotomy approach to perforated necrotizing enterocolitis: Is hypoxia-triggered "good angiogenesis" involved? Pediatr Surg Int 2000; 16(5–6):356–363.

81. Harberg FJ, McGill CW, Saleem MM, et al. Resection with primary anastomosis for necrotizing enterocolitis. J Pediatr Surg 1983; 18(6):743–746.

82. Cooper A, Ross AJ III, O'Neill JA Jr, et al. Resection with primary anastomosis for necrotizing enterocolitis: A contrasting view. J Pediatr Surg 1988; 23(1 Pt 2):64–68.

83. Singh M, Owen A, Gull S, et al. Surgery for intestinal perforation in preterm neonates: Anastomosis vs stoma. J Pediatr Surg 2006; 41(4):725–729.

84. Irish MS, Ragi JM, Karamanoukian H, et al. Prenatal diagnosis of the fetus with cystic fibrosis and meconium ileus. Pediatr Surg Int 1997; 12(5–6):434–436.

85. Escobar MA, Grosfeld JL, Burdick JJ, et al. Surgical considerations in cystic fibrosis: A 32-year evaluation of outcomes. Surgery 2005; 138(4):560–571; discussion 71–72.

86. Borowitz D, Irish MS, Glick PL. Prognosis and medical management of patients with meconium ileus. Pediatr Pulmonol 1996; 13:198–200.

87. Saltzman DA, Johnson EM, Feltis BA, et al. Surgical experience in patients with cystic fibrosis: A 25-year perspective. Pediatr Pulmonol 2002; 33(2):106–110.

88. Colombo C, Russo MC, Zazzeron L, et al. Liver disease in cystic fibrosis. J Pediatr Gastroenterol Nutr 2006; 43:S49–S55.

89. Lai HC, Kosorok MR, Laxova A, et al. Nutritional status of patients with cystic fibrosis with meconium ileus: A comparison with patients without meconium ileus and diagnosed early through neonatal screening. Pediatrics 2000; 105(1 Pt 1):53–61.

90. Gross K, Desanto A, Grosfeld JL, et al. Intra-abdominal complications of cystic fibrosis. J Pediatr Surg 1985; 20(4):431–435.

91. FitzSimmons SC, Burkhart GA, Borowitz D, et al. High-dose pancreatic-enzyme supplements and fibrosing colonopathy in children with cystic fibrosis. N Engl J Med 1997; 336(18):1283–1289.

92. Burke MS, Ragi JM, Karamanoukian HL, et al. New strategies in nonoperative management of meconium ileus. J Pediatr Surg 2002; 37(5):760–764.

93. Rescorla FJ, Grosfeld JL. Contemporary management of meconium ileus. World J Surg 1993; 17(3):318–325.

94. Ein SH, Shandling B, Reilly BJ, et al. Bowel perforation with nonoperative treatment of meconium ileus. J Pediatr Surg 1987; 22(2):146–147.

95. Rescorla FJ, Grosfeld JL, West KJ, et al. Changing patterns of treatment and survival in neonates with meconium ileus. Arch Surg 1989; 124(7):837–840.

96. Weber TR, Tracy TF Jr, Silen ML, et al. Enterostomy and its closure in newborns. Arch Surg 1995; 130(5):534–537.

97. Bower TR, Pringle KC, Soper RT. Sodium deficit causing decreased weight gain and metabolic acidosis in infants with ileostomy. J Pediatr Surg 1988; 23(6):567–572.

98. Mushtaq I, Wright VM, Drake DP, et al. Meconium ileus secondary to cystic fibrosis. The East London experience. Pediatr Surg Int 1998; 13(5–6):365–369.

Open Pyloromyotomy

Expert: Sigmund H. Ein, M.D.

QUESTIONS

1. **What steps can be taken to reduce the chance of wound infection?**

   The two best ways to reduce the chance of wound infection is to keep the incision away from the umbilicus and to use prophylactic antibiotics (Ancef or Clindamycin, if allergic to Penicillin).

2. **How should mucosal perforation be managed?**

   Having only had two mucosal perforations in 791 pyloromyotomies, I am not an expert on the management of this major intraoperative complication. The easiest way is to close the mucosal hole with a fine suture (4-0 silk in an interrupted fashion) and cover the closure (without closing the pyloromyotomy) with omentum (Graham Patch). The alternative is to close the entire pyloromyotomy in one or two layers (mucosa and thickened muscle) and then doing a second pyloromyotomy by rotating the pyloric stenosis upward (below the original pyloromyotomy) or on the posterior aspect. Either way, a nasogastric (NG) tube should be left in place to drain the stomach. Some leave it in place for 12 hours before removing it and feeding the baby; that seems a bit risky to me. The safest way is to leave the NG tube in place for 5 to 7 days and do a contrast study before removing it. A peritoneal drain is also a real consideration, treating it like the NG tube (not removing it until the leak has been radiologically proven healed).

3. **How should patients with persistent postoperative vomiting be managed?**

   In my experience, all postoperative pyloromyotomies vomit for a day or so. However, if the vomiting is longer than that, then one has to worry about an incomplete pyloromyotomy. In such instances, the baby is also seldom able to feed more than 45-60 cc Q3 H. If the above situation ensues, an upper gastrointestinal (UGI) contrast study is warranted. If the pyloromyotomy is incomplete (the stomach doesn't empty similar to the preoperative study) then either reoperation is indicated or, if available, Interventional Radiology may attempt to dilate the incomplete pyloromyotomy. If persistent postoperative vomiting occurs in spite of the stomach emptying (albeit slowly), drug therapy (e.g., Maxeran) may improve things. One must also rule out radiologically, in such cases, gastroesophageal reflux, which can usually be treated with medical therapy and rarely with operative repair.

4. **Does the choice of incision influence the rate of wound infection?**

   Yes, I believe so. The closer to the umbilicus, the greater the chance for a postoperative wound infection, prophylactic antibiotics notwithstanding.

5. **Should mucosal integrity be tested during the operation?**

   Probably. The few times I have seen a mucosal hole during pyloromyotomy, it has been immediately noticeable. However, nothing is 100%, so it does no harm to squeeze the usually dilated (with air) stomach after the pyloromyotomy to see if in fact the pyloromyotomy has been complete and also to see if there is a mucosal hole at the pyloromyotomy site.

6. **What intraoperative maneuvers are most important to ensure a myotomy is complete?**

   I think the most important maneuver to ensure a myotomy is complete is to make sure it is done completely. After 791 pyloromyotomies in 35 years, I am 100% convinced that this goal (no incomplete pyloromyotomies) can be very easily accomplished by making the pyloromyotomy from the pyloric vein of Mayo (just proximal to the white pyloric ring) distally, to the normal inner circular muscle fibers proximally, a pyloromyotomy of about 2 cm. Another maneuver that seems to be successful is to squeeze the large amount of residual air in the enlarged stomach distally through the successful pyloromyotomy.

Finally a third maneuver, which never appealed to me, is to wiggle the pyloric ring, after the pyloromyotomy, to make sure it is no long intact.

7. **In the hypochloremic, alkalotic infant, what levels of resuscitation of chloride and CO_2 are adequate for operation?**
I found over the years that the most important (sensitive) electrolyte for correction monitoring was the chloride. Everything else seemed to fall in place as the low chloride was corrected. Originally, I wanted the chloride to be corrected up to 95, but a paper by one of our pediatric anesthesiologists said that the baby was more safely corrected when his/her chloride was about 105. Furthermore, to quickly correct the hypochloremic alkalosis with a saline solution more concentrated than normal saline can lead to too rapid a shift in electrolytes, including driving potassium back into the cells, causing potential complications. There should never be a rush to correct the hypochloremic alkalosis in a baby with pyloric stenosis; the emergency is over when the diagnosis is made.

Repair of Duodenal Atresia

Expert: Brad W. Warner, M.D.

QUESTIONS

1. **What steps can be taken to avoid injury to the ampulla of Vater?**
The key to avoiding injury to the ampulla is maintaining a high level of awareness of potential injury during all steps of the repair. The duodenotomy should be performed on the anterolateral aspect of the proximal duodenal wall. Avoid any medial duodenal incisions. The same should be true for what part of a duodenal web to excise. One the duodenum has been opened, the gallbladder can be gently squeezed to help identify the ampulla. This may function better by simultaneously occluding the more proximal hepatic ducts with gentle finger manipulation. Alternatively, secretin can be administered to induce pancreatic secretion although this is rarely necessary.

2. **When should a dilated duodenum be tapered?**
This is an area of great controversy. In my opinion, if the proximal duodenal caliber is greater than four times the size of the distal duodenum, I would favor a tapering duodenoplasty. The exception would be that if it is technically difficult due to a shortened proximal bulb.

3. **What steps should be taken to avoid missing a coexisting intestinal atresia?**
A coexisting intestinal atresia must be excluded. This cannot be done preoperatively. I, therefore, insert a 5-Fr feeding tube into the distal duodenum and carefully inject saline after occluding the proximal duodenum with my fingers around the tube. It is relatively easy to follow the path of the injected saline through the entire small bowel and into the colon. The presence of normal appearing (dark) meconium in the colon is also reassuring that there is no significant small bowel atresia.

4. **What are the most common complications after repair of duodenal atresia?**
One of the most common problems after repair of a duodenal atresia is delayed gastric/duodenal emptying. This is heralded by persistently high volume, bilious NG aspirate, or intolerance of feeding. A water-soluble contrast study showing some passage of contrast into the distal bowel is reassuring that this should improve over time. If delayed emptying persists and/or a residual stenosis is identified on a contrast study, reoperation with revision of the anastomosis as well as a tapering of the duodenum would be warranted. I would not consider this until at least 6 weeks following initial operative repair.

5. **What are unusual complications you have seen following repair of duodenal atresia?**
One major, but unusual complication I have heard about is anastomotic dehiscence in face of an indwelling transanastomotic feeding tube. This tube in retrospect was fairly stiff and perhaps a bit larger than should have been. I am not a proponent of these tubes in routine duodenal atresia repairs and this underscores why.

I have had a patient that had severe, persistent duodenal atony despite anastomotic revision, and tapering. This ultimately responded to a Roux-en-Y duodenojejunostomy.

6. **Should a duodenojejunostomy be avoided if at all possible, even if it seems technically easier?**
I always prefer a duodenoduodenostomy, but an anastomosis to the jejunum would not be an unreasonable alternative. I have done this when the proximal and/or distal duodenum are fixed medially by the pancreas and cannot be brought together without tension. This may also occur in the rare situation whereby there is a significant gap distance between the duodenal ends.

7. **How would you manage a postoperative stricture at a duodeno-duodenostomy?**
In the absence of a significantly dilated proximal duodenum, endoscopic balloon dilation may be considered, depending on the skill and expertise of the surgeon and/or GI colleagues. In most situations, reoperation with revision of the anastomosis would be preferred, along with a tapering duodenoplasty. A Heinecke–Mikulitz type of incision is made laterally through the stricture and then closed transversely.

Repair of Small Intestinal Atresia

Expert: Sigmund H. Ein, M.D.

QUESTIONS

1. **When should a tapering enteroplasty be performed?**
A tapering enteroplasty should be performed when the small bowel proximal to the atresia is quite large. How large is "quite large"? If it looks like it needs to be tapered, it should be.

2. **What technique should be used to taper the small intestine?**
I tried the Bianchi procedure and found it technically challenging. I almost always just pleated (imbricate, turn in) the anti-mesenteric border and carried it proximally until the bowel was normal size. I found that technique worked well both technically and clinically. I was always concerned about excising (by hand or stapling) a long length of ante-mesenteric bowel, because it would leave a long suture line which ran into the anastomosis. If I were to taper the small bowel now, I would use the STEP procedure, which is simple, easy, and very amenable to stapling. The reason for using the STEP procedure is that it not only tapers the dilated and hypertrophied proximal small bowel, but it also lengthens the congenitally short small bowel, which is often found in these small bowel atresia babies.

3. **When is the proximal intestine too large to taper?**
I don't think the proximal intestine is ever too large to taper unless it is discolored, devascularized or of questionable viability, at which point it should be resected.

4. **How should distal small intestinal atresias be ruled out?**
They can be ruled out by visually and manually "running" (examining) the distal bowel, which will rule out atresias with a gap. To rule out atresias in continuity, but with an intrinsic obstruction from a web, the best way is to pass a soft catheter (small Foley) into

the distal bowel and/or inject saline. There will be a dilatation at the point of obstruction. If not, the saline will run all the way into the colon. Of course, a preoperative contrast enema can also rule out a colon atresia and even a distal ileal atresia. A saline enema apparatus can also be set up in the operating room using a Foley catheter taped in place in the rectum before the patient is anesthetized and the saline can then be allowed to run into the colon retrograde, after the abdomen is opened, and under direct vision.

5. **What technical steps help prevent postoperative anastomotic stricture?**
   The two ends of bowel being anastomosed must have a good blood supply, and the less amount of sutures the better. You don't need too wide an anastomosis to allow small bowel contents to pass through. If the proximal bowel is still wider than the distal bowel, a wide 1 inch side-to-side anastomosis can be made in a way that doesn't create a blind loop. On a few occasions when there were many atresias which I chose to preserve, after the anastomoses (with very few fine sutures), I threaded (pulled) through the entire small bowel a very fine silastic tube as a stent and brought it out the proximal jejunum as a tube jejunostomy in the left upper abdominal wall and similarly distally out an appendicostomy (after removing the appendix) in the right lower abdomen. Obviously, nothing can pass through this repaired small bowel because this is really a stent and it obstructs the tiny lumen. I removed it after 2 to 4 weeks and then did a small bowel contrast study.

6. **What unusual complications have you seen following repair of intestinal atresia?**
   None that come to mind, which is surprising. However, when I looked back at my 100 small bowel atresia patients for an answer, I was surprised to see three things:
   1. Small bowel atresia seems to happen in more than the reported 8% of gastroschisis babies.
   2. There seemed to be more multiple atresias than I remember.
   3. There seemed to be a high number of volvuli associated with small bowel atresia patients.

7. **After repair of multiple atresias how would you proceed if bowel function had not returned after 6 to 8 weeks?**
   I'd try to outline the entire gastrointestinal tract for patency with a contrast study from above, and if unsuccessful from below, or both ways. Unless the intestinal tract looks completely obstructed, I'd continue with proximal decompression of the GI tract (by nasogastric tube to suction, or gastrostomy to bedside bag), stimulation with Maxeran (Metaclopramide) and total parenteral nutrition. Even if the GI tract looks completely obstructed, at 6 to 8 weeks, I'd do the above and not rush in to reoperate for at least another month or so. The latter situation, of course, depends upon how tensely distended or not the abdomen is. The longer the baby acts completely obstructed (confirmed by clinical examination of the abdomen and radiological investigations), I would be more inclined to reoperate.

16 | Complications of Colon Surgery

Roshni Dasgupta, M.D. and Jacob C. Langer, M.D.

INFLAMMATORY BOWEL DISEASE

Children and adolescents with inflammatory bowel diseases (IBD) make up a growing proportion of patients requiring surgery in the non-neonatal age group. IBD remains a medically incurable condition with significant morbidity. There has been an increased incidence of pediatric inflammatory bowel disease in all developed countries (1). The etiology of inflammatory bowel disease remains a mystery, and is thought to be multifactorial with a combination of environmental, infectious, and genetic factors. The initial therapy for inflammatory bowel disease is medical, and with recent advances in medical therapy the overall need for surgery may be mitigated (2,3). Despite this, surgical therapy will continue to play an integral role for management of patients with intractable disease. The surgical approach for the two disease entities remains distinctly different. In ulcerative colitis, a curative plan is undertaken, while for Crohn's disease the goal is relief of symptoms and most surgeons employ a conservative surgical approach.

Children with inflammatory bowel disease are generally malnourished and have often undergone long-term therapy with immunosuppressants and steroids. These children have poor wound healing and therefore are prone to increased risk of complications after surgical procedures (4).

Ulcerative Colitis

A restorative proctocolectomy has become an elective treatment for patients with ulcerative colitis no longer responsive to medical therapy, growth retardation, delayed puberty, or serious medication side effects. In particular, patients have steroid-related complications including cataracts, osteoporosis, myopathy, and glaucoma (3). These complications appear to be significantly higher in the pediatric population than in adults (3). Toxic megacolon is an absolute indication for emergent operative intervention. Studies report that 25% of children with ulcerative colitis eventually require surgical intervention, a higher proportion in children who are steroid dependent or with pan-colitis (3,4).

The choice of ileo-anal reconstruction in children undergoing a proctocolectomy for ulcerative colitis is controversial. In adults, the ileo-anal pouch (IAP) reconstruction is generally the procedure of choice. However, many pediatric surgeons still advocate a straight ileo-anal anastomosis (5).

Ileo-Anal Pouch

The IAP offers many pediatric patients a cure for ulcerative colitis with preservation of anal continence. The IAP allows the creation of a reservoir and often negates night bowel evacuations and decreases the number of bowel movements per day. This operation is usually done in a staged manner with two or three stages dependent on the status of the patient. IAP can be performed with laparoscopic assistance or open (Fig. 1) (6). Postoperative complications in children undergoing IAP are very common, as most series report about a 50% complication rate regardless if the procedure was performed open or laparoscopically (7,8). These complications are best divided into early and late.

Early complications include wound infections, anastomotic leakage, pelvic abscess, and mechanical obstruction often related to ileostomy creation. These complications are generally thought to be related to immunosupression and long-term high dose corticosteroid therapy (5,9).

Late complications include small bowel obstruction (SBO), pouchitis, incontinence, and malignancy. There is a higher incidence of SBO in patients that have undergone IPA than would be expected, and the reasons for this remain unclear (7). Generally, these episodes of SBOs can generally be managed with conservative therapy without the need for operative intervention.

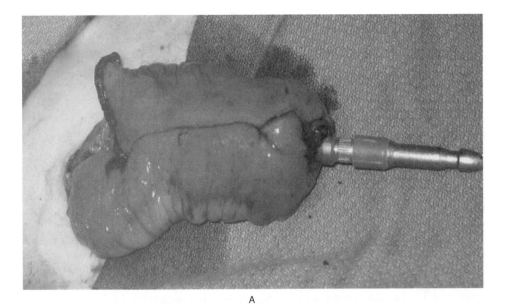

A

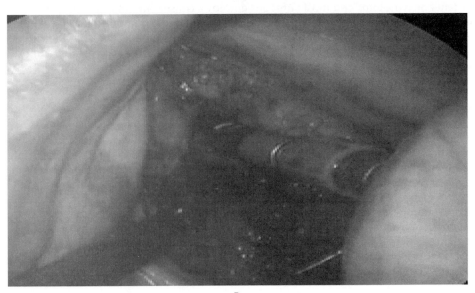

B

Figure 1   Laparoscopic assisted ileo-anal pouch procedure. (**A**) Extra-corporeal view of the ileo-anal pouch. (**B**) Laparascopic view of pouch.

Pouchitis, is an inflammatory complication with poorly understood cause. It is thought to be multifactorial in nature, with immune, bacterial overgrowth, and ischemic factors all playing a role (10). It is, however, more common in patients that have undergone IPA for ulcerative colitis than it is for those that undergo IPA for familial polyposis (11). Generally, the incidence of pouchitis runs about 30% of patients undergoing IPA for ulcerative colitis. The typical presentation of acute pouchitis includes malaise, fever, bloody diarrhea, arthralgia, and rashes. These episodes are generally treated with short courses of antibiotics and resolve quickly. Chronic pouchitis presents with intractable diarrhea, perineal excoriation, and malnutrition. This generally treated with antibiotics, topical or systemic steroids, 5-ASA, and immunosuppressants (10). Rarely does the pouch need to be resected.

Patients with final diagnoses of Crohn's disease and indeterminant colitis often have greater difficulties with chronic pouchitis and subsequent pouch failure (7). Pouch endoscopy is important in accurate diagnosis of inflammatory conditions of the pouch and can then guide appropriate therapy (11). Therefore preoperative investigations must be meticulous to rule out Crohn's disease, perhaps should include upper gastrointestinal (UGI) studies and even capsule endoscopy. In children, where there is a question of Crohn's disease the operation should likely be done in three stages to allow for histologic confirmation of the diagnosis.

Incontinence remains a long-term complication in patients postresection and reconstruction (7). Generally at least 30% of patients will have some element of incontinence which is primarily nocturnal (9,12,13). The reports of continence vary as there is no clear definition of continence and incontinence and often data are not accrued in a standardized fashion. In most cases, incontinence improves over time.

There have been sporadic case reports of adenocarcinoma in adults with ileal pouches, however no pediatric cases have been yet been noted, the youngest patient in the literature being 23 years of age (14,15). The chronic inflammatory nature of pouchitis may predispose patients to adenocarcinoma as most of these patients have no familial history of colon cancer or terminal ileitis. In patients that have a remnant of rectal cuff, annual surveillance for malignancy is essential.

The rates of infertility in patients who have undergone surgical procedures for ulcerative colitis are significantly greater than the general population (16,17). Studies have revealed that the ability to conceive prior to IAP is similar to that of the general population; however, this decreases significantly after IAP. A recent study revealed an infertility rate of 38.6% in patients with UC after IAP compared with 13.3% in patients managed medically (18). This is likely secondary to the deep pelvic dissection required in the procedure and the concomitant adhesions and potential damage to reproductive organs. Males undergoing IPA for UC may experience retrograde ejaculation and have erectile dysfunction in the postoperative period, but fertility rates have not been directly studied (19). Women with UC were also noted to have higher rates of spontaneous abortions and adverse pregnancy outcomes such as low birth weight, intrauterine growth retardation, preterm birth, and congenital anomalies as well as increased labor complications (17).

Straight EndoRectal Pull-Through

The straight endorectal pull (ERP) through was initially proposed by Ravitch and Sabiston and modified by Coran (20,21). The advantages of this procedure include a limited extra-rectal dissection, decreased risk of injury to the nerves and sphincter muscles and potentially lower risk of pouchitis. The distal ileum becomes distended over time and does develop a partial reservoir capacity (10). Complications reported with ERP include anastomotic leak, fistula, and wound infection. Studies that compare ERP to IPA show a similar complication rate with the primary difference being stool frequency, with children with straight ERP having significantly more bowel movements per day (5,12).

Crohn's Disease

Surgery only provides palliative relief of the symptoms and complications of Crohn's disease. The cumulative incidence of surgery in the pediatric population is noted to be 29% at 3 years postdiagnosis and 47% at 5 years postdiagnosis, this is similar to the incidence of surgery within the adult population (22,23). Patients that are at increased likelihood of requiring surgical intervention include those with poor growth at presentation, abscess or stricture development, increased serum anti-Saccharomyces cervisiae antibody (ASCA), and female gender (22,24). The most common indications for surgical intervention are abscess or fistula formation, refractory disease, growth retardation, and medication side effects.

Emergent surgery for Crohn's disease is relatively rare, compared to ulcerative colitis. Most pediatric patients have ileal disease that may or may not include the colon (10). Only about 10% of patients have exclusively colonic disease (25). Long-term recurrence is the norm for patients with Crohn's disease. Recurrence rates are as high as 60% and each subsequent bowel resection increases the risks of further nutritional compromise. Preservation of bowel length and relief of symptoms are the primary goals of surgical resection. Single localized sites of disease are amenable to resection; however, multiple areas may require strictureplasty to prevent extensive loss of bowel (10,26) (Fig. 2). Long segment colonic and perianal disease are often treated with a sub-total colectomy.

Postoperative complications are similar to those seen with ulcerative colitis and include SBO, abdominal and pelvic abscess, anastomotic strictures and leak, fistula formation, and

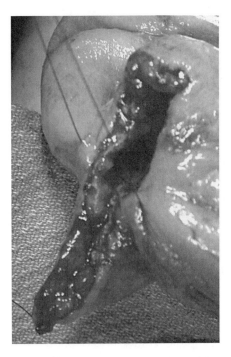

Figure 2   Stricturoplasty for Crohn's disease.

stoma complications (23). These complications are higher in patients who are malnourished and or on long-term steroid therapy (23). The incidence of colorectal malignancy is similar to that of ulcerative colitis and these patients should also undergo surveillance of all remaining colon (27).

Fertility rates in women with Crohn's disease were thought to be similar to the general population, however recent studies have shown that patients who have undergone surgery and particularly ileal resection, have decreased fertility rates compared to patients treated with medical therapy alone (17,28). Women with Crohn's disease are also at increased risk of adverse events during pregnancy and delivery. Males with Crohn's disease have decreased fertility; however, surgery intervention does not appear to be significant (17,29).

Hirschsprungs Disease

Hirschsprung disease (HSCR) occurs in approximately one in 5000 live born infants. The condition is characterized by the absence of ganglion cells within the myenteric and submucosal plexuses of the distal intestine. This developmental disorder of the enteric nervous system results in absent peristalsis in the affected bowel and the development of a functional intestinal obstruction.

The operative treatment for HSCR has progressed from Swenson's first description in 1949, where he recommended rectosigmoidectomy with preservation of the sphincters (30). This was initially done without a decompressing colostomy, however technical difficulties in small infants and the debilitated an malnourished state in which most infants presented caused most surgeons to adopt a multi-staged approach with the decompressive colostomy as the initial step (31). This multi-staged procedure had become the standard of care for several decades. Over the past decades, however with the evolution of minimal access surgery, the one-stage trans-anal and laparoscopic procedures have become increasingly popular.

The goals of surgical management for HSCR are to remove the aganglionic bowel and reconstruct the intestinal tract by bringing the normally innervated bowel down to the anus while preserving sphincter function. There have been many operations devised to accomplish these goals, but the most commonly performed at the present time are the Swenson, Duhamel, and Soave procedures. Although there have been many published series comparing these operations, none have been either prospective or controlled, and it is therefore difficult to determine if there are any significant advantages of one over the others.

The Swenson procedure consists of a low anterior resection of the rectum with an end-to-end anastomosis done by prolapsing the rectum and pulled-through bowel outside the anus.

A number of publications have documented excellent results from this approach, including a recent long-term follow-up of a large group of children that includes some of Swenson's original patients (32).

Duhamel in 1956 described a technique in which the native rectum is left in situ, and the normally innervated colon is brought behind the rectum in the presacral space (33). An end-to-side anastomosis is then done, and the two lumens are joined. Originally, this was accomplished by placing several clamps and cutting between them, but in recent years most surgeons use a linear stapler to accomplish this. This was originally described as an alternative to the Swenson procedure which minimized the pelvic dissection and maintained the integrity of the anterior rectal wall. Modifications to the original procedure have focused on the elimination of the rectal spur which can often cause difficulties with obstruction and stasis (34). The endorectal pull-through was first performed in the 1960s by Franco Soave (35). This operation was designed to avoid injury to pelvic vessels and nerves and protect the internal sphincter, all of which are theoretically at risk during the Swenson and Duhamel procedures. The operation consists of a mucosal proctectomy with preservation of the rectal muscular cuff, and the normally innervated colon is pulled through the muscular cuff and anastamosed just above the dentate line. In the original description, the pulled-through bowel was left hanging out for several weeks and relied on scarification of the two segments of intestine to support the anastomosis. Boley's modification of the Soave procedure, in which the anastomosis is done primarily, is employed by most surgeons today (36).

Early Postoperative Complications

The complications of surgery for HSCR include the general group of complications of any abdominal surgery, including bleeding, infection, injury to adjacent organs, and the risks of anesthesia. Those children who undergo a staged procedure with a preliminary stoma may experience stoma-specific complications including stricture, retraction, prolapse, and skin breakdown (37).

Anastomotic complications, although uncommon, can be seen after any of the pull-through procedures. Great care should be taken during the pull-through to prevent twisting of the anastomosis (Fig. 3). Anastomotic leak occurs infrequently, and can be avoided by close attention to adequate blood supply of the pulled-through bowel and to minimizing tension on the anastomosis. Although it has never been studied in a prospective fashion, the incidence of anastomotic leak in series of laparoscopic and transanal pull-throughs appears to be lower than that reported in the older literature of open pull-throughs. Strictures and retraction of the pull-through may also occur as a result of poor blood supply and tension. Anastomotic stricture is

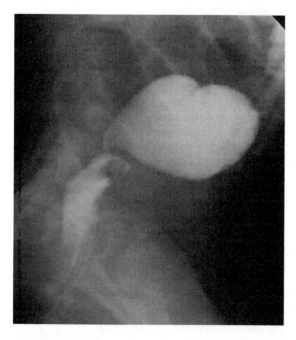

Figure 3   Anastomotic twist in trans-anal pull-through.

Table 1 Potential Causes of Late Complications Following
a Pull-through

Persistent obstructive symptoms
    Mechanical obstruction
    Persistent or acquired aganglionosis
    Colonic motility disorder
    Internal sphincter achalasia
    Stool-holding behavior

Incontinence
    Abnormal sphincter function
    Abnormal sensation
    "Overflow" incontinence due to constipation

Enterocolitis
    Obstruction
    Genetic or immunologic predisposition
    Abnormal mucin

also generally felt to be less common with the Duhamel procedure and in patients undergoing
a one-stage reconstruction. Perianal excoriation is seen in up to 50% of children undergoing
pull-through surgery, and tends to be more common in children with long-segment disease.

Late Complications
The long-term problems in children with HSCR include ongoing obstructive symptoms, incon-
tinence, and enterocolitis. Quite often an individual child may have a combination of problems.
The incidence of these problems varies in the literature, but ranges up to 50% in some series.
More recent publications report higher numbers, likely secondary to increased recognition of
these problems.

Obstructive Symptoms
Obstructive symptoms may take the form of abdominal distension, bloating, vomiting, or
ongoing severe constipation. Many of these children have postoperative symptoms that are
identical to the symptoms they initially presented with. In some cases, the child will have a
good response to surgery and then develop obstructive symptoms later, and in other cases the
child may not have any improvement in the postoperative period.
    The five major reasons for persistent obstructive symptoms following a pull-through are
listed in Table 1. These include mechanical obstruction, recurrent or acquired aganglionosis, disordered motility in the proximal colon or small bowel, internal sphincter achalasia, or functional
megacolon caused by stool-holding behavior (38).

Mechanical Obstruction
Mechanical obstruction may be the result of a stricture or a retained aganglionic spur from a
Duhamel procedure, which may fill with stool and obstruct the pulled-through bowel (Fig. 4).
The Duhamel procedure may also be complicated by a kink at the top of the anastomosis which
leads to obstruction. These complications can be identified by simple digital rectal examination
and a contrast enema. Although some strictures can be managed using repeated dilatations,
many require revision of the pull-through (39). Duhamel spurs can be resected from above
or managed by extending the staple line from below, with or without the aid of laparoscopic
visualization.

Persistent or Acquired Aganglionosis
Although rare, some children may have persistent aganglionosis. This may be due to pathologist
error (40), or a transition zone pull-through (41), and in some cases there may be ganglion cell
loss after a pull-through (41). It is imperative to do a rectal biopsy on the pulled-through bowel,
to determine whether there are normal ganglion cells present, and if there are not, most children
should undergo a repeat pull-through. This can be done using either a Soave or a Duhamel
approach (42,43).

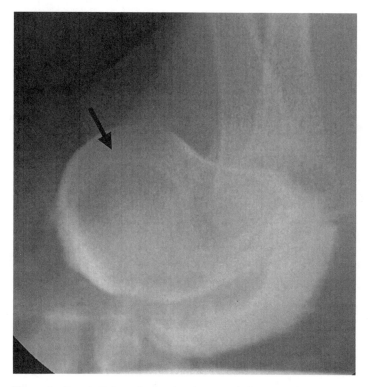

Figure 4   Spur in Duhamel procedure (*arrow pointing to spur*).

Motility Disorder

It is well recognized that children with HSCR may also have associated motility disorders, which may be focal (usually involving the left colon) or diffuse. In some cases, these abnormalities may be associated with histological abnormalities such as intestinal neuronal dysplasia (44). In children who have been shown not to have a mechanical obstruction and who have normal ganglion cells on rectal biopsy, investigations for motility disorders should be undertaken. This can include a radiological shape study, colonic manometry (45), and laparoscopic biopsies looking for intestinal neuronal dysplasia (46). If a focal abnormality is found, consideration should be given to resection and repeat pull-through using normal bowel. If the abnormality is diffuse, the appropriate treatment is medical including bowel management and the use of pro-kinetic agents.

Internal Sphincter Achalasia

Internal sphincter achalasia refers to the nonrelaxation of the internal anal sphincter that is present in all children with HSCR because they lack a normal recto-anal inhibitory reflex. However, in some children it may result in persistent obstructive symptoms. Traditionally, the treatment for this was internal sphincterotomy or myectomy, which is still recommended by many surgeons (47). Other authors have suggested the use of intrasphincteric botulinum toxin (48) (Fig. 5) or the application of nitroglycerine paste (49), both of which relax the sphincter in a reversible fashion. The advantage of the latter approaches is that they do not result in any permanent damage to the sphincter, and in most cases the obstructive symptoms from internal sphincter achalasia tend to resolve spontaneously over time and are gone in most children by the age of 5 years. In many cases, repeated injection of botulinum toxin or applications of nitroglycerine paste are necessary while waiting for resolution of the problem (50).

Functional Megacolon

There remain a group of children who do not have an identifiable cause for their symptoms and who do not respond to surgical or medical relaxation of the sphincter. Most of these children suffer from stool-holding behavior, and are best treated using a bowel management regimen consisting of laxatives, enemas, and behavior modification including support for the child and family.

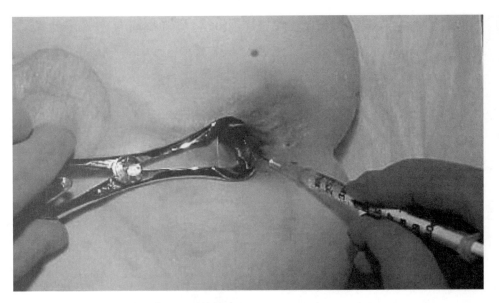

Figure 5   Intrasphincteric botulinum toxin injection.

In some severe cases of obstructive symptoms, the child may be best served by use of a cecostomy (51) and administration of antegrade enemas, or even by the creation of a proximal stoma.

An algorithm for the investigation and management of the child with obstructive symptoms is shown in Figure 6.

Incontinence
There are three main reasons for a child to be incontinent after a pull-through: abnormal sphincter function, abnormal sensation, or "overflow" incontinence due to constipation. Abnormal sphincter function may be due to sphincter injury during the pull-through or to a previous myectomy or sphincterotomy. A number of techniques exist for identifying this kind of injury,

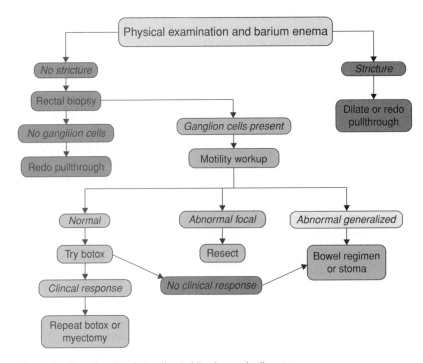

Figure 6   Algorithm for obstruction in Hirschprung's disease.

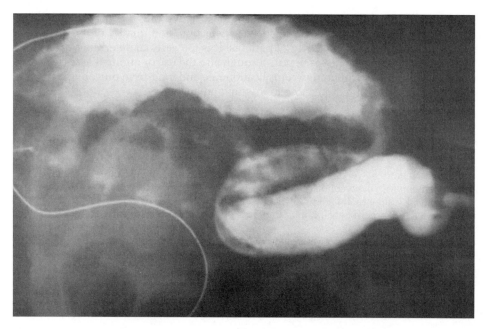

Figure 7 Contrast enema of enterocolitis, note thumbprint sign indicative of inflammation.

including anorectal manometry (52) and anal sonography (53). Abnormal sensation may take the form of either lack of sensation for a full rectum (which can also be identified using anorectal manometry), or injury to the transitional epithelium which permits differentiation between gas, liquid, and solid stool. This injury may occur during a pull-through, especially if the anastomosis is done too low.

Most children with incontinence after a pull-through have overflow of stool because of ongoing constipation. Once sphincter injury and a problem with sensation have been ruled out, the child should be worked up and treated for obstructive symptoms as described in the previous section.

Enterocolitis

As mentioned previously, enterocolitis may be a presenting feature of HSCR. However, it may also occur after surgical correction of the disease. Although the clinical features of enterocolitis are generally agreed upon (fever, abdominal distention, and diarrhea), a precise definition has not yet been developed (Fig. 7). There is, therefore, wide variation in the reported incidence of this problem postoperatively, with estimates ranging from 17% to 50%, calling into the question the specific clinical definition of enterocolitis (54). Enterocolitis also seems to be more common in children with longer segment disease and those with trisomy 21 (55). The absence of enterocolitis preoperatively does not ensure that the child will not develop enterocolitis in the postoperative period (56). The treatment of postoperative enterocolitis is largely symptomatic, and involves bowel rest with nasogastric drainage, intravenous fluids, broad-spectrum antibiotics, and decompression of the rectum and colon using rectal stimulation as well as irrigations. Minimization of the risk of enterocolitis can be accomplished by using prophylactic measures such as routine irrigations (57) or chronic administration of metronidazole, particularly in those who are thought to be at higher risk for this complication based on clinical history (58). Since enterocolitis is the most common cause of death in children with HSCR and can occur postoperatively even in patients who did not have it preoperatively, it is extremely important that the surgeon educate the family about the risk of this complication and urge early return to the hospital if the child should develop any concerning symptoms (59).

Long-Term Prognosis

Despite the relatively common occurrence of postoperative complications, there is evidence from long-term follow-up studies that most children with HSCR overcome these issues and do very well (60). Obstructive symptoms and incontinence seem to resolve with time, and that the risk of enterocolitis, in the absence of an ongoing obstructive cause, is almost eliminated after the first 5 years of life. Sexual function, social satisfaction, and quality of life all appear to be relatively normal in the vast majority of patients. It is too early to determine what effect newer approaches such as the single-stage pull-through and the use of minimal access surgical techniques will have on the postoperative complication rate and long-term outcome, but this is an important question that will require close follow-up and analysis.

REFERENCES

1. Logan RF. Inflammatory bowel disease incidence: Up, down or unchanged? Gut 1998; 42:309–311.
2. Escher JC, Taminiau JA, Nieuwenhuis EE., et al. Treatment of inflammatory bowel disease in childhood: Best available evidence. Inflamm Bowel Dis 2003; 9:34–58.
3. Hyams JS, Davis P, Grancher K, et al. Clinical outcome of ulcerative colitis in children. J Pediatr 1996; 129:81–88.
4. von Allmen D, Goretsky MJ, Ziegler MM. Inflammatory bowel disease in children. Curr Opin Pediatr 1995; 7:547–552.
5. Rintala RJ, Lindahl, H. Restorative proctocolectomy for ulcerative colitis in children—Is the J-pouch better than straight pull-through? J Pediatr Surg 1996; 31:530–533.
6. Simon T, Orangio G, Ambroze W, et al. Laparoscopic-assisted bowel resection in pediatric/adolescent inflammatory bowel disease: Laparoscopic bowel resection in children. Dis Colon Rectum 2003; 46:1325–1331.
7. Alexander F, Sarigol S, DiFiore J, et al. Fate of the pouch in 151 pediatric patients after ileal pouch anal anastomosis. J Pediatr Surg 2003; 38:78–82.
8. Larson DW, Dozois EJ, Piotrowicz K, et al. Laparoscopic-assisted vs. open ileal pouch-anal anastomosis: Functional outcome in a case-matched series. Dis Colon Rectum 2005; 48:1845–1850.
9. Wewer V, Hesselfeldt P, Qvist N, et al. J-pouch ileoanal anastomosis in children and adolescents with ulcerative colitis: Functional outcome, satisfaction and impact on social life. J Pediatr Gastroenterol Nutr 2005; 40:189–193.
10. Rice HE., Chuang E. Current management of pediatric inflammatory bowel disease. Semin Pediatr Surg 1999; 8:221–228.
11. Shen B, Lashner BA. Pouchitis: A spectrum of diseases. Curr Gastroenterol Rep 2005; 7:404–411.
12. Durno C, Sherman P, Harris K, Outcome after ileoanal anastomosis in pediatric patients with ulcerative colitis. J Pediatr Gastroenterol Nutr 1998; 27:501–507.
13. Rintala RJ, Lindahl HG. Proctocolectomy and J-pouch ileo-anal anastomosis in children. J Pediatr Surg 2002; 37:66–70.
14. Knupper N, Straub E, Terpe HJ, et al. Adenocarcinoma of the ileoanal pouch for ulcerative colitis-a complication of severe chronic atrophic pouchitis? Int J Colorectal Dis 2006; 21:478–482.
15. Hassan C, Zullo A, Speziale G, et al. Adenocarcinoma of the ileoanal pouch anastomosis: An emerging complication? Int J Colorectal Dis 2003; 18:276–278.
16. Hudson M, Flett G, Sinclair TS, et al. Fertility and pregnancy in inflammatory bowel disease. Int J Gynaecol Obstet 1997; 58:229–237.
17. Mahadevan U. Fertility and pregnancy in the patient with inflammatory bowel disease. Gut 2006; 55:1198–1206.
18. Johnson P, Richard C, Ravid A, et al. Female infertility after ileal pouch-anal anastomosis for ulcerative colitis. Dis Colon Rectum 2004; 47:1119–1126.
19. Tiainen J, Matikainen M, Hiltunen KM. Ileal J-pouch-anal anastomosis, sexual dysfunction, and fertility. Scand J Gastroenterol 1999; 34:185–188.
20. Ravitch MM., Handelsman JC. One stage resection of entire colon and rectum for ulcerative colitis and polypoid adenomatosis. Bull Johns Hopkins Hosp 1951; 88:59–82.
21. Coran AG, Sarahan TM, Dent TL, et al. The endorectal pull-through for the management of ulcerative colitis in children and adults. Ann Surg 1983; 197:99–105.
22. Gupta N, Cohen SA, Bostrom AG, et al. Risk factors for initial surgery in pediatric patients with Crohn's disease. Gastroenterology 2006; 130:1069–1077.
23. Patel HI, Leichtner AM, Colodny AH, et al. Surgery for Crohn's disease in infants and children. J Pediatr Surg 1997; 32:1063–1067; discussion 1067–1068.
24. Amre DK, Lu SE, Costea F, et al. Utility of serological markers in predicting the early occurrence of complications and surgery in pediatric Crohn's disease patients. Am J Gastroenterol 2006; 101:645–652.
25. Konno M, Kobayashi A, Tomomasa T, et al. Guidelines for the treatment of Crohn's disease in children. Pediatr Int 2006; 48:349–352.
26. Di Abriola GF, De Angelis P, Dall'oglio L, et al. Strictureplasty: An alternative approach in long segment bowel stenosis Crohn's disease. J Pediatr Surg 2003; 38:814–818.

27. Ribeiro MB, Greenstein AJ, Sachar DB, et al. Colorectal adenocarcinoma in Crohn's disease. Ann Surg 1996; 223:186–193.

28. Moser MA, Okun NB, Mayes DC, et al. Crohn's disease, pregnancy, and birth weight. Am J Gastroenterol 2000; 95:1021–1026.

29. Farthing MJ, Dawson AM. Impaired semen quality in Crohn's disease—Drugs, ill health, or undernutrition? Scand J Gastroenterol 1983; 18:57–60.

30. Swenson O, Rheinlander HF, Diamond I. Hirschsprung's disease: A new concept in etiology-operative results in 34 patients. N Engl J Med 1949; 241:551.

31. Gross RE. Congenital megacolon (Hirschsprung's disease). In Gross RE, ed. The Surgery of Infancy and Childhood. Philadelphia, PA: W.B. Saunders, 1953:330–347.

32. Sherman JO Snyder ME, Weitzman JJ, A 40 year multinational retrospective study of 880 Swenson Procedures. J Pediatr Surg 1989; 8:833–838.

33. Vrsansky P, Bourdelat D, Pages R. Principal modifications of the Duhamel procedure in the treatment of Hirschsprung's disease. Analysis based on results of an international retrospective study of 2,430 patients. Pediatr Surg Int 1998; 13:125–132.

34. Martin LW, Caudill DR. A method for elimination of the blind rectal pouch in the Duhamel operation for Hirschsprung's disease. Surgery 1967; 62:951–953.

35. Soave F. A new surgical technique for treatment of Hirschsprung's Disease. Surgery 1964; 56:1007–1014.

36. Weinberg G, Boley SJ. Endorectal pull-through with primary anastomosis for Hirschsprung's disease. Semin Pediatr Surg 1998; 7:96–102.

37. Nour S, Beck J, Stringer MD. Colostomy complications in infants and children. Ann Royal Coll Surg Engl 1996; 78:526–530.

38. Langer JC. Persistent obstructive symptoms after surgery for Hirschsprung disease: Development of a diagnostic and therapeutic algorithm. J Pediatr Surg 2004; 39:1458–1462.

39. Langer JC, Winthrop AL, Fitzgerald PG. Antegrade dilatation over a string for the management of anastomotic complications after a pull-through procedure. J Am Coll Surg 1996; 183:411–412.

40. Shayan K, Smith C, Langer JC. Reliability of intraoperative frozen sections in the management of Hirschsprung's disease. J Pediatr Surg 2004; 39:1345–1348.

41. White FV, Langer JC. Circumferential distribution of ganglion cells in the transition zone of children with Hirschsprung disease. Pediatr Dev Pathol 2000; 3:216–222.

42. Langer JC. Repeat pullthrough surgery for complicated Hirschsprung disease: Indications techniques and results. J Pediatr Surg 1999; 34:1136–1141.

43. Teitelbaum DH, Coran AG. Reoperative surgery for Hirschsprung's disease. Sem Pediatr Surg 2003; 12:124–131.

44. Schmittenbecher PP, Sacher P, Cholewa D, et al. Hirschsprung's disease and intestinal neuronal dysplasia—A frequent association with implications for the postoperative course. Pediatr Surg Int 1999; 15:553–558.

45. Pensabene L, Youssef NN, Griffiths JM, et al. Colonic manometry in children with defecatory disorders: role in diagnosis and management. Am J Gastroenterol 2003; 98:1052–1057.

46. Mazziottti MV, Langer JC. Laparoscopic full-thickness intestinal biopsies in children. J Pediatr Gastroenterol Nutr 2001; 33:54–57.

47. Abbas Banani S, Forootan H. Role of anorectal myectomy after failed endorectal pull-through in Hirschsprung's disease. J Pediatr Surg 1994; 29:1307–1309.

48. Langer JC, Birnbaum E. Preliminary experience with intrasphincteric botulinum toxin for persistent constipation after pull-through for Hirschsprung's disease. J Pediatr Surg 1997; 32:1059–1061.

49. Millar AJ, Steinberg RM, Raad J, et al. Anal achalasia after pull-through operations for Hirschsprung's disease—preliminary experience with topical nitric oxide. Eur J Pediatr Surg 2002; 12:207–211.

50. Minkes RK, Langer JC. A prospective study of botulinum toxin for internal anal sphincter hypertonicity in children with Hirschsprung's disease. J Pediatr Surg 2000; 35:1733–1736.

51. Chait PG, Shlomovitz E, Connolly BL, et al. Percutaneous cecostomy: Updates in technique and patient care. Radiology 2003; 227:246–250.

52. Zaslavsky C, Loening-Baucke V. Anorectal manometric evaluation of children and adolescents postsurgery for Hirschsprung's disease. J Pediatr Surg 2003; 38:191–195.

53. Kuwahara M, Iwai N, Yanagihara J, et al. Endosonographic study of anal sphincters in patients after surgery for Hirschsprung's disease. J Pediatr Surg 1999; 34:450–453.

54. Teitelbaum DH, Coran AG. Enterocolitis. Sem Pediatr Surg 1998; 7:162–169.

55. Caniano DA, Teitelbaum DH, Qualman SJ. Management of Hirschsprung's disease in children with trisomy 21. Am J Surg 1990; 159:402–404.

56. Hackam DJ, Filler RM, Pearl RH. Enterocolitis after the surgical treatment of Hirschsprung's disease: Risk factors and financial impact. J Pediatr Surg 1998; 33:830–833.

57. Marty TL, Seo T, Sullivan JJ, et al. Rectal irrigations for the prevention of postoperative enterocolitis in Hirschsprung's disease. J Pediatr Surg 1995; 30:652–654.

58. Elhalaby EA, Teitelbaum DH, Coran AG, et al. Enterocolitis associated with Hirschsprung's disease: A clinical histopathological correlative study. J Pediatr Surg 1995; 30:1023–1026; discussion 1026–1027.
59. Marty TL, Matlak ME, Hendrickson M, et al. Unexpected death from enterocolitis after surgery for Hirschsprung's disease. Pediatrics 1995; 96:118–121.
60. Yanchar NL, Soucy P. Long term outcomes of Hirschsprung's disease: The patients' perspective. J Pediatr Surg 1999; 34:1152–1160.

Ileoanal Pull-Through

Expert: Arnold G. Coran, M.D.

QUESTIONS

1. **What technical steps assist with the ileal segment that cannot reach the anus?**

    When doing an ileoanal pull-through, it is not uncommon for tension to develop as one is trying to reach the anus for the anastomosis, no matter what technique is used. Since our series of over 350 cases involves both a straight pull-through and a small pouch pull-through, if I encounter too much tension with one technique, I can often do the pull-through with less tension by switching to the other technique. This, of course, is done after the standard maneuvers for reducing tension have been used such as freeing all the lateral, avascular mesenteric attachments of the small bowel all the way up to the ligament of Treitz. Sometimes taking down the ligament of Treitz itself is necessary to relieve tension. It is interesting that the tension associated with a straight pull-through or a pouch pull-through is variable. Sometimes it is easier to bring a straight pull-through down, and sometimes it is easier to bring a pouch pull-through down; the advantage of having experience with both techniques.

2. **What strategies are important to prevent ileostomy complications?**

    I prefer to use a loop ileostomy placed in the right lower quadrant in all my patients. This allows better healing of the anastomosis. I usually close the ileostomy at about 10 weeks postoperatively, and discharge the patient the following day. The major complication of the loop ileostomy is partial ileal obstruction at the end of the proximal limb. This is always due to some edema at this site between the fourth and sixth postoperative day. It is always relieved by intubating the stoma for the day. I have never had to operate on any of these patients. I have not seen prolapse of the ileostomy because I always put a few tacking stitches between the ileostomy and the peritoneum before closing the abdomen.

3. **What technical strategies help limit postoperative bowel obstruction?**

    Although the literature has suggested a high incidence of postoperative adhesive bowel obstruction in ulcerative colitis, I have not encountered this high incidence. About 5% of our patients have needed an enterolysis. The "age old" question is how to prevent postoperative adhesions. This applies to postoperative adhesions seen after the surgery for ulcerative colitis as well as for many other conditions. Nobody has a good answer to this question.

4. **What are the most common complications following ileoanal pull-through and how can they be minimized or avoided?**

    The most common complications after a pull-through are in order of frequency:

    (a) Pouchitis when a pouch is used, which occurs in 20% to 25% of patients, and is usually managed with oral metronidazole, a few cases in which large pouches have been used may require pouch removal; I have never seen that in our series;

    (b) stricture of anastomosis; this is almost always managed by dilations in the office;

    (c) enteritis in cases of a straight pull-through; this is much less common than pouchitis, and is also managed with metronidazole;

    (d) retraction of the anastomosis; this is very rare if the anastomosis is not done under tension; this is usually heals but may lead to a significant stricture, which will require repeated dilations;

    (e) necrosis of the pull-through; this is extremely rare and, will require a redo pull-through;

(f) recto-vaginal fistula; this almost always occurs secondary to an anastomotic leak with abscess formation; repair of this will require an ileostomy plus a layered closure of the fistula;

(g) prolapse of the ileoanal pull-through; I have never seen this in any of our patients because the pull-through is always done with an endorectal technique in which two-thirds of the top of the rectal cuff is sutured to the ileal pull-through;

(h) erectile dysfunction in males, I have never seen this complication since I always use the endorectal technique and, thus, avoid the nervi eringentes.

5. What unusual complications have you seen following ileoanal pull-through?
All the complications that I have seen after a pull-through are mentioned in 4. However, one must consider a misdiagnosis of ulcerative colitis a complication. This has occurred in less than 5% of our patients. In each case, review of the original pathology confirmed the diagnosis of ulcerative colitis even though subsequent pathological evaluation of the pull-through ileum demonstrated Crohn's disease. All except a few of these patients required excision of the pull-through.

6. Are there contraindications to using an endorectal dissection in the ileo-anal pull-through?
There are no contraindications to using an endorectal dissection for the pull-through. In fact, this technique is preferable to the operation used by the adult colorectal surgeons, in which a low anterior anastomosis of the ileal pouch to the rectum is used, because in this latter operation much more rectal mucosa is left than is the case with endorectal technique. This is especially important when doing the operation for Familial Polyposis. Although the risk is small, the amount of the rectal mucosa left behind with the operation used in adults is at risk for the development of recurrent ulcerative colitis and for the development of carcinoma.

Laparoscopic Pull-Through for Hirschsprung's Disease

Expert: Jacob C. Langer, M.D.

QUESTIONS

1. How do you perform your initial biopsy to identify the transition zone?
Through an umbilical incision.

2. How do you initiate the muscosal dissection and how far above the dentate line do you begin?
I use four stitches to evert the anus (rather than a Lonestar retractor, which I find tears the tissue in a baby). I use a needle tip bovie on cutting to incise the mucosa, 5 mm above the dentate line in an infant (up to 1 cm in an older child).

3. How do you manage the detection of total colonic aganglionosis interaoperatively?
I do serial biopsies through the umbilical incision, and if the transition zone is in the small bowel I bring a loop ileostomy, consisting of normally innervated bowel, out through the umbilical incision.

4. How long is your muscular cuff?
Approximately 1 to 2 cm.

5. What are the most common complications after laparoscopic pull-through?
I don't do laparoscopic pull-throughs (I do transanal without laparoscopy). The most common complications are perineal excoriation in about 50%, narrowing of the cuff or anastomosis in about 10%, postoperative enterocolitis in about 25%.

6. What unusual complications have you seen?

Twisting of the pulled-through bowel in two patients. Umbilical wound infection in several patients. Interestingly, I have <u>not</u> seen an anastomotic leak since starting to do the transanal approach over 10 years ago.

7. **Are there still patients you would biopsy transanally after performing the rectal dissection?**
   No.

8. **Do you routinely dilate patients postoperatively? If so what is your protocol?**
   I see the child 1 to 2 weeks after the pull-through and calibrate the anastomosis either with a Hager dilator (in small children) or my finger (in larger children). I then see them and calibrate weekly for about 6 weeks, and then spread the visits apart. I do <u>not</u> have the parents routinely dilate unless I am concerned about narrowing when I do the calibration.

Open appendectomy

Robert Sawin, M.D.

1. **How would the incision be decided upon?**
   I almost always make my incision 1 to 2 cm caudad to McBurney's point, lateral to the edge of the rectus muscle, unless the maximum point of tenderness or a palpable mass is higher on the physical examination.

2. **What technical steps are important to reduce postoperative abscess formation?**
   Administration of broad-spectrum antibiotics preoperatively is essential. Complete aspiration of fluid from the right gutter, the pelvis, and the left side of the peritoneal cavity is important, regardless of whether antibiotic or saline irrigation is used. If irrigation is used, the patient should be placed in reverse Trendelenburg position to reduce the risk of abscess tracking cephalad in the gutter. Penrose drains placed in the right gutter and the deepest part of the pelvis can be brought out through the incision in cases of perforation.

3. **Should a purse-string suture be placed to imbricate the appendiceal stump?**
   I do place a purse-string, using Monocryl suture.

4. **What are the most common complications of open appendectomy?**
   Wound infection, intra-abdominal abscess, adhesive bowel obstruction, and antibiotic-associated colitis (Cc. dificile).

5. **What unusual complications have you seen following appendectomy?**
   Portal vein thrombosis (pyelophlebitis) and colo-cutaneous fistula.

6. **How would you initially manage a perforated and localized appendicitis with a 3.5 cm abscess and associated small bowel obstruction?**
   If the child was not toxic and older than 4 years, I would try percutaneous drainage of the abscess with a course of broad-spectrum antibiotics (Zosyn is our current drug of choice). If there was not definite improvement in the first 24 to 36 hours, then surgical treatment would be pursued.

7. **In the nonoperative management of localized yet perforated appendicitis with phlegmon, how do you determine the duration of antibiotic therapy? Do you prefer transition to oral antibiotics for a specific period of time after discharge?**
   A minimum of five days of in-hospital broad-spectrum intravenous antibiotic therapy is administered, after which discharge is based on whether the patient can tolerate oral feeding and oral pain medications. Intravenous antibiotics are continued for a minimum of 10 total days. Intravenous antibiotics are continued until the WBC is $\leq 11,000$. Oral antibiotics are not used in this setting.

17 | Complications of Surgery for Anorectal Malformations

Marc A. Levitt, M.D. and Alberto Peña, M.D.

Despite significant technical advances in the surgical repair of anorectal malformations, complications in the management of these patients are still common. The preoperative evaluation is vital, the definitive repair is fraught with potential complications, which often require a secondary procedure, and proper postoperative care, both in the short and long term, is an essential part of a patient's successful outcome. Complications are not isolated to patients with complex malformations, but include the entire spectrum of malformations, and in fact are quite common for the relatively benign malformations.

PREOPERATIVE EVALUATION AND NEWBORN MANAGEMENT

The preoperative evaluation essentially begins with a prenatal diagnosis, which is a rapidly improving area of technology. Accurate prenatal diagnosis may impact perinatal decisions and location for a baby's delivery, so that immediate newborn care can begin without delay. This is particularly important for babies with cloacal malformations and cloacal exstrophy. Most often, an anorectal malformation is not diagnosed prenatally. Once the baby is born, a protocol of evaluation is vital, including both clinical and radiologic assessment (1).

The correct newborn operation must be chosen, either a newborn pull-through or a colostomy, each of which has potential complications. In patients with cloacal malformations, there are unique problems that can occur with improper newborn treatment. In such patients, the clinician must recognize and manage hydrocolpos, perform a colostomy with avoidance of key pitfalls, and make a correct clinical diagnosis (2).

HYDROCOLPOS IN CLOACAL MALFORMATIONS

Failure to treat a hydrocolpos (Fig. 1) can result in obstruction of the urinary tract, prompting an unneeded urinary diversion, or lead to pyocolpos. Several techniques to drain a hydrocolpos can lead to difficulties. Catheterization of the common channel is unreliable as it may inadequately drain the vagina or vaginas if the catheter passes into the bladder. A plasty of the single perineal orifice may provide inadequate drainage particularly in cases of a long common channel. Dilatation of the common channel likewise may inadequately drain the dilated structures. A tube vaginostomy is most reliable and should be performed when the colostomy is created. The surgeon must also investigate whether there are two dilated hemivaginas, and drain both of them, either with separate tubes, or with one tube and creation of a window in the septum between the two vaginas.

If an infant with a cloaca is not growing well in the first weeks or months of life after the colostomy, it is most likely because a complicating problem has been missed. If the hydrocolpos is left undrained, patients may suffer from recurrent urinary tract infections, persistent acidosis, and failure to thrive. Failure to identify associated urologic problems such as vesicoureteral reflux may also be the cause. An incompletely diverting colostomy may lead to fecal contamination of the urinary tract.

In addition to management of a hydrocolpos, the surgeon must be thinking about the patient's gynecologic structures to prevent future problems (3,4). During the colostomy creation, during the definitive repair if a laparotomy is required, or during the colostomy closure, identifying and inspecting the gynecologic structures is vital. Patients may have many

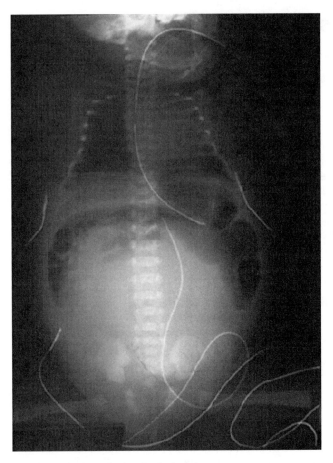

Figure 1 Radiograph showing hydrocolpos.

variations of Mullerian structure atresias or stenoses that can lead to future obstruction of menstrual flow, amenorrhea, and may affect their ability to conceive and carry a baby to term.

CLINICAL DIAGNOSIS

The diagnosis of most anorectal malformations is a clinical one. Once the perineum is inspected and the malformation identified, the correct newborn surgical intervention can be planned. For patients with evidence of rectoperineal fistula, a newborn or delayed pull-through can be performed without a colostomy. For infants with evidence of a rectourethral fistula (the most common anomaly in males), a colostomy is the recommended first step, prior to a future definitive reconstruction.

A single perineal orifice defines a cloaca, and if misdiagnosed, may lead to an unnecessary endocrinologic evaluation for "intersex." The hypertrophied clitoris that is sometime visible in cloacas can be confounding to a clinician not familiar with the external perineal appearance of a cloacal malformation. If the surgeon fails to make the correct diagnosis of a cloaca, they may be prompted to mobilize the rectum, and leave a urogenital sinus intact (Fig. 2). In such a case, a reoperation is required using a posterior sagittal approach, with rectal mobilization, and correction of the persistent urogenital sinus.

COLOSTOMY

Colostomy is an essential component of the newborn management of the majority of patients with anorectal malformations, and is a procedure with many preventable complications (5).

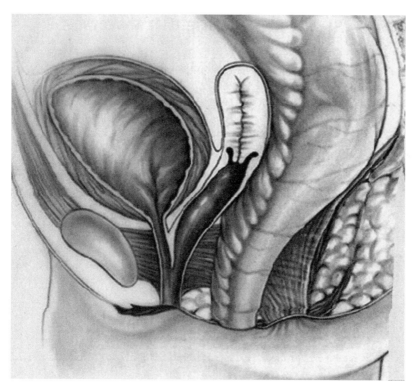

Figure 2 Pull-through only of rectum in a patient with a cloacal malformation, leaving the urogenital sinus untouched.

A colostomy placed too distally in the sigmoid can interfere with the future pull-through (Fig. 3). Colostomy prolapse is a significant problem, and occurs when the colostomy is created in a mobile portion of the colon (Fig. 4), or if a loop-type of colostomy is used. Colostomy prolapse is particularly problematic for patients with anorectal malformation who cannot afford to lose colon, as their capacity to form solid stool impacts their potential for fecal continence,

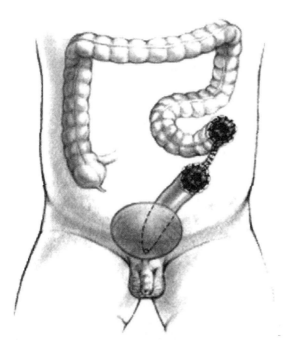

Figure 3 Colostomy created too distal in the sigmoid, which will interfere with the pull-through.

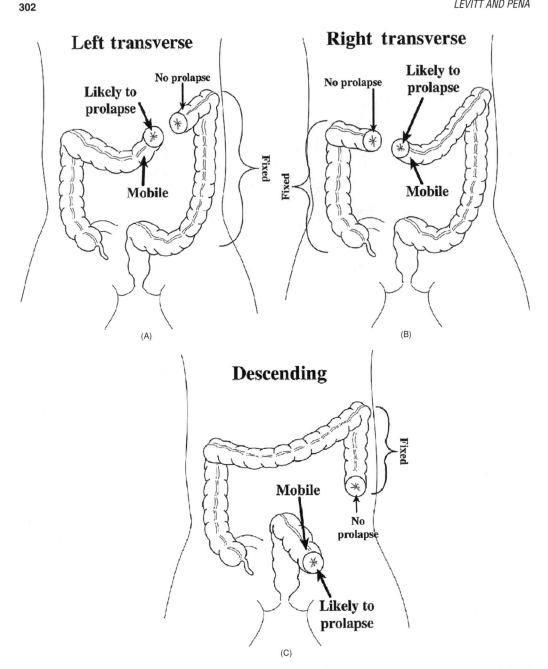

Figure 4 Colostomy prolapse can occur when the colostomy is placed in a mobile portion of the colon. (**A**) Left transverse, (**B**) right transverse and (**C**) descending.

and if incontinent, are more manageable with constipation, than with a tendency toward loose stools. Loop colostomies can lead to urinary tract infections from incomplete diversion of the fecal stream (Fig. 5) and fecal impaction in the distal colon. A Hartman procedure is problematic in patients with anorectal malformations, as there is no access for contrast studies to define the distal rectal anatomy, and these types of colostomies can lead to the development of mucoceles.

In a patient with an anorectal malformation, the stomas must be separated enough as to allow the stoma bag to cover only the proximal stoma, isolating the mucus fistula to prevent contamination, however, the stoma should not be separated more than necessary, so that a big laparotomy can be avoided at the time of colostomy closure. The opening of a sigmoidostomy

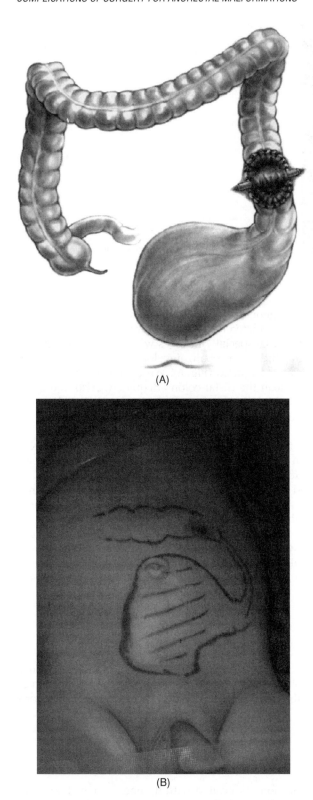

(A)

(B)

Figure 5 (**A**) Diagram of loop colostomy. (**B**) Picture of loop colostomy with distal fecaloma.

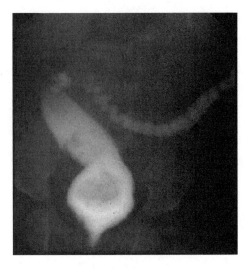

Figure 6 Transverse colostomy with distal microcolon and megarectosigmoid.

in the right upper quadrant can occur if the surgeon tries to find the transverse colon via a right upper quadrant incision and instead mistakes a dilated rectosigmoid for the transverse colon.

Patients with right transverse colostomies, especially in cases with a long time interval between the opening of the colostomy and the main repair, develop a characteristic distal microcolon followed by a more distal megarectosigmoid (Fig. 6). With tranverse colostomies it is also almost impossible to irrigate and clean the distal colon adequately. Also, the distal colostogram is difficult to do, as significantly high hydrostatic pressure is needed to show the precise anatomy. Finally, a longer colonic segment can allow for more resorption of urine and lead to acidosis.

Stricture of the colostomy is due to a technical problem in which the bowel suffers from ischemia due to an inadequate manipulation of the colon's blood supply. Dehiscences, infections, and sepsis aftercolostomy closure are also related to technical problems.

To avoid complications, the preferred colostomy seems to be one with separated stomas with the proximal end located just after the sigmoid comes off its left retroperitoneal attachment (5). The stomas should be separated enough to allow for the placement of a colostomy bag on the proximal stoma (Fig. 7). The proximal stoma must be located away from both the umbilicus and from the iliac crest, thus surrounded by a good portion of normal skin, so that the stoma bag can be easily adapted. The mucous fistula should be located medially and lower and should be fashioned tiny and flat to avoid prolapse, since it is only used for irrigations and diagnostic tests.

DISTAL COLOSTOGRAM

The purpose of the colostomy in addition to diversion of the fecal stream is for the performance of a distal colostogram to define the colorectal anatomy. Understanding the precise location of the distal rectum, and its relationship to the urinary tract, is vital to avoiding complications during the definitive repair (6).

DEFINITIVE REPAIR

The definitive repair has numerous complications associated with it, many of which are preventable with correct preoperative planning, and proper technique. Re-operative surgery is necessary for several of these complications, to alleviate pain, discomfort, and other sequelae.

It is clear that a patient's best chance for a good functional result is when the proper operation is performed during the first definitive procedure and complications are avoided (7). This is especially true in those patients born with a good prognosis defect. It is unfortunate when

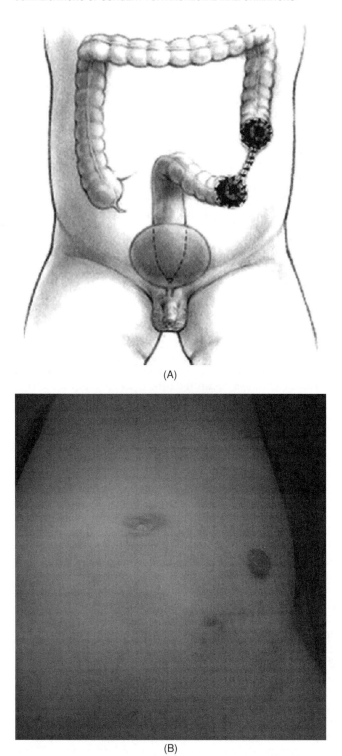

Figure 7 (**A**) Diagram of ideal colostomy. (**B**) Picture of ideal colostomy.

such patients end up with fecal or urinary incontinence, resulting from avoidable complications of the surgical repair.

Patients can sustain perioperative complications during or shortly after the first operation (7). The specific types of complication are described.

WOUND INFECTION

Wound infection of the posterior sagittal incision is very uncommon in the immediate postoperative period, but is more prevalent in the presence of a loop colostomy, which might not be completely diverting or in cases operated on without a colostomy. Fortunately, the infections usually affect only the skin and subcutaneous tissue and heal secondarily, without functional sequelae.

FEMORAL NERVE PALSY

Transient femoral nerve palsy can be observed, particularly in adolescent patients, and is a consequence of excessive pressure in the groin during the posteriorsagittal operation. This problem can be avoided by adequate cushioning of the patient's groin area.

RECTAL PROBLEMS

Patients can experience dehiscence, retraction, infection, and/or acquired atresia of the rectum related to technical problems during the pull-through. These are usually the result of excessive tension or inadequate blood supply. In addition, anal strictures may result when the prescribed protocol of dilatations is not followed.

Reoperation for these problems can be performed posterior sagittally. In cases of retraction, dehiscence, and acquired atresia, the rectum is usually located somewhere high in the pelvis surrounded by a significant amount of fibrotic tissue. Multiple fine silk sutures are placed in the rectal wall to exert uniform traction and facilitate a circumferential dissection of the rectum, trying to stay as close as possible to the rectal wall without injuring it. Bands and extrinsic vessels surrounding the rectum are divided and cauterized circumferentially until enough rectal length is gained as to place the rectum within the limits of the sphincter mechanism. Short ring-like rectal strictures can be treated with a Heineke-Mikulicz type of plasty. Strictures that are longer than 1 cm must be resected, with the rectum mobilized until the fibrotic portion can be removed, and a fresh nonscarred portion of rectum pulled down, creating a new anus.

Retraction, dehiscence, and acquired rectal atresias, are most likely due to inadequate mobilization of the rectum. During a primary procedure, the rectum, when seen posterior sagittally, is covered by a very characteristic white fascia that contains vessels to the rectum. The surgeon must dissect this fascia off the rectum remaining as close as possible to the rectal wall. Uniform traction provided by multiple fine silk sutures is imperative to facilitate this dissection. The intramural blood supply of the rectum is excellent; and the rectum can be dissected to gain significant length provided the rectal wall is not injured. The most likely cause for difficulty in dissection of the rectum is working outside of this fascia. Alternatively, dissection too close to the rectum, can injure the rectal wall, interfere with the intramural blood supply, and provoke ischemia. The result of all this is an incomplete mobilization, rectal ischemia, and a rectum to skin anastomosis performed under tension, which may explain most of these complications.

Rectal strictures are also most likely due to ischemia of the distal part of the rectum. When the rectum is correctly mobilized and the blood supply kept intact, it is extremely unlikely to see an anal stricture. Patients who fail to follow a protocol of dilatations can develop a thin fibrotic ring in the area of the anoplasty, which is easily treated either with an anoplasty or dilatations. A long narrow stricture is most likely due to rectal ischemia.

Some surgeons do not have their patients follow a protocol of anal dilatations. To avoid painful maneuvers to the patient, they follow a specific plan consisting of taking the patient to the operating room every week and under anesthesia performing forceful dilatations. Those dilatations can actually provoke lacerations in the anal verge, which then heal with scarring, only to be re-opened during the next forceful dilatation, leading ultimately to an intractable ring of fibrosis.

RECTO-URINARY AND RECTOVAGINAL FISTULAE

Patients may have various types of complications involving rectogenito-urinary tract fistulae. Fistulae can be *persistent* when the original recto-urethral fistula remains untouched during the main repair, even when the rectum was repaired. *Recurrent* fistulae may occur if the surgeon repaired the fistula but it re-opened. *Acquired* recto-urethral fistulae are those that are created during the repair of a benign malformation (6).

Acquired recto-vaginal fistula can occur during an attempted failed repair of a recto-vestibular fistula. Prior to the introduction of the total urogenital mobilization for cloaca repair, urethro-vaginal fistula was the most common and feared complication (8). In certain circumstances, the vagina can be rotated to try to prevent this complication but even with that maneuver, these fistulas can occur.

Persistent recto-urethral fistulae can occur in patients who were born with a recto-urethral bulbar fistula and underwent a repair that did not address the fistula. Surgeons following the old diagnostic approach may have performed an invertogram and found the bubble of rectal air close to the skin. This may have lead to an approach through the perineum, with identification of the rectum and subsequent pull-through and anoplasty. Since the surgeon was completely unaware of a low recto-urethral bulbar fistula, it was not repaired.

Recurrent recto-urethral fistulae may result if the fistula is closed, but the rectum is not mobilized adequately, leaving the anterior wall under tension. A dehiscence of the anterior rectal wall may explain the recurrence of the fistula. Also, leaving sutures in the rectum adjacent to the sutures in the urethra may lead to formation of a recurrent fistula. Consequently, an injured rectum that requires a repair to the anterior wall may create a situation for the development of a recurrent fistula. The same explanation may apply to recto-vaginal fistulae.

Acquired recto-urethral fistulae can occur in male patients who were born with recto-perineal fistulae if they undergo their first operation without the benefit of a Foley catheter in the urethra. During the mobilization of the anterior wall of the rectum, an unrecognized urethral injury can occur and, if not mobilized to leave normal rectal wall in front of the urethral injury, an acquired recto-urethral fistula will form.

Fistulous complications can be approached posterior sagittally. The posterior rectal wall should be opened and the fistulae identified and closed. The rectum then needs to be separated from the urinary tract or the vagina, and mobilized as so as to be sure that a completely normal anterior rectal wall is left in front of the urethral or vaginal suture line.

PERSISTENT UROGENITAL SINUS

A persistent urogenital sinus occurs in patients born with a cloacal malformation who underwent an operation in which the rectal component of the malformation was repaired, but the urogenital sinus was ignored (Fig. 2). Their reoperation can also be approached posterior sagittally. The rectum must be completely dissected and reflected out of the way. This allows exposure of the urogenital sinus, which can be repaired using the same technique that is employed during the treatment of a cloaca (9). Many such patients had an original diagnosis of a "recto-vaginal fistula" (10) and the true malformation, that of a cloaca, was not therefore recognized.

ACQUIRED VAGINAL ATRESIA

Complete fibrosis of the vagina due to excessive dissection can occur when a high vagina is mobilized. This is particularly problematic when the vagina is separated from the urethra during the repair of a cloacal malformation. The dissection of vagina from the urinary tract is not an easy maneuver, the vagina may become devascularized and as a consequence, patients develop ischemic vaginal atresia. This is why the development of the total urogenital mobilization has dramatically reduced this complication (8).

ACQUIRED URETHRAL ATRESIA

Acquired urethral atresia in cloaca patients can occur from devascularization of the pulled through or reconstructed neourethra. In male patients, it can occur when the urethra is accidentally transected during an attempt to repair an anorectal malformation. This complication most frequently occurs in males in whom the surgeon approaches the reconstruction posterior sagittally without a preoperative high pressure distal colostogram (6). To repair this problem, the

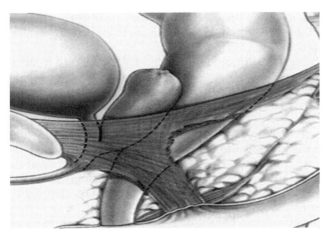

Figure 8   Posterior urethral diverticulum, representing the undissected former distal rectum.

rectum must be mobilized to expose the urethral area. Both urethral ends need to be identified, dissected, and mobilized to perform a tension free end-to-end anastomosis.

POSTERIOR URETHRAL DIVERTICULUM

This complication can occur when a retained portion of the rectum is left attached to the posterior urethra (Fig. 8). This complication can occur in patients born with a recto-urethral bulbar fistula repaired trans-abdominally. It is easy to understand that the surgeon was unable to reach the fistula site through the abdomen. Consequently, the rectum was amputated, leaving a piece of rectum attached to the urethra. This potential complication is also possible with a laparoscopic approach, particularly if the rectum reaches well below the peritoneal reflection.

These patients, are initially asymptomatic, but after years develop symptoms such as passage of mucous through the urethra, dribbling, orchioepididimitis, urinary tract infections, and urinary pseudo incontinence. In addition, we have seen one such patient who, after 30 years, developed an adenocarcinoma in the piece of rectum left attached to the urethra.

A posterior sagittal approach can be utilized to fix this problem, with mobilization of the rectum to expose the posterior aspect of the urinary tract, identification of the diverticulum, and dissection of it down to the urethra. The diverticulum can be separated from the urethra in the same manner as in a primary repair of anorectal anomalies with the urethra closed and the diverticulum resected.

OTHER UROLOGIC INJURIES

Significant urologic injuries such as transection of the bladder neck, transection of the urethra, injury to vas deferens, seminal vesicles, prostate, and ectopic ureters have occurred, usually when the posterior sagittal approach was performed without a good previous distal colostogram, and thus the precise anatomy was not known prior to the posterior sagittal dissection (6).

NEUROGENIC BLADDER

Neurogenic bladder in male patients with anorectal malformations is extremely unusual. In our series, we have only seen it in patients with a very abnormal sacrum or spine (11). If it does occur, it may represent a denervation of the bladder and bladder neck during the repair.

Patients with cloacal malformations are very different with regard to this subject. They often have a deficient emptying mechanism of the bladder. They do not have the typical "christmas tree" type of image of a neurogenic bladder seen in patients with a spina bifida but rather have a flaccid, smooth, large bladder that does not empty completely. Fortunately, most patients with cloacas have a very good bladder neck. The combination of a good bladder neck with a floppy, flaccid bladder, make these patients ideal candidates for intermittent catheterization, which keeps them completely dry (9).

Two exceptions to this rule exist. One is represented by patients that have a very long common channel, in which the hemivaginas as well as the rectum are attached to the bladder neck and after they are separated the patients are left with no bladder neck or a very damaged bladder neck. The second group is represented by a small number of cloaca patients that are born with separated pubic bones, who could be described as having a covered exstrophy (12). These patients have no bladder neck congenitally and they eventually require a continent diversion type of operation.

COMPLICATIONS OF THE LAPAROSCOPIC APPROACH TO ANORECTAL MALFORMATIONS

Long-term results and complications have not yet been described for the laparoscopic approach to imperforate anus, which is a relatively new approach, developed to avoid a laparotomy and to minimize the posterior sagittal incision (13). We have managed several complications from this approach performed at other institutions, and postulate the potential for others.

Avoidance of the perineal exposure afforded by the posterior sagittal approach can lead to inadvertent injuries, such as injury to the bladder neck, urethra, or to an ectopic ureter. Precise understanding of the anatomic relationships of the pelvis provided by the laparoscopic view is vital to avoid these problems.

Like with the former transabdominal approach (14), there is potential for leaving behind the distal rectal cuff, leading to a posterior urethral diverticulum, particularly for malformations below the peritoneal reflection, such a rectobulbar fistula.

Finally, to avoid rectal prolapse a pelvic hitch is employed (13). If this step is omitted, or done incorrectly, the incidence of prolapse will likely be significant. The laparoscopic approach also dissects the entire rectum, which may lead to more prolapse. With the avoidance of the posterior sagittal incision, the described laparoscopic operation omits several key steps of the posterior sagittal anorectoplasty (PSARP) that are very important to avoid prolapse (15), particularly tacking of the posterior rectal wall to the muscle complex.

RECTAL PROLAPSE

Rectal mucosal prolapse occurs following PSARP, with an incidence of 3% (15). It is more common in patients with higher malformations and with poor sacra and pelvic musculature. Significant prolapse may lead to ulceration, bleeding, and mucous production. It can interfere with anal canal sensation and thus impact a patient's functional prognosis.

Correction of prolapse can be performed transanally, with mobilization of redundant full thickness rectum, and redo-anoplasty. This is ideally done prior to colostomy closure. Sometimes, however, prolapse only develops after colostomy closure and in the presence of constipation. The repair of the prolapse in patients without a colostomy requires a strict pre-operative bowel preparation, insertion of a central line, nothing by mouth for seven days and administration of parenteral nutrition.

POSTOPERATIVE MANAGEMENT

The long-term concerns following surgery for anorectal malformations mainly involve a child's potential for bowel control. Most children have voluntary bowel movements, but a small percentage suffers from fecal incontinence despite a technically correct operation (11). Fecal incontinence may of course occur as a result of a technically incorrect operation. Such a patient must be identified, and may be a candidate for a reoperation. Constipation is a common sequelae following operations for anorectal malformations, and may lead to significant sequelae if not proactively managed.

FECAL INCONTINENCE

Reoperation to improve a patient's functional prognosis is indicated in several circumstances. During the first five years of our experience, re-operative surgery was performed on every patient we evaluated who underwent a repair at another institution and subsequently developed fecal incontinence. During those years, we hoped that the new posterior sagittal approach would give these patients an opportunity to recover bowel control. When the results were evaluated (16,17), only 30% of those patients experienced a significant improvement. Therefore, the indications for surgery were modified.

Presently, re-operation for fecal incontinence is recommended only for patients with very special criteria. It is for patients born with a malformation associated with a good prognosis, with a mislocated rectum. The rectosigmoid should be present, the sacrum normal, and the sphincter mechanism intact. In such cases, restoration of near normal anatomy may improve the functional outcome.

For these reoperations, the rectum is approached posteriorly. Multiple silk stitches are placed at the mucocutaneous margin in order to apply uniform traction to facilitate the dissection and mobilization of the rectum. A full rectal dissection and mobilization is performed, staying as close as possible to the bowel wall but avoiding injury. The limits of the sphincters, including the parasagittal fibers, muscle complex, and levator muscle are determined by electrical stimulation and the rectum is repositioned within it.

In some cases, the patient is found to have had colon, rather than rectum, pulled down to the anus. This is identified by the presence of a mesentery attached to the bowel. In such cases, the mesenteric fat should be trimmed from the last few centimeters of the rectum to allow for direct contact between the sphincter mechanism and the colonic wall. An anoplasty performed within the limits of the sphincter mechanism completes the reconstruction.

The number of patients that require a re-operation for fecal incontinence has decreased significantly over the years. This is likely due to the increased use of the posterior sagittal approach, which provides superior exposure and prevents the complete mislocation of the rectum seen with other techniques.

In the past, many patients underwent abdominal perineal pull-throughs with endorectal dissections of the rectosigmoid (14). This procedure essentially resulted in loss of the rectosigmoid. These patients do not suffer from constipation. Instead they suffer from increased colonic motility and a tendency to diarrhea. It took us several years to recognize this specific group of patients, and today revisional surgery is not offered to them, because it is clear that they never regain bowel control. They are provided with bowel management, with the goal of slowing down the colon, and emptying it daily with an enema (18). Fortunately, endorectal pull-throughs for anorectal malformations are rarely done and it is rather unusual to see these patients.

In addition to the above group, those patients born with a poor prognosis defect and fecal incontinence are also considered inappropriate candidates for re-operation. These patients typically have an abnormal sacrum, flat perineum, and poor sphincters. There is usually evidence that they were born with a high recto prostatic or recto bladder neck fistula, or a cloaca with a common channel longer than 3 cm. Their sacral ratio is almost always low, often less than 0.4. We do not re-operate on these patients, even if they have a completely mislocated rectum because they do not improve after re-operation. Instead they are offered a bowel management program (18) to prevent soiling and to keep them completely clean.

When revisional surgery for fecal incontinence is offered, the likelihood of the patient regaining bowel control is reviewed with the family. Even with those patients who are expected to improve, the bowel management program is implemented prior to surgery. If it turns out that the patient does not improve enough after reoperation to avoid enemas, the already tested bowel management is reinstituted.

SEQUELAE FROM CONSTIPATION

Constipation is the most common functional disorder observed in patients who undergo posterior sagittal anorectoplasty (11). Interestingly, the incidence of constipation is inversely related to the height of the anorectal malformation. This means that patients with the best prognosis for bowel control have the highest incidence of constipation. Patients with very poor prognosis, such as bladder neck fistula, have a rather low incidence of constipation.

Constipation seems to be related to the degree of preoperative rectal ectasia. Colostomies that do not allow cleaning and irrigation of the distal colon lead to megarectum. Transverse colostomies lead to a micro left colon with dilatation of the rectosigmoid. Loop colostomies allow for passage of stool and distal fecal impaction. It is clear that keeping the distal rectosigmoid empty and not distended from the time the colostomy is established, and proceeding with pull-through and subsequent colostomy closure as early as possible within several months, reduces the development of megarectosigmoid, and results in better ultimate bowel function.

A significant number of patients suffer from sequelae from the mismanagement of their constipation. Many patients are described as having "fecal incontinence" who actually have untreated severe constipation, chronic impaction. This condition is actually overflow pseudo-incontinence. These patients have several common features. All were born with a malformation with good functional prognosis, and all underwent a technically correct, successful operation. Postoperatively, they all had severe constipation that was not managed aggressively. They, therefore, developed megasigmoid and chronic fecal impaction, which develops into a vicious cycle. Adequate treatment of their constipation, with or without a sigmoid resection, (19) renders them fecally continent.

All patients in this pseudoincontinent group should undergo a "laxative test" to determine if they are fecally continent. First, large volume enemas are administered until the patient's colon is clean (disimpacted) as documented on a plain radiograph. Daily laxatives are then administered, increasing the amount each day until the amount necessary to produce colonic evacuation is determined. If the patient demonstrates the capacity to feel the stool in the rectum, reach the bathroom, have voluntary bowel movements and remain clean every day, the patient is continent. Such a patient can then be offered the option of continuing treatment with large quantities of laxative or undergoing a sigmoid resection (19) to make the constipation more manageable and thereby decreasing the laxative requirement.

This group of patients is extremely important to recognize. Some of these patients may be wrongly diagnosed as suffering from true fecal incontinence and some have even undergone re-operations such as gracilis muscle transfers or artificial sphincters that can actually make the patient worse. This problem should be suspected when one sees a patient that was born with a benign malformation, who underwent a technically correct operation, but was not treated correctly for constipation.

CONCLUSION

Unfortunately, despite great advances in pediatric surgical care, there remain a significant number of patients who undergo attempted anorectal repairs with significant complications, many of which are preventable. For good results, one must have a thorough understanding of the spectrum of anorectal malformations, employ proper newborn evaluation and management, utilize meticulous technique, and implement rigorous, careful postoperative management. These basic fundamentals need to be emphasized in the training of pediatric surgeons, so as to improve the outlook for children born with anorectal malformations.

REFERENCES

1. Shaul DB, Harrison EA. Classification of anorectal malformations—Initial approach, diagnostic tests, and colostomy. Semin Pediatr Surg 1997; 6(4):187–195.
2. Levitt MA, Peña A. Pitfalls in the management of newborn cloacas. Pediatr Surg Int 2005; 21(4):264–269.
3. Levitt MA, Stein DM, Peña A. Gynecological concerns in the treatment of teenagers with cloaca. J Pediatr Surg 1998; 33(2):188–193.
4. Warne SA, Wilcox DT, Creighton S, et al. Long-term gynecologic outcome of patients with persistent cloaca. J Urol 2003; 170(4):1493–1496.
5. Peña A, Krieger M, Levitt MA. Colostomy in anorectal malformations—a procedure with significant and preventable complications. J Pediatr Surg 2006; 41:748–756.

6. Hong AR, Rosen N, Acuña MF, et al. Urological injuries associated with the repair of anorectal malformations in male patients. J Pediatr Surg 2002; 37(3):339–344.

7. Peña A, Hong AR, Midulla P, et al. Reoperative surgery for anorectal anomalies. Sem Pediatr Surg 2003; 12(2):118–123.

8. Peña, A. Total urogenital mobilization—An easier way to repair cloacas. J Pediatr Surg 1997; 32(2):263–268.

9. Peña A, Levitt MA, Hong AR, et al. Surgical management of cloacal malformations: A review of 339 patients. J Pediatr Surg 2004; 39(3):470–479.

10. Rosen, NG, Hong AR, Soffer SZ, et al. Rectovaginal fistula: A common diagnostic error with significant consequences in girls with anorectal malformations. J Pediatr Surg 2002; 37(7):961–965.

11. Peña A, Levitt MA. Imperforate anus and cloacal malformations. In: Ashcraft KW, Holder TM, Holcomb W, eds. Pediatric Surgery. 4th ed. Philadelphia, PA: WB Saunders Col., 2005: 496–517.

12. Soffer SZ, Rosen NG, Hong AR, et al. Cloacal exstrophy: A unified management plan. J Pediatr Surg 2000; 35(6):932–937.

13. Georgeson KE, Inge TH, Albanese CT. Laparoscopically assisted anorectal pull-through for high imperforate anus—A new technique. J Pediatr Surg 2000; 35(6):927–931.

14. Kiessewetter WB. Imperforate anus. II—The rationale and technique of the sacroabdominoperineal operation. J Pediatr Surg 1967; 2:106–110.

15. Belizon A, Levitt M, Shoshany G, et al. Rectal prolapse following posterior sagittal anorectoplasty for anorectal malformations. J Pediatr Surg 2005; 40(1):192–196.

16. Peña A, deVries PA. Posterior sagittal anorectoplasty: Important technical considerations and new applications. J Pediatr Surg 1982; 17(6):796–811.

17. Peña A. Advances in the management of fecal incontinence secondary to anorectal malformations. In: Lloyd Nyhus, ed. Surgery annual. Connecticut: Appleton & Lange, 1990:143–167.

18. Peña A, Guardino K, Tovilla JM, et al. Bowel management for fecal incontinence in patients with anorectal malformations. J Pediatr Surg 1998; 33(1):133–137.

19. Peña A, El-Behery M. Megasigmoid—A source of pseudo-incontinence in children with repaired anorectal malformations. J Pediatr Surg 1993; 28(2):199–203.

Posterior Sagittal Anorectoplasty

Expert: Alberto Peña, M.D.

QUESTIONS

1. What are the most common complications associated with colostomy formation prior to repair of an anorectal malformation?

The most common complication is opening the colostomy too distal. This may result in the inability for the surgeon to pull the distal rectum down, due to the fact that the bowel is abnormally attached to the abdominal wall.

Another serious complication is the opening of a loop colostomy that is not totally diverting, allowing passage of stool into the distal limb and contaminating the urogenital tract, producing significant risk of urinary tract infection.

Colostomy Prolapse. This occurs, in our experience, in all those patients that receive a colostomy that was opened in a mobile portion of the colon. In the case of the descending colostomy, the proximal stoma usually does not prolapse (in a normally fixed colon) but the mucous fistula may prolapse because it belongs to the mobile portion of the colon, (the sigmoid). Colostomy prolapse sometimes is so severe that it produces ischemia of the most distal prolapsed part of the colon; the patient is at risk of losing a very important part of the colon and, therefore, water absorption capacity, with serious consequences for bowel control.

Colostomy Stricture. This is a consequence of a lack of good surgical technique. During the opening of a colostomy, one must be sure to have enough length of bowel to do a bowel-skin anastomosis under no tension. Also the closure of the wound must not compress the blood supply of the colon.

2. How can rectal prolapse following repair of anorectal malformations be avoided?

Rectal prolapse occurs in a significant number of patients (approximately 3%) operated on for an anorectal malformation. The main cause is that the patients do not have a normal sphincter mechanism. Therefore, the poorer the sphincter mechanism of the patient, the higher the incidence of rectal prolapse. To try to avoid rectal prolapse, one must avoid excessive dissection of the rectum. One must dissect only enough rectal length as to be able to reach the perineum with no tension. More dissection may affect the function of the rectum and also expose the patient to prolapse. In addition, we anchor the rectum to the posterior edge of the muscle complex with about four or five sutures. This may help to avoid prolapse. Patients operated laparoscopically, by definition, have a dissection of the entire rectum; we have seen a higher incidence of rectal prolapse.

3. **How should prolapse be managed if it occurs in these patients?**
   Prior to the colostomy closure, one is always obligated to see the result of the anoplasty. At that point, if the patient has "significant prolapse," the patient has the best opportunity to be repaired while still the colostomy is open. Because that way, the patient has no risk of infection and the entire procedure can be done on an ambulatory basis. We consider significant prolapse when the patient has more than 5 mm of prolapse and the caregiver tells us that the patient is bleeding frequently. In addition, there is significant wetness in the underwear. The operation that we perform consists of placing multiple sutures at the mucocutaneous junction of the anus and performing a circumferential incision peripheral to the silk stitches and dissecting full thickness approximately 2 cm of the rectum. At that point, we resect the excessive rectum and perform a new anastomosis with interrupted 5–0 or 6–0 Vicryl sutures.

4. **How can a megarectum following repair of an anorectal malformation be avoided?**
   We retrospectively studied the factors that determine the formation of a megarectum. We found, that a dilated rectum prior to the colostomy closure would translate directly into a more dilated rectum and severe constipation after the colostomy is closed. We also found that the opening of a transverse colostomy (which is still done by many surgeons all over the world), characteristically produces accumulation of mucus, and secretions from the colon into the distal bowel, producing severe megarectum. In addition, when a surgeon opens a transverse colostomy, it is impossible to irrigate the most distal part of the bowel and, therefore, the patient stays with the distal rectosigmoid full of meconium which contributes to creating a megarectum. After the pull-through has been done and the colostomy is closed, most patients with anorectal malformations suffer from a significant degree of hypomotility disorder of the rectosigmoid. Interestingly, that hypomotility disorder (translated into constipation), is more severe the lower the malformation. Therefore, one must expect that all patients would suffer from constipation. Constipation in patients with an anorectal malformation requires aggressive treatment. These patients need an amount of laxative much higher than what other constipated children need to empty the colon. Not giving the right amount of laxatives represents a problem because the patient will develop chronic fecal impaction. Constipation produces incapacity to empty the rectum. Incapacity to empty the rectum produces accumulation of stool, accumulation of stool produces dilatation of the colon, dilatation of the colon produces more constipation, and all of this becomes a vicious cycle that one must break. To avoid this, one must find out the amount of laxative that is adequate for the patient. That is determined by trial and error and taking X-ray films to monitor the amount of stool in the colon.

5. **What are your strategies for finding a high rectoprostatic fistula?**
   The rectobladder neck fistula is the highest of all defects and requires either a laparoscopy or laparotomy to separate the rectum from the bladder neck. The next "highest" malformation is a rectoprostatic fistula, and then comes the rectourethral bulbar fistula. Sometimes the rectoprostatic fistula is located very near the bladder neck so it becomes almost a bladder neck fistula. One should look at the high-pressure distal colostogram very carefully to plan the approach to division of the fistula. These patients need a meticulously, technically correct high-pressure distal colostogram in the lateral position that shows us where the tip of the coccyx is located and where the anal dimple is as marked with a lead marker. Looking at that perfect lateral film, one can see what to expect when we open posterior sagittally. Sometimes we find that the rectum is located too high as related to the coccyx; perhaps in those cases it would be better to find the rectum laparoscopically.

Looking at the high-pressure distal colostogram, one must have a very good idea in which direction to look for the rectum once we go deeper than the coccyx.

6. **What are your tricks for bringing down a very high rectum as in a rectobladder neck fistula?**

When one separates the rectum from the bladder neck, it is easy to appreciate that there is a long distance from the abdomen all the way to the perineum. Traditionally, surgeons learn in our general surgical training that one can sacrifice one of the main sources of blood supply of the colon (example: ileocolic), provided we preserve the other (middle colic and left colic) as well as the arcades of the blood supply of the colon. This rule should not be used when dealing with anorectal malformations because usually when the surgeons open a colostomy they end up sacrificing the arcades of the blood supply. What we have learned is that the distal rectum has an excellent intramural blood supply. Therefore, one can ligate the extrinsic blood supply of the rectum and the rectum usually survives, provided one can see directly that there is at least one good branch coming from the inferior mesenteric vessels to the rectosigmoid, and also provided that we do not injure the wall of the bowel. By doing that, we can gain enough length in the majority of cases for the rectum to reach the bottom. Ligating the inferior mesenteric vessels at the origin of the aorta assuming that the arcades would provide blood supply is a very risky maneuver, as I said, because usually the arcades were sacrificed before.

7. **Can a postoperative mucosal ectropion be repaired with simple local revision?**

I think that question was answered when we answered the question on how can rectal prolapse following repair of anorectal malformation be avoided?

Once the colostomy has been closed, if the patient has rectal prolapse we try to be a little bit more conservative in the indications to operate because those patients have a higher risk of retraction and infection. Therefore, we only operate on a prolapse when this is interfering with the quality of life of the patient. In other words, when the patient cannot ride a bicycle or cannot play sports because they produce bleeding, and when the wetness that produces the prolapse goes through the underwear, producing embarrassing events for the patient. Occasionally prolapse can interfere with anal canal sensation and the ability to squeeze the sphincter, and prolapse repair can improve bowel control in a patient who would have been expected to have good prognosis. The prolapse resection in patients without a colostomy is performed following specific precautions. We bring the patient to the hospital, the day before surgery prepare the entire gastrointestinal tract with GoLYTELY, perform the operation described above, and keep the patient n.p.o. for 7 days after the procedure. Parenteral nutrition is administered through a picc line. In other words, the repair is simple but the preoperative and postoperative care is not.

8. **Can you suggest an optimal toilet training regimen for the constipated toddler after repair of an anorectal malformation?**

Our philosophy concerning the medical management of patients with anorectal malformations is that all patients should be clean in the underwear after 3 years of age, either because they were born with a "good anorectal malformation" and, therefore, they have bowel control, or because, even when they were born with a "bad malformation," we keep them artificially clean with the implementation of a bowel management program. Our bowel management program is successful 95% of the time. Therefore, a small group of patients (less than 5%) will need a permanent colostomy because the bowel management does not work. At the present time, we can determine fairly accurately, the functional prognosis in most children, very early in life, based on the follow-up of over 2000 patients operated on by us with anorectal malformations. We believe it is extremely important to tell the parents (as early as possible) what is the final functional prognosis. For those patients that have a very bad prognosis, we do not bother trying to toilet train them, but we go straight into the bowel management program by the age of 3 years. For those patients who have a good prognosis, we keep trying toilet training because we know that they have a high chance to become toilet trained. For those patients that are in the middle of the spectrum, if they are not toilet trained by the age of 3, we may offer them bowel management on a temporary basis and every year we try to toilet train them because we know they have some chance to become toilet trained.

The toilet training process includes, to give three meals/day (no snacks) to try to create regularity in bowel movements; to be sure that the patient is not constipated and to establish a program of incentives for the child. The goal is to have one to two well-formed bowel movements per day. This bowel movement pattern is the easiest to translate into successful potty training.

There is a very interesting subgroup of patients that come for consultation to our clinic after they had the repair of a good prognosis type of anorectal malformation and they suffer from severe constipation. Those patients have a high chance to suffer from overflow pseudoincontinence, and just by disimpacting them first and then finding the amount of laxatives that make them empty the colon completely, it becomes obvious that they have been always continent except that they have never received an adequate treatment for their constipation. We say that these patients suffer from overflow pseudoincontinence.

9. **Is there a concern with the chronic use of milk of magnesia, senna, or Miralax?**
   Unfortunately we cannot answer those questions because we do not know. But we do know that if we do not give laxatives the patient will develop serious problems.

10. **How long do you use intravenous antibiotics after repair of a rectoprostatic urethral fistula? After repair of a rectoperineal fistula?**
    In both cases, we use intravenous antibiotics for 48 hours. When the patient was left with a Foley catheter, like in the recto-urethral then we administer oral prophylactic medication for the time that the catheter is in place. Also, if the patient has a urinary tract infection-predisposing factor such as vesicoureteral reflux, as soon as we stop the intravenous antibiotics we give prophylaxis for that specific reason.

18 | Complications of Hepatobiliary Surgery
Frederick M. Karrer, M.D.

Some of the most major operations performed by pediatric surgeons involve diseases of the hepatobiliary system. Consequently, complications are not unusual and attention to detail is crucial. Unlike adults, most of the diseases of the biliary tract in children are congenital in origin rather than acquired. Operations on the liver, on the other hand, are usually for acquired disease (i.e., tumors and trauma) just like adults.

BILIARY ATRESIA

Obliteration of the extrahepatic biliary tree usually presents with jaundice in the first few months of life in a previously healthy infant. Icterus leads to a work-up including laboratory studies, ultrasonography and possibly liver biopsy. The surgeon is usually then asked to confirm the diagnosis with an operative cholangiogram. If patency of the biliary tract (from the hepatic radicals to the duodenum) is demonstrated, biliary atresia is not present. Even if the ducts are minute, patency rules out biliary atresia and therefore other diagnoses must be entertained (e.g., neonatal hepatitis, cystic fibrosis, α-1-antitrypsin (AAT) deficiency, Alagille's syndrome) (1). In such instances, the cholangiocatheter is removed and a wedge liver biopsy obtained before closing. The most significant complication in this situation is one of misdiagnosis. Erroneous diagnosis of biliary atresia with performance of a Kasai procedure when the diagnosis is not biliary atresia, can lead to complete biliary obstruction, cholangitis, accelerated liver failure, and early liver transplantation or death (2). Several key points to avoid misdiagnosis and an unnecessary Kasai procedure from being performed are: (*i*) Preoperative evaluation should include a determination of the AAT level and phenotype. AAT deficiency patients have very tiny ducts that may not be well seen at cholangiography. A low AAT level or positive phenotype will prevent useless exploration. (*ii*) Evaluation of other clinical features such as peculiar facies (prominent forehead, pointed chin, and hypertelorism), heart murmur of pulmonic stenosis, butterfly vertebrae, or ophthalmologic findings of posterior embryotoxin can identify the patients with Alagille syndrome (paucity of the intrahepatic bile ducts), not biliary atresia (*iii*); (3) If on exploration, a normal-sized or enlarged gallbladder is found, then biliary atresia is unlikely, especially if the gallbladder contains green bile. (*iv*) Finally, if the distal common bile duct fills but not the proximal duct, beware! Attempt to encourage retrograde flow by occluding the distal duct during injection and use half-strength contrast. We prefer pinching with fingers to clamping, to avoid injury to the diminutive distal bile duct. If doubt exists, then the cholangiocatheter can be left in place and a formal cholangiogram performed in radiology with better image resolution (Fig. 1).

Failure to demonstrate biliary continuity is followed by performance of a Kasai portoenterostomy procedure. Even older patients (more than 100 days) can achieve benefit from the procedure, but the chances of success diminish with advancing age (4). The Kasai operation involves creation of a Roux-en-Y with retrocolic anastomosis to the amputated biliary remnant at the hilum of the liver, portoenterostomy. In approximately 15% of cases of biliary atresia, when the gallbladder and distal biliary tree are patent (obliteration proximally), then the gallbladder itself can be used as the drainage conduit, so called portocholecystostomy. This later procedure has the distinct advantage of almost completely eliminating the complication of cholangitis [*infra vide*] (5). The sphincter of Oddi provides a competent barrier to bacterial contamination of the porta which is an inherent flaw of Kasai's operation. Some surgeons have chosen not to use the gallbladder, opting for a standard Kasai anastomosis, due to concerns about the ability of the minute common duct to handle the bile output. Anxiety about adding backpressure against the already challenged biliary ductules can be ameliorated by leaving a catheter in the

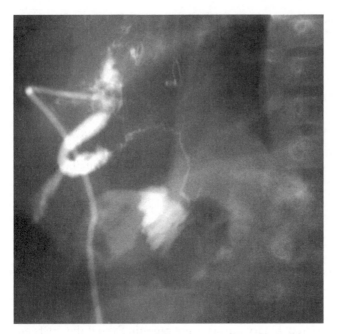

Figure 1 Intraoperative cholangiogram of a two-month-old cholestatic female showing hypoplastic bile ducts.

fundus of the gallbladder to decompress until the bile duct is capable of handling the drainage (6) (Fig. 2).

Cholangitis

The presence of enteric bacteria combined with poor bile flow and partial biliary obstruction is a perfect recipe for cholangitis. Almost every infant experiences at least one episode during the first year, and some have recurrent bouts. Cholangitis may be manifested by fever, jaundice, and sometimes, acholic stools. Laboratory investigation usually shows a leukocytosis (with a left shift), elevated serum bilirubin and hepatic enzymes (especially alkaline phosphatase and gamma glutamyl transferase). The clinical and laboratory changes may lag however, so that fever in biliary atresia patients is assumed to be cholangitis in the absence of another explanation. Intravenous broad spectrum antibiotics are started immediately since the potential consequences of bile shutdown are so dire. Untreated cholangitis can result in complete shutdown of bile flow and permanent liver damage. We use imipenum-cilastin (Primaxin®)

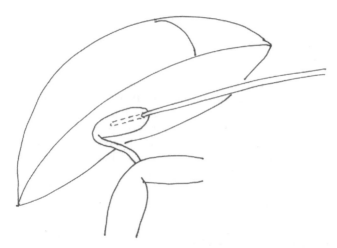

Figure 2 The success of a "gallbladder Kasai," portocholecystostomy, is improved if a small catheter is left in the gallbladder for decompression during the early postoperative period.

and add aminoglycosides if fever persists. Prophylactic antibiotics during the first year may be effective for the prevention of cholangitis (7), but we usually reserve them for the repeat offenders. For recalcitrant cases, systemic steroids can help by decreasing inflammation and increasing bile flow (8). We use a high dose, short duration regimen, but others have reported use of low dose of prednisone over months postoperatively (9). Neither of these regimens has been subjected to randomized controlled trial. The establishment of the Biliary Atresia Research Consortium, a NIH-funded study group of eight pediatric centers, has taken on this question as one of the first initiatives. Hopefully, this will lead to answers to this and other questions in the management (and etiology) of biliary atresia patients (10).

Biliary Conduits and Valves

Early modifications (e.g., Kasai hepatic portoenterostomy II and Suruga) utilized exteriorization to decompress the biliary conduit and to monitor the quantity and quality of bile flow (11). Unfortunately, in the presence of portal hypertension these enterostomies frequently became a liability due to stomal hemorrhage. Consequently, these modifications have been abandoned. Other authors sought to reduce or eliminate cholangitis by interposing an anti-reluxing valve between the liver and the alimentary tract. While conceptually attractive, the evidence for the effectiveness of intussusception valves has been mixed. A number of modifications of Kasai's original operation have been proposed, but none have been conclusively shown to have any significant benefit over the standard procedure in long-term follow-up (Fig. 3) (12).

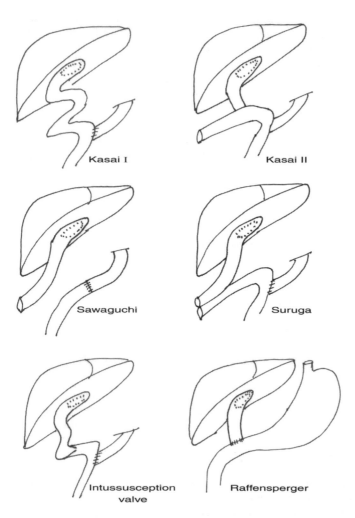

Figure 3 Many modifications of Kasai's original description were described. All were intended to reduce the number and severity of cholangitis events, but none proved to be durable or without unintended consequences.

Failure to Drain Bile

In spite of a technically satisfactory procedure, about 10% of babies never drain bile after Kasai's operation, or drain bile for only a very limited interval. In the past, attempts to establish bile flow led to repeated explorations with deeper dissection or scoring of the hilum. In general, success rates with re-excision have been extremely low if the first procedure was done correctly by an experienced pediatric surgeon. The development of jaundice in a child who cleared jaundice after the Kasai operation should however generate an investigation to discover a mechanical reason, for instance, obstruction of the Roux-en-Y, peri-hilar bile cyst/abscess, or intrahepatic biloma. Abdominal ultrasound and an iminodiacetic acid (IDA) scan may identify correctable causes of jaundice, but the vast majority of children will have no identifiable cause. Exploration without identifiable obstruction is rarely if ever successful in the long term. The concern about undirected exploration is that reoperations make subsequent liver transplantation more difficult, bloodier and higher risk (13). Consequently, we have no longer recommended reoperation unless the baby clearly had well-established bile drainage, cleared the jaundice, and then develops sudden bile shutdown with evidence of obstruction (14). Antibiotics and choleretic agents such as corticosteroids and usodeoxycholic acid may stimulate some bile flow in the early phases after bile shutdown (15). Ursodiol has a choleretic, cholelitholytic, and hepatoprotective effect that may be particularly valuable in this population (16).

Portal Hypertension

Some degree of hepatic fibrosis is present in every infant with biliary atresia, even at the time of initial diagnosis. In the majority, the fibrosis is progressive, leading to cirrhosis in many in spite of a "successful" Kasai procedure. One consequence of progressive fibrosis and cirrhosis is the development of portal hypertension. Portal hypertensive complications from both extrahepatic and intrahepatic causes will be covered later. (page 323)

Malabsorption and Fat Soluable Vitamin Deficiency

Bile salts are necessary for absorption of fat. Even in successful cases of biliary atresia, normal bile salt excretion, and therefore fat absorption, is not accomplished for several months. The diminished bile acids results in incomplete micelle formation and poor absorption of fats particularly long-chain triglycerides. Median-chain triglycerides (MCT) are more readily absorbed since they can be transported directly into the portal circulation without the need for micelle formation and transport via the lacteals. Therefore, formulas containing fat as MCT are preferred, e.g., Progestamil, Portagen, and Alimentum (17,18). In those children who are unable to take sufficient calories by mouth, nocturnal enteral feeds can be added via nasogastric feeding tube to supplement their nutrition (19).

Fat-soluble vitamin absorption is compromised as well and without supplementation, deficiencies of vitamin A, D, E, and K can occur (20). Vitamin A deficiency is manifest by night blindness (nyctalopia) and has been documented in the biliary atresia population (21). Rickets, with susceptibility for fractures, has also been seen from vitamin D deficiency (22). Vitamin E has several important functions, but shortage can result in loss of reflexes and delayed gross motor development (23). Finally, the role of vitamin K in production of coagulation factors VII, IX, and X results in significant coagulopathy when there is insufficient absorption (24). Each of these require, at least monitoring of serum levels, and usually supplementation.

Liver Failure/Cirrhosis

In about two-thirds of the patients with biliary atresia, the combination of cholestasis and ongoing fibrosis leads to cirrhosis, portal hypertension, and liver failure. This usually leads to referral for liver transplantation. Prior to the availability of liver replacement, over half of the patients with biliary atresia were dead by age 5 (25). The common indications for liver transplantation are (*i*) portal hypertensive complications, (*ii*) growth failure and (*iii*) synthetic failure (e.g., jaundice, coagulopathy, hypoalbuminemia). The management of these complications can directly influence the outcome of the liver transplant. Treatment of portal hypertensive complications is covered later (page 315). The treatment of growth failure includes special formulas, supplemental enteral feedings, and sometimes intravenous hyperalimentation. In the face of growth retardation, supplementation by nocturnal or continuous nasogastric feedings will often correct the nutritional caloric deficit. In some patients, growth cannot be improved even with enteric

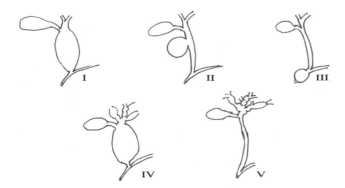

Figure 4 Classification of choledochal cyst. Types I and IV are the most common.

supplementation and in these circumstances, intravenous hyperalimentation may be required in the short term while awaiting urgent liver replacement.

In the presence of hepatic synthetic failure (jaundice, coagulopathy, and hypoalbumine-mia), there is little that can be done to improve the liver function short of transplantation. Oral vitamin K supplementation is standard but, with advancing liver failure, becomes less and less effective and parenteral vitamin K may be required (26). The importance of nutritional supplementation has already been discussed but again, as hepatic function wanes, the ability of the liver to synthesize proteins falls off. The technical details and complications of liver transplantation will be covered in Chapter 23.

CHOLEDOCHAL CYST

Choledochal cysts are the result of congenital maldevelopment of the biliary tract that can involve cystic dilation of both the intra- and extrahepatic bile ducts. There are several varieties of choledochal cyst (Fig. 4), but the most common are type I fusiform extrahepatic cysts, type V intrahepatic cysts also called Caroli's disease and type IV which is a combination of types I and V with both intra- and extra-hepatic cysts (27). Patients with type I choledochal cyst classically present with jaundice, pain, fever, and a mass. Some are discovered incidentally by prenatal ultrasonography. Untreated, all patients are at risk for development of cholangitis, pancreatitis, biliary cirrhosis, and malignancy. Malignant degeneration and the development of cholangiocarcinoma is 20 times higher than the population at large in long-term follow-up (28).

Internal Drainage

Historically, two operative procedures were commonly used for type I choledochal cyst; internal drainage and primary excision. Internal drainage procedures drain the cyst directly into the duodenum or jejunum (choledochocysto-duodenostomy or choledochocysto-jejunostomy, respectively). The complications of these procedures consist of anastomotic stricture, cholangitis, biliary stasis and stone formation, pancreatitis, and cholangiocarcinoma. The incidence of these complications was 34% to 58% (29). The explanation for this high complication rate is that failure to excise the diseased ductal tissue results in anastomosis to the cyst wall, which is largely composed of scar. Consequently, the anastomosis is prone to stricture resulting in stasis of bile in the unresected cyst which promotes cholangitis and stone formation. More importantly, the susceptibility to malignancy is not reduced by simple internal drainage (30). The incidence of cholangiocarcinoma in the residual cyst is significant over time and once present, resection for cure is rare (31).

Total Excision

Complete excision of the choledochal cyst with reconstruction utilizing a Roux-en-Y anastomosis to the common hepatic duct, hepaticojejunostomy, is the preferred technique (32). This procedure accomplishes the desired goals of good mucosa to mucosa approximation for the anastomosis and near-total elimination of the premalignant cyst. Total excision of the choledochal cyst is not without hazard however. Complications include bile leak, stricture and stone formation, recurrent cholangitis, pancreatitis or pancreatic fistula, and vascular injury (33). Bile leak is generally a minor complication seen in only a few patients and only in the acute postoperative phase. Leakage from the anastomosis is usually minor and temporary. A small closed suction drain left at the time of operation will permit conservative management until the leak completely ceases. Stricture at the anastomosis is rarely seen after complete cyst excision and Roux-en-Y reconstruction. Since the common hepatic duct is usually dilated at the level of transection owing to partial obstruction, anastomosis to the bowel is relatively straightforward. Consequently, the rate of stricture, cholangitis, and stone formation is quite low. The exception is the situation in which total excision is not possible because the cyst extends into the intrahepatic ducts (Type IV). In these cases, the anastomosis is to diseased tissue and so the development of a stricture is not unexpected.

In many patients with choledochal cyst, there is a long common channel between the pancreatic duct and common bile duct. The pancreatico-biliary junction is therefore more cephalad than normal. Consequently, distal dissection of the choledochal cyst requires special care to avoid injury to the anomalous junction. Damage or ligation of the pancreatic cyst can result in recurrent pancreatitis or pancreatic fistula. If there is any doubt, intraoperative cholangiography can help identify this junction. In practice, we typically leave a tiny portion of the distal choledochal cyst and oversew this remnant proximal to the junction with the pancreatic duct. There is little concern over leaving this small portion since the harmful toxic bile acids are no longer in contact.

The most concerning and immediately life-threatening complication of surgery for choledochal cyst is injury to the hepatic vasculature. Very large, type I cysts and those that have been associated with significant inflammation from recurrent cholangitis are especially problematic. The cyst wall can be extremely thick and densely adherent to the hepatic artery and portal vein. Attempts to completely excise these cysts can result in accidental injury, with hemorrhage or interruption of vascular supply to the liver. To prevent these complications, Lilly proposed dissection within the wall of the cyst, leaving a posterior outer shell overlying the vessels (34). This technique uses a plane within the cyst wall and allows the diseased inner lining and mucosa to be stripped out, much like the mucosectomy used in an endorectal pullthrough (Fig. 5).

Once the cyst or its inner lining are excised, reconstruction is accomplished by standard Roux-en-Y drainage. Accurate mucosa to mucosa approximation is required to reduce complications of bile leak and enteric fistula to a minimum. Some have recommended interposition of a jejunal segment, hepatico duodenostomy, but there is not statistical evidence to show any advantage (32). Laparoscopic techniques have also been described, but there are no controlled

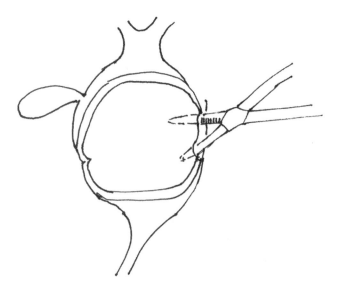

Figure 5 Internal technique for choledochal cyst resection. The cyst is opened on the presenting surface transversely and a plane developed between the inner lining and the outer wall. This technique avoids injury to the underlying portal vein and hepatic artery.

trials (35). Attempting to perform this procedure laparoscopically is a major undertaking requiring advanced skills. The penalty for a strictured biliary anastomosis or for vascular injury could be lifelong. The cosmetic and short-term recovery advantages of a laparoscopic approach need to be carefully weighed by the surgeon, family, and patient.

It is felt that the chronic exposure to the toxic bile acids that results from biliary stasis causes repeated injury to the biliary epithelium and in the long term promotes the development of cholangiocarcinoma. Thus, if the cyst, or its inner lining are excised/excluded then we believe the risk of choloangiocarcinoma is eliminated. No examples of malignancy developing in such a patient exists. On the other hand, retention of portions of the cyst that are partially or wholly intrahepatic is a gamble. If the intrahepatic cysts are confined to one lobe, then hepatectomy theoretically eliminates the risk of malignancy. The risk of a major hepatic resection must then be balanced against the risk of subsequent development of cholangiocarcinoma. Unfortunately, there is insufficient data to accurately make that assessment. Consequently, we feel that an acceptable alternative is to recommend ursodeoxycholic acid (ursodiol) and regular follow-up hepatic enzyme determinations. Ursodiol has many potentially beneficial effects; a choleretic effect that may reduce stasis and reduce time of exposure of the biliary epithelium (16). It also has a cytoprotective property, protecting cholangiocytes against the cytotoxicity of hydrophobic bile acids (36,37). Finally, the demonstrated litholytic properties may be beneficial to dissolve stones or prevent stones in patients with retained intrahepatic cysts (38,39). If hepatic enzyme levels remain elevated in a patient with retained intrahepatic cyst confined to one lobe, serious consideration to lobectomy should be given. If hepatectomy is not an option because of bi-lobar disease, then liver transplantation is the only option.

PERFORATION OF THE BILE DUCTS

Spontaneous perforation of the extrahepatic biliary tree is a rare condition seen in newborns. The perforation is most commonly at the junction of the cystic duct and common duct and is thought to represent a congenital weakness in the wall of the bile duct resulting in rupture. The infant usually presents with mild jaundice, irritability, failure to thrive, and sometimes ascites. The leaking bile forms a pseudocyst in the subhepatic space or may leak freely leading to biliary ascites. The diagnosis may be made with ultrasonography and IDA scanning. Ultrasound examination shows an ill-defined cystic collection in the hilum of the liver and may demonstrate ascites (40). IDA images usually show extravasation of the radionucleide into the subhepatic space. Treatment involves exploration, intraoperative cholangiography and simple drainage, and rarely bile duct reconstruction. The most feared complication of this disease is damage to the minute common bile duct. Consequently, conservative management is with drainage alone with a subhepatic drain and a cholecystostomy. After a cholangiocatheter is placed into the gallbladder, contrast injection will accurately identify the site of perforation. Since the catheter will often remain in place until the leak has sealed, take some extra time to ensure that it is well secured and properly positioned. Sometimes sludge or inflammation gives the radiographic appearance of a partially or completely obstructed distal common bile duct. Still, the inflamed hilum should not be dissected (41). To do so risks inadvertent injury of the duct or the hepatic vasculature. The area should be widely drained since inadequate drainage can result in later infection. The catheter left in the gallbladder can be used for later cholangiopraphy to document healing of the perforation and patency of the distal duct. If the obstruction of the distal common duct is severe or does not resolve over time, Roux-en-Y hepaticojejunostomy reconstruction may be required (42).

PORTAL HYPERTENSION

Hypertension in the portal venous system is a result of obstruction to flow. The restriction may be either suprahepatic (e.g., hepatic vein thrombosis), intrahepatic (e.g., cirrhosis) or prehepatic (e.g., portal vein thrombosis). The most important clinical consequence of portal hypertension is esophageal variceal hemorrhage. Esophageal varices are the consequence of the development of portosystemic collaterals between the portal vein, left gastric vein, and short gastric veins to the submucosal plexus in the esophagus. The esophageal varices then drain via the azygous/hemiazygous system into the superior vena cava. Because the distal esophageal veins are very superficial, they are susceptible to rupture.

Esophageal Variceal Hemorrhage

Bleeding from varices can be sudden and severe and can quickly lead to hypovolemia, anemia, and shock. Fortunately in children, variceal bleeding is usually well tolerated and stops spontaneously before complications of shock occur (43). Still, supportive treatment with intravenous volume replacement, transfusion, and close monitoring in a critical care setting are required. Bleeding can be controlled initially by pharmacologic means (e.g., vasopressor or octreotide) but ultimate control will usually require invasive procedures (44). For the majority, endoscopy is the first-line method chosen. Not only does endoscopy offer diagnostic visualization of the bleeding source, but also control by band ligation or sclerosis. The two techniques have roughly equal efficacy however, banding appears to be associated with fewer complications (45). Complications include fever, esophageal ulceration, stricture formation, and dysmotility.

The next most invasive technique to control esophageal variceal hemorrhage is transjugular intrahepatic portosystemic shunting (TIPPS). This radiologic technique creates a shunt between the portal vein and the hepatic vein by deploying an expandable metallic wall stent within the liver. It has had limited application in small children due to the miniature size of the vessels and also because in children, extrahepatic portal vein thrombosis is frequently the cause of the portal hypertension (46). TIPPS is also associated with a high incidence of stenosis of the shunt. Many can be reopened with ballooning techniques, but still frequent surveillance and dilations are required. Probably the best use of TIPPS is in the somewhat older child with end-stage liver disease, as a bridge to transplantation. Most children with end-stage liver disease should be referred early for listing for liver transplantation and endoscopic means used to control their variceal bleeding (47–49).

Portosystemic Shunts

With the success of liver transplantation and endoscopic methods to manage variceal hemorrhage, shunt procedures are much less commonly performed. The most common indication currently is for patients with portal vein thrombosis (PVT). This eliminates many of the commonly used shunts (e.g., portocaval) because the portal vein is not available for bypass. The shunts now in favor: Mesocaval, Warren (distal splenorenal), and Meso-Rex each have different advantages and disadvantages.

The mesocaval shunt was popularized by Clatworthy and modified by others. Most often it is now performed as an H-type mesocaval shunt using a synthetic graft (e.g., PTFE) or vein graft. Relatively easy to construct, the technical details are nonetheless very important. It is a nonselective shunt so might be associated with a greater incidence of encephalopathy, at least theoretically. There are insufficient patient numbers or studies however to make a definitive judgment.

The distal splenorenal (Warren) shunt was designed to reduce the complication of encephalopathy by maintaining portal flow and only decompressing the sinistral portion of the portal circulation thereby effectively eliminating esophageal varices. Unfortunately, over time, collateralization results in decompression of the entire portal circulation and the potential for encephalopathy rises.

The Meso-Rex shunt is a relatively new technique which was specifically developed for circumstances of portal vein thrombosis. It relies upon the fact that the intrahepatic portal vein remains patent even in patients with portal vein thrombosis. Therefore, bypass from the portal circuit (usually superior mesenteric vein) to the left branch of the portal vein re-established normal prograde portal flow. The procedure is technically demanding and requires removal of the left internal jugular vein for use as a conduit, but series of small numbers of patients have demonstrated good decompression of portal pressure and no evidence of encephalopathy (50).

All of these procedures and others are technically demanding, tedious, and potentially dangerous. Complications include intraoperative bleeding, thrombosis, and stenosis. Fortunately, for this group of patients PVT the liver function is usually preserved so they usually do not have coagulopathy. In fact, it is sometimes recommended to add aspirin for short-term anticoagulation to prevent early thrombosis. Stenosis is a purely technical problem prevented only by meticulous attention to detail and avoidance of twisting or kinking of the vessels. We still use a continuous suturing technique but avoid excessive tension by the assistant which can lead to "purse-stringing" of the anastomosis.

CHOLELITHIASIS AND CHOLECYSTITIS

The incidence of cholelithiasis and cholecystitis in children is increasing. This trend is the result of a combination of factors: (i) improved survival of infants and children with serious illnesses, (ii) complicated medical interventions (total parenteral nutrition, bowel resections, etc.), (iii) increasing obesity in children and lipid dysregulation, and (iv) improved ability to detect stone disease of the gallbladder. Laparoscopic techniques have largely replaced open cholecystectomy even though there are no randomized controlled clinical trials of laparoscopic versus open cholecystectomy in children. Still, the laparoscopic techniques result in less trauma, reduced pain, shorter hospital stay, and improved cosmetic result which have clear advantages. Laparoscopic cholecystectomy is now the gold standard (51).

Laparoscopic cholecystectomy is a very common operation in adults and is becoming more frequently required in children (52). It might follow then that the complication rate among pediatric surgeons would be increased, but this does not seem to be the case. Part of the explanation may be that, in general, the anatomy is more straightforward. Children tend not to have the thick, chronically inflamed gall bladders that are common place in adults. They also are, on balance, thinner so anatomic details are not obscured in layers of adipose tissue. Nonetheless, understanding of the potential complications and the avoidance of them is important, as well as their management when they occur.

A complete review of the indications for proceeding to operation are beyond the scope of this section. Given that, it is important to note that an important part of prevention of complications is sufficient preoperative preparation. Patients should have fluid balance restored by adequate intravenous hydration, sepsis controlled by administration of intravenous antibiotics, and underlying conditions investigated and treated before proceeding to the operating room. The timing of cholecystectomy deserves some attention as well. It is generally recommended to intervene early, within 72 hours of the onset of symptoms (53). Operating later is associated with increased difficulty due to edema/inflammation and consequently complications are more likely due to obfuscation of the anatomy. The more common and serious complications seen after laparoscopic cholecystectomy are bile duct injury, bile leak, bleeding, and trocar injuries.

The key to avoidance of bile duct injury during cholecystectomy is careful dissection and correct interpretation of the anatomy. The most common cause of injury to the common bile duct is misidentification of the biliary anatomy. The following steps are suggested to minimize this risk:

1. Use of a 30° telescope.
2. Initiation of dissection on the gallbladder with division of the peritoneum on the infundibulum and extension of the dissection ventrally on the gallbladder as far as possible anteriorly and posteriorly.
3. Exposure of the strictures in the hepatobiliary triangle by interior and lateral traction on the infundibulum.
4. Clear identification of the cystic artery and cystic duct extending to the gallbladder before ligation and transection, so called "critical view" (54).
5. Use of operative cholangiography if clear anatomic identification is not possible.
6. Avoidance of diathermy anywhere close to the common duct.

Most bile duct injuries are not diagnosed during the operation. Cystic duct leaks identified at operation can be addressed directly with ligation. If bile leak is identified later, it can be diagnosed by endoscopic retrograde cholangiopancreatography and if no major ductal disruption is found, it can be stented endoscopically (55). For partial duct lacerations, the best treatment is primary repair with fine absorbable suture and drainage. Complete ductal transections usually will require Roux-en-Y hepaticojejunostomy. If the operating surgeon is not comfortable with such a procedure, then consultation intraoperatively with a surgical colleague is recommended (56). Missed injuries often present days to weeks later with vague symptoms or with classic symptoms of jaundice and bile peritonitis. A high index of suspicion is necessary to avoid delay in diagnosis. Vascular injuries are similarly often the result of misinterpreted anatomy. The frequency of anomolus arterial supply to the gall bladder and liver is high (57). Hemorrhage can obscure vision and lead to inaccurate application of clips or ill-advised use of cautery. Unintended ligation/coagulation at the right hepatic artery or other accessory replaced arteries can result in hepatic ischemia and late intrahepatic bile strictures. Overzealous dissection around the common bile duct can lead to ischemia and stricture.

REFERENCES

1. Moore TC. Biliary atresia and related conditions (Chapter 8). In Moore TC (ed) Challenges in Pediatric Surgery. Austin: RE Landes, 1994:109–129.
2. Lilly J. The surgery of biliary hypoplasia. J Pediatr Surg 1976; 11:815–821.
3. Quiros-Tejiera RE, Ament ME, Heyman MB, et al. Variable morbidity in Alagille syndrome: A review of 43 cases. J Pediatr Gastroenterol Nutr 1999; 29(4):431–437.
4. Davenport M, Piricelli V, Farrant P, et al. The outcome of the older (> or = 100 days) infant with biliary atresia. J Pediatr Surg 2004; 39(4):575–581.
5. Lilly JR. Hepatic portocholecystostomy for biliary atresia. J Pediatr Surg 1979; 14(3):301–304.
6. Lilly JR, Stellin G. Catheter decompression of hepatic portocholecystostomy. J Pediatr Surg 1982; 17(6):904–905.
7. Bu LN, Chen HL, Chang CJ, et al. Prophylactic oral antibiotics in prevention of recurrent cholangitis after the Kasai portoenterostomy. J Pediatr Surg 2003; 38:590–593.
8. Karrer FM, Lilly JR. Corticosteroid therapy in biliary atresia. J Pediatr Surg 1985; 20(6):693–695.
9. Escobar MA, Jay CL, Brooks RM, et al. Effect of corticosteroid therapy on outcomes in biliary atresia after Kasai portoenterostomy. J Pediatr Surg 2006; 41(1):99–103.
10. Shneider BL, Brown MB, Haber B, et al. A multicenter study of the outcome of biliary atresia in the United States, 1997 to 2000. J Pediatr 2006; 148(4):432–435.
11. Lilly JR, Starzl TE. Liver, Gallbladder and Extrahepatic Bile Ducts. In Welch KJ (ed), Complications of Pediatric Surgery: Prevention and Management. Philadelphia, PA: WB Saunders, 1982:237–255.
12. Karrer FM, Lilly JR, Stewart BA, et al. Biliary atresia registry, 1976 to 1989. J Pediatr Surg 1990; 25(1):1076–1080.
13. Rivilla F, Vazques J, Ros Z, et al. Reoperation in biliary atresia. Cir Pediatr 1989; 2(3):110–113.
14. Ohi R. Biliary atresia. A surgical perspective. Clin Liver Dis 2000; 4(4):779–804.
15. Meyers RL, Book LS, O'Gorman MA, et al. High-dose steroids, ursodeoxycholic acid, and chronic intravenous antibiotics improve bile flow after Kasai procedure in infants with biliary atresia. J Pediatr Surg 2003; 38:406–411.
16. Angulo P. Use of ursodeoxycholic acid in patients with liver disease. Curr Gastroenterol Rep 2002; 4(1):37–44.
17. Ng VL, Balistreri WF. Treatment options for chronic cholestasis in infancy and childhood. Curr Treat Options Gastroentrol 2005; 8:419–430.
18. Novy MA, Schwarz KB. Nutritional considerations and management of the child with liver disease. Nutrition 1997; 13(3):177–184.
19. Francavilla R, Miniello VL, Brunetti L, et al. Hepatitis and cholestasis in infancy; clinical and nutritional aspects. Acta Paediatr Suppl 2003; 91(441):101–104.
20. Andrews WS, Pau CM, Chase HP, et al. Fat soluable vitamin deficiency in biliary atresia. J Pediatr Surg 1981; 16(3):284–290.
21. Ferenchak AP, Gralla J, King R, et al. Comparison of indices of vitamin A status in children with chronic liver disease. Hepatology 2005; 42(4):782–792.
22. Sokol RJ. Fat soluable vitamins and their importance in patients with cholestatic liver diseases. Gastroentrol Clin North Am 1994; 23(4):673–705.
23. Sokol RJ. Vitamin E and neurologic deficits. Adv Pediatr 1990; 37:119–148.
24. Mager DR, McGee PL, Furuya KN, et al. Prevalence of vitamin K deficiency in children with mild to moderate chronic liver disease. J Pediatr Gastroenterol Nutr 2006; 42(1):71–76.
25. Izant RJ Jr, Akers DR, Hays DM, et al. Biliary Atresia Survey. Proceedings of Surgical Section. Elk Grove Village, IL: American Academy of Pediatrics, 1965.
26. Pereira SP, Shearer MJ, Williams R, et al. Intestinal absorption of mixed micellar phyllaquinone (vitamin K1) is unreliable in infants with conjugated hyperbilirubinemia: Implications for oral prophylaxis of vitamin K deficiency bleeding. Arch Dis Child Fetal Neonatal Ed 2003; 88(2):113–118.
27. Todani T, Watanabe Y, Narusue M, et al. Congenital bile duct cysts: Classification, operative procedures and review of thirty-seven cases including cancer arising from choledochal cyst. Am J Surg 1977; 134(2):263–269.
28. Lilly JR, Ohi R. Complication of surgery for biliary atresia and choledochal cysts. In: deVries PA, Shapiro SR, eds. Complications of Pediatric Surgery. New York: Wiley Medical, 1982:155–166.

29. Lister J. Liver and biliary tree (chapter 5). In Lister J (ed) Complication in Paediatric Surgery. London: Bailliere Tindall, 1986:161–170.
30. Metcalfe MS, Wemyss-Holden SA, Maddern GJ. Management dilemmas with choledochal cysts. Arch Surg 2003; 138:333–339.
31. deVries JS, deVries S, Aronson DC, et al. Choledochal cyst: Age of presentation, symptoms and late complications related to Todani's classification. J Pediatr Surg 2002; 37(11):1568–1573.
32. Flanigan PD. Biliary cysts. Ann Surg 1975; 182(5):635–643.
33. Li MJ, Feng JX, Jin QF. Early complications after excision with hepaticoenterostomy for infants and children with choledochal cysts. Hepatobiliary Pancreat Dis Int 2002; 1(2):281–284.
34. Lilly JR. Total excision of choledochal cyst. Surg Gynecol Obstet 1978; 146:254–256.
35. Le DM, Woo RK, Sylvester K, et al. Laparoscopic resection of type 1 choledochal cysts in pediatric patients. Surg Endosc 2006; 20(2):249–251.
36. Paumgartner G, Beuers U. Ursodeoxycholic acid in cholestatic liver disease: Mechanisms of action and therapeutic use revisited. Hepatology 2002; 36:525–531.
37. Stiehl A, Benz C, Sauer P. Mechanism of hepatoprotection action of bile salts in liver disease. Gastroenterol Clin North Am 1999; 28:195–209.
38. Ros E, Navarro S, Bru C, et al. Ursodeoxycholic acid treatment of primary hepatolithiasis in Caroli's syndrome. Lancet 1993; 342:404–406.
39. Salvioli G, Salati R, Lugli R, et al. Medical treatment of biliary duct stones: Effect of ursodeoxycholic acid administration. Gut 1983; 24:609–614.
40. Lilly JR, Weintraub WH, Altman RP. Spontaneous perforation of the extrahepatic bile duct and bile peritonitis in infancy. Surgery 1974; 75:664–673.
41. Prevot J, Babut JM. Spontaneous perforations of the biliary tract in infancy. Prog Pediatric Surg 1971; 3:187.
42. Spigland N, Greco R, Rosenfeld D. Spontaneous biliary perforation: Does external drainage constitute adequate therapy? J Pediatr Surg 1996; 31(6):782–784.
43. Fonkalsrud EW. Treatment of variceal hemorrhage in children. Surg Clin North Am 1990; 70(2):475–487.
44. Ryckman FC, Alonso MH. Causes and management of portal hypertension in the pediatric population. Clin Liver Disease 2001; 5(3):789–818.
45. Price MR, Sartorelli KH, Karrer FM, et al. Management of esophageal varices in children by endoscopic variceal ligation. J Pediatr Surg 1996; 31(8):1056–1059.
46. Zargar SA, Javid F. Khan BA, et al. Endoscopic ligation compared with sclerotherapy for bleeding esophageal varices in children with extrahepatic portal venous obstruction. Hepatology 2002; 36(3):666–672.
47. Poddar U, Thapa BR, Singh K. Band ligation plus sclerotherapy versus sclerotherapy alone in children with extrahepatic portal venous obstruction. J Clin Gastroentrol 2005; 39(7):626–629.
48. Huppert PE, Astfalk W, Brambs HJ, et al. Transjugular intrahepatic portosystemic shunt in children. Initial clinical experiences and literature review. Rofo 1998; 168(6):595–603.
49. Huppert PE, Goffette P, Astfalk W, et al. Transjugular intrahepatic portosystemic shunts in children with biliary atresia. Cardiovasc Intervent Radiol 2002; 25(6):484–493.
50. Dasgupta R, Roberts E, Superina RA, et al. Effectiveness of Rex shunt in the treatment of portal hypertension. J Pediatr Surg 2006; 41(1):108–112.
51. Kim PC, Wesson D, Superina R, et al. Laparoscopic cholecystectomy versus open cholecystectomy in children: Which is better? J Pediatr Surg 1995; 30:971–973.
52. Waldenhausen JHT, Benjamin DR. Cholecystectomy is becoming an increasingly common operation in children. Am J Surg 1999; 177:364–367.
53. Lo CH, Liu CL, Fan STY, et al. Prospective randomized study of early versus delayed laparoscopic cholecystectomy for acute Cholecystitis. Ann Surg 1998; 227(4):461–467.
54. Strasberg SM, Hartl M, Soper NJ. An analysis of the problem of biliary injury during laparoscopic cholecystectomy. J Am Coll Surg 1995; 180:101–125.
55. Katsinelos P, Paroutoglou G, Beltsis A, et al. Endobiliary endoprosthesis without sphincterotomy for treatment of biliary leakage. Surg Endosc 2004; 18:165–166.
56. Connor S. Garden OJ. Bile duct injury in the era of laparoscopic cholecystectomy. Br J Surg 2006; 93:158–168.
57. Skandalakis JE, Gray SW, Rowe JS, eds. Anatomical Complications in General Surgery, Chapter 6, Biliary Surgery. New York: McGraw Hill Book Co, 1983:125–145.

Kasai Portoenterostomy

Expert: R. Peter Altman, M.D.

QUESTIONS

1. **How do you decide if you are in the correct plane of the portal plate?**
   Assuming the extrahepatic biliary system is continuous, which it usually is, I mobilize the atretic gallbladder from its bed and identify and dissect the common bile duct remnant toward the duodenum. I then divide the common bile duct which enables me to identify the plane between the fibrotic bile duct and the portal vein. The dissection is continued cephalad using sharp and blunt dissection. Q-tips are ideal as blunt dissectors. The dissection is carried proximally until the bifurcation of the portal vein is identified. There are usually two or three tributaries of the portal vein at this level. These are controlled either by careful cautery or with fine ties. Once these venous tributaries are divided, the plane between the fibrous tissue at the porta and the portal vein become clear. The portal plate is dissected taking care to remain outside the liver parenchyma. After the portal plate is identified, double-armed sutures (6-0 PDS) are placed at the lateral margins of the plate and the fibrous tissue plug is transected.

2. **What steps do you take to mobilize the liver?**
   For the routine Kasai procedure it is not necessary to mobilize the liver. Formerly, I mobilized the liver for reoperations. Since we rarely do reoperate (see below) we leave the liver in situ for the performance of Kasai portoenterostomy. The disadvantage of liver mobilization is postoperative ascites which outweighs the theoretical advantage gained by extensive liver mobilization. For exposure of the porta hepatis, I ask that an assistant scrub for the case to provide retraction. Alternatively, a fixed retractor can be used in some circumstances.

3. **It is necessary to perform a nipple valve for the portoenterostomy?**
   We reviewed our experience with over 400 cases, most of whom had either vented or valved conduits. Using the Cox formula for multivariate analysis we learned that neither vent nor valve had any statistically significant effect on outcome. Therefore, we no longer valve nor vent the conduit.

4. **What are the most common complications of a Kasai portoenterostomy?**
   In our experience, complications after the Kasai portoenterostomy have been remarkably few. That is assuming that cholangitis is not considered a "complication" of the operation. We have not experienced any cases of intraoperative bleeding. Several patients have developed postoperative small bowel obstruction secondary to adhesions. We emphasize careful, meticulous closing of the small bowel mesentery after conduit construction. That is essential to avoid postoperative internal hernia and small bowel obstruction.

5. **What unusual complications of Kasai portoenterostomy have you encountered?**
   Because we close the end of the conduit and construct an end-to-side bilienteric anastomosis, it is important that the anastomosis be placed precisely at the junction of the turned-in jejunum. In several patients we constructed the anastomosis too proximal. As a result there was redundancy distal to the anastomosis. Over time, the distal closed end of the jejunal conduit filled with bile which had no access to the GI tract. The patient presented with a fluid (bile) filled mass. Management required reoperation and jejunojejunostomy (conduit-conduit) assuring that there could be no recurrence.

6. **What preoperative factors help reduce complications?**
   We try to emphasize an expeditious work-up and timely operative treatment. We rely on percutaneous liver biopsy and discourage repeated liver function tests which rarely contribute much new information. When we see a patient who is younger than 9 weeks, a technetium IDA scan is recommended. Diagnosis after 9 weeks may preclude nuclear

scanning because of the need to pretreat with phenobarbital for 5 days. Our objective is to do the Kasai before 10 weeks of age.

7. What causes cholangitis?

I don't pretend to know although I suspect that intestinal reflux into the conduit contributes as does the interruption of lymphatics resulting from the portal dissection. Perhaps the most important factor is bile stasis. We know from our experience with vented conduits that bile flow was not brisk until several months after the operation. Stagnant bile, as with any other system, is vulnerable to infection.

8. Do postoperative antibiotics prevent cholangitis?

They may. Following portoenterostomy, we rely on oral antibiotics for at least 2 years in hopes that they will reduce the incidence and severity of postoperative infection, if not prevent it entirely. We use sulfamethoxazole/trimethoprim (Bactrim) suspension at a dose of 2.5 mg trimethoprim given once per day for this purpose. If there is break through infection, the patients are hospitalized and treated with parenteral antibiotics.

9. Is there a role for early re-exploration for failure of bile flow?

That question is frequently asked. If the first operation is done by an experienced pediatric surgeon, I do not recommend re-exploration for early failure feeling that if the fibrous tissue at the porta is divided at the optimal location, there is nothing to be gained by retransection. In the early days, I felt differently and I was much more liberal with re-exploration. As I got more and more experience with the technical aspects of the operation and in view of the fact that liver transplantation is a viable option in most centers, I feel that, if a second operation is indicated, it should be a liver transplant. We have not re-explored a patient at our center for more than 20 years.

10. How long should the Roux-en-Y jejunostomy be?

We use about 45 cm without incident. I am not aware of any data that indicates that an alternative length would not be acceptable.

11. Should steroids be administered postoperatively?

While many of the studies are underpowered statistically, there are data suggesting that steroids improve postoperative bile flow. Currently, we start steroids in the first postoperative week, as soon as the patient is tolerating oral feedings. Our protocol uses prednisolone liquid and begins with a dose of 2 mg/kg/day divided into two doses. The prednisolone is tapered off over the first 4 to 6 weeks after surgery.

12. Is there a role for phenobarbital postoperatively?

We do not see a role for phenobarbital, however, we put our patients on ursodiol (Actigall) routinely. Patients remain on ursodiol (10–15 mg/kg/dose BID) for several years.

Excision of Choledochal Cyst

Expert: Frederick C. Ryckman, M.D.

QUESTIONS

1. How should the common bile duct be managed distal to the choledochal cyst?

One of the critical elements in the dissection of a choledochal cyst is the management of the distal common bile duct. Critical information relating to the safety of this step is achieved through the use of an intraoperative cholangiogram. This investigation helps define the location of the pancreatic duct and possible long common channel anatomy which might complicate distal duct and cyst closure. When undertaking open choledochal cyst resection, I prefer to open the anterior choledochocyst wall after completing the circumferential dissection of the cyst to confirm the internal anatomy demonstrated on the cholangiogram. Closure of the distal duct is then undertaken under direct vision using multiple interrupted dissolving 4.0 monofilament sutures. When this dissection is undertaken using laparoscopic techniques, superior traction of the distal cystic elements will allow dissection of the retroduodenal and intrapancreatic portion of the cyst. Knowledge of the distal cyst anatomy and the location of the pancreatic duct is critical in these cases as open internal visualization is more difficult. Staple or Endoloop closure of the distal duct it is then possible. Retention of the distal cyst remnant at the time of cyst closure can result in redevelopment of a choledochal cyst within the superior margin of the pancreatic head. This is not only prone to progressive enlargement, but also contains abnormal mucosa with its tendency for metaplastic or neoplastic degeneration.

2. **How should the anastamosis be performed in a patient when the cyst extends into both hepatic ducts?**
   Management of the proximal choledochal cyst is often complex. This decision is complicated by the tendency of the extrahepatic normal proper hepatic ducts to dilate related to distal obstruction. This is accentuated in the left proper hepatic duct as it traverses the Rex recess in an extrahepatic location. The critical element here is deciding the level of transaction to allow anastomosis to an area of normal mucosa. This can be identified by direct opened inspection of the bile duct. It is my preference to open the proximal cyst in the region of the anatomic common bile duct which allows direct visual identification of inflow hepatic radicals and assessment of the biliary mucosal integrity. In most cases reconstruction at the level of the bifurcation incorporating a single common cuff is possible. If mucosal integrity cannot be assured at that level further proximal dissection can be undertaken. This is limited on the right proper hepatic duct by the rather early intrahepatic passage of the right anterior and posterior ductal elements. On the left, the extended extrahepatic Rex recess portion of the left proper hepatic duct can be more easily accessed in its location superior and slightly posterior to the portal vein. Even in cases where individual hepatic duct reconstruction must be undertaken, the lumen of the duct is rarely so small that it requires internal stenting for drainage. Our duct reconstruction technique includes the placement of multiple interrupted monofilament nonpermanent 5.0 or 6.0 sutures with their knots on the external anastomotic surface.

3. **What technique of Roux-en-Y formation reduces complications?**
   Our Roux-en-Y technique has been formulated in an attempt to prevent reflux of enteric contents and provide for an obstruction free anastomosis. We perform the Roux-en-Y anastomosis at the first significant arcade distal to the ligament of Treitz. We use a 35-cm retrocolic isoperistaltic Roux and reconstruct the anastomosis as an end to side reconstruction. In an effort to prevent enteric reflux, multiple seromuscular sutures are placed between the inflow jejunal limb and the Roux limb to establish a narrow angle of inflow. We have avoided the use of ante-colic limbs in an effort to decrease the risk of inferior displacement by the colon and traction on the anastomotic site.

4. **What strategies should be performed in the patient with pericystic inflammation?**
   A variety of alternative management strategies can be performed in a patient with severe pericystic inflammation. It is fortunate that the combination of early diagnosis and appropriate antimicrobial treatment for cholangitis has decreased the incidence of severe pericholecystic inflammation. However, in cases where this still occurs, the technique initially described by Lilly and associates is helpful. The technique involves employing a submucosal dissection throughout the posterior element of the choledochal cyst where the posterior wall is juxtaposed to the hepatic artery and the portal vein. The submucosal dissection allows the maintenance of the posterior elements of the choledochal cyst overlying the portal vein preventing operative injury. Careful attention must be paid at the proximal anastomosis to be sure that the anterior wall of the portal vein is not incorporated into the posterior anastomotic sutures when complete dissection of the vein from the bile duct system has not been completed.
   In cases where severe cholangitis has complicated the choledochal cyst, we would recommend appropriate antibiotic administration for the treatment of cholangitis accompanied by a transhepatic biliary drainage catheter if necessary to decrease inflammation prior to undertaking the definitive resection. Although uncommon, injury to the portal vein

during this dissection step has resulted in both portal vein thrombosis and severe portal hypertension as well as permanent injury requiring liver transplantation.

5. **What are the most common complications following resection of a choledochal cyst?**
   The most common complication not previously discussed is anastomotic stenosis. Technical elements to avoid anastomotic stenosis include the prevention of a peri anastomotic leak which often leads to an anastomotic stricture. It is our preference to undertake this anastomosis in an end to side fashion using multiple absorbable, interrupted, nonpermanent monofilament 5-0 or 6-0 sutures with the knots on the external anastomotic surface. The size of the bile duct is large enough that an intraductal stent for external stenting is rarely, if ever, necessary. Prevention of leakage by appropriate and precise suture placement would minimize the tendency toward stricture formation. Peri anastomotic inflammation caused by even a small biliary leak has a tendency to aggravate stricture formation leading to anastomotic stenosis.

   It is our practice to do follow up minimally invasive imaging (ultrasound) at approximately 3 months to define the absence of stricture and we usually repeat this image again at 1 year following surgical reconstruction.

19 | Complications of Surgery of the Spleen

Kurt D. Newman, M.D. and Todd A. Ponsky, M.D.

INTRODUCTION

Splenic Structure and Function

The role of the spleen has eluded physicians since ancient times. The significance of the spleen has only been understood for the last 50 years. The spleen has three major functions: fetal hematopoiesis, maintenance of immune function, and mechanical blood filtration (1).

The mechanism of splenic function is closely tied to its anatomic structure. The spleen is encapsulated by the visceral peritoneum. The splenic artery, from the celiac trunk, and the short gastric arteries, from the left gastric and the left gastroepiploic arteries, contribute the arterial blood supply to the spleen. Arterial blood enters the white pulp, which is mostly lymphoid tissue. Within this tissue, the blood passes through a network of arteries lined by macrophages, T-lymphocytes, and plasma cells. The blood is then directed through follicles of B-lymphocytes. The contact of the antigens within these cells allows immune recognition and initiates an immune response. Specifically, as blood passes through the B-lymphocyte follicles in the white pulp, the antigens are recognized and antibodies, IgM, are formed. In addition to IgM, opsinizing proteins, tuftsin, and properdin, are also produced.

The blood leaves the white pulp and crosses the marginal zone, a sheet of T-lymphocytes, into the red pulp. Here, the blood enters one of two routes: the "closed circulation" through endothelial-lined capillaries into the venous system or the "open circulation" into the Billroth's cords, which comprise a macrophage lined reticular meshwork. As blood passes through the open circulation, aged and damaged cells and debris are filtered and engulfed by the splenic phagocytes. Aged erythrocytes, which have lost their pliancy, are unable to squeeze through the narrow slits of the red pulp meshwork unlike normal erythrocytes, which maintain their pliability and are able to slide through (1,2).

As mentioned above, the spleen serves a hematopoetic function in the fetus. With the exception of children with certain anemic diseases, the hematopoetic function of the spleen typically ceases at 5 months of age.

Indications for Splenectomy

Splenectomy was first described by Sutherland and Burghard in 1910 (3). In this case, the splenectomy was performed for hereditary spherocytosis (HS). As the understanding of the immunologic function of the spleen has grown, we are more aware of the potential risk resulting from its removal. Therefore, splenectomy is limited to specific indications, either elective or traumatic.

Elective Indications

The elective indications for splenectomy include severe hemolytic anemia, immune cytopenia, metabolic storage disease, and secondary hypersplenism (4). Some common indications are discussed below.

Immune Thrombocytopenic Purpura

Immune thrombocytopenic purpura (ITP) is one of the most common elective indications for splenectomy in children and the most common in adults with an incidence of 14,000 cases per year (5). In this autoimmune disease, the spleen produces antiplatelet antibodies that sequester and destroy platelets. Children with platelet counts less than 20,000 cells/μL or those children with conditions that pose a high risk for bleeding are treated with medical therapy. If the thrombocytopenia is refractory to medical therapy or relapses after initial response, splenectomy is indicated. Splenectomy leads to a complete and permanent in response in 65% of children (6).

Hereditary Spherocytosis

Hereditary spherocytosis is an autosomal dominant inherited hemolytic anemia that results from a deficiency of spectrin, an erythrocyte cytoskeletal protein. The rigidity of these cells and their spherical shape leads to sequestration in the endoreticular meshwork of the spleen. Splenectomy is currently the treatment of choice for children with HS. Moderate-to-severe HS is an absolute indication for splenectomy. This hereditary anemia is cured in 90% of children following splenectomy. To decrease the chance of overwhelming post-splenectomy sepsis (OPSS), splenectomy in these children is usually postponed until after the fourth or fifth year of life.

Sickle Cell Disease

Children with this hemoglobinopathy have sickle-shaped cells that can become sequestered in the reticuloendothelial system of the spleen leading to severe anemia. Most sickle cell patients will never require a splenectomy. Typically, a child will be considered for splenectomy in the face of two minor splenic sequestration crises or one major crisis. These crises result from the acute sequestration of red blood cells in the spleen that can result in left upper quadrant pain, severe anemia, and/or hypotension. These children must receive adequate preoperative hydration.

β-Thalassemia

β-thalassemia is another inherited hemoglobinopathy that occasionally requires splenectomy. The abnormal hemoglobin causes the erythrocyte to take an aberrant shape that causes it to be sequestered by the spleen. Splenectomy is indicated in these children when there is a marked increase in the need for blood transfusions, a reticulocyte count exceeding 10%, or severe or symptomatic hypersplenism. Improving medical therapies such as desferoxamine and bone marrow transplantation are reducing the need for splenectomy (1).

Other Indications

Gaucher's disease is an autosomal recessive disorder caused by a β-glucosidase deficiency. This deficiency leads to a buildup of glucocerebroside in the reticuloendothelial system leading to splenomegaly. The resulting hypersplenism often leads to pancytopenia. Splenectomy is considered in patients with severe or symptomatic splenomegaly or pancytopenia. Recently, there have been encouraging results with enzyme replacement therapy with macrophage-targeted glucocerebrosidase in children with type 3 Gaucher's disease. This will hopefully decrease the number of splenectomies needed in these children.

Lymphoma and angiosarcoma are splenic tumors that rarely necessitate splenectomy. Angiosarcoma typically presents with rupture and lymphoma typically presents as metastatic disease from another primary site.

Most cysts and abscesses do not require splenectomy. Occasionally splenic cysts may require a partial splenectomy if the cyst becomes very large or leads to splenic rupture. Most abscesses resolve with antibiotics or antifungal agents.

Overall, hypersplenism accounts for 5% to 50% of all splenectomies; trauma, 10% to 30%; incidental to other surgery, 20% to 36%; and malignancy, 19% to 34% (7).

EVOLUTION OF THERAPY

Traumatic Splenic Injury

The spleen is the most frequently injured intra-abdominal organ in children. While appropriate therapy has been debated for the last 30 years, it has become generally accepted that the majority of children with blunt splenic injuries can be treated with nonoperative management. Children with blunt splenic trauma have better outcomes when managed nonoperatively, with success rates reported between 50% and 60% (8). According to the American Pediatric Surgical Association (APSA) Trauma Committee, 2.5% of children with isolated spleen injury require operative intervention (9,10). Immediate operative intervention for blunt splenic trauma is indicated in those children with hemodynamic instability. Emergency splenectomy should be performed through a midline incision. The spleen should be mobilized and delivered into the surgical wound by dividing the lateral reflection. All attempts should be made to preserve splenic tissue by splenorrhaphy or partial splenectomy except in the face of an unstable patient, severe fragmentation, or interruption of the blood supply (1,11).

Partial Splenectomy Versus Total Splenectomy

The movement toward splenic salvage is not only seen in traumatic injury, but also in elective resections. While most conditions mentioned above will require a total splenectomy, the efficacy of partial splenectomy has been studied in certain conditions. Nonparasitic cysts that are symptomatic or over 5 cm in diameter should be removed by partial splenectomy or near-total cystectomy "decapsulation." Studies have looked at the efficacy of partial splenectomy in patients with thalassemia, but are inconclusive and need further evaluation (12). Patients with Gaucher's disease who were treated with partial splenectomy have had recurrent hypersplenism (13).

Laparoscopic Splenectomy Versus Open Splenectomy

In 1991, the first successful laparoscopic splenectomy was performed. Laparoscopic splenectomy is now accepted by some as the standard technique for certain conditions. Several studies have demonstrated less morbidity, accelerated postoperative recovery, decreased postoperative pain, and improved postoperative pulmonary function but increased cost (5,14,15). Once a contraindication to laparoscopic splenectomy, massive splenomegaly can now be treated with a hand-assisted laparoscopic approach. The two absolute contraindications for a laparoscopic splenectomy are severe cardiopulmonary disease and hepatic cirrhosis with portal hypertension. Previous abdominal surgery is a relative contraindication (14).

COMPLICATIONS

Although a generally safe procedure, splenectomy can be associated with significant morbidity and mortality. Much of the risk associated with splenectomy is related to the pre-existing conditions of the children. Children with ITP, for example, will have thrombocytopenia and thus a higher propensity to bleed. Morbidity rates for open splenectomy have ranged from 15% to 61% and mortality rates between 6% and 13% in published reports. Laparoscopic splenectomy morbidity and mortality rates range from 0% to 15% and 0% to 5%, respectively. Selection bias makes it difficult to compare these outcomes given that the more critical children, such as trauma victims, will usually undergo an open procedure (16).

Hemorrhage

The incidence of major intraoperative bleeding during splenectomy approximates 1% to 5% making this the most frequent intraoperative complication. Hemorrhage is common in traumatic splenectomies. In children with massive hemorrhage or hemodynamic instability, a total splenectomy may be the safest option as opposed to splenic preservation.

Bleeding is the most common indication for conversion from laparoscopic splenectomy to open splenectomy (16). During elective splenectomy, the most common reasons for intraoperative bleeding are coagulopathy or technical error including vessel injury during dissection or loss of a surgical tie. Bleeding related to coagulopathy can be minimized by administering clotting factors or platelets prior to or during the operation. Platelet transfusion is typically reserved for counts less than 10,000 cells/μL (5). Slow bleeding in a coagulopathic patient can often be controlled with thrombotic agents such as thrombin, gelfoam, or absorbable fabric (Surgicel). The splenic ligaments, i.e., the splenocolic, splenophrenic, and splenorenal ligaments are typically avascular. In children with portal hypertension, however, these ligaments may be highly vascular and should be divided with care. The short gastric vessels within the gastrosplenic ligament should be divided between clamps and not with cautery. A potential pitfall during laparoscopic splenectomy is injury to the splenic vessels while encircling the hilum. This can be avoided with prudent inspection of all sides of the hilum. Rotation of the position of the laparoscope at this step will improve visualization of the posterior vessels. If bleeding does occur from a torn vessel, immediate pressure can be applied with the grasper to allow time for suction and planning of proper ligation. Bleeding from a capsular tear can be controlled by applying direct pressure or coagulation with an argon beam coagulator (17). Paramount to a safe laparoscopic splenectomy is good judgment of when to convert to an open approach. Delay in conversion from laparoscopic to open splenectomy in the face of hemorrhage may have catastrophic consequences.

336 NEWMAN AND PONSKY

Postoperatively, bleeding may occur due to persistent thrombocytopenia. The hemoglobin level should be checked on postoperative day 1 and daily hemoglobin levels should be ordered if blood loss is suspected. Any change in hemodynamics or urine output should alert the surgeon to potential ongoing blood loss.

Pancreatic Injury

The pancreas is at particular risk for injury during splenectomy given its proximity to the splenic hilum. Pancreatic injury occurs in 1% to 3% of open splenectomies (17). Dissection as close to the spleen as possible may minimize injury to the pancreas, stomach, or any other surrounding structures. In the case of brisk bleeding from the splenic hilum, the pancreas is often injured when clamps are hurriedly placed on the bleeding vessel. Some have advocated the routine use of manual tamponade of hilar bleeding until the anatomy can be clearly identified and the pancreas safeguarded. Most pancreatic injuries can be managed by ligation of injured ducts and closed drainage. Severe pancreatic injury may require a distal pancreatectomy with closed drainage. Inadequate repair of an injury or an unrecognized injury may lead to pancreatitis and/or a pancreatic fistula. Postoperative fluid collections below the left diaphragm should raise the suspicion of a pancreatic leak and the collection should be drained percutaneously and sent for an amylase level. If the drain amylase level is normal, the drain can be removed. If the drain amylase level is high, a pancreatic leak is confirmed and the drain should remain in place to maintain a controlled fistula. Frequent drain amylase levels should be obtained. Drains should remain in place until output has ceased or the amylase level returns to normal. Initially, children should remain with nothing by mouth and be placed on total parental nutrition to decrease pancreatic secretions. The role of octreotide or somatostatin in the treatment of pancreatic fistulas is still under debate (18). Some have recommended up to 6 months of conservative fistula management before returning to the operating room for surgical repair or internal drainage. Endoscopic retrograde cholangiopancreatography may help identify the location of pancreatic injury and define the ductal anatomy (19).

Persistent Postoperative Thrombocytopenia

In children with ITP, the platelet level should begin to increase by the second postoperative day following splenectomy. Persistent or recurrent thrombocytopenia following splenectomy should alert the surgeon to the possibility of a missed accessory spleen or splenosis. Failure of improvement or recurrent thrombocytopenia following splenectomy occurs in 20% to 25% of patients (5,20).

Missed Accessory Spleens

Fifteen to thirty percent of children will have at least one accessory spleen. It is crucial to identify these accessory spleens when performing a splenectomy for a hematological disorder. A missed accessory spleen, although initially small in size, can compensate enough to cause recurrent disease. These accessory spleens can often be found in the splenocolic, splenophrenic, and splenorenal ligaments, splenic hilum, mesentery, or omentum. Careful examination of all these structures is crucial to prevent recurrent disease. During the performance of laparoscopic splenectomy, it is advisable to remove accessory spleens as soon as they are identified. Accessory spleens may be left in place during exploration for splenic trauma as their compensatory function may be helpful.

Splenosis

Another potential cause of persistent or recurrent thrombocytopenia is splenosis. Splenosis is re-implanted splenic tissue following splenic rupture. This tissue may attain compensatory function and result in recurrent disease. Splenosis has been reported in 48% to 66% of children (16). Meticulous examination for splenosis following careful splenic removal is critical. If a missed accessory spleen or splenosis is suspected, a technetium liver-spleen scan can be performed. Any indication of splenic activity may necessitate re-exploration and removal of the missed splenic tissue. In children with delayed recurrence of thrombocytopenia following splenectomy, a CT scan may demonstrate enlarged, compensated splenic tissue.

Postoperative Thrombocytosis

In normal children, the spleen sequesters 30% of circulating platelets (7). Following splenectomy, platelets are no longer sequestered by the spleen resulting in a rise in the number of circulating platelets immediately following surgery. This thrombocytosis usually peaks between postoperative days 7 and 10 (17). The incidence of thrombotic events in these children, however, is rare. Early postoperative ambulation should be encouraged but antiplatelet or anticoagulant medications are unnecessary.

Thrombosis of the Portal Venous System

Both open and laparoscopic splenectomy is associated with portal venous system thrombosis. Several studies have demonstrated an incidence of 6.3% to 10% as diagnosed by ultrasonography (21,22). Adults seem to have a higher incidence of thrombosis due to the fact that splenectomy is more likely performed for malignancy. A study by Ikeda suggests that laparoscopic splenectomy results in a higher incidence of portal venous thrombosis. When the authors compared open splenectomy versus laparoscopic splenectomy, over half of the laparoscopic patients (55%) had CT evidence of thrombosis while the open splenectomy patients had only a 19% thrombosis rate. The authors suggest that changes in intrabdominal pressure due to insufflation and the extra length of the splenic vein stump during staple closure result in the higher incidence during laparoscopic splenectomy (23).

Overwhelming Postsplenectomy Sepsis

Removal of the spleen predisposes children to OPSS. OPSS is septicemia, meningitis, or pneumonia that is typically fulminant and can occur several days postoperatively or years following splenectomy (24). Without the protective immune function of the spleen against encapsulated organisms such as *Streptococcus penumoniae*, *Neisseria meningitides*, or *Hemophilus influenzae*, children who have undergone splenectomy have a 4.4% chance of morbidity from OPSS with a 2.2% mortality rate. The incidence of OPSS in children is highest in infancy and is four times that of adults (24).

Prevention of OPSS is best achieved with immunization and education. Preoperative vaccination with *Streptococcus pneumoniae* and *Hemophilus influenzae* vaccines is suggested in most patients. Ideally, vaccination should occur 2 to 4 weeks preoperatively and every 5 years postoperatively. Children who have undergone emergency splenectomy should be vaccinated postoperatively prior to discharge from the hospital. Because the current vaccine for *Neisseria meningitides* does not contain serotype B, the most common strain in North America, there is a debate regarding its routine use in asplenic children.

Many advocate routine prophylaxis with penicillin for several years following splenectomy, especially in children younger than 5 years of age (2). Parents and children should be informed of the increased risk of infection and the potential presenting symptoms.

Subphrenic Abscess

The onset of fever in a child approximately 1 week following splenectomy may indicate the formation of intra-abdominal abscess. There is a 4% to 8% incidence of subphrenic abscess formation following splenectomy (16). CT scan or ultrasound will usually confirm the diagnosis. Subphrenic abscesses are best treated with drainage and intravenous antibiotics. Drainage can usually be performed percutaneously. If percutaneous drainage is not possible, the abscess can be drained by either an open intraperitoneal or extraperitoneal approach. Fluid from the collection should be sent for an amylase level to rule out pancreatic leak. If a leak is confirmed, a drain should be placed and managed as discussed above.

Pleural Effusion

Occasionally a fluid collection may develop in the left pleural space. In most cases, these effusions are sympathetic effusions that resolve spontaneously and require no intervention. However, patients who develop respiratory compromise or fever or in whom there is continued expansion of the fluid collection, drainage is recommended. Fluid should be sent for culture, gram stain, and amylase level. These effusions, along with atelectasis and pneumonia, make pulmonary compromise the most common postoperative complication from splenectomy (10–18%). Recent reports suggest significantly decreased pulmonary complications in laparoscopic splenectomies compared to open splenectomies (17).

Wound Complications

Wound complications are not uncommon for this operation. These complications are usually related to the children's pre-existing conditions. Specifically, children with thrombocytopenia may develop a wound hematoma. These wounds usually should be opened and drained to prevent the formation of an infected hematoma. Furthermore, these children are often taking steroids which not only decrease their immunity, thereby predisposing them to wound infections, but high dose steroids may prevent proper wound healing and dehiscence may occur. Postoperatively, the surgical wound should be inspected once or twice daily for erythema or drainage.

CONCLUSION

The recent understanding of splenic function has allowed us to appreciate the importance of the spleen, especially in children. Realizing its immunoprotective role, surgeons have become more selective when deciding to remove the spleen. The trend toward splenic salvage in trauma has become accepted within the pediatric population and is now gaining popularity in the adult arena. While simultaneously working to minimize the number of splenectomies performed for trauma in children, surgeons are also working to minimize the invasiveness of those splenectomies that are performed. Laparoscopic splenectomy is becoming more popular in the elective setting. With the advancement of technology and our understanding of splenic function and structure, children who undergo splenectomies are going home sooner, and having less postoperative complications. Nonetheless, complications from splenectomy will occur and the surgeon must be prepared to recognize and treat these outcomes.

REFERENCES

1. Schiller M. The spleen. In: O'Neill J, Rowe MI, Grosfeld JL, et al. eds. Pediatric Surgery. 5th ed. St. Louis: Mosby—Year Book, 1998:1545–1554.
2. Beauchamp RD, Holzman MD, Fabian TC. Spleen. In: Townsend CM, ed. Sabiston Textbook of Surgery. 16th ed. Philadelphia, PA: W.B. Saunders Co., 2001;1144–1163.
3. Sutherland G, Burghard F. The treatment of splenic anemia by splenectomy. Lancet 1910; 2:1819.
4. French J, Camitta BM. The spleen. In: Behrman RE, ed. Nelson Textbook of Pediatrics. 16th ed. Philadelphia, PA: W.B. Saunders Co., 2000;1526–1530.
5. Katkhouda N, Mavor E. Minimal access surgery: Laparoscopic splenectomy. Surg Clin North Am 2000; 80:1285–1297.
6. George JN, Woolf SH, Raskob GE, et al. Idiopathic thrombocytopenic purpura: A practice guideline developed by explicit methods for the American Society of Hematology. Blood 1996; 88:3–40.
7. Sumaraju V, Smith LG, Smith SM. Infectious complications in asplenic hosts. Infect Dis Clin North Am 2001; 15:551–565.
8. Nix JA, Costanza M, Dale BJ, et al. Outcome of the current managment of splenic injuries. J Trauma 2001; 50:835–842.
9. Stylianos S. Evidence-based guidelines for resource utilization with isolated spleen or liver injury. J Pediatr Surg 2000; 35:164–169.
10. Stylianos S. Guidelines for the treatment of children with blunt spleen or liver injury. In: Mattei P, ed. Surgical Directives: Pediatric surgery, Philadelphia, PA: Lippincott, Williams and Wilkins, 2003:123–127.
11. Gaines BA. Abdominal and pelvic trauma in children. Crit Care Med 2002; 30:S416–423.
12. Al-Salem AH, Al-Dabbous I, Bhamidibati P. The role of partial splenectomy in children with thalassemia. Eur J Pediatr Surg 1998; 8:334–338.
13. Bar Maor JA. Partial splenectomy in Gaucher's disease: Follow-up report. J Pediatr Surg 1993; 28:686.
14. Janu PG, Rogers DA, Lobe TE. A comparison of laparoscopic and traditional open splenectomy in childhood. J Pediatr Surg 1996; 31:109–113.
15. Minkes RK. Laparoscopic versus open splenectomy in children. J Pediatr Surg 2000; 80: 699–701.
16. Friedman RE, Phillips EH. Laparoscopic splenectomy, In: Ponsky J, ed. Complications of Endoscopic and Laparoscopic Surgery. Philadelphia, PA: Lippincott-Raven Publishers, 1997:159–170.
17. Silver D. Complications of coagulation and splenectomy, In: Greenfield LJ, ed. Complications in Surgery and Trauma. 2nd ed. Grand Rapids: J.B. Lippincott Co., 1990:200–202.

18. Li-Ling J, Irving M. Somatostatin and octreotide in the prevention of postoperative complications and the treatment of enterocutaneous pancreatic fistulas: A systemic review of randomized controlled trials. Br J Surg 2001; 88:190–199.

19. Keith RG. Pancreatic ductal disruptions leading to pancreatic ascites, or pancreatic pleural effusions. In: Cameron J, ed. Current Surgical Therapy. St. Louis: Mosby, Inc., 2001:547–549.

20. Di Paolo JA, Buchanan GR. Immune thrombocytopenic purpura. Pediatr Clin N Am 2002; 49:911–928.

21. Skarsgard E, Doski J, Jaksic T, et al. Thrombosis of the portal venous system after splenectomy for pediatric hematologic disease. J Pediatr Surg 1993; 28:1109–1112.

22. Hassn AM, al-Fallouju FM, Ouf TI, et al. Portal vein thrombosis following splenectomy. Br J Surg 2000; 87:367–368.

23. Ikeda M, Sekimoto M, Takiguchi S, et al. High incidence of thrombosis of the portal venous system after laparoscopic splenectomy. Ann Surg 2005; 241:208–216.

24. Singer DB. Postsplenectomy sepsis. In: Rosenberg HS, Bolande RP, eds. Perspectives in Pediatric Pathology. Chicago, IL: Year Book Medical Publishers, 1973:285–311.

25. Howdieshell TR, Heffernan D, Dipiro JT. Therapeutic Agents Committee of the Surgical Infection Society. Surgical infection society guidelines for vaccination after traumatic injury. Surg Infect 2006; 7(3):275–303.

Splenectomy and Splenic Salvage

Expert: Steven Stylianos, M.D.

QUESTIONS

1. **What is your strategy for postoperative prophylaxis after splenectomy?**

   Daily oral penicillin prophylaxis is recommended through childhood. Aggressive diagnostic and therapeutic action is mandated for all possible bacterial infections in splenectomized children. Recently, a panel of experts conducted a thorough review of published literature, as well as information posted on the internet at the websites of the U.S. Centers for Disease Control and Prevention, among others. MEDLINE was searched for the period 1966–2004 using relevant terms including "splenectomy," in combination with "vaccine" and "immunization." The Cochrane database was searched also. Reference lists were cross referenced for additional relevant citations.

   After splenectomy, it is recommended that all persons aged 2 to 64 years receive 23-valent pneumococcal vaccine and meningococcal vaccine, with *Hemophilus influenzae* type B vaccine administered to high-risk patients as well. Vaccination should be given 2 weeks before elective splenectomy, or 2 weeks after emergency splenectomy. A booster dose of pneumococcal vaccine is recommended after 5 years; no re-vaccination recommendation is made for meningococcal or *Hemophilus influenzae* type B vaccine. There are limited data on the use of vaccines after injury. This document brings together a disparate literature of variable quality into a discussion of the infectious risks after injury relevant to vaccine administration, a summary of safety and adverse effects of vaccines, and evidence-based recommendations for vaccination (25).

2. **Is a liver/spleen scan necessary to detect accessory spleens prior to elective splenectomy for hematologic disease?**

   A thorough search of the abdomen, performed during elective splenectomy, should suffice. Laparoscopic techniques should allow for more effective surveillance of the abdomen and detection of accessory spleens.

3. **Does postoperative thrombocytosis following splenectomy need to be treated?**

   Postoperative thrombocytosis following splenectomy is clinically unimportant in terms of morbidity and requires no treatment other than that for the primary condition.

4. **What technical strategy works best to prevent postoperative bleeding following a procedure for splenic salvage?**

   Compression of the repaired spleen by wrapping with Vicryl mesh.

5. **Is there a role for splenic embolization via pediatric interventional radiology as an adjunct in splenic salvage attempts?**

Splenic embolization is being used with increasing frequency in adults with blunt splenic injury depending on signs of continued hemorrhage or the presence of higher grade injuries. The largest series in teenagers is soon to be published from the University of Maryland Cowley Shock/Trauma Center. This report of 44 patients indicates that the procedure is safe and effective in this age group.

6. **Do you routinely obtain a gallbladder ultrasound prior to splenectomy for sickle cell disease?**

Routine gallbladder ultrasound is obtained prior to splenectomy for sickle cell disease. Cholecystectomy is added to the operative procedure for splenectomy when indicated.

7. **How would you proceed in the postoperative evaluation for a missed accessory spleen?**

A sulfur colloid isotope scan will be helpful if there is a large accessory spleen. An abdominal CT with i.v. contrast should provide better spatial resolution even in the setting of smaller splenic moieties.

20 | Complications in Pediatric Surgical Oncology

Kyriacos Panayides, M.D. and Richard J. Andrassy, M.D.

Childhood malignancy is a relatively rare event with an approximate incidence of 1 in 500 by the age of 15 years (1). The survival for children with cancer has dramatically improved over the last 20 years. Approximately 70% to 80% of children with cancer will be alive for 5 years after diagnosis (2). Many of the advances in the treatment of childhood cancers have been through development of intensive chemotherapy and radiotherapy regimens. The complexities of modern oncologic care have mandated a multidisciplinary approach to patient care. The pediatric surgical oncologist plays an important role in the multidisciplinary management of pediatric cancers and therapy is constantly evolving. Although the surgical removal of solid tumors and management of the surgical complications remain important aspects of pediatric surgical oncology, surgeons involved in the care of children and adolescents with malignancies face a variety of new problems and complications related to the therapy and supportive care. The surgeon must naturally be familiar with medical management of malignancies, the problems that may arise as a result of therapy and the appropriate role of surgical intervention in their management. While chemotherapy and radiation continue to improve, there are associated complications related to toxicity and varied drug use that may lead to the need for surgical intervention. This chapter will focus on some of the commonly seen complications of the management of pediatric oncology patients.

COMPLICATIONS OF VASCULAR ACCESS

Vascular access is the most frequent surgical procedure for the pediatric surgical oncologist. Thus, these relatively routine procedures are fraught with the highest number of complications. The need for multiple chemotherapeutic drugs, antibiotics, parenteral nutrition, fluid management, and blood drawing frequently requires surgically placed central catheters. Immunosuppression, frequent access, and multiple lines increase the risk of complications.

There are three general types of catheters requiring surgical support. The standard percutaneous, nontunneled central venous catheter (CVC) is used for short-term access in patients, or for patients with contraindications to tunneled, long-term CVCs, such as sepsis. These are placed using the Seldinger technique and the size may range from 4 French to 8 French. Most are double or triple lumen CVCs so that multiple antibiotics or fluids can be administered. We frequently use antibiotic impregnated catheters in these patients since some studies indicate a decrease in catheter-related bloodstream infections (3–5). The second general category is the external tunneled CVC, first described by Broviac in 1973 (6). This is a flexible silicone tube with a Dacron cuff that may be placed by the Seldinger technique or by cut-down. In addition to possible infection or thrombosis, these catheters may be dislodged, broken, or the cap dislodged with the possibility of bleeding or air embolism.

The third general type of indwelling device is the totally implanted, subcutaneous ports. These catheters are most frequently placed by the Seldinger technique with a subcutaneous pocket to place the reservoir. These are well tolerated by children and have less of a problem with dislodgement or breakage, but do require a second procedure for removal. These allow long-term intermittent use with minimal care between use episodes.

Complications related to these catheters are related to technical problems in the operating room, mechanical problems after insertion, thrombotic problems, and infection/sepsis (7) (Table 1).

Catheter-related infections and occlusions associated with long-term central venous access were the most common complication reported with the use of vascular access devices in the Children Cancer Study Group prospective analysis of venous access (8).

Table 1 Common Central Venous
Catheter Complications

1. Placement
   (a) Pneumothorax/hemothorax
   (b) Arterial puncture
   (c) Hematoma
   (d) Malpositioning
2. Mechanical
   (a) Breakage
   (b) Dislodgement
   (c) Kinking or impingement
3. Thrombotic
   (a) Thrombus in catheter
   (b) Venous occlusion
4. Infectious
   (a) Local wound infection
   (b) Bactermia/ sepsis

Placement of an indwelling device in a patient who is, or becomes, immunocompromised or may have bacteremia at the time of placement will always be risky. The need for vascular access versus the possible complications is always reviewed preoperatively. Infectious complications that occur weeks after placement are frequently caused by the patient being colonized or by breaks in catheter care. Catheter-related infections may also be related to infection at the site of entry with migration of the pathogen along the catheter, hub site infections from breaks in sterile technique, or hematogenous seeding of the catheter (7). The catheter should be placed under operative, sterile conditions, and any manipulation of the catheter should likewise be under sterile technique. This has been shown to be effective in clinical trials at our institution (9). Other studies (3–5), have demonstrated that the use of antimicrobial-impregnated catheters may reduce the risk of catheter-related bloodstream infections. Catheters inserted in the subclavian vein have a lower incidence of infection than catheters inserted in the femoral vein (i.e., 1.2 infections per 1000 catheter-days with subclavian vein catheterization versus 4.5 infections per 1000 catheter-days with femoral vein catheterization) (10).

Catheter hubs must be disinfected prior to each use and antibiotic ointments around the catheter avoided. The use of antibiotic ointment promotes the development of antibiotic-resistant bacteria (11), increases the colonization rate by fungi (12), and has not been shown to decrease the risk of catheter-related infections (13). Recent studies assessing the efficacy of an antimicrobial dressing impregnated with chlorhexidine gluconate (BioPatch, Johnson and Johnson, Somerville, New Jersey, U.S.A.) have been promising, but have not been studied in children at this time (14,15). Despite these precautions and sterile techniques, infectious complications remain the leading cause of nonelective removal (8).

Mechanical and technical complications of central venous access are also quite common. The most common technical problems include; arterial puncture, hematoma, pnemothorax/hemothorax, and malpositioning of the catheter. Mechanical problems include; breakage, thrombotic blockage, kinking, and impingement by the clavicle or first rib. Subclavian vein and internal jugular vein catheterization have similar complications. Subclavian vein catheterization has a higher risk of pneumothorax. The femoral site carries the highest risk of mechanical and infectious complications and therefore the subclavian vein or internal jugular vein should be the locations of choice for long-term CVCs (see Table 2) (7).

The incidence of mechanical complications increases with inexperience, multiple previous catheters, failed attempts, scarring or anatomical anomalies (16). Insertion of a CVC by a physician who has performed greater than 50 catherizations results in significantly fewer complications (17).

Patients with indwelling CVCs are at high risk for catheter-related thrombosis. The clinical incidence of thrombosis is not evident since not all thromboses cause catheter occlusion or embolize. The risk of catheter-related thrombosis depends on the insertion site. Merrer and colleagues reported a 21.5% thrombosis rate in patients with femoral venous catheters and only a 1.9% rate in those with subclavian vein catheters (18). Another study showed that internal

Table 2 Frequency of Mechanical Complications, According to the Route of Catheterization

Complication	Frequency		
	Internal Jugular	Subclavian	Femoral
	Percent		
Arterial puncture	6.3–9.4	3.1–4.0	9.0–15.0
Hematoma	<0.1–2.2	1.2–2.1	3.8–4.4
Hemothorax	NA	0.4–0.6	NA
Pneumothorax	<0.1–0.2	1.5–3.1	NA
Total	6.3–11.8	6.2–10.7	12.8–19.4

Source: From Ref. 7.

jugular venous catheters had an approximately four times higher risk of thrombosis than with subclavian catheters (19). This has not been our known experience. Catheter occlusions caused by thrombosis may be cleared by utilizing thrombolytics, such as urokinase or tPA, although this frequently is not successful. The majority of CVCs placed by our pediatric surgeons at MD Anderson Cancer center are by the percutaneous subclavian route.

Solid Tumors

Complications arising from the surgical management of solid tumors do occur, but they may be minimized with precise and meticulous surgical technique. Infection, minor bleeding, and damage to adjacent structures are inherent risks to any surgical procedure. More specific complications may be explored by considering the type of tumor being resected; notably neuroblastoma and nephroblastoma.

Neuroblastoma

Neuroblastoma is the most common childhood extracranial solid tumor, affecting 1 in 7000 children younger than 5 years of age (20). The biology and stage of the tumor defines the treatment that is given (21–25). However, surgery remains a cornerstone of treatment in the disease. Neoadjuvant chemotherapy has made surgical resection technically more feasible and has improved local control and survival (26–28). Neuroblastoma may develop from any neural crest-derived tissue; however, most are located in the retroperitoneum (29). The location of the tumor (i.e., retroperitoneal versus thoracic) will have slightly different anatomic complications, but we will focus on retroperitoneal tumors. In the literature, surgical complication rates for patients with neuroblastoma have ranged from 3% to 57% (30).

Complications from the treatment of neuroblastoma can be divided into early and late (Table 3). The most common early complications include the requirement for nephrectomy and injury to vasculature structures, including renal vessels, aorta, and inferior vena cava. These complications are due to the tumor's invasive behavior and propensity to encase major organs and vascular structures. Shamberger et al. report a 14.9% nephrectomy/renal infarction rate among 349 patients with large primary tumors crossing the midline or distant metastasis during surgery for local control. In their study, reasons for nephrectomy included direct involvement of the kidney by adjacent tumor (33%), clinical impression that the tumor was a Wilms' tumor (21%), renal vessels could not be separated from the tumor (19%), extensive tumor surrounding the kidney (15%), postoperative renal infarction (8%), marked decrease in unilateral renal function after chemotherapy (2%), and position of the tumor posterior to the kidney and vena cava making resection without nephrectomy impossible (2%). In addition, the risk of nephrectomy was 25% in patients treated with initial resection versus only 10% in patients undergoing resection after chemotherapy ($P = 0.12$: OR, 2.32) (26). Renal involvement has been correlated with large size of the primary, lymph node involvement, an undifferentiated histological pattern (31), and N-MYC status. Nakagawara et al. describe a higher rate of nephrectomy in patients with N-MYC amplification versus those without (82% versus 7%) (32).

Injury to major vessels is the next most common early complication seen during the treatment of neuroblastoma. Canete et al. describe a series of 78 patients undergoing neuroblastoma resection where 1.3% (1/78) suffered a major vascular injury to the inferior vena

Table 3 Early and Late Complications in Neuroblastoma
Treatment

Early
  A. Anatomic
    1. Requirement for nephrectomy
    2. Major vessel injury
  B. Mechanical
    1. Ileus
    2. Bowel obstruction secondary to adhesions
    3. Bowel obstruction secondary to intussusception
  C. Medical
    1. Higher transfusion requirement (PRBC)
    2. Higher postoperative infection rate
    3. Greater need for nutritional support
  D. Other
    1. Increase in pain consultation
    2. Hypertension
    3. Chyle leak
    4. Diarrhea
    5. Pleural effusion
Late
    1. Renal atrophy
    2. Renovascular hypertension
    3. Acute renal failure
    4. Pneumonia
    5. Pulmonary hemorrhage
    6. Cardiomyopathy
    7. Cardiomyositis
    8. Vertebral deformity
    9. Liver dysfunction
  10. Hearing loss
  11. Goiter
  12. Hypothyroidism
  13. Growth retardation
  14. Second cancer

Abbreviation: PRBC, Packed red blood cells

cava (33). Careful dissection around vascular structures may minimize intraoperative injury, but more than often, injuries to vessels do not become apparent until the early postoperative period. Tanabe et al. report a series of 58 patients where 10% developed renal impairment postoperatively diagnosed by the onset of oliguria or anuria, and angiography or ultrasonography (34). Moreover, Barrette et al. report a 27% rate of renal atrophy secondary to ischemia/thrombosis of the renal artery (3 out of 11 patients) discovered postoperatively (35). In summary, extreme care should be taken when mobilizing vessels in pediatric patients, since the vessels are more fragile than those of adult vessels and excessive traction may lead to intimal damage. Despite this meticulous attention in the operating room, this complication is not always avoidable.

Mechanical complications may occur postoperatively. This may take the form of an ileus or pseudo-obstruction or an actual intestinal obstruction secondary to adhesions or intussusception. Occasional ileus may be inevitable after intraabdominal or retroperitoneal surgery. Management of this problem includes placement of nasogastric tube, maintaining the patient NPO, and keeping the blood electrolytes normal. The ileus should resolve in 3 to 5 days once the nasogastric tube drainage decreases in amount, the abdomen becomes much softer, and the child passes flatus. In addition to adhesions causing a bowel obstruction after surgery, one unique complication after retroperitoneal surgery is the small intestine intussusception causing a bowel obstruction. On average, this is seen on the fourth postoperative day and may be diagnosed by ultrasonography (36). Pumberger and colleagues report a bowel obstruction reoperation rate of 8% in 110 children requiring a retroperitoneal tumor resection. Furthermore, postoperative intussusception is responsible for 5% to 15% of all postoperative intestinal obstructions requiring surgical revision and represents 1.4% to 14/5% of the total number of intussusceptions

(37). The treatment of this complication is usually reoperation due to the fact that the intussusceptum and intussuscipiens are both small bowel, therefore, making hydrostatic reduction ineffective. The awareness of this rare complication will not only make a more timely diagnosis, but embark on timely management and less patient suffering.

More intense medical protocols have also caused serious complications in the treatment of neuroblastoma. For instance, Cantos and colleagues compared complications in patients undergoing a more intensive Children's Oncology Group (COG) protocol A3973 for Stage 4 neuroblastoma versus the less intensive protocols of the Children's Cancer Group (CCG) 3891 and the Pediatric Oncology Group (POG) 9341. Of note, the intraoperative transfusion rate was higher in the COG A3973 protocol (86% versus 45%, $P = 0.0019$), the postoperative infection rate was higher (32% versus 3%; $P = 0.02$), and other postoperative issues such as nutritional support were higher (45% versus 3%, $P = 0.0001$). Complications such as increased pain consultation, hypertension, chyle leak, diarrhea, and pleural effusion were also higher in the COG A3973 protocol, but did not reach clinical significance. Since the survival rate was higher in the COG A3973 protocol and the recurrence was significantly lower, these postoperative complications were deemed acceptable (30).

Since many advances in childhood cancer have occurred in the last 20 years, more children are surviving, hence, the physician is experiencing more late complications of treatment than in the past. These include, but are not limited to, renal and hepatic impairment, endocrine disorders, growth impairment, cardiac and pulmonary impairment, fertility issues, and second malignancy. When looking at late complications after surgery in patients with neuroblastoma, Kuroda and colleagues report a treatment-associated morbidity rate of 15.0% in nonadvanced infantile patients, 42.1% in advanced infantile patients, and 33.3% in advanced older patients. As discussed above, renovascular problems were most frequently seen (especially after intraoperative radiation) along with pulmonary problems, cardiac problems, second cancers, thyroid dysfunction, vertebral deformity, and growth retardation (38).

Nephroblastoma (Wilms' Tumor)

Renal tumors are the second most common abdominal tumors in children and Wilms' tumor is the most common malignant renal tumor in children (5–8% of childhood cancers) (39). Just as in neuroblastoma, multimodal therapy over the last two decades has made inoperable tumors operable, and has improved outcomes in patients with Wilms' tumors. The postoperative complications in the treatment of Wilms' tumors is almost identical to that of neuroblastoma. The only major difference is the rare need for contralateral nephrectomy of a normal kidney due to the excessive dissection of the renal vessels and subsequent injury or thrombosis. The National Wilms' Tumor Study still advocates routing exploration of the contralateral, supposedly normal, kidney, and a few groups have advocated that today's imaging modalities are sensitive enough to possibly not require this routine exploration. Nevertheless, the introduction of standardized surgical procedures and preoperative chemotherapy has reduced the rate of surgical complications (40,41). To assist in prevention of complications when treating Wilms' tumor, one must be aware of the risk factors of the tumor that may lead to complications. Those risk factors include (a) advanced local tumor at time of diagnosis, (b) intravascular tumor extension, and (c) the resection of other organs at the time of the nephrectomy (42–45). According to Ritchey and colleagues, the complication rate of Wilms' tumor excision was 12.7%. The most common complications included intestinal obstruction, extensive hemorrhage, wound infection, and vascular injury (40) (Table 4).

The aforementioned complications are decreased when compared to the previous National Wilms' Tumor Study and this may be due to the use of preoperative chemotherapy for patients deemed to be at high risk for complications. This decrease in surgical complications in patients receiving preoperative chemotherapy has also been documented by the International Society of Pediatric Oncology (41). The results of prospective studies illustrating a relationship between preoperative chemotherapy and the decrease of surgical complications are still needed. Other complications that have been seen include bowel injury and superior mesenteric artery injury when a large tumor invades these structures.

Complications will be pronounced if there is local recurrence of a Wilms' tumor. As a result, local recurrence is a prognostic factor associated with poor outcomes (42). To help prevent local occurrence the surgeon has to be meticulous with respect to two areas: 1) avoid presence of microscopic tumor at the margin of surgical resection (46), and 2) avoid intraoperative tumor

Table 4 Common Complications in Treatment
of Wilms' Tumor

1. Intestinal obstruction	5.1%
2. Extensive hemorrhage	1.9%
3. Wound infection	1.9%
4. Vascular injury	1.5%
5. Other	2.3%
	12.7%
• Complications in Table 3 also occur	

Source: From Ref. 40.

spillage (increases local recurrence 3.7 times) (42). If this can be accomplished in a safe manner, the risk of complications and local recurrence will lessen.

COMPLICATIONS OF MEDICAL THERAPY REQUIRING SURGICAL EVALUATION

Medications administered in the treatment of childhood malignancies have considerable toxicities. Sequelae of many of these toxicities have surgical implications of which the pediatric surgeon must be aware. The diagnosis of potential complications can be extremely difficult in this patient population due to the immunosuppression of antineoplastic therapy. Not only does this make the children more prone to the morbidity and mortality of infectious cause that normally would be contained by an intact immune response, but it also may mask signs and symptoms and alter blood values which may delay diagnosis. In addition, thrombocytopenia and coagulopathy are also common in children receiving treatment for malignant disease. All of the above factors can converge to make the evaluation of acute surgical conditions in the child with malignancy a difficult problem. Focus will be placed on the three most common complications of medical therapy requiring surgical evaluation: 1) neutropenic enterocolitis, 2) acute pancreatitis, and 3) venoocclusive disease (VOD) of the liver (Table 5).

Neutropenic enterocolitis, also known as typhilitis, is an acute life-threatening condition characterized by transmural inflammation of the small and/or large intestine in patients who are severely immunosuppressed and is especially seen in children receiving induction chemotherapy for acute leukemia. The most common location for the inflammation is the terminal ileum and cecum. Mortality rates have been reported as 5% to 100%, with averages around 40% to 45% (47). Clinical symptoms include acute abdominal pain (usually right-sided), nausea and vomiting, fever, watery or bloody diarrhea, abdominal distention, hematemesis, and anorexia. These symptoms usually occur 10 to 14 days after the initiation of cytotoxic chemotherapy and the patients are profoundly neutropenic (absolute neurophil count or ANC < 100 cells/mm^3) (48). The differential diagnosis of this condition must include acute appendicitis and pseudomembranous enterocolitis. Diagnostic imaging is extremely useful in assisting with the diagnosis. At our institution, we prefer abdominal CT scanning which will usually show bowel wall (especially cecal) thickening, inflammation, and presence of peritoneal fluid. Other institutions have also been proponents of CT scanning over ultrasound in the diagnosis of typhilitis; therefore, it is now the diagnostic procedure of choice (49). The need to avoid unnecessary laparotomy is paramount because these patients often have poor physiologic reserve and poor wound healing properties. The majority of these cases can be managed by bowel rest, intravenous fluid resuscitation, fluid and electrolyte management, total parenteral nutrition, serial abdominal radiographs, intravenous broad spectrum antibiotics, and serial physical examinations. Shamberger and colleagues examined the medical and surgical management of neutropenic enterocolitis in children with leukemia and recommended the following criteria for surgical

Table 5 Common Complications of
Medical Therapy Requiring Surgical
Evaluation

1. Neutropenic enterocolitis (typhilitis)
2. Acute pancreatitis
3. Venoocclusive disease of the liver

management: 1) persistent gastrointestinal bleeding after resolution of neutropenia and correction of coagulopathy, 2) evidence of perforation, 3) clinical deterioration despite maximal supportive management, suggesting uncontrolled sepsis, and 4) development of symptoms of an intraabdominal process, which, in the absence of neutropenia, would require surgery (50) (Table 6).

Unless otherwise indicated, the complication of neutropenic enterocolitis should be treated nonoperatively to give the patient the best chance of survival.

Acute pancreatitis is also a reasonably common recognized complication of antineoplastic therapy. Pancreatitis may be caused by a myriad of medications, but in the oncologic field, L-asparaginase administration, and corticosteroid use predominate. This condition should be suspected in virtually every cancer patient complaining of abdominal pain to prevent missing or delaying the diagnosis. The spectrum of disease is wide ranging from a mild self-limiting course to a severe fulminant disease with multisystem organ failure. The diagnosis is usually made by an appropriate history including risk factors such as offending medications, by an appropriate physical exam eliciting severe epigastric tenderness, and by elevated amylase and lipase levels. It should be noted, however, that with L-asparaginase-associated pancreatitis, serum amylase, and lipase levels may not be as high as in other cause of acute pancreatitis (51).

The management of acute pancreatitis is rarely surgical. Supportive management includes oxygen if needed, nothing by mouth, intravenous fluids, maintaining normal electrolytes, discontinuing possible pancreatitis-inducing medications, and total parenteral nutrition or postpyloric feeds. Surgical indications include pancreatic abscess, infected pseudocyst, symptomatic pseudocyst, and extensive infected pancreatic necrosis in the face of clinical deterioration (52,53). Just as in neutropenic enterocolitis, surgery should be avoided in acute pancreatitis secondary to antineoplastic therapy.

Lastly, high-dose chemotherapy and bone marrow transplantation can lead to venoocclusive disease of the liver. VOD is due to damage to the endothelium of hepatic venules and centrilobular hepatic necrosis. This insult causes remodeling which, in turn, leads to fibrosis and occlusion of central hepatic veins (54). Patients with VOD present with right upper quadrant pain, weight gain, and ascites. Clinical criteria for the diagnosis of VOD in patients undergoing bone marrow transplantation include: (a) jaundice or serum bilirubin greater than 2 mg/dL, (b) hepatomegaly, (c) right upper quadrant pain, (d) ascites, and (e) unexplained weight gain (55,56). The diagnostic finding on ultrasonography is the reversal of flow in the portal and hepatic veins. A critical aspect of this disease is that once it occurs, the probability that other systems will fail increases dramatically, and potentially fatal multiorgan system failure may occur. Children with Wilms' tumor are particularly susceptible to VOD after high-dose chemotherapy. Czuderna and colleagues report a series of 206 patients with Wilms' tumor treated with actinomycin-D and vincristine. Of these 206 patients, 10 (4.9%) developed clinical criteria for VOD (57). Other than surgical intervention for diagnostic biopsy, management of VOD is supportive.

Second Malignancy

Children who have previously been treated for cancer have a higher risk of developing a second malignancy later on in life. This is likely due to the carcinogenic effects of chemotherapy and radiotherapy given for the first cancer plus the patient's natural genetic predisposition (58). Approximately one in every 640 individuals in the United States between the ages of 20 and 39 years is a survivor of childhood cancer (59). It is extremely difficult to predict which patient will develop a second cancer and when they will do so because the information we have about the long-term effects of chemotherapy and radiotherapy is based on treatments from many years ago. The types and doses of therapies have changed, therefore, the long-term effects

Table 6 Operative Indications in Neutropenic Enterocolitis

1. Persistent GI bleeding (neutropenia and coagulopathy corrected)
2. Bowel perforation
3. Clinical deterioration on maximal supportive management (suggesting uncontrolled sepsis)
4. Development of intraabdominal process which would require surgery (in the absence of neutropenia)

Abbreviation: GI, Gastrointestinal.

Table 7 Cumulative Incidences of Subsequent Malignant Neoplasms at 20 years

Hodgkin disease	7.6%
Soft-tissue sarcoma	4.0%
Bone sarcoma	3.3%
Leukemia	2.1%
CNS cancer	2.1%
Neuroblastoma	1.9%
Non-Hodgkin lymphoma	1.9%
Kidney tumors	1.6%
Average	3.2%

Source: From Ref. 70.

have probable changed as well. According to the Childhood Cancer Survivor Study (CCSS), the cumulative incidence of subsequent malignant neoplasms (SMN) 20 years from the time of original cancer diagnosis is 3.2% overall. The incidence varies by diagnostic subgroups with neuroblastoma and kidney tumors 1.9% and 1.6%, respectively (60) (Table 7).

Upon analyzing the above data, it appears most individuals will not experience SMN in the first 20 years after cancer diagnosis. These numbers are expected to rise as the cohort group followed by the CCSS ages further; however, these data are not yet available. In addition to genetics, radiation plays a major role in the development of second cancers. Most commonly, these are osteosarcomas of the affected bone (61). Other tumors including breast cancer have been described after chest irradiation for Hodgkin's disease in females (62). The younger age at time of treatment (63) and radiation doses greater than 40 Gy (64) in patients treated for Hodgkin's disease both increase the risk of a second malignancy. Independent risk factors for SMN (adjusted for radiation exposure) include (a) female gender, (b) original cancer diagnosed at a younger age, (c) original diagnosis of Hodgkin's disease or soft-tissue sarcoma, and (d) exposure to alkylating agents (60). Even though safety and efficacy trials of all treatments given are studied and the risk of second cancer is present, one must not sacrifice survival from the original cancer in order to decrease subsequent malignancy. A solution of balance must be found: one that meets the patient's medical needs (i.e., cancer cure) and one that meets the family's emotional needs (i.e., avoid devastation of second cancer).

SUMMARY

The number of possible surgical complications in pediatric surgical oncology are too numerous to mention in their entirety in this chapter. However, the common ones can be classified into vascular access complications, complications associated with major solid tumors such as neuroblastoma and Wilm's tumor, medical complications requiring surgical evaluation, and the appearance of second cancers. Knowing when to expect and how to treat these complications is important, but learning to prevent them is crucial. Nevertheless, prevention is not always possible and complications are inevitable and must not be thought of as failures.

In conclusion, the role of the pediatric surgical oncologist has changed over the last twenty years. The surgeon provides vital services in the multi-disciplinary care of children and adolescents with malignant disease. Survival of children with malignancy continues to improve and tailored therapy will reduce the incidence of complications.

REFERENCES

1. Ries LA, Hankey BF, Miller BA, et al., eds. Cancer Statistics Review 1973–1988. NIH Publication No. 91–278. Bethesda, MD: NIH, 1991:13(2):53–58.
2. Mertens AC, Yasui Y, Neglia JP, et al. Late mortality experience in five-year survivors of childhood and adolescent cancer: The Childhood Cancer Survivor Study. J Clin Oncol 2001; 19:3163–3172.

3. Raad I, Darouiche R, Dupuis J, et al. Central venous catheters coated with minocycline and rifampin for the prevention of catheter-related colonization and bloodstream infections: A randomized, double-blind trial. Ann Intern Med 1997; 127:267–274.

4. Maki DG, Stolz SM, Wheeler S, et al. Prevention of central venous catheter-related bloodstream infection by use of an antiseptic-impregnated catheter: A randomized, controlled trial. Ann Intern Med 1997; 127:257–266.

5. Veenstra DL, Saint S, Sullivan SD. Cost-effectiveness of antiseptic-impregnated central venous catheters for the prevention of catheter-related bloodstream infection. JAMA 1999; 282:554–560.

6. Broviac JW, Cole JJ, Scribner BH. A silicone rubber atrial catheter for prolonged parenteral alimentation. Surg Gynecol Obstet 1973; 136:602–606.

7. McGee DC, Gould MK. Preventing complications of central venous catheterization. N Engl J Med 2003; 348(12):1123–1133.

8. Wiener ES, McGuire P, Stolar CJH, et al. The CCSG prospective study of venous access devices: An analysis of insertions and causes of removal. J Pediatr Surg 1992; 27:155–164.

9. Raad I, Hohn DC, Gilbreath BJ, et al. Prevention of central venous catheter-related infections by using maximal sterile barrier precautions during insertion. Infect Control Hosp Epidemiol 1994; 15:231–238.

10. Merrer J, De Jonghe B, Golliot F, et al. Complications of femoral and subclavian venous catheterization in critically ill patients: A randomized controlled trial. JAMA 2001; 286:700–707.

11. Zakrzewska-Bode A, Muytjens HL, Liem KD, et al. Mupirocin resistance in coagulase-negative staphylococci, after topical prophylaxis for the reduction of colonization of central venous catheters. J Hosp Infect 1995; 31:189–193.

12. Flowers RH III, Schwenzer KJ, Kopel RF, et al. Efficacy of an attachable subcutaneous cuff for the prevention of intravascular catheter-related infection: A randomized, controlled trial. JAMA 1989; 261:878–883.

13. Maki DG, Band JD. A comparative study of polyantibiotic and iodophor ointments in prevention of vascular catheter-related infection. Am J Med 1981; 70:739–744.

14. Garcia R, Jendresky L. Adding a chlorhexidine patch to the IHI bundle: Goal zero in reducing central line-associated bacteremia. Am J Infection Control 2006; 34(5):6–41.

15. Garland JS, Alex CP, Mueller CD, et al. A randomized trial comparing povidone-iodine to a chlorhexidine gluconate-impregnated dressing for prevention of central venous catheter infections in neonates. Pediatr 2001; 107(6):1431–1437.

16. Mansfield PF, Hohn DC, Fornage BD, et al. Complications and failures of subclavian-vein catheterization. N Engl J Med 1994; 331:1735–1738.

17. Sznajder JI, Zveibil FR, Bitterman H, et al. Central vein catheterization: Failure and complication rates by three percutaneous approaches. Arch Intern Med 1986; 146:259–261.

18. Merrer J, De Jonghe B, Golliot F, et al. Complications of femoral and subclavian venous catheterization in critically ill patients: A randomized controlled trial. JAMA 2001; 286:700–707.

19. Timsit JF, Farkas JC, Boyer JM, et al. Central vein catheter-related thrombosis in intensive care patients: Incidence, risk factors, and relationship with catheter-related sepsis. Chest 1998; 114:207–213.

20. Ries LA, Eisner MP, Kosary CL, et al. SEER Cancer Statistics Review, 1975–2002. Bethesda, MD: NIH, 2002.

21. Maris JM. The biologic basis for neuroblastoma heterogeneity and risk stratification. Curr Opin Pediatr 2005; 17(1):7–13.

22. Weinstein JL, Katzenstein HM, Cohn SL. Advances in the diagnosis and treatment of neuroblastoma. Oncologist 2003; 8(3):278–292.

23. Castel V, Garcia-Miguel C, Malero A., et al. The treatment of advanced neuroblastoma. Results of the Spanish Neuroblastoma Study Group (SNSG) studies. Eur J Cancer 1995; 31 A(4):642–625.

24. Kushner BH, LaQuaglia MP, Bonilla MA, et al. Highly effective induction therapy for stage 4 neuroblastoma in children over 1 year of age. J Clin Oncol 1994; 12(12):2607–2613.

25. Cheung NV, Heller G. Chemotherapy dose intensity correlates strongly with response, medical survival and median progression-free survival in metastatic neuroblastoma. J Clin Oncol 1991; 9(6):1050–1058.

26. Shamberger RC, Smith El, Joshi VV, et al. The risk of nephrectomy during local control in abdominal neuroblastoma. J Pediatr Surg 1998; 33:161–164.

27. Rubie H, Plantaz D, Coze C, et al. Localized and unresectable neuroblastoma in infants: Excellent outcome with primary chemotherapy. Med Pediatr Oncol 2001; 36:247–250.

28. Kishner BH, Wolden S, LaQuaglia MP, et al. Hyperfractionated low-dose radiotherapy for high-risk neuroblastoma after intensive chemotherapy and surgery. J Clin Oncol 2001; 19:2821–2828.

29. Cotterill SJ, Pearson AD, Pritchard J, et al. Clinical prognostic factors in 1277 patients with neuroblastoma: Results of the European Neuroblastoma Study Group Survey 1982–1992. Eur J Cancer 2000; 36:901–908.

30. Cantos MF, Gerstle JT, Irwin MS, et al. Surgical challenges associated with intensive treatment protocols for high-risk neuroblastoma. J Pediatr Surg 2006; 41:960–965.

31. Albregts AE, Cohen MD, Galliani CA. Neuroblastoma invading the kidney. J Pediatr Surg 1994; 29:930–933.
32. Nakagawara A, Ikeda K, Yokoyama T, et al. Surgical aspects of N-myc oncogene amplification of neuroblastoma. Surgery 1988; 104:34–39.
33. Canete A, Jovani C, Lopez A, et al. Surgical treatment for neuroblastoma; complications during 15 years' experience. J Pediatr Surg 1998; 33:1526–1530.
34. Tanabe M, Ohnuma N, Iwai J, et al. Renal impairment after surgical resection of neuroblastoma. J Pediatr Surg 1996; 31:1252–1255.
35. Barrette S, Bernstein ML, Leclerc J-M, et al. Treatment complications in children diagnosed with neuroblastoma during a screening program. J Clin Oncol 2006; 24:1542–1545.
36. Niu ZB, Hou Y, Wang CL. Postoperative intussusception in children: A review of 14 cases. Chin Med Sci J 2005; 20:265–267.
37. Pumberger W, Pomberger G, Wiesbauer P. Postoperative intussusception: An overlooked complication in pediatric surgical oncology. Med Pediatr Oncol 2002; 38:208–210.
38. Kuroda T, Saeki M, Honna T, et al. Late complications after surgery in patients with neuroblastoma. J Pediatr Surg 2006; 41:2037–2040.
39. Blakely ML, Ritchey ML. Controversies in the management of Wilms' tumor. Semin Pediatr Surg 2001; 10:127–131.
40. Ritchey ML, Shamberger RC, Haase GM, et al. Surgical complications after primary nephrectomy for Wilms' tumor: Report from the National Wilms' Tumor Study Group. J Am Coll Surg 2001; 192:63–68.
41. Godzinski J, Tournade MF, de Kraker J, et al. Rarity of surgical complications after post-chemotherapy nephrectomy for nephroblastoma. Experience of the International Society of Pediatric Oncology. Eur J Pediatr Surg 1991; 26:610–612.
42. Shamberger RC, Guthrie KA, Ritchey ML, et al. Surgery-related factors and local recurrence of Wilms' tumor in National Wilms' Tumor Study IV. Ann Surg 1999; 229:292–297.
43. Shamberger RC, Ritchey ML, Haase GM, et al. Intravascular extension of Wilms' tumor. Ann Surg 2001; 234:116–121.
44. Ritchey ML, Kelalis PP, Haase GM, et al. Preoperative therapy for intracaval and atrial extension of Wilms' tumor. Cancer 1993; 12:4104–4110.
45. Ritchey ML, Kelalis PP, Breslow N, et al. Surgical complications after nephrectomy for Wilms' tumor. Surg Gynecol Obstet 1992; 175:507–514.
46. Breslow N, Sharples K, Beckwith BJ, et al. Prognostic factors in non-metastatic, favorable histology Wilms' tumor: Results of the Third National Wilms' Tumor Study. Cancer 1991; 68:2345–2353.
47. Jain Y, Arya LS, Kataria, R. Neutropenia enterocolitis in children with acute lymphocytic leukemia. Pediatr Hematol Oncol 2002; 17: 99–103.
48. Angel CA, Rao BN, Wrenn E Jr., et al. Acute appendicitis in children with leukemia and other malignancies: Still a diagnostic dilemma. J Pediatr Surg 1992; 27:476–479.
49. Hobson MJ, Carney DE, Molik KA, et al. Appendicitis in childhood hematologic malignancies: Analysis and comparison with typhilitis. J Pediatr Surg 2005; 40:214–219.
50. Shamberger RC, Winstein HJ, Delorey MJ, et al. The medical and surgical management of typhilitis in children with acute nonlymphocytic (myelogenous) leukemia. Cancer 1986; 57:603–609.
51. Sadoff J, Hwang S, Rosenfeld D, et al. Surgical pancreatic complications induced by L-asparaginase. J Pediatr Surg 1997; 32:860–863.
52. Rau B, Uhl W, Buchler MW, et al. Surgical treatment of infected necrosis. World J Surg 1997; 21:155–161.
53. Hartwig W, Maksan SM, Foitzik T, et al. Reduction in mortality with delayed surgical therapy of severe pancreatitis. J Gastrointest Surg 2002; 6:481–487.
54. Crawford JM. The Liver. In: Cotran RS, ed. Robbins Pathologic Basis of Disease. 6th ed. Philadelphia: WR Saunders and Company, 1999:874–875.
55. Bisogno G, de Kraker J, Weirich A, et al. Veno-occlusive disease of the liver in children treated for Wilms' tumor. Med Pediatr Oncol 1997; 29:245–251.
56. D'Antiga L, Baker A, et al. Veno-occlusive disease with multi-organ involvement following actinomycin-D. Eur J Cancer 2001; 37:1141–1148.
57. Czauderna P, Katski K, Kowalczyk J, et al. Venoocclusive liver disease (VOD) as a complication of Wilms' tumor management in the series of consecutive 206 patients. Eur J Pediatr Surg 2000; 5: 300–303.
58. Knudsen AG. Cancer genetics. Am J Med Gen 2002; 111:96–102.
59. National Cancer Policy Board: Weiner SL, Simone JV, Hewitt M, eds. Childhood Cancer Survivorship: Improving Care and Quality of Life. Washington, DC: National Academy of Sciences, 2003:32.
60. Robison LL, Green DM, Hudson M, et al. Long-term outcomes of adult survivors of childhood cancer: Results from the Childhood Cancer Survivor Study. Cancer 2005; 104(11 suppl):2557–2564.
61. Hawkins MM, Wilson LM, Burton HS, et al. Radiotherapy, alkylating agents, and risk of bone cancer after childhood cancer. J. Natl. cancer Inst. 1996; 88:270–278.

62. Travis LB, Hill DA, Dores GM, et al. Breast cancer following radiotherapy and chemotherapy among young women with Hodgkin disease. J Am Med Assoc 2003; 290:465–475.

63. Swerdlow AJ, Barber JA, Hudson GV, et al. Risk of second malignancy after Hodgkin's disease in a collaborative British cohort: The relation to age at treatment. J Clin Oncol 2000; 18:498–509.

64. Tucker MA, Meadows AT, Boice JD Jr, et al. Leukemia after therapy with alkylating agents for childhood cancer. J Natl Cancer Inst 1987; 78:459–464.

Resection of Wilms' Tumor

Expert: Jay L. Grosfeld, M.D.

QUESTIONS

1. What technical steps are important to prevent tumor rupture?

One of the most important steps in avoiding tumor rupture in instances of Wilms' tumor is to provide an adequate transperitoneal incision. Flank incisions are to be avoided. We prefer a large transverse supraumbilical incision. A bilateral subcostal approach is acceptable as well. We rarely use a thoracic extension. The latter may be necessary for very large upper pole tumors that displace the diaphragm superiorly. In more recent years, this subset might be a tumor that we would opt for biopsy and preoperative chemotherapy.

Recognizing that significant tumor spillage may have an adverse effect on tumor relapse and outcome makes it essential to take those steps necessary to reduce the risk of tumor spill. Careful entry into the retroperitoneal space by mobilization of the colon and its mesentery off the tumor provides good exposure for left-sided tumors. Elevating the pancreas may also be useful in gaining good exposure. The colon and duodenum are mobilized by a Kocher maneuver on the right to gain adequate exposure. Although it is preferable to obtain control of the vessels at the renal hilum early in the dissection, this may not always be possible in instances of a large tumor. Early control of the blood supply (taking the vein first to avoid potential entry of tumor cells into the vena cava) may reduce blood loss during the dissection. We double tie the aortic and vena caval sides of the vessels and also tie the tumor side to prevent potential tumor spill and then divide the vessels between the ties. In the presence of a very large tumor that obscures the hilum – that may have to wait. For upper pole tumors, the adrenal gland should be taken enbloc with the tumor. This can be avoided in instances of lower pole lesions. This helps gain access to the posterior and superior portions of the tumor that are adherent to the diaphragm where the risk of tumor rupture may be higher. Although it is unusual for Wilms' tumor to invade the diaphragm – dense adherence can lead to tumor rupture and taking a small portion of the diaphragm may avoid injury to the tumor capsule and avoid spillage.

Preoperative imaging should identify cases where the tumor has extended into the ureter (urothelial extension) and renal vein (vascular extension). Making sure that you gain control of the vena cava above and below the renal vein with vascular loops allows you to "fish out" the attached tumor extension if it is localized to the immediate area of the renal vein. More extensive venous extension superiorly into the retrohepatic vena cava and atrium (identified by proper imaging) may benefit from preoperative chemotherapy before attempting operative intervention. In some instances, the intravascular tumor will disappear, in others it may shrink and "back out" of the atrium into the abdominal portion of the vena cava avoiding the need for cardiopulmonary bypass. The ipsilateral ureter is divided close to the bladder in all cases. In instances where the tumor extends down the ureter, careful palpation can often identify its most distal location. If there is any question about extension into the bladder (a very rare event) cystoscopy can be performed. While most Wilms' tumors are resectable, occasionally, the tumor may be densely adhered to local structures. In the majority of cases, this does not correlate with local invasion and it is usually unnecessary to do major en-bloc resections of other organs and structures where tumor spill may occur and a higher postoperative complication rate has been noted. Under these circumstances, it is better to carefully biopsy the tumor and some perirenal and periaortic lymph nodes (for adequate staging), close the abdomen and treat with chemotherapy and come back for a second look resection.

2. **How should tumor extension into the renal vein be managed?**
   See above.

3. **When is it necessary to perform a thoracic extension of an abdominal incision during resection of a Wilms' tumor?**
   See above.

4. **What factors would lead you to consider neoadjuvant therapy?**
   Preoperative neoadjuvant chemotherapy has become the primary method of treatment for Wilms' tumor in Europe. It has been used extensively in the SIOP studies. The original thesis is that it would reduce the incidence of tumor rupture and operative complications. Both chemotherapy and radiation tend to shrink the tumor and "toughen" the tumor capsule. Despite this precaution, the rate of tumor spill in the SIOP studies is approximately 3% and postoperative complications occurred in 8%. Although tumor spill is not a study indicator in the NWTS in the United States, a tumor spill rate of 12% to 20% was noted in early studies. Methods we have used to avoid tumor spill have been mentioned above. There are downsides to primary chemotherapy use including administration of potentially harmful drugs to patients with benign lesions or other renal tumors unresponsive to the antineoplastic agents typically used for Wilms' tumor. These patients represented 5% of the cases in the SIOP studies.

    Despite the fact that primary surgical resection is the method of choice in managing Wilms' tumor in this country, there are certain situations where neoadjuvant chemotherapy is very useful and frequently employed. Most pediatric surgeons would be comfortable using neoadjuvant treatment for patients that require preservation of renal parenchyma. This would include children with a solitary kidney, horseshoe kidney, and instances of bilateral Wilms' tumor. As we noted previously, for patients with intravascular extension of Wilms' tumor, preoperative chemotherapy may eradicate the tumor in a few, shrink it in many, and have it "back out" of the atrium in some, thus reducing the need for cardiopulmonary bypass. There is another uncommon subset of patients that might benefit from neoadjuvant therapy—the Stage 4 patient with pulmonary metastases with significant respiratory distress. In these instances, with neoadjuvant treatment the lung metatsases would shrink (some would disappear) and permit the child's respiratory condition to improve and withstand a laparotomy.

    With the SIOP group now employing a needle biopsy to determine the correct diagnosis before administering chemotherapy, it seems reasonable to selectively extend the use of this approach to children with massive tumors identified as being adherent to surrounding structures and organs on modern imaging studies. Tumors >10.0 cm have been identified as having an increased risk for rupture and complications. Adequate tissue for histological diagnosis and genetic studies to identify children with loss of heterozygosity (LOH) at 1p and 16q which might alter the chemotherapy would be important considerations.

5. **What are the most common complications following resection of a Wilms' tumor?**

6. **What unusual complications have you seen following the resection of a Wilms' tumor?**
   Aside from the typical postoperative atelectasis and a rare wound infection (<1.0%), the most common complication following resection of a Wilms' tumor is postoperative adhesive bowel obstruction. This may occur early or late. The incidence in the NWTS studies is 6.9%. Intraoperative hemorrhage has been observed in approximately 5% of cases with only one death attributable to this complication. Injuries to other organs occur in about 1% and vascular injuries to the vena cava, aorta or rarely the superior mesenteric artery in 1.5% of cases.

   I have personally had a few interesting complications—one was a pulmonary tumor embolus following removal of a Wilms' tumor affecting the left kidney with extension into the vena cava. The child survived following cardiopulmonary bypass and pulmonary embolectomy. He is a long-term survivor now in his late 20s. Another interesting case was a child who developed evidence of early bowel obstruction and was explored on the fifth postoperative day and had a postoperative small bowel intussusception. Simple reduction resolved the problem. A third patient develop severe ascites following resection of a large, left-sided, upper pole Wilms' tumor that extended to the diaphragm and near the esophageal hiatus. We assumed this was related to division of lymphatics under the diaphragm during the dissection and treated the child with TPN, and somatosatin. After 3 weeks the situation resolved. We had one boy that developed acute appendicitis 4 days after resection of a Wilms' tumor. Fortunately, he was not perforated at operation. This was in the prelaparoscopy days.

7. In the era of new generation CT scanners, have you had an unexpected finding when exploring the contralateral kidney?

We used to explore (expose and palpate) the opposite kidney routinely—searching for a second lesion. We have had one instance that we found a small nodular mass on the surface of the kidney that we biopsied and it turned out to be a nephrogenic rest. More recent data from the NWTS suggest that with contemporary modern imaging techniques, it may be unnecessary to do this in the current era. Lesions as small a 1.0 cm have been identified, and as in our case—most of these are nephrogenic rests.

Resection of Neuroblastoma

Expert: Andrew M. Davidoff, M.D.

QUESTIONS

1. Is it important to excise the wound from a previous biopsy site?

No. Unlike for many sarcomas, nonrhabdomyosarcoma soft tissue sarcomas, in particular, in which excising a prior biopsy site is important, this is not the case for neuroblastoma, generally, a highly chemosensitive tumor. I am not aware of any cases in the published literature of neuroblastoma recurrence in the skin or soft tissues through which a biopsy was obtained. Nevertheless, I do excise prior open biopsy sites routinely, but for strictly cosmetic reasons. I do not make an effort to record or recall the specific site through which a percutaneous tru-cut biopsy was performed, if that was the method for obtaining diagnostic material.

2. What steps can be taken to avoid nephrectomy during resection of a retroperitoneal neuroblastoma?

Every effort should be made to avoid nephrectomy when resecting a retroperitoneal neuroblastoma. Patients with favorable clinical characteristics and tumor biology generally have an excellent outcome regardless of the completeness of resection while patients with unfavorable clinical characteristics and tumor biology need intensive multimodality therapy for which normal renal function is required in order to receive the full recommended doses. Thus, in neither circumstance should a nephrectomy be purposefully performed in order to attempt to get a gross total resection. Rarely, kidneys are removed because of a mistaken diagnosis of Wilms' tumor. Careful assessment of the preoperative imaging and completion of the laboratory evaluation, including urinary catecholamines if the diagnosis is in question, should help avoid this occurrence.

Because intraabdominal neuroblastoma often grows into the renal hilum, encasing the renal vessels, kidney loss, either during surgery or as a long term functional outcome (see discussion of "disappearing kidney" below), is not an uncommon occurrence, particularly in patients with high risk disease. This complication may occur in upward of 15% of cases and occurs due to injury to the renal vasculature rather than to the kidney itself. This can be either inadvertent ligation and division of the renal artery and/or vein, injury to either of these vessels that cannot be successfully repaired, or due to trauma to the artery or vein from torque that results in a loss of blood flow and subsequent renal infarction.

It is, therefore critical to identify both the renal artery and vein early in the course of an operation. This is best done by identifying their takeoff from the aorta and inferior vena cava and following the course of these vessels out to the renal hilum, dividing the encasing tumor on top of the vessels and then freeing them along their circumference and length. Great care must be taken when removing tumor from behind the renal vein not to apply torque to the artery while retracting the tumor mass.

I administer renal-dose dopamine during these cases, although I am not sure that it helps. In cases where a kidney appears to become dusky due to torque on the renal artery, some have advocated intramural lidocaine in an attempt to break the spasm of the artery, although I am not certain of the effectiveness of this maneuver either. Torque on the aorta itself can also impair blood flow to the contralateral renal artery. In addition, the surgeon should be aware that there may be multiple renal arteries supplying a given kidney. The preoperative imaging can often help identify this circumstance although careful dissection along the aorta at the time of surgery should reveal anatomic variations.

3. **How should extension of neuroblastoma into the neural foramen be managed?**
   Extension of neuroblastoma into the neural foramen is a fairly common occurrence, especially with thoracic primaries. In general, there is rarely an indication to remove the tumor extension surgically, as the risks of resecting this residual disease appear to outweigh the benefits. Patients with favorable clinical characteristics and tumor biology have an excellent oncologic and neurologic prognosis despite leaving some gross residual disease in the neural foramen. Patients with unfavorable clinical characteristics and tumor biology will receive intensive multimodality therapy, which is a critical component of successful treatment.

   Tumor extension into the neural foramen and spinal canal that causes acute neurologic deterioration may be most appropriately treated by emergent surgical resection, approached via a laminotomy.

4. **What steps do you perform to avoid injury to intraabdominal visceral vessels?**
   Intraabdominal neuroblastoma, particularly with unfavorable biology, has a propensity for encasing the visceral vessels. A critical step for avoiding injury to these vessels is their identification before they pass through the tumor, most often at their take-off from the aorta. As with the renal arteries, discussed above, this should be done as early as possible during the course of an operation. The tumor on the anterior surface of the artery can then be incised along the length of the vessel and the tumor then removed piecemeal after freeing the circumference of the artery. It is very difficult to identify the artery by simply dissecting into the middle of the tumor. Some surgeons advocate the use of CUSA or intraoperative ultrasound to help in the identification and preservation of the visceral vessels; I have no personal experience with either technique.

5. **What is the cause of a disappearing kidney after neuroblastoma resection?**
   "Disappearing kidney" is the phrase used to refer to atrophy of a kidney felt to have been due to vascular injury at the time of surgery. However, the consequence of this traumatic injury is generally not noted until later in a patient's clinical course, often months later, when a follow-up or re-staging imaging study, generally a CT scan, demonstrates a diminutive or completely absent kidney. The exact etiology for this complication is not well understood but is believed to involve spasm and/or intimal disruption of the renal artery due to excessive manipulation, particularly torque, on the vessel when trying to expose and resect lymphadenopathy from behind the renal vein or artery. Clearly, the intimate relationship of the tumor and the encased vessel plays a significant role in the pathophysiology of this entity, as the kidney can be mobilized and manipulated, along with its artery, extensively during other surgical procedures, such as a partial nephrectomy without inciting spasm of the artery and subsequent renal atrophy.

6. **What is the most common complication during resection of a neuroblastoma?**
   There are a wide range of significant potential complications, discussed below, that depend on a variety of factors including the inherent biology of the tumor, the location of the tumor, and the skill, experience and aggressiveness of the operating surgeon. Overall, I believe that vascular injuries are probably the most common, significant complications that occur during the resection of a neuroblastoma.

7. **What unusual complications occur following resection of a neuroblastoma?**

Attempting to achieve a gross-total resection of a neuroblastoma can be among the most challenging operations that a pediatric surgeon performs. The list of significant complications associated with such a procedure is extensive, with several studies in the literature reporting a complication rate of >40% for resection of a neuroblastoma and an incidence of peri-operative mortality of around 2% to 3%. The types of complications that can occur are generally site-specific, and although they are not necessarily "unusual" or unique to neuroblastoma resection, they occur with a greater frequency during this type of procedure. A brief list of the site-dependent complication is as follows:

Thoracic: Horner's syndrome (injury to the stellate ganglion), pleural effusion, chylothorax (disruption of the thoracic duct).

Abdominal: diarrhea (from denervation of the bowel), intestinal obstruction (perioperative or late), nephrectomy/renal atrophy, vascular injury, chylous ascites (lymphatic disruption), and ureteral injury.

Pelvic: vascular injury, nerve injury—sciatic nerve palsy, urinary and fecal incontinence, neurogenic bladder, erectile dysfunction, leg weakness or nerve root injury (L4-S1).

Paraspinal: hematoma within the spinal canal.

21 | Complications of Laparoscopic and Thoracoscopic Surgery

Garret Zallen, M.D.

INTRODUCTION

The New Frontier

Miniature access surgery has been one of the biggest advances in surgical technique in the last 30 years. What was initially limited to a few procedures, with poor visualization, extraordinarily long cases, and outcomes that were fraught with complications, has now been adapted to almost every area in surgery and with outcomes often superior to open techniques. This explosion in applicability and volume has been due to the incredible pace at which technology has been developed to allow the surgeon to perform operations that were once felt to be science fiction. This technology has required the surgeon to learn completely new skill sets and with that has come entirely new conditions that create errors and complications.

Since Hippocrates' time, the surgeon and the patient were in direct contact, either by sight or touch. With the creation of robotic surgery it is now possible for the surgeon to never lay a hand on the patient. While this represents an extreme of the consequences of technology, miniature access surgery has created a whole new paradigm to which the surgeon must adapt. Our neural network at first clashes with this new set of sensory inputs, or often lack of input. The surgeon must adapt to the loss of haptic feedback (direct touch), the loss of the third dimension, magnified views, an unstable and changing horizon, and the failure of any of the equipment that is bringing information to his or her brain. It is as if we are being thrust into an environment for which our bodies are not designed to handle, an environment akin to a hostile wilderness, like a climber trying to summit Everest. We exist in an environment where our minds and body were never designed to work. Yet we adapt to these conditions, or in surgical parlance, we adapt through a process called the learning curve.

Into Thin CO_2

The analogy of surviving in the wilderness helps to analyze and categorize the errors that occur in miniature access surgery. Just like there are errors that occur in base camp, on the ascent and on the descent, the surgeon can make errors that occur before the incision, during the operation, or after the operation is completed. Proper planning of an operation is vital, but more important is the ability to change that plan.

In order to plan an operation, the surgeon must have the experience and knowledge to create that plan. This brings us to the first area where errors occur—that is, experience. Prior to operating, the surgeon needs to gain the skills necessary to be successful. The concept of the learning curve within surgery began to gain traction with the advent of laparoscopy. A search of PubMed shows the first discussions of the learning curve in relation to surgical technique began in the early 1990s. These review papers dealt with the incidence of complications during laparoscopic cholecystectomies and the apparent decrease as the surgeon performed greater numbers of these cases. Why this discussion had not occurred with the advent of new open surgical operations is not entirely clear, but a plausible explanation is the total unfamiliarity we had with the world of laparoscopy. So how do we gain experience in this new technique of operating? "See one, do one, teach one" no longer applied as it was not so much the operation that was being learned, but how to actually operate.

Currently we have training programs that teach miniature access techniques. In theory we are supposed to be proficient by the time we graduate. But are we? The concept of proficiencies that graduates must demonstrate during their training may answer this question, but unfortunately nature does not adjust her difficulty level to match that of the climber, nor does the case adjust for the surgeon. Training attempts to predict the future, to give us the skills to safely operate on what we predict we will encounter. You would never climb Mt. Everest as your first hike, nor would you do a thoracoscopic repair of a congenital diaphragmatic hernia as your first miniature access case. Clearly, training is essential to error reduction. However, it cannot prevent errors.

But what of the learning curve? How does a surgeon prevent undertaking a case that seems straightforward only to get rapidly out of control because of patient factors that could not be predicted? It is impossible. Everyone would agree that driving home from work is a simple task, but throw an unexpected blizzard and ice storm in the mix and it becomes a harrowing experience. Some errors cannot be prevented with experience. However, experience teaches us when it is time to pull over and stop driving. Likewise the experienced surgeon has the sense to know when it is time to open or stop—a skill that can never be measured by any proficiency test. Perhaps that is the true learning curve.

The Climb

To reach the summit the climber must know the route. In order for a surgeon to perform a successful operation he or she must know the anatomy. The advent of miniature access surgery has created a new set of anatomy—two dimensional. The disconnect between three-dimensional structure and a limited angle of view, not to mention variations in anatomy, can lead to errors. We have all been in situations where we see what we expect to see, but our expectations have distorted reality. An example of this is the surgeon who is confused by the anatomy of the biliary system, but "knows" the cystic duct must be what he/she is looking at and divides the common duct. How does this happen? In wilderness terms this is referred to as bending the map (1). Taking information from the environment that seems to be incongruent with the map but projecting expectations on what is in view until the reality is bent to match one's mental map. This happens to lost hikers all the time, and to surgeons as well. Miniature access surgery creates an environment that makes this even easier than open surgery. The lack of three dimensions and a horizon that is relative (turning the camera) can be disorienting. Add that to the fact that many pediatric operations are done on babies who have anomalous anatomy, allowing bending the map to be an easy step to make.

There are ways to avoid making known errors. The camera should always be held at the correct angle to the horizon. Angled scopes can provide different views of the anatomy which may help clarify structures. Moving the scope from one trocar to another for a different view can also help give a different perspective. Preoperative imaging may be important to help create a map in the baby with anomalous anatomy where no map may exist. Finally, knowing when one is lost and admitting it may prevent disaster. Asking for help from a different set of eyes, spending more time defining the anatomy, or converting to a different technique are all good to do when the map does not match the landscape.

PRINCIPLES OF COMPLICATION AVOIDANCE DURING LAPAROSCOPY AND THORACOSCOPY

Exposure and Space

Having made the analogy to wilderness survival to cover the basic principles, it is time to discuss the considerations specific to pediatric laparoscopy. One of my mentors used to say "that surgery should be easy"—if it is not, then you are not doing it right. What he was alluding to is that unless there is proper exposure even the most experienced surgeon will struggle. Laparoscopy in children is hampered by the same principles as an adult, but on a much smaller scale. It is often necessary to work in a space smaller than a coffee cup. For this reason careful preoperative planning of camera placement and port placement is necessary. Some of the common planning errors that occur in pediatric miniature access surgery are poor patient selection, improper patient positioning, improper trocar alignment, improper equipment, and improper equipment settings. While some would argue that every patient is a candidate for miniature access surgery, common sense would dictate that certain patients may benefit from open procedures. Due to their size, pediatric patients can be positioned in a variety of manners on the operating room table (transverse, stirrups, at the foot of the table, etc.). Planning a position that will create operator, patient, and monitor in a straight line will facilitate a smoother operation. Likewise a small infant may need to be raised off the table on a platform to allow the operator's hands to get low enough on the table to work in the anterior abdomen or chest. Positioning the patient to optimize exposure and movement of the surgeon during the miniature access procedure and not a "compromise" position that will allow an open operation will lead to the greatest chance of success. The pediatric surgeon needs to be aware of the size of instruments that will function optimally—5 mm versus 3 mm. Correct trocar placement is essential to a smooth operation. The surgeon needs to have a mental map of what lies beneath and place his or her trocars appropriately. However, when things are not as planned, trocars may need to be moved, a difficult maneuver as it requires admitting that the original plan was faulty. This is an essential skill to learn—our plans do not always match what we find. Understanding these planning steps will help minimize errors and hopefully complications.

Trocars

Trocar insertion, placement, and type of trocar are essential to the successful completion of an operation. More frequent than causing a disaster, improper trocar placement may cause unnecessary frustration. Some types of trocars have big heads and will hit the adjacent trocar, hampering movement of the instruments. For this reason, in little babies it is sometimes more feasible to insert instruments directly into the chest or abdomen, without the use of a trocar. This is most successful if the patient is thin and there are going to be minimal or no instrument exchanges, such as in a pyloromyotomy.

Insertion of the trocars is the time during the operation where most of the catastrophic complications can occur. Great vessel injury occurs in about 0.05% of trocar insertions and the mortality rate from these injuries is up to 20% (2). For this reason, insertion should not be taken lightly and of all parts of the operation should be performed by someone with significant experience. There are several techniques for the initial trocar insertion: Veress needle, semi-open, open with a Hassan trocar, infra-umbilical, and trans-umbilical. Furthermore, there are multiple types of trocars: cutting, blunt, radial expanding, and optical trocars. Generally speaking, when there are multiple ways to accomplish something in surgery, this means that none of them are perfect. In the case of trocar insertion this is indeed the case and every method of insertion above has been paired with the different trocar systems and all have an inherent risk (3). For this reason, experience in trocar placement is necessary, but more important is the ability to quickly react to vessel injury and having the facilities necessary to manage these injuries. Just like a mountain climber should know how to self arrest during a fall, a laparoscopic surgeon must know how to quickly gain access to and control these injuries.

There are a few things that can be done to help minimize the risk of trocar insertion. The insertion of the umbilical trocar can be the most hazardous portion of the case, as it is often accomplished without direct visualization. However, an understanding of the anatomy of the abdominal cavity can help minimize serious vascular injury. The aorta and vena cava bifurcate at or just inferior to the level of the umbilicus; therefore, a trocar inserted straight down risks injury to these structures. A trocar inserted in a more tangential and lateral direction avoids these two structures. Once the umbilical trocar is inserted, the rest of the trocars can be inserted under direct visualization. Using trans-illumination in a semi-dark room can show the location of vessels in the abdominal wall and help prevent hemorrhage from placing trocars through these vessels, especially the epigastric vessels. When inserting a trocar under vision, it should be inserted in a tangential direction—parallel to the floor once the tip has penetrated the peritoneum and the tip should always be kept in the field of vision. Using both hands helps prevent the trocar from plunging into a loop of bowel. In little infants the abdominal wall is so thin and elastic that unless the initial stab wound is stretched with a hemostat, the trocar can collapse the abdominal wall into the field of view and make visualization difficult. Finally, securing a trocar to the abdominal wall not only helps prevent the risk of reinsertion, but it also saves a lot of time and frustration. There are several techniques to accomplish this. I prefer to use a small piece of a Foley catheter that is fitted like a doughnut around the trocar and sutured to the skin with a nylon suture.

Energy Sources

Minimally invasive procedures have become feasible largely because we can control blood vessels with a variety of energy sources from monopolar cautery, harmonic energy, and tissue sealing instruments. Unfortunately, all of these instruments spread energy past the area of interest and in the case of monopolar cautery can arc to tissue remote from the surgical site. For these reasons, the surgeon must be knowledgeable of the various types of energy sources and be able to adjust the energy levels according to the size of the patient. Due to the size constraints of pediatric patients, a common error is to not have the entire "active" surface of the energy source in the field of view and to inadvertently injure adjacent tissue. For this reason, it is imperative to have the whole "active" portion of the instrument visible. Also, using the lowest effective settings avoids collateral damage and arcing potential. When using devices that are designed to act as a cutting tool as well as a dissecting tool, such as the harmonic scalpel, it is important to either allow time for the tips of the instrument to cool or to cool the tips on either the liver or abdominal wall prior to grabbing or dissecting bowel. Failure to cool the instrument prior to dissecting or holding a piece of bowel after activation can result in thermal injury to the bowel and possible delayed perforation.

Another area where errors occur is a system problem. Some of these energy sources require the use of a foot pedal. This requires surgeons to not only employ the use of both of their hands, but their foot as well—the equivalent of rubbing your stomach, patting your head, and hopping up and down on one foot. While this is possible, it adds an additional layer for error. It is not uncommon for someone to not release the "on" pedal when the cutting is done and, furthermore, to hit the "on" switch inadvertently as it is out of the field of vision. More instruments with hand control are being manufactured, but even this is not foolproof and inadvertent triggering still occurs. Further study into the ergonomics and cognitive awareness needs to be done. Likewise, safety system research needs to be advanced by manufacturing companies.

CO_2 Insufflation

Exposure is the key to any successful operation. In open operations this is accomplished by large incisions and retractors. Laparoscopy relies on good camera angles and adequate insufflation. The instillation of CO_2 accomplishes the goal of providing exposure in a noncombustible environment. While lots of attention has been directed toward CO_2 absorption and its potential physiological effects (4–6), most of these papers deal with theoretical consequences and in practice there are very little deleterious effects. However, there are several instances where improper insufflation can cause significant harm. The first relates to the pressure of the insufflation. Most insufflators are pre-set to 15 mmHg. This pressure is appropriate for most laparoscopy, except perhaps for very small infants and those with significant cardiac anomalies. When these settings are used for thoracoscopy, however, it can create a tension physiology. Therefore, the surgeons must be aware of the settings and the function of their equipment. To make matters worse, some will re-set to 15 mmHg of pressure if they are turned off and restarted during a case. Systems where the surgeon is in direct control of these systems via a sterile touch panel screen may be safer.

Perhaps the most devastating complication of insufflation is a gas embolus. There are multiple reports of gas embolus from CO_2 entering an open vein such as during a liver resection (7,8). Even more devastating is the direct insufflation of CO_2 into a vein such as the patent umbilical vein in a neonate. These events can be fatal and rapid recognition is essential. Loss of end-tidal CO_2, sudden hypotension, tachycardia, or cardiac arrest may be due to gas embolus. Standard measures such as patient position with the left side down and head down and aspiration of the right atrium via central line may be life saving. When these events occur, insufflation should be immediately stopped and ACLS measures initiated. A cardiac echo will help make the diagnosis. Specific measures to help prevent these instances include careful placement of the initial umbilical trocar in the newborn to avoid umbilical vein insufflation, conversion if there is a large open vein that is susceptible to gas insufflation and a high index of suspicion followed by a rapid response and resuscitation.

COMPLICATIONS OF LAPAROSCOPY

Laparoscopic Appendectomy

The laparoscopic appendectomy is the most common laparoscopic procedure performed by the pediatric surgeon. While all of the above general considerations are relevant to this procedure, there are some specific complications that are inherent to this operation. The most common is injury to the bowel due to the large amount of inflammation and phlegmon. I feel this complication can be almost entirely prevented if the surgeon adopts the strategy of not always operating to remove the appendix. This may seem strange, but remember the analogy of the mountain climber—no one would climb Everest if they knew a blizzard was coming. Likewise, when the surgeon encounters a phlegmon and the appendix is difficult to identify, let alone dissect, then he or she should stop the operation, place a drain, and treat with broad spectrum antibiotics and return when the "weather" is better. Failure to do this may result in injury to the bowel during dissection, removal of something other than the appendix or leaving a long appendiceal stump. The latter can actually lead to "stump appendicitis" and the need for a second appendectomy. Some surgeons advocate nonoperative management of ruptured appendicitis to begin with, followed by an interval appendectomy.

Laparoscopic Pyloromyotomy

Few operations strike fear in the hearts of pediatric surgeons like that of the laparoscopic pyloromyotomy. It takes a relatively easy open operation and creates an operation that requires a very specific skill set. But once these skills are mastered, it brings the operation back down to a very simple and expedient operation. There are essentially three unique steps to the operation and each has a set of complications. The first step is grasping the duodenum. Duodenal injuries can occur if the duodenum is only partially grasped and the grasper crushes the sidewall of the duodenum. This can cause an immediate perforation or more worrisome it can cause a delayed perforation due to eventual necrosis. To help prevent this complication a gentle and full grasp of the duodenum should be undertaken. A second instrument inserted through the midline trocar can help push the duodenum into the grasper.

The second step is the incision of the pylorus. Perforation of the mucosa can occur during this step. The use of a disposable knife that has distinct cutting depths is optimal. Care should be taken not to start the incision distal to the pyloric ring and carried too proximal on the stomach. A preoperative ultrasound can help determine the depth of the incision that is safe based on the thickness of the pylorus.

Once the incision is made, the third step is spreading the thickened muscle to split the hypertrophied pylorus. There are several types of laparoscopic pyloric spreaders that can be employed. The mistake to avoid at this step is inserting the spreader too deeply in the incision and perforating the mucosa, or to spread too distally and tear the duodenal mucosa. At times the safer maneuver is to grasp both sides of the pylorus with each of the graspers and gently tear the last millimeter of the incision. When in doubt to extend the myotomy distally, avoid the temptation. Incomplete myotomies do not usually occur distally and you may end up injuring the duodenal mucosa. Inflating the stomach can help detect leaks, but it is not foolproof. A leak after a myotomy is serious, but if missed can be devastating. If the baby is not acting normally, becomes distended, drops its urine output, becomes tachycardic, or displays other unexpected symptoms, it needs to be evaluated for a leak and possibly re-explored.

The biggest step to avoiding complications from a laparoscopic pyloromyotomy begins prior to the operation. The diagnosis is usually made via ultrasound. Often these are done at referring institutions that do not routinely perform ultrasounds on babies. In my experience I have seen more than one false-positive report. I feel most of these ultrasounds need to be re-done or at least re-read by a pediatric radiologist. Doing a myotomy on a normal pylorus is a recipe for perforation, especially when the baby did not need the operation in the first place.

Laparoscopic Splenectomy

Laparoscopic splenectomy is usually performed for enlargement of the spleen due to a chronic hemolytic condition caused by one of the various types of hemoglobinopathies or splenic platelet sequestration. In both cases, the spleen may be very large and this can present the greatest challenge for safe removal. In order to prevent significant hemorrhage from loss of control of the hilar vessels, proper exposure is paramount. As was outlined earlier, this is an operation where the patient needs to be positioned to optimize laparoscopic exposure, not a "compromise position in case you need to open." An almost lateral decubitus position provides the best exposure. With optimal exposure, injury to the pancreas and stomach can be more easily avoided.

The choice of energy sources for division of vessels is also important. The use of a Ligasure™ or a similar device provides the optimal sealing of larger vessels up to 7 mm. The use of a stapler is also effective, but care must be taken to avoid injury to the underside of the splenic vein when dissecting around the hilar vessels and placing the stapler. Finally, once the spleen has been dissected free, it must be safely removed. There have been reports of devastating intra-abdominal injury when a morcellator was used and the protective bag was breached (9). I feel that removing the spleen piecemeal with a blunt instrument is the safest. This step may take longer than the actual disection, but avoids creating a complication after the difficult part of the case is completed—the so-called descent phenomenon.

Splenic and/or portal vein thrombosis has been reported after laparoscopic splenectomy. In the adult literature, rates as high as 50% have been reported (10,11). In the pediatric population, it would seem to be a much more rare complication. Avoiding this complication is still not well understood and treatment of children following laparoscopic splenectomy to prevent this complication is also not understood at this time. What is clear is that the earlier the treatment, the better the response. Therefore, if the patient develops any symptoms of mesenteric vein thrombosis, a prompt evaluation followed by anticoagulation therapy is warranted if the evaluation reveals clot.

Laparoscopic Nissen Fundoplication

The development of the laparoscopic technique for the Nissen fundoplication was one of the operations that catapulted laparoscopic surgery in children into the mainstream. Greeted with great enthusiasm, the popularity of this operation has uncovered a number of potential complications and a whole chapter could easily be devoted to this operation alone. There are four essential steps to this operation that are unique. The first is dissection of the short gastric vessels from the spleen. The choice of energy sources varies, but should not be taken lightly. While these vessels in children are small and significant hemorrhage is not common, transfer of energy to the stomach and subsequent perforation from thermal injury can easily occur. For this reason, the vessels should be divided as far from the stomach as possible and using the minimal amount of energy needed to safely divide the vessels. If there is inadvertent spread of thermal energy to the gastric wall, this should be over-sewn as the damage is usually more extensive than it appears and perforation will likely occur. Injury to the spleen can also occur during this portion of the operation and can be avoided by good exposure and gentle traction on the short gastric vessels.

The second step is dissection around the esophagus. This step is usually straightforward, but can become complicated if the angle of dissection is too cephalad. In this case, the dissection ends up going into the mediastinum and potentially into the pleural space. Taking care to dissect in a more right to left direction and not "upwards" will help prevent this. More worrisome, however, is the risk of hepatic vascular injury. It is not uncommon to encounter a replaced left hepatic artery coursing nearly across the pars flaccida, right in the way of the retro-esophageal dissection. While it can be tempting to divide this vessel, this could lead to hepatic injury. Usually, gentle retraction of the vessel allows for a safe dissection. If this cannot be accomplished, placement of another instrument to aid in retraction can be helpful.

The third step is closure of the hiatus. The stitch that sutures the left and right Crura together used to carry the nickname of the "dysphagia" stitch. In fact, if this is placed too tightly it can cause dysphagia by constricting the esophagus. In order to prevent this, use of an appropriately sized bougie in the esophagus to prevent narrowing is essential. The size of the bougie is debatable and there are several methods described to choose the appropriate size. A rule that can be applied is selecting a bougie equal in size to the child's thumb. Finally, appreciation of the location of the aorta posterior to this stitch can help prevent injury to the descending aorta.

The final step is completing the wrap. This can also be done over a bougie to prevent the wrap from being too tight. Data have clearly shown that a wrap does not have to be tight to prevent reflux, but tight wraps can lead to more cases of postoperative dysphagia (12). Placement of the sutures for the wrap is important in that they create the longest possible intra-abdominal esophagus and that they are not tied so tightly that they cause ischemia of the stomach with resultant perforation.

As in any operation, complications can occur, but delayed recognition can be devastating. The standard postoperative course for a laparoscopic Nissen should be smooth. If the patient experiences symptoms such as significant pain, distension, fever, tachycardia, then a prompt evaluation should be undertaken. The use of a contrast upper GI series can be helpful to demonstrate a perforation and leak, but normal study should not be interpreted as proof that all is well. If there is any question, then it is often better to go back to the operating room and look in the abdomen. Perforations caught early and treated have a much better outcome.

COMPLICATIONS OF THORACOSCOPY

The invention of thoracoscopy actually pre-dates the use of laparoscopy. This was made possible by the fact that the rigid thorax provides a space for visualization without the need for insufflation. This fundamental difference gives thoracoscopy a unique set of complications and challenges. In pediatric patients, the use of single lung ventilation may not be possible due to size constraints. In fact I have found the use of bronchial blockers or double lumen tubes to be an unnecessary use of time. Instead, excellent visualization can be achieved by insufflating into the chest using a closed system of trocars. One must be careful not to insufflate at pressures above 6 to 8 mmHg to avoid tension pnuemothorax physiology. Just as in laparoscopy, the surgeons must be aware of the settings of their equipment and make sure that presets do not exceed this desired pressure.

Placement of trocars can also be a source of complications. Just as in the peritoneal cavity, the pleural space is a potential space and injury to the lung can occur if bladed trocars are used or if previous surgeries or infection have fused the pleural space. For this reason, the use of blunt or nonbladed trocars for entry may be the safest method. Once the chest is accessed, a thorough knowledge of thoracic anatomy is essential. I think that the chest, specifically the hilum of the lung, can be one of the easiest places to bend the map as it can be difficult to visualize the anatomy. Since the thorax is a rigid space, the surgeon must be aware of the types of equipment that will fit into that space. For instance, the endo-GIA stapler will not fit in the chest of a one-year-old. For that reason, the hilar vessels and bronchus must be divided using a different device. Furthermore, the angles in the chest do not always allow for stapling even when the chest is large enough.

Thoracoscopic Lung Biopsy and Lobectomy

Thoracoscopic lung biopsy has become the operation of choice for almost all lung biopsies. It provides an excellent tissue sample with a minimum incision. As mentioned earlier, a good knowledge of anatomy is essential and so is good preoperative imaging, especially if there are specific targets. Nodules for biopsy need to be peripheral or large enough that they will be visible when the lung collapses. Small nodules can sometimes be "palpated" using a laparoscopic grasper. If a nodule cannot be located, then a small incision and insertion of a finger through the chest wall may help identify the target without making a full thoracotomy incision. Biopsy of hilar lesions is not a common problem in children, but should be undertaken with care.

Lobectomy can be safely performed thoracoscopically. A recent large series demonstrated the feasibility and safety of this procedure (13). Previously it was felt that the operation could not be performed if there was not a complete fissure. With the use of a Liga-sure™ or other sealing device, the fissure can be safely divided and the hilar structures located and divided. When resecting an upper or right middle lobe it is recommended that prior to dividing a bronchus, the bronchus be compressed with a grasper and the lung inflated to make sure that the bronchus going to the lower lobe(s) is not being divided. When dividing major pulmonary vasculature, loss of control of a vessel can be catastrophic. For this reason, using a device that seals, but does not divide, can help prevent division of a vessel before it is entirely sealed across.

Thoracoscopic Treatment of Parapneumonic Effusions

As in mountain climbing where there may be many ways to reach the summit, in the treatment of parapneumonic effusions there are multiple treatment paths. These effusions can be treated with antibiotics alone, tube thoracostomy, fibrinolytics, thoracoscopy, and thoracotomy. Different treatment plans have been put forth based on the composition of the fluid, the duration of the effusion, or the quality of the fluid—loculated or nonloculated. The data show, however, that early thoracoscopic drainage of parapneumonic effusions is the most expeditious route to recovery (14). In fact, choosing the wrong treatment may be the first error in delaying recovery. Unlike most other thoracoscopies where the pleural space is free, entry into the pleural space can be the most challenging part of the operation. Blunt entry into the chest followed by careful and patient blunt dissection with the scope and insufflation until there is enough room to see and get a second port in is usually successful. During this dissection it is important to keep the scope pressed to the chest wall while it is swept back and forth to avoid injuring the lung. Unlike in adults where the fibrinous rind is often densely adherent to the lung, in children it can usually be peeled easily from the visceral pleura. In the instance where it cannot be, care should be taken to avoid tearing into the lung parenchyma. It is not essential to remove all of the peel as long-term lung entrapment from these "rinds" is very uncommon in children. Finally, once the chest has been debrided, the scope should be switched to a different port to provide an alternative point of view. Significant areas can be missed if only one view port is utilized.

While not specific to this procedure, chest tubes can be a significant source of morbidity in children. Even though thoracoscopy provides excellent visualization for the placement of a chest tube, if the tube is not sutured into place securely it can easily become dislodged and malpositioned. Due to the small size of the chest tube, many of the connectors from the suction containers do not fit well. I have seen too many pneumothoraces created by air leaking into the system from poorly fitting connectors. Taking the time to find the right connector can save several days in the hospital, not to mention many phone calls and preventable stress. Also, due to the thinness of the chest wall in children, air can leak through the chest wall. For this reason, it is important to place a good occlusive dressing over the chest tube. Since most chest tubes are placed through a port site during thoracoscopy, the hole in the chest wall goes straight into the pleural space instead of being tunneled over a rib or two. If this is a concern, the muscle can be closed where the port traversed the chest wall, and using the same skin incision, a new tunnel can be made superior to the previously closed hole, creating a tunneled chest tube tract.

CONCLUSION

When asked why he decided to climb Mt. Everest, Sir Edmond Hillary famously replied—"because it was there." This is the same reason why we often use new technology; because we can. Care must be taken, however, when new technology is applied in the field of surgery to ensure that the ends are justified, not just the means. Laparoscopy and thoracoscopy have indeed proven to be effective and often superior techniques to open procedures, but have created a whole new set of complications and issues. Continuing to study the root causes of these errors is essential for good outcomes. However, in any system, there is a defined set of failures that cannot be avoided despite the best of efforts. For this reason, avoiding mistakes is a noble task, but the greater task is to recognize when errors have occurred and correcting them or asking for help from someone who can. It is the later characteristic, responsibility, and duty that define the great surgeon.

REFERENCES

1. Gonzales L. Deep Survival. W.W. Norton & Company, 2003; 143–162.
2. Roviaro GC, Varoli F, Saguatti L, et al. Major vascular injuries in laparoscopic surgery. Surg Endosc 2002; 16(8):1192–6. Epub 2002 May.
3. Vilos GA, Ternamian A, Dempster J, et al. Laparoscopic entry: A review of techniques, technologies, and complications. J Obstet Gynaecol Can 2007; 29(5):433–465.
4. Ciftci O, Elemen L, Elemen F, et al. Laparoscopic surgery: Does it increase the probability of atrial and ventricular arrhythmias in children? Surg Laparosc Endosc Percutan Tech 2008; 18(2):173–17.
5. McHoney M, Mackinlay G, Munro F, et al. Effect of patient weight and anesthetic technique on CO_2 excretion during thoracoscopy in children assessed by end-tidal CO_2. J Laparoendosc Adv Surg Tech A 2008; 18(1):147–151.
6. O'Malley C, Cunningham AJ. Physiologic changes during laparoscopy. Anesthesiol Clin North Am 2001; 19(1):1–19.
7. Schmandra TC, Mierdl S, Hollander D, et al. Risk of gas embolism in hand-assisted versus total laparoscopic hepatic resection. Surg Technol Int 2004; 12:137–143.
8. Schmandra TC, Mierdl S, Bauer H, et al. Transoesophageal echocardiography shows high risk of gas embolism during laparoscopic hepatic resection under carbon dioxide pneumoperitoneum. Br J Surg 2002; 89(7):870–876.

9. Milad MP, Sokol E. Laparoscopic morcellator-related injuries. J Am Assoc Gynecol Laparosc 2003; 10(3):383–385.
10. Miniati DN, Padidar AM, Kee ST, et al. Portal vein thrombosis after laparoscopic splenectomy: An ongoing clinical challenge. JSLS 2005; 9(3):335–338.
11. Brink JS, Brown AK, Palmer BA, et al. Portal vein thrombosis after laparoscopy-assisted splenectomy and cholecystectomy. J Pediatr Surg 2003; 38(4):644–647.
12. Bowrey DJ, Peters JH. Current state, techniques, and results of laparoscopic antireflux surgery. Semin Laparosc Surg 1999; 6(4):194–212.
13. Albanese CT, Rothenberg SS. Experience with 144 consecutive pediatric thoracoscopic lobectomies. J Laparoendosc Adv Surg Tech A 2007; 17(3):339–341.
14. Kurt BA, Winterhalter KM, Connors RH, et al. Therapy of parapneumonic effusions in children: Video-assisted thoracoscopic surgery versus conventional thoracostomy drainage. Pediatrics 2006; 118(3):e547–e553. Epub Aug 14, 2006.

Laparoscopic Cholecystectomy

Expert: Thom E. Lobe, M.D.

QUESTIONS

1. **Should routine intraoperative cholangiography be performed during laparoscopic cholecystectomy in children and adolescents?**
   I do not believe that routine cholangiography is essential today, so long as you are clear on your anatomy and there is neither a history nor clinical suggestion of stone disease. If the anatomy is uncertain as a result of inflammation, congenital anomaly, or the presence of abundant fat in the tissue overlying the ducts, making them more susceptible to injury, a cholangiogram should be performed. Similarly, if there is a history of stones, jaundice, or a large duct is observed, a cholangiogram should be performed to look for residual stones.

2. **What technical steps help prevent injury to the common bile duct?**
   Good retraction of the fundus and infundibulum so that the ducts are well displayed will help. The peritoneum overlying the ducts from cystic duct to its junction with the common duct (including viewing the common duct proximal and distal to the junction) should be sufficient to minimize the risk of injury. In addition, I never use a device with energy in my dissection of the ducts. The ducts can be displayed easily with a minimum of hemorrhage without using electrocautery or another energy source that is likely to cause thermal injury if it accidentally contacts the duct while the energy is applied.

3. **How should patients with coexisting common bile duct stones be managed?**
   This depends on the experience of the surgeon. If a surgeon is inexperienced, the best option is to perform the laparoscopic cholecystectomy and perform the cholangiogram to confirm that the stones have not passed. An ERCP can be performed after the patient recovers. Depending on the surgeon's skill and expertise, a cholodochotomy can be performed through which an infant cystoscope or small flexible scope can be passed to inspect and instrument the ducts. Many stones can be simply "pushed" into the duodenum. Others require removal with a stone basket. When neither of these options work, a "t" tube can be left as an access for the interventional radiologists after the patient recovers from the surgery.

4. **Do you favor the fundus down approach versus a Triangle of Calot initial dissection?**
   I routinely begin at the Triangle of Calot.

5. **Should acute cholecystitis be "cooled off" prior to performance of a laparoscopic cholecystectomy?**
   I believe that this is an old school approach. The standard of care in many centers includes operating for acute disease. The morbidity is less and the patient recovers sooner.

6. **In the era of minimally invasive surgery, how should asymptomatic cholelithiasis be managed in the otherwise healthy child?**

   My preference is to leave the patient alone unless there are justifiable symptoms.

7. **How would you manage the inflamed and scarred gallbladder, where you judged further dissection in the Triangle of Calot too risky?**

   When scarring is severe or the anatomy is confusing, a cholangiogram is essential. If I do not believe that I can perform a cholecystectomy using laparoscopy, I will consider converting to an open case. My goal in this situation is to prevent further stone formation and to eliminate the possibility of inflammation due to cholecystitis. I use my cholangiogram as a guide so that I can attempt to divide the cystic duct safely. One option is to open the gallbladder along its longitudinal axis and the strip the mucosa as one does with a cholodochal cyst. If the cystic duct cannot be ligated, it may be over sewn at its junction with the gallbladder taking care to not capture the common duct. The inflamed seromuscular wall can be left in place so long as the mucosa has been removed.

Laparoscopic Nissen Fundoplication

Expert: George W. Holcomb, M.D., M.B.A.

QUESTIONS

1. **What technical steps help avoid slippage of the Nissen fundoplication?**

   Our group has been very interested in transmigration of the fundoplication wrap as, in our experience, over 90% of the patients requiring a re-do fundoplication require it because of transmigration rather than the wrap falling apart. Between 2000 and 2002, we mobilized the esophagus extensively in order to create what we felt was an adequate length of intra-abdominal esophagus. In doing so, however, we found a 12% incidence of transmigration of the fundoplication wrap postoperatively. In 2002, we changed to minimal mobilization of the esophagus as well as placement of esophagocrural sutures to help obliterate this potential space for transmigration of the wrap. These two maneuvers resulted in a reduction in our transmigration rate to 5%. This was presented at APSA in 2006 and subsequently published in *Journal of Pediatric Surgery* (42:25–30, 2007). Thus, we feel that minimal mobilization around the esophagus and keeping the phrenoesophageal barrier intact along with placement of four esophagocrural sutures at 8 o'clock, 11 o'clock, 1 o'clock, and 4 o'clock are all helpful maneuvers to reduce transmigration of the fundo-plication wrap.

2. **How should the greater curvature blood vessels be divided?**

   In my opinion, it is mandatory to divide the short gastric vessels in order to create a tension-free Nissen fundoplication. In patients up to 4 or 5 years of age, this ligation and division can be accomplished with an instrument connected to cautery. Our preference is to use the Maryland dissecting instrument connected to cautery and use the tip of the instrument much like a sharp bovie. Others use the hook cautery for this purpose. After about 5 years of age, we generally use the harmonic scalpel for this purpose.

3. **What intraoperative steps reduce the chance of the fundoplication being too tight?**

   The first step was mentioned above in that it is important to divide the short gastric vessels so that the fundoplication wrap is "loose" and "floppy," which really means that the wrap is tension free. Secondly, it is important that the suture line of the fundoplication lies at approximately 10 or 11 o'clock. A suture line that lies at 10 or 11 o'clock means that less fundus has been brought posterior to the esophagus and more has been brought anterior. This helps reduce the anterior compression of the esophagus as well as anterior angulation of the esophagus, which can occur if too much fundus is posterior to the esophagus. Finally, it is vital to use a bougie. In patients under 15 kg, we have created a table (*Journal of Pediatric Surgery* 37:1664–1666, 2002) in which the bougie size is determined by the patient's weight. This is a simple method of finding an adequate size bougie for this purpose. In over 500 fundoplications, I have only had to perform an esophageal dilation on one child following the initial fundoplication. Therefore, I believe that such a table and the use of a bougie helps eliminate the problem of dysphagia from a fundoplication that is too tight.

4. What unusual complications have you seen?

With a technique that has been standardized over 15 years, I cannot remember any unusual complications. As previously mentioned, the usual complications are transmigration of the fundoplication wrap. In fact, only one patient between 2000 and 2007 who has required a re-do fundoplication has not had transmigration of the fundoplication wrap. I do know of one patient who required a splenectomy for bleeding at the time of fundoplication, but I have not seen this complication personally.

5. Are there technical steps of the operation that can reduce the chance of retching?

This is a very difficult question to answer. I believe there are probably two etiologies to retching. One is acute distention of the stomach which can be managed with lower volume feedings over a longer period of time. In our experience, retching does not seem to occur very much in the neurologically normal child or baby. If it does, it seems to resolve over time. This is mainly a problem in the neurologically impaired child who also has a gastrostomy so it is often possible to try lower volume feedings over a longer time. Occasionally, it can be helpful to try continuous tube feedings up to 24 hours a day to see if this helps the problem. The second etiology arises in the central nervous system related to the neurologically impaired children. In such patients, they often will not respond to smaller volume and tube feedings. We have tried a number of medications such as Reglan or Erythromycin without much success. We have also tried Periactin (2 mg/5 cm^3; 1 mg BID to start) which has been helpful in a few patients. Finally, if the patient has a gastrostomy, the gastrostomy can be vented at the time of feedings or retching with some amelioration of the symptoms.

6. Are there any special considerations in the child with a V-P shunt? With activities?

There are no real special considerations in a child with a V-P shunt other than to be sure that the shunt is not injured at the time of the fundoplication. However, often there will be some adhesions around the shunt in the upper abdomen which need to be lysed for adequate visualization. Where the shunt is actually placed in the abdomen can be important. Some neurosurgeons place it in the midline; others place it on the right or left side. If you are able to work with your neurosurgeon and ask him/her to place it on the right side over the liver, it is usually out of the way. If it is placed in the left upper quadrant, it can often be in the way of your visualization. In the patient with the V-P shunt, antibiotics should be administered preoperatively and for 1 to 2 days postoperatively. There are no special considerations with the child with ascites, although obviously the reason for the development of the ascites can be important in figuring out if there will be any bleeding problems or problems that develop that are related to the underlying condition.

Laparoscopic Appendectomy

Expert: Carroll M. Harmon, M.D., Ph.D.

QUESTIONS

1. How should division of the appendix from the cecum proceed if the inflammation extends to the base of the appendix?

I will often use the gastrointestinal load of the endoGIA stapler and take a centimeter or so of cecum along with the appendix. This might require more than one firing of the stapler. Normally for most pediatric patients the vascular load is best for the base of the appendix. Laparoscopic ileocectomy is also on option.

2. **Should inflamed and adherent omentum be resected with the appendix?**
   In many cases of acute appendicitis the omentum is adhered to the inflamed appendix but is easy to "peel" off. It is not actually sealing a perforation. However, if it appears that the omentum is patching a perforation or that the wall of the appendix beneath the omentum is gangrenous, it is possible and appropriate to divide the tongue of omentum and leave this in place as an appendiceal patch. The omentum can be divided using a variety of techniques including hook or scissor monopolar cautery or one of several sealing devices such as the Ligasure (Covidien), Sonosurg (Olympus), or Harmonic Shears (Ethicon). Usually, omental adherence involves the distal half of the appendix and therefore the attached omentum does not interfere with the dissection through the mesoappendix and to the base of the appendix.

3. **What steps should be taken if the bag ruptures during removal of the appendix from the umbilical trocar site?**
   Specific steps should be taken to avoid bag rupture. First, if a 12-mm trocar has been used at the umbilicus, many inflamed appendices can be extracted safely through the trocar without using an endo bag. If an endo bag is needed and there is difficulty in extracting the bag and appendix, we often enlarge the facial opening by sliding a grove director through the skin incision and under the linea alba both proximally and distally and slide a #11 blade scalpel in the groove of the grooved director such that the sharp edge cuts the facia, under direct laparoscopic visualization. Using this maneuver to enlarge the incision typically results in easy extraction of the bagged appendix. If, however, the bag does rupture and the appendix falls back into the peritoneal cavity, then the appendix should be quickly found and grasped and held or moved to a lateral location, such as lateral to the cecum. The umbilical skin incision, if necessary, and the umbilical facial opening can be enlarged as described above. The surgeon's index finger can also be inserted through the umbilical trocar site to assist with dilation of the opening. Another endo bag device should then be placed back into the peritoneal cavity through the enlarged umbilical site to retrieve the appendix.

4. **What intraoperative steps can be taken to prevent intra-abdominal abscess formation?**
   Intraoperative maneuvers that definitively prevent postoperative intra-abdominal have not been clearly defined by rigorous clinical research. Though there continues to be debate as to whether laparoscopic appendectomy for perforated appendicitis has a higher incidence of postoperative intra-abdominal abscess risk, our own published study did not show this in children. Therefore, I recommend laparoscopic appendectomy for both acute and complicated appendicitis. Steps that *might* help to lower the rate of postoperative intra-abdominal abscess formation include appropriate timing of preoperative antibiotics, avoidance of perforating a gangrenous, nonperforated appendix (handle the mesoappendix during manipulation and dissection), retrieval and extraction of an appendicolith, aspiration of purulent fluid, saline irrigation of the right lower quadrant with aspiration of irrigation fluid, and use of an extraction bag. There are no compelling data to argue for leaving an intraperitoneal drain to lessen the incidence of intra-abdominal abscess.

5. **Does the muscle layer need to be closed on all trocar sites?**
   I always close the facia at the umbilical trocar site. A 12-mm trocar or cannula is typically used at this site for introduction of a stapling device and for appendiceal extraction. The other two trocar sites for the typical appendectomy are 4 or 5 mm. We typically use a radial dilation cannula system (STEP, Covidien) for our 12- and 5-mm access devices. After removal, the diameter of the facial defect is significantly smaller than 12 or 5 mm. Therefore, in thin children, I recommend at least closing the anterior abdominal wall musculature for 4 or 5 mm sites. I do not routinely close these sites in children with a thick subcutaneous layer. Though we have experienced a few 3 to 5 mm trocar site hernias in infants (not for appendicitis) who have only had skin closure, I am not aware of any symptomatic 3 to 5 mm trocar site hernias in older children in our large pediatric endosurgery practice.

6. **What unusual complications have you seen during performance of a laparoscopic appendectomy?**

Fortunately, I have not experienced any memorable significant complications during laparoscopic appendectomy. I have had near misses with trocar-related bowel injury in children who have had previous open abdominal operations. I have had significant meso-appendiceal bleeding that was recognized and dealt with laparoscopically. I recently had a case of ruptured appendicitis with an extruded appendicolith in an 8 year old who had previously had an endo-rectal pull through for Hirschsprung disease. The abscess and appendicolith were very low against the right rectal side wall and much more distal than would be typical with an intact peritoneal lining of the pouch of Douglas. I treated the patient with antibiotics and then performed a very difficult laparoscopic interval appendectomy.

7. **Is there a clear role for irrigation, perforated appendix or not?**

To my knowledge, there are no definitive clinic research data available to support a clear role for peritoneal irrigation for appendicitis.

8. **What is your preferred method for dividing the meso-appendix? Is it age/vessel size related?**

The meso-appendix can be divided very easily with monopolar hook cautery across all ages and patient sizes. This simple device can be used quite effectively as a dissector, coagulator, and tissue divider. In unusual circumstances, such as an extraordinarily thick mesentery, an endo-GIA stapler can be used; however there can be some bleeding from the staple line, even with the vascular load. Other devices can be used such as the Ligasure or Sonosurg, but these increase expense without distinct advantage over monopolar cautery. Simple ligation with a 2-O tie of silk or vicryl using intracorporeal tying works fine as well.

Laparoscopic Hernia Repair

Expert: Felix Schier, M.D.

QUESTIONS

1. **What technical steps should be emphasized to prevent recurrence?**

Inguinal hernias are not equivalent to open inguinal rings. And open inguinal rings are not identical to inguinal hernias. There are hernias with closed internal inguinal rings and there are open internal inguinal rings without hernia. This has been observed for many years in open surgery and is analogous with the phenomenology of recurrences. In only a third of recurrences the internal inguinal ring in fact is again fully open. It is partially open in approximately 25%, has only a small opening in 21%, and is even completely closed in 18%.

In addition, there were four different further aspects of recurrences.

1. In our experience, recurrences occurred mostly on the right side, even when adjusted for the predominance of right-sided hernias. The reason is unknown to us. Possibly this has to do with the fact that in the majority of our surgeons the right hand is the dominant one and that in right-sided hernias surgeons tend to start suturing laterally and proceed medially until they finally approach the cord structures and the epigastric vessels. There might be a reluctance to come too close, resulting in a mechanically weak area medially. On the left side, surgeons with a dominant right hand tend to start suturing medially, where the crucial structures lay, and proceed laterally with the suturing.

2. Recurrences occur mostly in boys, even when adjusted for the statistical predominance of boys with inguinal hernias.

   This effect is related to aspect number 1 and may best be explained by the surgeon's inhibition to come too close to the vas and the epigastric vessels.

3. Virtually all recurrences occur medially, next to the vas and the epigastric vessels, almost never laterally.

4. In direct hernias, recurrences will frequently occur if only the peritoneum is sutured.

With the laparoscopic approach, direct hernias are more frequently seen than with the open approach, with the laparoscopic picture probably being the more realistic representation (Rare inguinal hernia forms in children. F. Schier, J. Klizaite. *Pediatr Surg Int* 20: 748–752, 2004). Initially, in direct hernias we simply sutured the peritoneum at the opening. This resulted in approximately 70% recurrences. Now, we incise the peritonum, expose the underlying anatomy with the lateral extension of the opening, remove the occasional lipoma, and first close the defect with two to three slow-absorbable sutures and then close the peritoneum on top with a running suture. This completely stopped all recurrences in direct hernias.

There are a few recurrences from knots coming apart. We observed laparoscopists pulling both suture ends of closed knots *not* in the level of the knot but slightly outwards, toward the surgeon, resulting in much less force exerted unto the knot and in the risk of a loose knot.

In most recurrences, however, the original knot or suture is still visible and intact. A reopening is found between the knot and the epigastric vessels/vas deferens. Obviously a weak spot had been left between knot and vessels.

Our consequence therefore was to include a good bite of tissue from *medially* to the epigastric vessels and include this into the knot. Esthetically this will not look as elegant as a suture and a knot confined to tissue exclusively from the area *lateral* to the epigastric vessels, but it reduces the rate of recurrences (unfortunately not to 0%).

2. What technical steps are important to avoid injury to the vas and vessels?

Injury to the vas and the epigastric vessels is not a problem in reality. An injury to the vas we have never seen. The tissue/peritoneum on top of the epigastric vessels is so loose that it can be easily lifted with a forceps or needle holder and moved left and right in order to clearly identify the underlying vas.

This also is the case with the epigastric vessels. The covering peritoneum is not as mobile as over the vas. Still, it can be lifted and the needle safely negotiated around the vessels. Again, we have never seen a bleeding from an epigastric vessel (possibly at the price of a few recurrences).

Concern has been raised whether the knot might jeopardize testicular perfusion. We performed a perfusion study and did not find any restrictions in testicular perfusion after laparoscopic inguinal hernia repair.

3. By what approach is recurrence following laparoscopic repair managed?

Again by laparoscopy. First, the view is much better than with the open approach. In practically all recurrences there are no visible traces from the previous intervention, except for the sutures. Second, in only a third of recurrences the internal inguinal ring is in fact again fully open. It is partially open in approximately 25%, has only a small opening in 21%, and is even completely closed in 18%. Thus, in only slightly more than half of recurrences there is a true opening to be closed. In the remainder there is only a small opening just wide enough to permit passage of fluid, or no opening at all. It is by no means technically more demanding to close the opening in a recurrence than in a primary case. The vessels are as easy to identify as before.

"Recurrences" without an opening are a problem in 18% of cases. The problem also exists in adult patients. An underlying lipoma might mimick a hernia. In adult patients a few law suits have originated from this dilemma. The accusation was to have operated on the wrong side and to have caused an unnecessary recurrence.

4. What are the most common complications and how can they be avoided?

There are three common complications.

1. Most discussed are recurrences. We feel that a recurrence rate of 3% to 4% is realistic. The less traumatic the minimally invasive approach is, the more recurrences it will have. The more traumatic the open approach, the less recurrences it will have. At the moment, the recurrence risk is minimized by including tissue into the knot from medially of the epigastric vessels. The knot will look more voluminous but results in fewer recurrences. Furthermore, we would recommend adding one or two more sutures if there is the least doubt about the mechanical quality of the first suture. There

are two psychological obstacles to a second or third suture. Only one suture looks elegant and quick. A second or third suture would relinquish this effect. Laparoscopic suturing is more tedious than open suturing. A laparoscopist will therefore think a second longer about a second suture. However, both effects should be ignored as much as possible.

2. Rarely there is a herniation of omentum into the umbilical trocar site. In these cases the umbilical suture was insufficient, obviously.

3. Surprisingly, hydroceles—our primary concern—almost never occur. If a hydrocele occurs, we puncture it once or twice, without further sequelae. Primary hydroceles, in contrast, have been treated by closure of the internal inguinal ring, in an identical fashion to hernia repair. We had an unacceptably high number of recurrences with this approach, and do not offer it to parents any more.

5. **Would any specific defect, or size of defect, prompt the use of prosthetic material? How about in recurrent situations? In athletic adolescents?**

We have no experience with prosthetic material. Also, in athletic adolescents we would not dare to simply suture the internal inguinal ring, out of fear that the mechanical strength would not suffice. Our maximum age for simple suture closure of the internal inguinal ring in inguinal hernia is approximately 13 years.

In fact, we have operated with this technique on a few adults, a few men (none athletic) and a few females up to the age of 36 years (one among them very active in track-and-field-sports at an Olympic level). A recurrence occurred in a man with Hunter syndrome, none in the females. In all of these patients we had applied at least three sutures. Interestingly, the Hunter patient (a 26-year-old male) had had a direct and an indirect hernia. The recurrence occurred at the site of the previous indirect hernia which was only closed with a single suture. There was no recurrence, however, at the site of the direct hernia which had to be closed layer-by-layer with several sutures.

A major—and favorable—difference between the open and laparoscopic approach in inguinal hernia is re-recurrence. We saw several patients with multiple recurrences, up to five recurrences. The maximum was one patient who had been operated on 18 times for recurrences (!), always in the open technique. This virtually does not occur with the laparoscopic technique. If a recurrence occurs after laparoscopy, it is closed again laparoscopically, and this, as a rule, will be the last procedure for the patient. Re-recurrences after laparoscopy are extremely rare.

Laparoscopic Pyloromyotomy

Expert: George W. Holcomb, M.D., M.B.A.

QUESTIONS

1. **How should the procedure be performed when the patient's umbilicus is not healed?**

Usually, patients with pyloric stenosis present after 10 to 14 days of life. In most cases, the umbilical stump has dried and healed without evidence of complications. If the umbilical stump is still "wet", in our experience, this does not mean that a laparoscopic pyloromyotomy with insertion of an umbilical cannula cannot be performed. Ancef (25 mg/kg) is administered. The umbilicus is thoroughly cleansed with a Q-tip soaked in Betadine followed by prep and drape in a standard fashion. Next, I like to take cautery and coagulate the contents of the "wet" umbilicus to help obliterate any bacteria. Whether or not this helps is unclear. However, with the combination of cleansing the area with Betadine and cauterization of the contents, we have not had an increased incidence of infection in such a patient. Usually, there is an umbilical fascial defect present so it is quite easy to gently introduce the 5 mm cannula.

2. **How should mucosal perforation be managed?**

If a mucosal perforation is noted, then the surgeon has the option of either converting to an open operation or repairing it laparoscopically. In my opinion, the right lateral "stab" incision should be extended and an open exploration performed. The mucosal defect is closed, the seromuscular myotomy is also reapproximated and a pyloromyotomy is performed away from this original pyloromyotomy. It is not necessary to perform the second pyloromyotomy on the back side of the pylorus, but it should be performed away from the original one.

Another option is to repair it laparoscopically which has been performed successfully. However, it is my feeling that once a mistake is noted with a laparoscopic operation, in most cases, conversion to an open operation should be done to take care of the problem. It is much better to convert rather than make a second mistake.

3. **Is there a reliable test to detect mucosal perforation intraoperatively?**
Our usual technique is to ask the anesthesiologist to introduce a red rubber catheter following completion of the pyloromyotomy and instill 30 to 60 cm^3 of air into the stomach to test for a mucosal leak. Whether or not this is helpful to detect occult leaks, which are not readily apparent, is unclear. However, it is a means of trying to detect mucosal perforation intraoperatively rather than being surprised when the baby exhibits peritoneal signs postoperatively.

4. **What strategies should be applied to avoid mucosal perforation?**
It is important to remember that the hypertrophied pyloric musculature is thickest in the center of the pylorus and decreases in depth as one approaches each end. Therefore, it is important to initially spread in the center of the myotomy which, in turn, helps break the hypertrophied muscle fibers adjacent to this site. It is also important not to have the edge of the pyloric spreader underneath the muscle as this can lead to injury to the submucosa and entry into the mucosa. Also, it is important to spread less vigorously as one approaches each end of the pyloromyotomy as the thickness of the musculature does decrease at each end. It is also important to realize that the myotomy that is performed laparoscopically is probably smaller than the one performed open. What this means is that the large myotomy that was performed with the open technique was probably not needed. One technique that I use in unclear cases is to measure the length of the myotomy that has been performed and compare it to the results found on the ultrasound. This measurement is performed by cutting a silk suture to a known size and placing it along the myotomy to measure it fairly accurately. If the ultrasound and intraoperative measurements are similar in length, then I do not extend the myotomy further. On the other hand, if there is more than 3 to 4 mm difference between the measured myotomy and the ultrasound findings, then it is not unreasonable to spread a little more at each end.

5. **Do 3 mm trocar sites need to be closed?**
These stab incisions do not need to be closed and the fascia of these stab incisions does not need to be closed either. Our usual technique is to approximate the skin with steri-strips. We have not noticed any problems with this approach.

6. **What are the most common complications following laparoscopic pyloromyotomy?**
The complications that one can see include wound infection, a "bump" formed under one of the stab incisions, an incomplete myotomy, and mucosal perforation. Wound infection occurs in approximately 1% of cases. This can usually be managed with antibiotics and local care. It is unclear what the "bump" under one of the incisions actually is. On occasion, there can be a very small tongue of omentum that has become incarcerated in one of these sites. Having re-explored a couple of patients in whom this stab incision technique has been utilized for other conditions, a tongue omentum can be seen, but this finding cannot be seen. Incomplete myotomy and mucosal perforation also occur approximately 1% of the time.

7. **In suspected cases of incomplete myotomy, does the minimally invasive approach change your management by prompting laparoscopic "inspection" of the myotomy sooner than you might reoperate if the original approach was open?**
In our experience, we have had two patients out of approximately 500 who developed an incomplete myotomy (we have also just had one perforation which was managed

laparoscopically). Therefore, we do not have a large experience with reoperation. In fact, these two incomplete myotomies were managed by balloon dilation and resolved. Therefore, I believe initial balloon dilation is probably the appropriate technique rather than a re-myotomy.

Thoracoscopic Lobectomy

Expert: Craig T. Albanese, M.D.

QUESTIONS

1. What is the best way to manage an incomplete fissure?
An incomplete fissure can be "completed" using either an endo-GIA stapler (USSC, Norwalk, CT) or the Ligasure vessel sealing device (Valleylab, Boulder, CO). The stapler is used for large patients, the Ligasure for the majority of our pediatric patients. I like to use the 5-mm Ligasure that has the curved tips. It works well for lung tissue and significant air leaks from the cut surface are not common. If there is absolutely no fissure, one must start at the pulmonary artery and trace its course and create a fissure that way, again with either a stapler or the Ligasure.

2. How is a prolonged postoperative air leak managed?
This management is no different than open thoracic surgery. It depends on one's definition of "prolonged" but I recommend tube thoracostomy drainage (on or off suction is debatable but I prefer suction) and time. I usually wait 2 weeks before going to the next step, which would be pleurodesis. I do not believe there is a perfect way or agent for pleurodesis—one can use mechanical methods such as bleomycin, talc, or others. Certainly, if there is a massive amount of leak early postoperatively, the presumptive diagnosis is a bronchopleural fistula and I would reoperate in this case.

3. What instruments are used for vessel division and how does the size of the vessel influence your choice? Are the newer 2 mm vascular staples useful?
I divide all vessels that are less than 5 to 7 mm with the Ligasure. If a vessel in a child is larger than this, instead of upsizing a port to a 12 mm, I will use suture ligation and/or 5 mm clips. In large children/adolescents where the vessels are all greater than 7 mm, I use the vascular endo-GIA placed through a 12-mm valved port. I have not used the newer 2-mm vascular staples.

4. What is the most difficult lobe to resect and what are the technical difficulties inherent in those resections?
The upper lobes are the most difficult to resect because of the poor access to lobar hilar structures. There is a risk of inadvertently ligating or injuring the vasculature and bronchus to the adjacent lower lobe.

One must start with the division of the superior pulmonary vein. This will expose the main pulmonary artery trunk. The arterial segmental vessels are serially ligated from front to back. One will also be able to complete the fissure during this vascular dissection and then the bronchus will be exposed.

5. What are the most common complications occurring following thoracoscopic lung resection?
Transient air leak is the most common complication. Bleeding can occur from scar/adhesions in those patients who have had previous bouts of pneumonia or infections in their lung masses. This usually does not necessitate transfusion or conversion to an open thoracotomy but it does extend the time for the procedure.

6. What unusual complications have you seen following thoracoscopic lung resection?
None that I would classify as unusual.

7. **What is your technical preference for bronchial division/closure?**
   In small children, I divide the bronchus sharply with scissors and then suture ligate it with absorbable suture material. In large patients, I divide and seal it with a vascular endo-GIA stapler.

8. **Is there a role for intraoperative fibrin sealants?**
   Perhaps. Fibrin glue was shown in one study (Ann Thorac Surg 75:1587, 2003) to lessen peripheral air leaks after lobectomy. Fibrin glue may be beneficial to use when one has to surgically complete a fissure.

Thoracoscopic Repair of Esophageal Atresia

Expert: Craig T. Albanese, M.D.

QUESTIONS

1. **What technical steps are important to prevent stricture?**
   I adhere to the same principles as I would for open surgery; try to avoid tension (which is difficult in this clinical scenario), avoid disrupting the distal esophageal blood supply as much as possible, and I do not use silk sutures since they have been shown to have a higher rate of stricture. I also do not like the stiff knots that are created with PDS and Prolene, so I use an absorbable suture (Vicryl).

   One must be aware that the surgical view is magnified and "gaps" appear larger than they really are. Thus, I believe there is a tendency to put too many sutures in the anastomosis and this can lead to stricture.

2. **Does it matter if an esophageal leak occurs intrapleurally?**
   No. The leak matters, not the location. Hence, adequate control (drainage) of the leak is important.

3. **What technical steps can be achieved thoracoscopically to prevent a recurrent fistula?**
   First, do not use a titanium clip to ligate the fistula. One can interpose fibrin glue, pleura (hard to do), or a biological mesh between the esophageal anastomosis and the ligated stump of the tracheal fistula.

4. **Does the anastomosis need to be drained with an intrapleural tube?**
   Not in all cases. This is pure operator judgment. In cases where I believe there may be a reasonable chance for a leak, I place an intrapleural tube. In all other cases, I do not insert a tube.

5. **What are the most common complications occurring after repair of esophageal atresia thoracoscopically?**
   The complications are no different than those encountered during an open procedure. There is a slightly higher incidence of stricture but the numbers are still too small to say for sure. This might be due to the placement of too many sutures or inadequate esophageal mobilization.

6. **Can you suggest when an "experienced" minimal access surgeon should attempt thoracoscopic EA repair?**
   One should be comfortable suturing and performing intracorporeal knot tying in very small spaces. It is best to ensure that one can perform these tasks in a small baby who needs a fundoplication before tackling this procedure. I highly recommend being proctored/assisted by someone experienced in this procedure. It is also critical that one has the support of our pediatric anesthesiology colleagues. One needs to know that the oxygen saturations will not be 100% (more like 92–95%) and the end-tidal carbon dioxide levels will be above normal (can be around 60 Torr or higher). These are not clinically harmful numbers and do not need to be aggressively corrected intraoperatively. If one tries to

attain "normal" numbers by increasing the tidal volumes, one will lose operating domain due to lung expansion and will not be able to complete the procedure thoracoscopically due to inadequate exposure of the posterior mediastinum.

7. **A postoperative day #7 esophagram shows a significant leak. What factors would lead you to reoperation versus nonoperative management?**
   In general, most anasotomotic leaks seal without operative intervention, using tube drainage, antireflux medication, and time. The only time I would consider reoperating is a massive (akin to complete dehiscence) leak very early (first 2 or 3 days) postoperatively.

22 | Complications in Pediatric Trauma

Steven Stylianos, M.D., Michael G. Vitale, M.D., and Richard H. Pearl, M.D.

INTRODUCTION

The development of pediatric expertise within regional trauma systems has led to advances in triage and transport of seriously injured children to facilities prepared for the unique challenges of these patients (1). Despite these advances, many serious and often life-threatening complications of both the host response to injury and the treatment rendered can occur. We will focus on specific treatment-related complications of common abdominal and orthopedic injuries. Complex critical care issues such as multi-system organ failure, "adult" respiratory distress syndrome, systemic inflammatory response syndrome, and neurotrauma complications are beyond the scope of this chapter (2).

ABDOMINAL INJURY

The treatment of children with major abdominal injuries has changed significantly in the past two decades. Surgical restraint has been the theme in recent years and increased awareness of the anatomic patterns and physiologic responses characteristic of pediatric trauma has resulted in the successful nonoperative treatment of many abdominal solid organ injuries. Our colleagues in adult trauma care have acknowledged this success and applied many of the principles learned in pediatric trauma to their patients (3,4).

Important contributions have been made in the diagnosis and treatment of children with abdominal injury by radiologists and endoscopists. The resolution and speed of computed tomography (CT), screening capabilities of focused abdominal sonography for trauma (FAST), and the percutaneous, angiographic, and endoscopic interventions of nonsurgeon members of the pediatric trauma team have all enhanced patient care and improved outcomes. Each section of this chapter will focus on common blunt injuries and unique aspects of care in children.

Spleen and Liver Injury

The spleen and liver are the organs most commonly injured in blunt abdominal trauma, with each accounting for one-third of the injuries. Nonoperative treatment of isolated splenic and hepatic injuries in stable children is now a standard practice. Controversy exists regarding the utility of CT grading as a predictor of outcome in liver and spleen injury (5–8). Recently, the APSA Trauma Committee has defined consensus guidelines for resource utilization in hemodynamically stable children with isolated liver or spleen injury based on CT grading (Table 1). Prospective application of these guidelines resulted in treatment conformity with safe reduction in resource utilization (9,10). The decision to operate for spleen or liver injury, which should be made by the attending surgeon, is best based on evidence of continued blood loss, such as low blood pressure, tachycardia, decreased urine output, and falling hematocrit. The rates of successful nonoperative treatment of isolated blunt splenic and hepatic injury now exceed 90% in most pediatric trauma centers and adult trauma centers with strong pediatric commitment (9–12).

Surgeons unfamiliar with current treatment algorithms for blunt splenic injuries in children occasionally question the nonoperative approach. This is important because the majority of seriously injured children are treated outside the dedicated pediatric trauma centers. While several adult trauma services have reported excellent survival rates for pediatric trauma patients, analysis of treatment for spleen and liver injuries reveals an alarmingly high rate of operative treatment (11,13–15). It is possible that trauma surgeons, influenced by their past

Table 1 Consensus Guidelines for Resource Utilization in Children with Isolated Spleen or Liver Injury

CT Grade	I	II	III	IV
ICU days	None	None	None	1 day
Hospital stay (day)	2	3	4	5
Predischarge imaging	None	None	None	None
Postdischarge imaging	None	None	None	None
Activity restriction[a] (wk)	3	4	5	6

[a] Return to full contact, competitive sports (i.e., football, wrestling, hockey, lacrosse, mountain climbing, etc.) should be at the discretion of the individual pediatric trauma surgeon. The proposed guidelines for return to unrestricted activity include "normal" age-appropriate activities
Abbreviations: CT, computed tomography; ICU, intensive care unit.

experience with adult patients, are more likely to favor operative treatment than their pediatric surgical colleagues. Adult trauma surgeons caring for injured children must consider the anatomic, immunologic, and physiologic differences between pediatric and adult trauma patients and incorporate these differences into their treatment protocols. The major concerns are related to the potential risks of increased transfusion requirements, missed associated injuries, and increased length of hospital stay. Each of these concerns has been shown to be without merit (9,10,16–21).

Missed Associated Abdominal Injuries

Advocates of surgical intervention for splenic trauma cite their concerns about missing associated abdominal injuries if no operation is performed. Morse and Garcia reported successful nonoperative treatment in 110 of 120 children (91%) with blunt splenic trauma, of whom 22 (18%) had associated abdominal injuries (18). Only three of these 120 patients (2.5%) had gastrointestinal injuries and each was found at early celiotomy done for a specific indication. There was no morbidity from missed injuries or delayed surgery. Similarly, a review of the NPTR from 1988 to 1998 revealed 2977 patients with solid abdominal visceral injury; only 96 (3.2%) had an associated hollow viscus injury (19). Higher rates of hollow viscus injury were observed in assaulted patients and those with multiple solid visceral injury or pancreatic injury. Differences in mechanism of injury may account for the much lower incidence of associated abdominal injuries in children with splenic trauma. There is no justification for an exploratory celiotomy solely to avoid missing potential associated injuries in children.

Complications of Nonoperative Treatment

Nonoperative treatment protocols have been the standard for most children with blunt liver and spleen injury during the past two decades. The cumulative experience gained allows us to evaluate both the benefits and risks of the nonoperative approach. Fundamental to the success of the nonoperative strategy is the early, spontaneous cessation of hemorrhage. Transfusion rates for children with isolated spleen or liver injury have fallen below 10% confirming the lack of continued blood loss in the majority of patients (9,10,12,20). Despite many favorable observations, isolated reports of significant delayed hemorrhage with adverse outcome continue to appear (22,23). Shilyansky et al. reported two children with delayed hemorrhage 10 days after blunt liver injury (24). Both children had persistent right upper quadrant (RUQ) and right shoulder pain despite normal vital signs and stable hematocrits. The authors recommended continued in-house observation until symptoms resolve. Recent reports described patients with significant bleeding 38 days after Grade II spleen injury and 24 days after Grade IV liver injury (23,25). These rare occurrences create anxiety in identifying the minimum safe interval prior to resuming unrestricted activities.

Routine follow-up imaging studies have identified pseudocysts and pseudoaneurysms following splenic injury (7,12,26,27). Splenic pseudoaneurysms often cause no symptoms and appear to resolve with time (27). The true incidence of self-limited, post-traumatic splenic pseudoaneurysms is unknown, as routine follow-up imaging after successful nonoperative treatment has been largely abandoned. Once identified, the actual risk of splenic psuedoaneurysm rupture is also unclear. Angiographic embolization techniques can successfully treat these lesions obviating the need for open surgery and loss of splenic parenchyma (7,12). Splenic pseudocysts can achieve huge size leading to pain and gastrointestinal disturbance. Simple percutaneous aspiration leads to a high recurrence rate. Laparoscopic excision and marsupialization are highly effective.

SEQUELAE OF DAMAGE CONTROL STRATEGIES

Even the most severe solid organ injuries can be treated without surgery if there is prompt response to resuscitation (28). Most spleen and liver injuries requiring operation are amenable to simple methods of hemostasis using a combination of manual compression, direct suture, and topical hemostatic agents. In young children, the sternum can be divided rapidly to expose the suprahepatic or intrapericardial inferior vena cava (IVC). Children will tolerate clamping of the IVC above the liver as long as their blood volume is replenished. With this exposure, the liver and major perihepatic veins can be isolated and the bleeding controlled to permit direct suture repair or ligation of the offending vessel.

The early morbidity and mortality of severe hepatic injuries are related to the effects of massive blood loss and replacement with large volumes of cold blood products. The consequences of prolonged operations with massive blood product replacement include hypothermia, coagulopathy, and acidosis. Although the surgical team may keep pace with blood loss, life-threatening physiologic and metabolic consequences are inevitable and many of these critically ill patients are unlikely to survive once their physiologic reserves have been exceeded. A multi-institutional review identified exsanguination as the cause of death in 82% of 537 intraoperative deaths at eight academic trauma centers (29). The mean pH was 7.18 and mean core temperature was 32 °C prior to death. Moulton et al. reported survival in only 5 of 12 (40%) consecutive operative cases of retrohepatic vascular or severe parenchymal liver injury in children (30).

Maintenance of physiologic stability during the struggle for surgical control of severe bleeding is a formidable challenge even for the most experienced surgical team, particularly when hypothermia, coagulopathy, and acidosis occur. This triad creates a vicious cycle in which each derangement exacerbates the others and the physiologic and metabolic consequences of the triad often preclude completion of the procedure. Lethal coagulopathy from dilution, hypothermia, and acidosis can rapidly occur (31).

Increased emphasis on physiologic and metabolic stability in emergency abdominal operations has led to the development of staged, multi-disciplinary treatment plans, including abbreviated laparotomy, perihepatic packing, temporary abdominal closure, angiographic embolization, and endoscopic biliary stenting (32–34). Asensio et al. reported 22 patients with Grade IV or V injuries treated between 1992 and 1997 (35). Mean blood loss was estimated at 4.6 liters and mean packed red cell transfusion was 15 units. Ten patients were packed at the first operation. Fifteen patients had postoperative angiographic embolization in an attempt to control hemorrhage. Survival was 92% in 13 Grade IV patients and 78% in 9 Grade V patients.

Abbreviated laparotomy with packing for hemostasis allowing resuscitation prior to planned re-operation is an alternative in unstable patients where further blood loss would be untenable. This "damage control" philosophy is a systematic, phased approach to the management of the exsanguinating trauma patient (36–38). The three phases of damage control are detailed in Table 2. Although controversial, several resuscitative endpoints have been proposed beyond the conventional vital signs and urine output, including serum lactate, base deficit, mixed venous oxygen saturation, and gastric mucosal pH. Once patients are rewarmed, coagulation factors replaced, and oxygen delivery optimized, the patient can be returned to the operating room for pack removal and definitive repair of injuries. A review of nearly 700 adult patients treated by abdominal packing from several institutions demonstrated hemostasis in 80%, survival of 32% to 73% and abdominal abscess rates of 10% to 40% (39,40). Although abdominal packing (PACKS) with planned re-operation has been utilized with increasing

Table 2   "Damage Control" Strategy in the Exsanguinating Trauma Patient

Phase 1	Abbreviated laparotomy for exploration, control of hemorrhage and contamination, packing and temporary abdominal wall closure
Phase 2	Aggressive ICU resuscitation, core rewarming, optimize volume and oxygen delivery, correction of coagulopathy
Phase 3	Planned re-operation for packing change, evacuation and definitive repair of injuries, abdominal wall closure

Abbreviation: ICU, intensive care unit.

frequency in adults during the past two decades, there is little published experience reported in children (38,41–48). Nevertheless, we feel that this technique has a place in the management of children with massive intra-abdominal bleeding, especially after blunt trauma.

We reported a 3-year-old child who required PACKS for a severe liver injury, making closure of the abdomen impossible (42). A Silastic "silo" was constructed to accommodate the bowel until the PACKS could be removed. The patient made a complete recovery. The combined technique of PACKS and a silo allowed time for correction of the hypothermia, acidosis, and coagulopathy without compromise of respiratory mechanics. A recent review reported 22 infants and children with refractory hemorrhage (ages 6 days to 20 years) who were treated with PACKS (43). The anatomic site of hemorrhage was the liver and/or hepatic veins in 14, retroperitoneum and/or pelvis in 7, and the pancreatic bed in 1. Primary fascial closure was accomplished in 12 (55%) patients, whereas temporary skin closure or prosthetic material was used in the other 10. PACKS controlled hemorrhage in 21 of 22 (95%) patients. Removal of PACKS was possible within 72 hours in 18 (82%) patients. No patient rebled after PACKS removal; however, two patients died with PACKS in place. Seven patients (32%) developed an abdominal or pelvic abscess. All were successfully drained by laparotomy (six patients) or percutaneously (one patient). Six of the seven patients with abdominal sepsis survived. Overall, 18 patients (82%) survived. Two deaths were due to multi-system organ failure, one succumbed to cardiac failure from complex cardiac anomalies, and one death was from exsanguination after blunt traumatic liver injury. There were no differences in the volume of intraoperative blood product transfusion, time to initiate PACKS, physiologic status, or type of abdominal closure between survivors and nonsurvivors.

While the success of abdominal packing is encouraging, it may contribute to significant morbidity such as intra-abdominal sepsis, organ failure, and increased intra-abdominal pressure. Adams et al. evaluated fluid samples from 28 patients with abdominal packing and found peritoneal endotoxin and mediator accumulation even when cultures were sterile (49). The authors concluded that laparotomy pad fluid accumulating after damage control laparotomy can contribute to neutrophil dysfunction by enhancing neutrophil respiratory burst and inhibiting neutrophil responses to specific chemotactic mediators needed to fight infection. Thus, the known propensity of such patients to both intra-abdominal and systemic infection may be related to changes in neutrophil receptor status and effector function related to accumulation of inflammatory mediators in the abdomen. Early washout, repetitive packing, and other efforts to minimize mediator accumulation deserve consideration.

It is essential to emphasize that the success of the abbreviated laparotomy and planned re-operation depends on an early decision to employ this strategy prior to irreversible shock. A staged operative strategy for unstable patients represents advanced surgical care and requires sound surgical judgment and expertise. Abdominal packing, when employed as a desperate, last-ditch resort after prolonged attempts at hemostasis have failed, has been uniformly unsuccessful. Physiologic and anatomic criteria have been identified as indications for abdominal packing. Most of these have focused on intraoperative parameters including pH (~7.2), core temperature (<35 °C), and coagulation values (prothrombin time > 16 seconds) in the patient with profuse hemorrhage requiring large volumes of blood product transfusion.

The optimal time for re-exploration is controversial because neither the physiologic endpoints of resuscitation nor the increased risk of infection with prolonged packing is well defined. The obvious benefits of hemostasis provided by packing are also balanced against the potential deleterious effects of increased intra-abdominal pressure on ventilation, cardiac output, renal function, mesenteric circulation, and intra-cranial pressure. Timely alleviation of the secondary "abdominal compartment syndrome" may be a critical salvage maneuver for patients. Temporary abdominal wall closure at the time of packing can prevent the abdominal compartment syndrome. We recommend temporary abdominal wall expansion in all patients requiring packing until the hemostasis is obtained and visceral edema subsides.

A staged operative strategy for unstable trauma patients represents advanced surgical care and requires sound judgment and technical expertise. Intra-abdominal packing for control of exsanguinating hemorrhage is a life-saving maneuver in highly selected patients in whom coagulopathy, hypothermia, and acidosis render further surgical procedures unduly hazardous. Early identification of patients likely to benefit from abbreviated laparotomy techniques is crucial for success.

Abdominal Compartment Syndrome

The abdominal compartment syndrome is a term used to describe the deleterious effects of increased intra-abdominal pressure (50). The "syndrome" includes respiratory insufficiency from worsening ventilation/perfusion mismatch, hemodynamic compromise from preload reduction due to IVC compression, impaired renal function from renal vein compression as well as decreased cardiac output, intra-cranial hypertension from increased ventilator pressures, splanchnic hypoperfusion, and abdominal wall overdistention. The causes of intra-abdominal hypertension in trauma patients include hemoperitoneum, retroperitoneal, and/or bowel edema and use of abdominal/pelvic packing. The combination of tissue injury and hemodynamic shock creates a cascade of events, including capillary leak, ischemia-reperfusion, and release of vasoactive mediators and free radicals, which combine to increase extra-cellular volume and tissue edema. Experimental evidence indicates significant alterations in cytokine levels in the presence of sustained intra-abdominal pressure elevation (51,52). Once the combined effects of tissue edema and intra-abdominal fluid exceed a certain level, abdominal decompression must be considered.

The adverse effects of abdominal compartment syndrome have been acknowledged for decades; however, abdominal compartment syndrome has only recently been recognized as a life-threatening yet potentially treatable entity (33,53). The measurement of intra-abdominal pressure can be useful in determining the contribution of abdominal compartment syndrome to altered physiologic and metabolic parameters (54–56). Intra-abdominal pressure can be determined by measuring bladder pressure. This involves instilling 1 mL/kg of saline into the Foley catheter and connecting it to a pressure transducer or manometer via a three-way stopcock. The symphysis pubis is used as the zero reference point and the pressure measured in cmH_2O or mmHg. Intra-abdominal pressures in the range of 20 to 35 cm H_2O or 15 to 25 mmHg have been identified as an indication to decompress the abdomen. Many prefer to intervene according to alterations in other physiologic and metabolic parameters rather than a specific pressure measurement. Chang et al. reported 11 adult trauma patients with abdominal compartment syndrome in whom abdominal decompression improved preload, pulmonary function, and visceral perfusion using pulmonary artery catheters and gastric tonometry (55).

Experience with abdominal decompression for abdominal compartment syndrome in children is limited (28,38,43,53,56–58). Nonspecific abdominal CT findings in children with abdominal compartment syndrome include narrowing of the IVC, direct renal compression or displacement, bowel wall thickening with enhancement, and a rounded appearance of the abdomen (57). Neville et al. reported the use of patch abdominoplasty in 23 infants and children, of which only three were trauma patients (58). These authors found that patch abdominoplasty for abdominal compartment syndrome effectively decreased airway pressures and oxygen requirements. Failure to respond with a decrease in airway pressures or FiO_2 was an ominous sign in their series. Several authors have found that abdominal decompression resulted in decreased airway pressures, increased pO_2, and increased urine output in children with abdominal compartment syndrome (53,56). Many materials have been suggested for use in temporary patch abdominoplasty including silastic sheeting, Goretex® sheeting, intravenous bags, cystoscopy bags, ostomy appliances, and various mesh materials. The vacuum pack technique, recently used in adults, seems promising (37,48).

Biliary Leaks

Nonoperative management of pediatric blunt liver injury is highly successful but is complicated by a 4% risk of persistent bile leakage (59,60). Radionuclide scanning is recommended when biliary tree injury is suspected (61). Delayed views may show a bile leak even if early views are normal. Several reports have highlighted the benefits of endoscopic retrograde cholangiopan-creatography (ERCP) with placement of transampullary biliary stents for biliary duct injury following blunt hepatic trauma acknowledging that while ERCP is invasive and requires conscious sedation, it can pinpoint the site of injury and allow treatment of the injured ducts without open surgery (33,62–64). Endoscopic transampullary biliary decompression is a recent addition to treatment for patients with persistent bile leakage. The addition of sphincterotomy during ERCP for persistent bile leakage following blunt liver injury has been advocated to decrease intrabiliary pressure and encourage internal decompression (60,62). It is important to note that endoscopic biliary stents may migrate or clog and require specific treatment.

Complications of Pancreatic Injury

Injuries to the pancreas are uncommon with estimated ranges from 3% to 12% in children sustaining blunt abdominal trauma. Pancreatic disruption in children occurs most often from sudden compression injuries of the abdomen. Bicycle and playground injuries predominate and presentation is often delayed up to 48 hours. Serum amylase is elevated in the majority of children with traumatic pancreatitis, but the level and the duration of elevation is not always an indicator of severity of illness or of subsequent pseudocyst formation. Similarly, early abdominal CT findings can underestimate the severity of pancreatic injury.

Pseudocysts occur in 38% to 78% of children with traumatic pancreatitis. Spontaneous resolution of pseudocysts occurs in about 50% of cases and is best monitored by serial ultrasound examinations (65,66). The high rate of spontaneous resolution of post-traumatic pseudocysts in children reflects the absence of underlying ductal obstruction. The differentiation of peripancreatic fluid collections from mature pseudocysts by abdominal CT and sonography may also influence the success rate for post-traumatic pseudocysts. Percutaneous catheter drainage, when effective, can replace cystenterostomy and external drainage. Potential advantages include relief of gastrointestinal obstructive symptoms-related compression by the pseudocyst, early resolution prior to cyst wall maturation needed for internal drainage procedures, and avoidance of a major surgical procedure.

Eight children with post-traumatic pseudocysts have had successful percutaneous drainage without complication or recurrence in two earlier reports (65,66). Catheters were removed in a mean of 28 days (range 10–50 days). Some children can be followed as outpatients with serial sinograms prior to catheter removal. In contrast, Rescorla et al. reported failure of percutaneous drainage in three of four children with traumatic pancreatic pseudocysts, but ERCP revealed disruption of the main pancreatic duct in all three children with failed percutaneous drainage (67).

The advances in percutaneous techniques by invasive radiologists have led to excellent results with minimal risks. Percutaneous drainage of pancreatic pseudocysts should be attempted to avoid major abdominal surgery and general anesthesia, the risk of anastomotic suture line breakdown, and the sequelae of delayed enteral nutrition. Operation is indicated when catheter drainage is unsuccessful.

Persistent drainage from pancreatic duct injuries is another challenging problem in which ERCP can be helpful. The demonstration of a major duct injury should lead to prompt surgical intervention. A recent report emphasized the safety and efficacy of ERCP in six children with a significant blunt pancreatic ductal trauma, each of whom was treated with subsequent spleen-sparing distal pancreatic resection (68). ERCP can lead to serious complications during acute pancreatic inflammation and should only be performed by skilled endoscopists familiar with pediatric equipment and technique.

Individual centers frequently report small patient numbers, which makes it difficult to evaluate their results critically. Recently, two centers (Toronto and San Diego) reported their experiences with divergent methods of managing blunt traumatic pancreatic injuries in a series of reports (69–73). Canty and Weinmanreported 18 patients with major pancreatic injuries over a 14-year period (71). Distal pancreatectomy was performed on eight patients (44%). In 5 of 6 patients, with either proximal duct injuries or injuries missed on initial CT scan, a pseudocyst developed. In two other children who had minimal initial symptoms and no admission CT scan performed, pseudocysts also occurred. Of the seven pseudocysts, two resolved and five were treated by cyst-gastrostomy. The remaining two patients, treated more recently, had ERCP with duct stenting, which resulted in resolution of symptoms and complete healing. These authors concluded that distal pancreatic injuries should be treated with distal pancreatectomy and proximal injuries with observation. Reports from Dallas (74) and Seattle (75) also favor early distal pancreatectomy for transection to the left of the spine to shorten hospital stay. However, long-term complications of operation, including intestinal obstruction and endocrine and exocrine dysfunction, were not assessed. Additional conclusions were that pseudocysts should be observed or drained by cyst-gastrostomy and pancreatic duct/ampulla stent placement by ERCP was safe and effective in cases where pancreatic duct disruption is suspected, acknowledging that CT scanning is suggestive but not always diagnostic for the type and location of pancreatic injury. (69–71).

The experience from Toronto is markedly different (72). A summary comparing the San Diego and Toronto protocols is depicted in Table 3. The striking differences in these series are the 100% diagnostic sensitivity of CT scanning in Toronto versus 69% in San Diego and the 44% operative rate in San Diego versus 0% in Toronto. A subsequent study provided long-term follow-up on patients with pancreatic duct transections (73). Complete follow-up was available in nine. Four (44%) developed pseudocysts, of which three were drained percutaneously. The mean hospital stay was 24 days. All recovered. Follow-up CT scans in eight of nine patients revealed atrophy of the distal pancreas in six and completely normal glands in two. There was no exocrine or endocrine dysfunction (mean follow-up 47 months).

Several therapeutic strategies including early ERCP intervention for diagnosis and treatment with ductal stenting (68,70), the use of somatostatin to decrease pancreatic secretions and promote healing (76), and magnetic resonance cholangiopancreatography (MRCP) as a diagnostic tool (77) require further study prior to wide application.

ABDOMINAL TRAUMA—SUMMARY

Recent advances in the delivery of trauma and critical care in children have resulted in improved outcome following major injuries. Clinical experience and published reports have documented the safety of nonoperative treatment of children with solid organ injuries, and recent radiologic and endoscopic contributions have reduced the need for diagnostic or therapeutic laparotomy. In addition, complications of operative and nonoperative treatment after spleen, liver, and pancreas injury are now best treated with a multidisciplinary approach drawing on the expertise of surgeons, endoscopists, and diagnostic/interventional radiologists. Although the trend is in this direction, the pediatric surgeon should remain the physician-in-charge in the multidisciplinary care of critically injured children. *The decision not to operate is always a surgical decision.*

COMPLICATIONS IN ORTHOPEDIC TRAUMA

Though in many ways children are more resilient to injury than adults, the unique anatomy and physiology of children place them at risk for a number of complications. Certain fractures, for example, have a particular predilection for complications. Hip fractures in children are associated with a high rate of avascular necrosis, particularly when the fracture occurs close to the physis. The open physis of the proximal femur creates a watershed area where blood supply is tenuous and easily interrupted. These fractures are true orthopedic emergencies and require urgent management to reduce the likelihood of this devastating complication. Distal femoral fractures classically result in a growth arrest in approximately 30% of cases. Proximal tibial fractures may appear to be benign injuries but the distal fragment may displace posteriorly and disrupt the popliteal vessels; compartment syndromes occur in 5% to 10% of these injuries. Open fractures and compartment syndromes require urgent diagnosis and treatment, and are the most common surgical emergencies following injury to the musculoskeletal system in children.

OPEN FRACTURES

Open fractures account for approximately 3% of all children's fractures, with regional referral centers reporting even higher incidence (78). Wound classification continues to be based on the Gustillo–Anderson system (79). Type I fractures are generally low-energy injuries with a wound less than 1 cm in length. With a wound more than 1 cm, fractures are classified as Type II as

Table 3 A Comparison of Two Protocols in the Management of Blunt Injuries to the Pancreas in Children

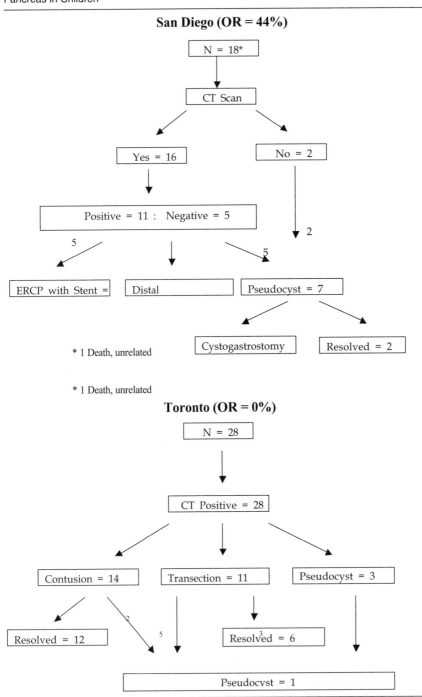

Abbreviations: CT, computed tomography; OR, odds ratio.

long as there is no significant contamination or soft tissue disruption. Contaminated wounds, avulsions, and wounds with marked fracture instability are classified as Type III, as are wounds that require flap coverage (Type IIIB) and wounds with neurovascular disruption (Type IIIC). Management of open fractures in children is similar to treatment in adults. Generally speaking, all open fractures (with the possible exception of low-energy injuries to the hand) require urgent operative irrigation and debridement. Tetanus should be administered when appropriate and

IV antibiotics should also be administered. The role of wound cultures in the emergency room remains controversial and is generally not performed at our institution (80). Early operative stabilization of open fractures facilitates the management of multiply injured children and external fixation continues to be the gold standard. Intramedullary fixation has several limitations in children including subsequent growth problems secondary to insertion through an open physis and interference in the tenuous blood supply when placed in an anterograde manner through the proximal femur. Small diameter flexible titanium intramedullary rods avoid some of these problems and are increasingly being used in the treatment of diaphyseal fractures. Any laceration in the area of a joint should be viewed with high suspicion. If the laceration violates the joint capsule, the joint may be seeded with skin flora resulting in joint sespis. X-rays should be carefully inspected for air within the joint, which is the sine qua non of an "open joint". Additionally, sterile saline may be injected into the joint to assess if the laceration communicates with the joint. If there is any doubt, the child should be taken for urgent irrigation and debridement (open or arthroscopic) to avert the consequences of joint sepsis.

COMPARTMENT SYNDROME

Definition and Pathophysiology

Though compartment syndrome occurs most commonly following tibial diaphyseal injuries and forearm fractures, this potentially devastating complication may occur following injuries to almost any area including the hand, foot, arm, thigh, and buttocks. Furthermore, though fracture is the most common cause, compartment syndrome may occur after contusion, burns, surgery, and even vigorous exercise. Compartment syndromes develop when hemorrhage and soft tissue edema result in a build-up of pressure in the compartment bound by the various inelastic osteofascial boundaries present in each extremity. As pressure builds, venous outflow becomes obstructed which serves to catalyze the cycle of intracompartmental edema, pressure buildup, and tissue damage. Capillary and arteriolar flow ceases when intracompartmental pressures exceed systolic pressures and tissue ischemia and necrosis ensue. Irreversible injury begins within 6 hours of ischemia. Ischemic ("Volkmann's") contracture is the permanent deformity and loss of function that occurs following muscle and nerve necrosis.

Diagnosis

Pain, pressure, pulselessness, paresthesia, and pallor are the "Five P's" of compartment syndrome, but changes in sensation and blood flow indicate that significant tissue injury has already occurred. Pain out of proportion to injury is the earliest sign that should prompt further evaluation, but, admittedly, pain is difficult to quantify in young children. Pain with passive stretch of the hand or ankle should also raise suspicion, but, again, physical findings are not always reliable in children. Compartment syndromes may have a delayed onset, and one recent review of compartment syndromes in children suggests that increasing requirement for analgesic medication is the most sensitive sign of impending compartment syndrome (81). Compartment syndrome should be ruled out in any unresponsive, unreliable, or uncooperative patient (e.g., head trauma, drug, or alcohol intoxication) who has sustained significant trauma to an extremity. Likewise, the diagnosis of compartment syndrome should be considered in any child with significant injury to an extremity.

There are a number of other situations in which acute compartment syndrome may develop. Children with known bleeding dyscrasias are at particular risk, there are reports of compartment syndrome even after very minor injury. Compartment syndromes have been reported as a complication of treatment with MAST trousers (82). Rapid systemic resuscitation can also cause secondary extremity compartment syndrome (SECS) in otherwise uninjured extremities (83). Though rare, SECS is associated with high mortality, and compartment pressures should be monitored in any patient with severe diffuse edema following resuscitation.

Intracompartmental Compartment Pressure Measurement

Direct intracompartmental compartment pressure measurement can accurately quantify and diagnose compartment syndrome. This should be thought of as a confirmatory test; if there is significant clinical suspicion, compartment pressures are best measured in the operating room prior to definitive treatment so as not to delay care. Pressures can be easily measured in the operating room by attaching a 18-gauge needle to an arterial line. A number of commercially available devices accurately measure compartment pressure, and Whitesides has described a method to quickly measure compartment pressures using items commonly available in any emergency room (84). It is critical that compartment pressures are measured in all compartments in the affected extremity (e.g., anterior, lateral, deep posterior, and superficial posterior in the tibia). Compartment syndromes of the foot require a high index of suspicion, and compartment pressures should be measured in any crush injury as contractions may result from unrecognized, subacute compartment, which may be limited to just one or two of the nine individual compartment in the foot (85).

There is some variability in the definition of compartment syndrome as measured by compartment pressures. Normal resting muscle pressures are less than 5 mmHg. Most authors agree that emergent fasciotomy is indicated when compartment pressures reach 30 mmHg, or within 10 to 30 mm of diastolic pressure (86,87). Fasciotomies must address all involved compartments, with wounds generally left open for several days until swelling subsides.

CONCLUSION

Current attention on reduction of medical errors is an opportunity for all medical specialties to critically analyze results within the entire specialty and not just at one facility. Specialty-driven quality improvement initiatives will be attractive to funding sources and should lead to consensus guidelines. The impact of developing clinical guidelines on quality of care and costs can be significant. Consensus guidelines will have direct economic relevance while bringing order and conformity to patient management resulting in optimal utilization of resources while maximizing patient safety. The rapidly changing health care environment has put new pressures of accountability on physicians. There is a great need and opportunity to apply evidence-based methodology in pediatric trauma care and pediatric surgery in general to enhance the care for our patients (88,89). Specialty-wide outcomes research and evidence-based studies will allow pediatric surgeons to proactively define optimal care, reduce complications, and enhance both physician and patient satisfaction.

ACKNOWLEDGMENT

This work was supported in part by the Arnold P Gold Foundation.

REFERENCES

1. Potoka DA, Schall LC, Gardner MJ, et al. Impact of pediatric trauma centers on mortality in a statewide system. J Trauma 2000; 49:237–245.
2. Calkins CM, Bensard DD, Moore EE, et al. The injured child is resistant to multiple organ failure: A different inflammatory response? J Trauma 2002; 53:1058–1063.
3. Hoff WS, Holevar M, Nagy KK, et al. Practice management guidelines for the evaluation of blunt abdominal trauma. J Trauma 2002; 53:602–615.
4. Malhotra AK, Fabian TC, Croce MA, et al. Blunt hepatic injury: A paradigm shift from operative to nonoperative management in the 1990s. Ann Surg 2000; 231:804–813.
5. Potoka DA, Schall LC, Ford HR. Risk factors for splenectomy in children with blunt splenic trauma. J Pediatr Surg 2002; 37:294–299.
6. Hackam DJ, Potoka D, Meza M, et al. Utility of radiographic hepatic injury grade in predicting outcome for children after blunt abdominal trauma. J Pediatr Surg 2002; 37:386–389.
7. Mehall JR, Ennis JS, Saltzman DA, et al. Prospective results of a standardized algorithm based on hemodynamic status for managing pediatric solid organ injury. J Am Coll Surg 2001; 193:347–353.
8. Moore EE, Cogbill TH, Jurkovich GJ. Organ injury scaling: Spleen and liver (1994 revision). J Trauma 1995; 38:323–324.
9. Stylianos S and the APSA Trauma Committee. Evidence-based guidelines for resource utilization in children with isolated spleen or liver injury. J Pediatr Surg 2000; 35:164–169.

10. Stylianos S and the APSA Trauma Study Group. Prospective validation of evidence-based guidelines for resource utilization in children with isolated spleen or liver injury. J Pediatr Surg 2002; 37:453–456.

11. Mooney DP, Birkmeyer NJO, Udell JV. Variation in the management of pediatric splenic injuries in New Hampshire. J Pediatr Surg 1998; 33:1076–1080.

12. Wilcox JJ, Lovvorn HN, Schropp KP, et al. Nonoperative management of splenic trauma in children: Failure, complications, and pseudoaneurysms. J Pediatr Surg 2003 personal communication.

13. Frumiento C, Vane DW. Changing patterns of treatment for blunt splenic injuries: A 11-year experience in a rural state. J Pediatr Surg 2000; 35:985–989.

14. Rhodes M, Smith S, Boorse D. Pediatric trauma patients in an "adult" trauma center. J Trauma 1993; 35:384–393.

15. Keller MS, Vane DW. Management of pediatric blunt splenic injury: Comparison of pediatric and adult trauma surgeons. J Pediatr Surg 1995; 30:221–225.

16. Pearl RH, Wesson DE, Spence LJ. Splenic injury: A five year update with improved results and changing criteria for conservative management. J Pediatr Surg 1989; 24:428–431.

17. Lynch JM, Ford H, Gardner MJ. Is early discharge following isolated splenic injury in the hemodynamically stable child possible? J Pediatr Surg 1993; 28:1403–1407.

18. Morse MA, Garcia VF. Selective nonoperative management of pediatric blunt splenic trauma: Risk for missed associated injuries. J Pediatr Surg 1994; 29:23–27.

19. Nance ML, Keller MS, Stafford PW. Predicting hollow visceral injury in the pediatric blunt trauma patient with solid visceral injury. J Pediatr Surg 2000; 35:1300–1303.

20. Shafi S, Gilbert JC, Carden S. Risk of hemorrhage and appropriate use of blood transfusions in pediatric blunt splenic injuries. J Trauma 1997; 42:1029–1032.

21. Miller K, Kou D, Stallion A, et al. Pediatric hepatic trauma: Does clinical course support intensive care unit stay? J Pediatr Surg 1998; 33:1459–1462.

22. Goettler CE, Stallion A, Grisoni ER, et al. Delayed hemorrhage after blunt hepatic trauma. J Trauma 2002; 52:556–559.

23. Fisher JC, Moulton SL. Nonoperative management and delayed hemorrhage following pediatric liver injury. J Pediatr Surg 2004; 39:619–622.

24. Shilyansky J, Navarro O, Superina RA, et al. Delayed hemorrhage after nonoperative management of blunt hepatic trauma in children: A rare but significant event. J Pediatr Surg 1999; 34:60–64.

25. Brown RL, Irish MS, McCabe AJ, et al. Observation of splenic trauma: When is a little too much? J Pediatr Surg 1999; 34:1124–1126.

26. Norotsky MC, Rogers FB, Shackford SR. Delayed presentation of splenic artery pseudoaneurysms following blunt abdominal trauma: Case reports. J Trauma 1995; 38:444–447.

27. Frumiento C, Sartorelli K, Vane DW. Complications of splenic injuries: Expansion of the nonoperative theorem. J Pediatr Surg 2000; 35:788–791.

28. Pryor JP, Stafford PW, Nance ML. Severe blunt hepatic trauma in children. J Pediatr Surg 2001; 36:974–979.

29. Hoyt DB, Bulger EM, Knudson MM. Death in the operating room: An analysis of a multi-center experience. J Trauma 1994; 37:426–432.

30. Moulton SL, Lynch FP, Canty TG. Hepatic vein and retrohepatic vena caval injuries in children: Sternotomy first? Arch Surg 1991; 126:1262–1266.

31. Watts DD, Trask A, Soeken K, et al. Hypothermic coagulopathy in trauma: Effect of varying levels of hypothermia on enzyme speed, platelet function, and fibrinolytic activity. J Trauma 1998; 44:846–854.

32. Denton JR, Moore EE, Codwell DM. Multimodality treatment for Grade V hepatic injuries: Perihepatic packing, arterial embolization, and venous stenting. J Trauma 1997; 42:964–968.

33. Yang EY, Marder SR, Hastings G, et al. The abdominal compartment syndrome complicating nonoperative management of major blunt liver injuries: Recognition and treatment using multimodality therapy. J Trauma 2002; 52:982–986.

34. Kushimoto S, Arai M, Aiboshi J, et al. The role of interventional radiology in patients requiring damage control laparotomy. J Trauma 2003; 54:171–176.

35. Asensio JA, Demetriades D, Chahwan S. Approach to the management of complex hepatic injuries. J Trauma 2000; 48:66–69.

36. Shapiro MB, Jenkins DH, Schwab CW, et al. Damage control: Collective review. J Trauma 2000; 49:969–978.

37. Barker DE, Kaufman HJ, Smith LA, et al. Vacuum pack technique of temporary abdominal closure: A 7-year experience with 112 patients. J Trauma 2000; 48:201–207.

38. Vargo D, Sorenson J, Barton R. Repair of Grade VI hepatic injury: Case report and literature review. J Trauma 2002; 53:823–824.

39. Cogbill TH, Moore EE, Jurkovich GJ. Severe hepatic trauma: A multicenter experience with 1335 liver injuries. J Trauma 1998; 28:1433–1438.

40. Hirshberg A, Mattox KL. Planned re-operation for severe trauma. Ann Surg 1995; 222:3–8.

41. Rotondo MF, Schwab CW, McGonigal MD. Damage control: An approach for improved survival in exsanguinating penetrating abdominal injury. J Trauma 1993; 35:375–383.

42. Stylianos S, Jacir NN, Hoffman MA, et al. Pediatric blunt liver injury and coagulopathy managed with packs and silo. J Trauma 1990; 30:1409–1410.

43. Stylianos S. Abdominal packing for severe hemorrhage. J Pediatr Surg 1998; 33:339–342.

44. Evans S, Jackson RJ, Smith SD. Successful repair of major retrohepatic vascular injuries without the use of shunt or sternotomy. J Pediatr Surg 1993; 28:317–320.

45. Horwitz JR, Black T, Lally KP. Venovenous bypass as an adjunct for the management of a retrohepatic venous injury in a child. J Trauma 1995; 39:584–585.

46. Davies MRQ. Iatrogenic hepatic rupture in the newborn and its management by pack tamponade. J Pediatr Surg 1997; 32:1414–1419.

47. Strear CM, Graf JL, Albanese CT, et al. Successful treatment of liver hemorrhage in the premature infant. J Pediatr Surg 1998; 33:849–851.

48. Markley MA, Mantor PC, Letton RW, et al. Pediatric vacuum packing wound closure for damage-control laparotomy. J Pediatr Surg 2002; 37:512–514.

49. Adams JM, Hauser CJ, Livingston DH, et al. The immunomodulatory effects of damage control abdominal packing on local and systemic neutrophil activity. J Trauma 2001; 50:792–800.

50. Saggi BH, Sugerman HJ, Ivatury RR, et al. Abdominal compartment syndrome. J Trauma 1998; 45:597–609.

51. Oda J, Ivatury RR, Blocher CR, et al. Amplified cytokine response and lung injury by sequential hemorrhagic shock and abdominal compartment syndrome in a laboratory model of ischemia-reperfusion. J Trauma 2002; 52:625–632.

52. Rezende-Neto JB, Moore EE, de Andrade MVM, et al. Systemic inflammatory response syndrome secondary to abdominal compartment syndrome: Stage for multiple organ failure. J Trauma 2002; 53:1121–1128.

53. Sharpe RP, Pryor JP, Gandhi RR, et al. Abdominal compartment syndrome in the pediatric blunt trauma patient treated with paracentesis: Report of two cases. J Trauma 2002; 53:380–382.

54. Hobson KG, Young KM, Ciraulo A, et al. Release of abdominal compartment syndrome improves survival in patients with burn injury. J Trauma 2002; 53:1129–1134.

55. Chang MC, Miller PR, D'Agostino R, et al. Effects of abdominal decompression on cardiopulmonary function and visceral perfusion in patients with intra-abdominal hypertension. J Trauma 1998; 44:440–445.

56. DeCou JM, Abrams RS, Miller RS, et al. Abdominal compartment syndrome in children: Experience with three cases. J Pediatr Surg 2000; 35:840–842.

57. Epelman M, Soudack M, Engel A, et al. Abdominal compartment syndrome in children: CT findings. Pediatr Radiol 2002; 32:319–322.

58. Neville HL, Lally KP, Cox CS. Emergent abdominal decompression with patch abdominoplasty in the pediatric patient. J Pediatr Surg 2000; 35:705–770.

59. Bass BL, Eichelberger MR, Schisgall MR. Hazards of non-operative therapy of hepatic trauma in children. J Trauma 1984; 24:978–982.

60. Scioscia PJ, Dillon PW, Cilley RE. Endoscopic sphincterotomy in the management of posttraumatic biliary fistula. J Pediatr Surg 1994; 29:3–6.

61. Sharif K, Pimpalwar AP, John P, et al. Benefits of early diagnosis and preemptive treatment of biliary tract complications after major blunt liver trauma in children. J Pediatr Surg 2002; 37:1287–1292.

62. Sharpe RP, Nance ML, Stafford PW. Nonoperative management of blunt extrahepatic biliary duct transection in the pediatric patient. J Pediatr Surg 2002; 37:1612–1616.

63. Church NG, May G, Sigalet DL. A minimally invasive approach to bile duct injury after blunt liver trauma in pediatric patients. J Pediatr Surg 2002; 37:773–775.

64. Moulton SL, Downey EC, Anderson DS. Blunt bile duct injuries in children. J Pediatr Surg 1993; 28:795–797.

65. Bass J, DiLorenzo M, Desjardins JG. Blunt pancreatic injuries in children: The role of percutaneous external drainage in the treatment of pancreatic pseudocysts. J Pediatr Surg 1988; 23:721–724.

66. Burnweit C, Wesson D, Stringer D. Percutaneous drainage of traumatic pancreatic pseudocysts in children. J Trauma 1990; 30:1273–1277.

67. Rescorla FJ, Cory D, Vane DW. Failure of percutaneous drainage in children with traumatic pancreatic pseudocysts. J Pediatr Surg 1990; 25:1038–1042.

68. Rescorla FJ, Plumley DA, Sherman S. The efficacy of early ERCP in pediatric pancreatic trauma. J Pediatr Surg 1995; 30:336–340.

69. Jobst MA, Canty TG, Lynch FP. Management of pancreatic injury in pediatric blunt abdominal trauma. J Pediatr Surg 1999; 34: 818–824.

70. Canty TG, Weinman D. Treatment of pancreatic duct disruption in children by an endoscopically placed stent. J Pediatr Surg 2001; 36:345–348.

71. Canty TG, Weinman D. Management of major pancreatic duct injuries in children. J Trauma 2001; 50:1001–1007.

72. Shilyansky J, Sen LM, Kreller M, et al. Non-operative management of pancreatic injuries in children. J Pediatr Surg 1998; 33:343–349.

73. Wales PW, Shuckett B, Kim PC. Long-term outcome of non-operative management of complete traumatic pancreatic transection in children. J Pediatr Surg 2001; 36:823–827.

74. Meier DR, Coln CD, Hicks BA, et al. Early operation in patients with pancreas transection. J Pediatr Surg 2001; 36:341–344.

75. McGahren ED, Magnuson D, Schauer RT, et al. Management of transection of the pancreas in children. Aust NZ J Surg 1995; 65:242–246.

76. Boman-Vermeeren JM, Vermeeren-Walters G, Broos P, et al. Somatostatin in the treatment of a pancreatic pseudocyst in a child. J Pediatr Gastroenterol Nutr 1996; 23:422–425.

77. Soto JA, Alvarez O, Munera F, et al. Traumatic disruption of the pancreatic duct: Diagnosis with MR pancreatography. Am J Roentgenol 2001; 176:175–178.

78. Mann DC, Rajmaira S. Distribution of physeal and nonphyseal fractures in 2650 long-bone fractures in children aged 0–16 years. J Pediatr Orthop 1990; 10:713–716.

79. Gustilo RB, Anderson JT. Prevention of infection in the treatment of one thousand and twenty-five open fractures of long bones: Retrospective and prospective analyses. J Bone Joint Surg Am 2002; 84-A:682.

80. Kreder HJ, Armstrong P. The significance of perioperative cultures in open pediatric lower-extremity fractures. Clin Orthop 1994; 302:206–212.

81. Bae DS, Kadiyala RK. Acute compartment syndrome in children: Contemporary diagnosis, treatment, and outcome. J Pediatr Orthop 2001; 21:680–688.

82. Aprahamian C, Gessert G. MAST-associated compartment syndrome: A review. J Trauma 1989; 29:549–555.

83. Tremblay LN, Feliciano DV. Secondary extremity compartment syndrome. J Trauma 2002; 53:833–837.

84. Whitesides TE, Heckman MM. Acute compartment syndrome: Update on diagnosis and treatment. J Am Acad Orthop Surg 1996; 4:209–218.

85. Manoli A. Compartment syndromes of the foot: Current concepts. Foot Ankle 1990; 10:340–344.

86. Heckman MM, Whitesides TE. Histologic determination of the ischemic threshold of muscle in the canine compartment syndrome model. J Orthop Trauma 1993; 7:199–210.

87. McQueen M. Acute compartment syndrome. Acta Chir Belg 1998; 98:166–170.

88. Hardin WD, Stylianos S, Lally KP. Evidence-based practice in pediatric surgery. J Pediatr Surg 1999; 34:908–913.

89. Stylianos S. Outcome studies and practice guidelines in trauma. Sem Pediatr Surg 2002; 11:36–41.

23 | Complications of Pediatric Transplantation

Stephen P. Dunn, M.D. and Nikolai A. Bildzukewicz, M.D.

INTRODUCTION

Solid organ replacement therapy has now become standard for the treatment of children with heart, liver, intestinal and renal failure. In 2007, 543 liver and 727 renal transplants were performed in children across the United States. Early recovery from solid organ transplantation is the best predictor of long-term survival. A foundation of solid surgical technique underlies the success of all transplant procedures.

Due to the inherent technical difficulties as well as the often small patient size in the pediatric population, complications are common following solid organ transplantation. Surgical complications frequently impair graft function and may ultimately lead to the demise of the patient. These complications are also very expensive, significantly increasing total hospital costs (1). Thus, it is essential to promptly diagnose and treat these problems to minimize morbidity and mortality.

The goal of this chapter is to provide a broad overview as well as some detail regarding common, technical complications of solid organ transplantation in children. Familiarity with common complications is useful not only to pediatric surgeons but also to other physicians as these patients are often seen in their local communities for follow-up care. The focus of this chapter will be complications pertinent to hepatic and renal transplantation, the most common solid organs transplanted in patients younger than 18 years. The reader is encouraged to pursue further reading on each of these subjects for a more precise understanding of the management of these complications. The management of these events continues to evolve as improvements in diagnosis and treatment are implemented.

LIVER TRANSPLANTATION

Liver transplantation continues to be one of the most demanding procedures performed in pediatric patients. A precisely performed operative procedure, good graft function, and aggressive treatment of postoperative complications are fundamental to successful outcomes for these children. Most children require liver transplantation at an early age and most have had prior abdominal surgery. These characteristics increase the technical difficulty of these procedures.

Before discussing postoperative complications, a word on technical variant allograft and expanded-criteria donors is necessary to frame the role they play in regard to postoperative complications.

Technical Variant Grafts

Recently, the use of hepatic grafts has expanded to include reduced, split, and living-related donors. These technical variant grafts were originally advocated to expand the donor pool, and they are now the most common transplant allograft type in children. With this expansion, however, comes an increased risk for postoperative vascular and biliary complications.

With the exception of living-donor hepatic grafts, technical variant grafts are associated with a poorer recipient prognosis when compared to whole organ transplants (2). The cause of increased mortality associated with these grafts may be related in part to the higher acuity of these patients. Except for recipients of living-donor grafts, recipients of technical variant grafts have an increased PELD (Pediatric End Stage Liver Disease) score when compared to recipients of whole organs. This suggests that the health of the recipient may be one of the main contributors to post-transplant outcome in technical variant graft recipients. Technical variant grafts have been shown to be the most significant variable for late graft loss following transplantation (3).

Technical variant grafts are created by division of a whole donor liver into smaller portions, and this presents additional complexity for vascular reconstruction. Typical arterial reconstruction for a right lobe graft is donor right hepatic artery to recipient hepatic artery. Portal reconstruction is typically from the donor right portal vein branch to the recipient main portal vein. For a left lateral segment graft, the left branch of the portal vein and left branch of the hepatic artery are the typical inflow vessels. The left lateral segment artery can be quite small, often measuring only two to three millimeters in size. The importance of using visual magnification in reconstructing these vessels is emphasized.

Preservation of the recipient vena cava is a common adjunct to reconstruction of these segmental or technical variant grafts. This results in a so-called piggyback configuration in which the liver is sewn onto the recipient vena cava with an anastomosis of the donor hepatic veins directly to the recipient inferior vena cava.

Bile duct reconstruction in technical variant grafts is almost always to a Roux-en-Y limb of jejunum. Most children do not require a long Roux-en-Y segment as this may adversely affect nutrition as well as drug absorption. Roux-en-Y limbs of 20 cm are deemed adequate by many pediatric transplant surgeons. Stent placement across the biliary anastomosis is not standard due to the difficulty in removing the stent as well as the high incidence of stone formation around the stent if left in place.

An obvious risk factor for surgical complications of technical variant graft procedures is size discrepancy. If the graft is too small, there may be inadequate hepatic function and acute portal hypertension. If the graft is too big, there may be respiratory compromise. Attempted abdominal closure may result in impairment of perfusion of the graft. The optimal size relationship of the graft to the recipient body weight is 0.8% to 6%. This may be accurately estimated by preoperative assessment with volumetric CT scanning of the potential donor.

Expanded-Criteria Donors

The need for a greater number of donor organs has resulted in the increased recovery of livers from donors previously considered marginal. The organs of these expanded-criteria donors may function well and be lifesaving in their recipients. However, the recipient's overall risk as well as the risk of postoperative complications is increased when an expanded-criteria donor is used. Similarly, donation after cardiac death has also been pursued as an additional source of donor organs. Currently, liver transplantation has a 1.85-fold increased risk of failure in recipients of organs from donation after cardiac death (4). Ischemic biliary injuries are also associated with organs from these donors.

Primary Nonfunction

Primary hepatic nonfunction is a serious complication following liver transplantation in which the allograft does not provide primary hepatic support for the recipient. This uncommon, life-threatening complication occurs in 1% to 6% of patients, and presents early in the postoperative period (5). Primary nonfunction, if left untreated, results in multiorgan injury, cerebral edema, and brain death. The allograft must be replaced promptly.

The cause of primary nonfunction is poorly understood. Risk factors can be divided into donor, transplant, and recipient factors. Laboratory values that have been identified in donor populations where the risk of primary nonfunction is increased include elevations in prothrombin time and serum sodium levels. The presence of allograph steatosis (especially greater than 60% macrovesicular steatosis) has also been identified as a significant risk factor. In addition, preexisting donor conditions such as anemia, hypoxia, and hypotension requiring vasopressor support may also play a role. In terms of operative risk factors, primary nonfunction is associated with prolonged cold ischemic times as well as technically difficult vascular anastomoses. Postoperative hypotension and vascular thrombosis in the recipient also increase the risk for primary nonfunction. The incidence of this complication in living-related transplants is less than 2% suggesting that donor quality may be an important contributor to the higher incidence of primary nonfunction in cadaveric transplantation.

Primary nonfunction is more highly associated with technical variant grafts. This may be due to an increase in cold ischemic time associated with back table dissection or division of the allograft. An attempt to do more of these recoveries with in situ division while maintaining perfusion has been advocated (6).

Characteristically, the patient with primary nonfunction will quickly become ill, developing marked coagulopathy and encephalopathy. Laboratory evaluation usually reveals marked elevation of serum ammonia, liver transaminases (aspartate aminotransferase (AST) and alanine aminotransferase (ALT) greater than 5000), and a marked prolongation in the prothrombin time (international normalized ratio (INR) greater than 2.5). This coagulopathy will manifest clinically as intra-abdominal bleeding or bleeding from the operative wound and all skin puncture sites. This is usually associated with hemodynamic instability, which then progresses rapidly to acute renal failure and eventual cardiovascular collapse. The patient's mental status usually remains obtunded in the early postoperative period and progresses to hepatic coma. Immediate allograft replacement is indicated. In cases where transaminases rise and prolongation of the prothrombin time is more modest without other evidence of end organ injury, careful observation with supportive care has been successful. However, all of these patients should be treated as if retransplantation is necessary and should be given priority status on the waiting list for retransplantation. Immediate allograft replacement has been successful in these cases. Primary nonfunction is one of the leading causes of retransplantation in children, occurring in 16% to 30% of transplant recipients (7,8).

Vascular Complications

Vascular complications are common following pediatric liver transplantation. When compared to adults, children are at greater risk for vascular complications, principally, due to smaller vessel diameter. These complications may be either arterial or venous, and they typically present early in the postoperative period. Problems include both stenosis and thrombosis of the hepatic artery, portal vein, hepatic veins, and inferior vena cava. Their prompt recognition and treatment is essential to minimize morbidity and ensure long-term graft survival. Some of the more common complications are discussed later.

Hepatic Artery Thrombosis

The most common and serious postoperative complication in pediatric liver transplantation leading to graft failure is hepatic artery thrombosis. Failure to recognize hepatic artery thrombosis will result in graft failure as well as decreased patient survival. It accounts for 10% to 33% of all causes of liver retransplantation (7,8). In the past, hepatic artery thrombosis occurred in approximately 40% of pediatric transplant recipients, carrying with it a mortality of 50% to 58% (9). With advances in microsurgical techniques, now only 5% of patients develop hepatic artery thrombosis during the first 30 days following transplantation (10).

The single most important contributing factor to hepatic artery thrombosis is the technical difficulty of adequately providing good arterial flow. Additional risk factors include a history of smoking, prolonged cold ischemia time, size discrepancy between donor and recipient vessels, prior liver transplant, cytomegalovirus (CMV) infection, and acute rejection within the first postoperative week (11). A postoperative hypercoagulable state may also increase the risk of hepatic artery thrombosis. In addition to smaller arterial size, children also have lower mean arterial pressures, putting them at greater risk of thrombosis.

The adequacy of hepatic artery reconstruction can normally be determined in the operating room by evidence of blood flow in the recipient vessel. This can be assessed by direct observation and by Doppler evaluation. The experienced transplant surgeon is rarely misled by the adequacy of arterial perfusion of the graft.

Clinical presentation varies widely in patients with hepatic artery thrombosis, which may manifest acutely, or be chronic and indolent in its course. If minor, patients may exhibit mild elevations of liver enzymes. If severe, they may present with acute liver failure progressing eventually to fulminant hepatic necrosis. This is marked by markedly elevated liver enzymes, worsening coagulopathy, and mental status changes.

Resultant biliary problems are also frequent, especially biliary leaks. Blood flow to the biliary anastomosis is dependent on the hepatic artery. If this blood flow is compromised, the anastomosis can break down, resulting in bile leakage. If hepatic artery thrombus formation follows a more chronic course, biliary strictures or even hepatic abscesses may form. Some patients may remain asymptomatic owing to a well-developed collateral arterial supply (12). To help avoid this dreaded complication, routine Doppler ultrasound examination of the hepatic allograft should be performed within 24 hours of the procedure, and any failure to identify hepatic arterial waveform should lead to immediate angiographic investigation or surgical exploration.

Immediate operative intervention with thrombectomy is required for acute hepatic artery thrombosis. This is frequently successful, especially when the return to the operating room identifies a technical problem that can be corrected. Careful thrombectomy of the recipient hepatic artery with embolectomy catheters, excision of the damaged portions of the vessels with a second anastomosis, and the addition of anticoagulation is usually successful in maintaining patency of the artery and salvaging the graft. Balloon angioplasty as well as endoluminal stent placement are useful adjuncts for late presentations (12). Hyperbaric oxygen may also play a role in stabilizing patients with hepatic artery thrombosis as well as delaying the need for retransplantation (13).

In an attempt to prevent hepatic artery thrombosis, postoperative administration of various medications and blood products is used at most centers. Our own preference is to use fresh frozen plasma to restore more normal coagulation parameters as well as an antiplatelet agent (aspirin) daily for patients with platelet counts over 50,000. This approach addresses the deficiency of antithrombin III in the immediate post-transplant period. This regimen has been associated with an extremely low rate of hepatic artery thrombosis. Other centers routinely place patients on low molecular weight heparin or dextran in the postoperative period (14).

Numerous prophylactic approaches have been taken to try and improve the success of hepatic artery reconstruction. The initial efforts were directed at long aortic conduits taken from the donor that were placed in an infrarenal location. Over time, it was found that this was not beneficial and led to a higher rate of thrombosis, in part due to accumulation of thrombus in the size-discrepant aortic conduit. Celiac reconstruction has been advocated using proximal reconstruction of the donor celiac artery to the recipient celiac axis. This is only possible with whole organ transplantation or in technical variant grafts where the celiac axis is preserved with the segmental graft. As mentioned earlier, all vascular anastomoses should be performed under magnification, either with loupes or with the operating microscope as an aid to technical perfection.

The risk of hepatic artery thrombosis has been shown to be increased in whole liver grafts when compared to reduced-size, technical variant grafts (15). With the advent of living-donor as well as in situ split-liver transplantation, primary end-to-end reconstruction of the hepatic artery using fine microvascular techniques has been associated with a lower rate of thrombosis, thus confirming that precise surgical technique is the foundation of successful hepatic artery reconstruction (14).

Portal Vein Thrombosis

Portal vein thrombosis is a relatively uncommon complication of hepatic transplantation. It has a frequency of 1% to 4%. Portal vein size, anatomic positions, decreased portal vein flow, and the type of graft used in reconstruction are all considered risk factors for portal vein thrombosis (16). It is also seen more frequently in recipients with prior portal vein thrombosis as well as those with previous portal vein operations.

Portal vein thrombosis can present early or late in the postoperative period. It is sometimes clinically silent, or it may present with mild elevations in hepatic function tests with worsening ascites. It can also present with signs and symptoms of portal hypertension including splenomegaly and bleeding from esophageal varices (17). Failure to diagnose and treat portal vein thrombosis can lead to graft failure.

Doppler ultrasound is the imaging modality of choice if portal vein thrombosis is suspected clinically. Magnetic resonance angiography is a good second option. Other tests that may be used include transhepatic portography and mesenteric angiography. These interventional radiologic techniques can not only confirm but can also treat portal venous thrombosis.

Once diagnosed, immediate attempts at revascularization should be made with reexploration and open thrombectomy (using balloon embolectomy catheters), but long-term success is limited. In some cases, segmental portal vein resection may be necessary. Percutaneous approaches with portal vein thrombectomy, balloon angioplasty, or thrombolysis are also possible but may be complicated by postoperative hemorrhage. Mesocaval shunting may be necessary to control bleeding or ascites. Postshunt encephalopathy is a common complication of this approach. In rare cases where the child has received a whole organ transplant and the left branch of the portal vein remains patent, a mesoportal shunt may be successful. Eventually, graft replacement via retransplantation may be required to treat the complications associated with portal vein thrombosis.

A few methods have been described to help reduce the incidence of portal vein thrombosis. One of the most common indications for liver transplantation in children is biliary atresia. The portal vein in these patients is frequently small and hypoplastic, and there has been a compensatory increase in hepatic arterial blood flow. Experience has demonstrated that dissection of the portal vein toward the confluence of the superior mesenteric vein and splenic veins with anastomosis to the more dilated portion of the portal vein creates better inflow to the recipient portal vein (18). For technical variant grafts, rotation of the left lateral segment graft approximately 90 degrees counterclockwise around the long axis of the body creates a better orientation of the portal vessels and less kinking of the anastomosis. In spite of these technical precautions, thrombosis still occurs. Underlying coagulopathy is generally considered to contribute to this complication. Anticoagulation is not usually given specifically for prophylaxis of portal venous thrombosis, but to the extent that it is used to prevent hepatic artery thrombosis, the portal vein anastomosis probably benefits.

Hepatic Vein Outflow Obstruction

Hepatic vein obstruction is an extremely rare complication following pediatric liver transplantation. Whole organ transplantation usually involves caval replacement and therefore the hepatic veins are not at great risk. Also, triangulation of the caval side of the hepatic vein-to-caval anastomosis in the piggyback configuration used for segmental grafts creates a large anastomosis that infrequently fails.

Hepatic vein outflow obstruction is usually a result of kinking of the suprahepatic cava or hepatic-caval anastomosis. This can occur when the graft is relatively small for the child as the graft may not sit securely in the right upper quadrant. Careful orientation of the graft at the time of implantation is required to avoid this complication.

Hepatic vein obstruction typically presents with hepatomegaly, graft dysfunction, and hepatocyte injury manifested by rapidly rising hepatic enzymes. Splenomegaly and massive ascites are common. Doppler ultrasound will show poor venous outflow in these circumstances. Immediate reoperation is required, and revision of the caval anastomosis may be necessary to restore hepatic vein outflow. Retransplantation is indicated if the allograft injury is severe.

Inferior vena cava thrombosis is rare. In whole liver transplants, it occurs at either the superior or inferior caval anastomosis. A higher incidence is reported with the piggyback technique. Risk factors for inferior vena caval thrombosis include intraoperative technical difficulties, the use of intravascular catheters, and compression of the inferior vena cava by surrounding fluid collections (19). In children, it may be clinically silent except for the presence of increased lower extremity edema. Doppler ultrasound and MR angiography are the studies of choice. If diagnosed late, inferior vena cava thrombosis is not easily treated. The thrombosis is usually extensive, extending from the suprarenal cava to the hepatic veins. Replacement of the cava is theoretically possible but is not usually indicated due to the relatively mild symptoms of venous hypertension in most children.

Hemorrhage

Hemorrhage is avoidable in most instances. Intraoperative blood loss in hepatic transplantation is common with an average transfusion requirement equaling one or more of the patient's total blood volume per case. Hemorrhage is more often related to coagulopathy in children with hepatic failure. Nevertheless, careful operative technique usually results in a relatively dry operative field by the completion of the procedure, especially if the transplanted liver is functioning adequately. Severe intraoperative bleeding may be a manifestation of diffuse intravascular coagulation. The most accurate measure of abnormalities of coagulation intraoperatively is thromboelastography. Empiric treatment of intraoperative hemorrhage with Factor VII or Amicar has been successful (20). It should be noted that there is a higher risk of vascular thrombosis when these agents are used.

Clinically, post-transplant hemorrhage presents as excessive bloody drainage from perihepatic drains, a dropping hematocrit, decreased urine output, and/or hypotension. Reoperation is required for any of these signs. At reoperation, surgical bleeding is the rule rather than the exception. Correction is usually straightforward. Hemorrhage in the setting of poor graft function is alarming for medical bleeding and may be a manifestation of primary graft non-function. In these cases, management of the coagulopathy with attempts to find a replacement allograft is the best approach.

Biliary Complications

Complications of the biliary reconstruction are the most common problems seen following pediatric liver transplantation. Most occur within the first 3 months postoperatively, but they may be seen several months or even years after the procedure. Overall, the incidence in whole organ transplantation is 6% to 8%. It is 10% to 16% in reduced-size transplants and 15% to 20% in living-related transplants. These complications include bile leaks, bile duct strictures, intrahepatic bile duct injuries with segmental stenosis and biliary lakes, and biliary sludge or cast syndrome. Percutaneous management of these complications is successful 89% of the time (21).

As mentioned earlier, bile duct problems are a common complication in patients with hepatic artery thrombosis. The interruption of hepatic artery blood supply results in bile duct injury due to the critical requirement of the biliary tree for nutrient arterial blood flow. This is especially seen in the early postoperative period where arterial interruption may cause injury to the hepatic parenchyma, but almost always is associated with a slightly delayed necrosis of portions of the extrahepatic bile ducts. This usually results in a bile leak with biloma formation. Other significant risk factors for biliary complications include the mode of hepatic artery reconstruction, CMV infection, intrapulmonary shunting, and ABO incompatible transplantation (22). In addition, the presence of more than one bile duct in the allograft has been shown to increase the incidence of biliary complications following liver transplantation in children (23).

Clinically, bile leaks present as bile noted in operative drains. These leaks are common in segmental or technical variant grafts. Most small leaks arise from the raw surface of the divided liver, and they typically stop within a few days of diagnosis. Leaks which continue beyond this time are abnormal and may require operative intervention. Investigations which may be helpful in decision making are cholescintigraphy (HIDA) scans and retrograde drainage studies. These better define the site of the leak and the adequacy of the biliary drainage. Immediate reoperation is not always necessary if it can be inferred from clinical information that the leak is small and well drained.

Once an indication for retransplantation, the majority of bile leaks are now managed nonoperatively with the use of percutaneous transhepatic biliary stents. Initial drainage of the biloma and antibiotic therapy for the associated infection are the most appropriate initial therapies. Failure of conservative management or a major disruption of the anastomosis mandates an immediate retransplantation (24).

Biliary obstruction is usually the result of a stricture in the ductal system. Biliary strictures occurring within the first postoperative month are usually the result of technical surgical errors. Late bile duct strictures are usually the result of impaired blood flow, but they may occur in the absence of measurable hepatic artery thrombosis. Most of the strictures occur at the cut margin of the liver where the bile duct is transected during the hepatic division. Intrahepatic strictures are uncommon when the hepatic artery is patent. There is a higher incidence of strictures noted in reduced-size and living-related transplants (25).

Like biliary leaks, obstruction can usually be treated nonoperatively (26). Initial treatment of these anastomotic strictures is most commonly by percutaneous transhepatic stent placement. In some cases, temporary stent placement alone is successful. It has been our approach to reoperate on cases after temporary stent placement and revise the hepaticojejunostomy by performing a stricturoplasty. This has proven successful in almost all cases with a very low incidence of recurrence.

Intrahepatic bilomas or bile lakes are a late manifestation of bile duct injury. They present as cholangitis and are associated with an infected intrahepatic fluid collection. Polymicrobial infection is common. These bilomas are associated with hepatic artery thrombosis in most cases. Percutaneous drainage may be used as a temporizing measure. Long-term management may require segmental hepatic resection or retransplantation. Identification and treatment of the proximal bile duct stricture associated with these lesions is usually not successful.

Bile sludge syndrome or biliary cast syndrome is a complication due to graft ischemia or graft preservation injury. Repeated endoscopic retrograde cholangiopancreatography (ERCP) irrigation and balloon clearance of sludge may maintain graft function and prevent biliary obstruction. Most children do not have a biliary tree that is accessible by ERCP as their biliary drainage is to a Roux-en-Y limb of jejunum. Allograft replacement may be necessary if cholangitis or biliary obstruction becomes unmanageable.

Infectious Complications

Intra-abdominal Abscess

Intra-abdominal abscess formation is a risk for all children receiving a liver transplant. Contamination of the operative field is common due to enterotomies made during the hepatectomy, the creation of the Roux-en-Y limb of jejunum, and spillage of bile from the donor or recipient organ. Most of these abscesses are caused by gram-negative bacteria, but they may also be due to gram-positive organisms or yeast. Broad spectrum perioperative coverage is common as are attempts to eliminate fluid collections with wide surgical drainage. Undrained blood or fluid provides an excellent, nutrient-rich environment for bacterial growth. Bile leaks may lead to intra-abdominal abscess if they are not recognized and drained.

Intra-abdominal abscesses characteristically present with fever and other signs of infection including an elevated white blood cell count and bacteremia. The majority is diagnosed with CT scanning. The use of intravenous antibiotics along with percutaneous drainage has replaced operative exploration in most cases.

RENAL TRANSPLANTATION

Introduction

Children present with end stage renal disease from the newborn period to adolescence. The underlying pathology ranges from those unique to the newborn to those that are more commonly found in adults. Transplantation of the small child is almost always deferred until an optimal size for living-related or cadaveric transplantation is achieved. The ability to fit an adult kidney within the child's abdomen is frequently the ultimate consideration. Living-related donor transplantation has the best graft outcome for children, with a 93% 1-year and 75% 5-year graft survival rate (27). After size considerations, bladder or urologic considerations present the most unique problems for childhood renal transplantation. An adequate, low-pressure, continent reservoir for urine, which can be catheterized, is necessary.

Surgical complications are the most common complications following renal transplantation in children, and they often lead to significant morbidity (28). These complications following include delayed graft function or acute tubular necrosis (ATN), vascular thrombosis, urinary leak or obstruction, vesicoureteral reflux, and lymphocele (29–34). The risk of complications is highly associated with specific patient groups or allograft characteristics. The risk of ATN increases with increased warm and cold ischemic time. Vascular complications are more common in smaller children where the recipient vessels may be small or there may be pressure on the graft from a tight abdominal closure (35). A small allograft may twist causing vascular obstruction due to kinking of the vessels. Urologic complications are more common in children with bladder abnormalities or reconstructed urine reservoirs (28). Ureteral ischemia may cause failure of the ureteroneocystostomy or ureteroureterostomy resulting in urine leak or ureteral obstruction (28). As in hepatic transplantation, prompt recognition and treatment of these complications is important to maximize patient and graft survival.

Acute Tubular Necrosis

ATN is a clinical syndrome characterized by oliguria in a well-perfused kidney. Immediate function of the transplanted kidney with a brisk diuresis is generally expected after transplantation. Minimal or no urine output suggests the possibility of allograft dysfunction which may be due to ATN or a number of other causes. The incidence of ATN is low in living-donor transplantation, thus demonstrating the nearly negligible impact of cold storage on renal function when cold storage times are short and the allograft is otherwise healthy. Prolonged cold storage is associated with an extremely high rate of ATN. Organs recovered from donation after cardiac death also have an increased rate of ATN due to donor warm ischemia prior to recovery.

In the early post-transplant period, low or absent urine output is addressed by a treatment algorithm. Establishing patency of the urine drainage catheter is the initial step. Hemodynamic parameters are then assessed and interventions made to optimize perfusion of the renal allograft. Doppler ultrasound examination of the transplanted kidney is performed to assess allograft blood flow, the ureter, and bladder. Diuretics may be given when indicated to determine if flow of urine can be established. A urinary fractional sodium excretion assessment is performed if urine is available for assessment prior to diuretic administration. If perfusion is good, the ureter is not obstructed or leaking, and the drainage catheter is patent, ATN is likely. A radionucleotide excretion study will support the diagnosis. Renal biopsy is helpful in excluding other causes of graft dysfunction such as accelerated acute rejection. Other pathologic mechanisms are suspected as time from transplant without diuresis increases.

Reducing intravenous fluids to one-third of maintenance requirements and performing dialysis when indicated are the standard treatments for ATN. ATN will usually resolve with recovery of adequate renal function if the recipient can be supported with dialysis and no further renal injury occurs. In the past, rejection of the nonfunctioning renal allograft decreased the recovery of these organs. Many programs now use a long acting polyclonal antilymphocyte antibody to prevent rejection when there is evidence of ATN.

Vascular Thrombosis

The renal allograft has an arterial and a venous anastomosis to recipient vessels. The iliac artery and vein, or the aorta and vena cava, are the typical recipient vessels to which the donor renal artery and vein are attached. The renal allograft is typically placed into the right iliac fossa. Access to recipient vessels is readily available using an extraperitoneal approach. Some have advocated an intra-abdominal approach in smaller children, but an extraperitoneal approach is almost always possible. Intra-abdominal allograft placement increases the likelihood of intraperitoneal complications, especially postoperative adhesions which can lead to intestinal obstruction (30).

Vascular complications are usually associated with a large kidney in a small child. Experience is most helpful in situating the donor graft to optimize vascular reconstruction. The left kidney is typically used due to its longer vein. This positions the renal vein posteriorly when placed in the right iliac fossa. The renal artery then must pass either over this vein or around it to join the recipient iliac artery or aorta. Attention to the potential competition for space and an attempt to optimize location is required with this type of reconstruction. It is frequent that the donor renal vein has to be shortened to avoid kinking. The renal artery must be sewn to its recipient vessel without vessel angulation. If an extraperitoneal approach has been used, graft movement is unusual. The adequacy of vascular reconstruction is easily assessed in the operating room. It is always better to remove the kidney, reperfuse it with cold preservation fluid, and then start again than to accept a tenuous vascular reconstruction. Thrombosis of the artery or vein almost always results in graft loss. Proper positioning of the graft and careful vascular reconstruction are the best methods to prevent vascular thrombosis.

Suspected vascular thrombosis may be diagnosed by Doppler ultrasound, CT angiography, or by a nuclear medicine blood flow study. Immediate return to the operating room is necessary in order to salvage the graft. Thrombectomy, cold perfusion of the kidney with vascular reconstruction, and heparinization of the recipient may be successful at times, but many grafts have already suffered catastrophic injury at diagnosis. Graft nephrectomy is the usual treatment in an obviously necrotic graft.

Urinary Complications

Many children requiring a renal transplant have had obstructive uropathy as the cause of their renal failure. Prior surgical procedures may have left the retroperitoneum scarred. The bladder is frequently abnormal and augmentation of the bladder may have been performed. It is best to have carefully planned the urinary reconstruction prior to transplantation. The presence of an experienced pediatric urologist to assist with urinary reconstruction is desirable.

Obstruction of the urinary catheter with blood after transplantation is a common and vexing problem in children. Overdistention of a small, unused bladder may result in intravesicle bleeding and care should be used when distending the bladder prior to reconstruction. When bleeding from the bladder occurs, irrigation catheters may be necessary. Transurethral placement may not be possible due to the large caliber of these catheters. A suprapubic catheter may be necessary in addition to a transurethral catheter in these circumstances. Irrigation of the bladder catheter is the first step in clearing the catheter of blood. Sterile water is used to induce red cell lysis. Small volumes of sterile water with aspiration of the instilled amount are repeated until the fluid returned is no longer grossly bloody. This approach is usually successful.

Obstruction of the ureter is associated with ureteral necrosis. The ureteral blood supply is segmental, but interruption of the blood supply to the lower pole of the kidney frequently causes ischemia to the ureter. Careful attention to lower pole perfusion is necessary during vascular reconstruction in order to avoid ureteral ischemia. The ureteral blood supply may also be interrupted by dissection in the triangle of tissue between the ureter and the lower pole of the kidney. Ureteral obstruction can be treated temporarily by percutaneous tube nephrostomy. Shoker et al. demonstrated that early use of percutaneous nephrostomy significantly improved graft survival and reduced the incidence of further complications (36). Placement of a ureteral stent by cystoscopy is usually unsuccessful. Reoperation for ureteral obstruction is almost always required with revision of the ureteroneocystostomy.

A urinary leak following ureteroneocystostomy may occur for several reasons. The ureter may become dislodged from the bladder tunnel, or the ureter may become necrotic due to ischemia causing disruption of the ureteroneocystostomy. The bladder itself may rupture at the site of the ureteral implantation. Urinary leaks usually manifest as decreased urine output with increased output from perinephric drains. Urinary leaks usually require reexploration with revision of the ureteroneocystostomy. The use of a ureteral stent placed at the time of revision is beneficial.

Vesicoureteral reflux is relatively common in children due to obstructive uropathy. Most surgeons will remove the nonfunctioning kidneys along with their ureters in an attempt to decrease the rate of postoperative urinary tract infection. This complication is due to the reflux of urine into dilated remnant ureters. A nonrefluxing ureteroneocystostomy is always desirable but especially so in these circumstances. A higher rate of graft loss due to reflux and upper tract infection is documented in these cases. Reimplantation of the ureter is performed in cases of post-transplant vesicoureteral reflux.

Lymphocele

Lymphoceles are collections of lymphatic fluid in the retroperitoneal tissues near the transplanted allograft. Dissection of perivascular lymphatic vessels near the iliac vessels, aorta, or vena cava with subsequent lymphatic leak is the usual cause. Lymphoceles may be asymptomatic, or they may cause obstruction of the ureter. Ultrasound will demonstrate the fluid collection and may document partial ureteral obstruction. Dynamic excretion as demonstrated by a radionucleotide function study can provide further evidence of ureteral obstruction. Lymphoceles are successfully treated 50% of the time with percutaneous catheter drainage and sclerotherapy (36). In other cases, open or laparoscopic marsupialization of the lymphocele to the peritoneal cavity is curative.

REFERENCES

1. Ammori JB, Pelletier SJ, Mathur A, et al. Financial implications of surgical complications in pediatric liver transplantation. Pediatr Transplant 2008; 12:174–179.
2. Diamond IR, Fecteau A, Millis JM, et al. Impact of graft type on outcome in pediatric liver transplantation: A report from studies of pediatric liver transplantation (SPLIT). Ann Surg 2007; 246(2):301–310.
3. Sieders E, Peeters PM, TenVergert EM, et al. Graft loss after pediatric liver transplantation. Ann Surg 2002; 235(1):125–132.
4. Organ Donation Breakthrough Collaborative. http://www.organdonationow.org (Oct 17, 2007).
5. D'Alessandro AM, Knechtle SJ, Chin LT, et al. Liver transplantation in pediatric patients: Twenty years of experience at the University of Wisconsin. Pediatr Transplant 2007; 11:661–670.
6. Yersiz H, Renz JF, Farmer DG, et al. One hundred in situ split-liver transplantations: A single-center experience. Ann Surg 2003; 238(4):496–507.
7. Jain A, Mazariegos G, Kashyap R, et al. Pediatric liver transplantation: A single center experience spanning 20 years. Transplantation 2002; 73(6):941–947.
8. Uribe M, Buckel E, Ferrairo B, et al. Pediatric liver retransplantation: Indications and outcome. Transplant Proc 2007; 39:609–611.
9. Mazzaferro V, Esquivel CO, Makowka L, et al. Hepatic artery thrombosis after pediatric liver transplantation: A medical of surgical event? Transplantation 1989; 47:971–977.

10. Settmacher U, Stange B, Haase R, et al. Arterial complications after liver transplantation. Transpl Int 2000; 13:372–378.

11. Vivarelli M, Cucchetti A, La Barba G, et al. Ischemic arterial complications after liver transplantation in the adult: Multivariate analysis of risk factors. Arch Surg 2004; 139:1069–1074.

12. Moray G, Boyvat F, Sevmis F, et al. Vascular complications after liver transplantation in pediatric patients. Transplant Proc 2005; 37:3200–3202.

13. Mazariegos GV, O'Toole K, Mieles LA, et al. Hyperbaric oxygen therapy for hepatic artery thrombosis after liver transplantation in children. Liver Transpl Surg 1999; 5(5):429–436.

14. Goss JA, Shackleton CR, McDiarmid SV, et al. Long-term results of pediatric liver transplantation: An analysis of 569 transplants. Ann Surg 1998; 228(3):411–420.

15. Sieders E, Peeters PM, TenVergert EM, et al. Graft loss after pediatric liver transplantation. Ann Surg 2002; 235(1):125–132.

16. Buell JF, Funaki B, Cronin DC, et al. Long-term venous complications after full-size and segmental pediatric liver transplantation. Ann Surg 2002; 236(5):658–666.

17. Millis JM, Seaman DS, Piper JB, et al. Portal vein thrombosis and stenosis in pediatric liver transplantation. Transplantation 1996; 62(6):748–754.

18. Broniszczak D, Szymczak M, Kaminski A, et al. Vascular complications after pediatric liver transplantation from the living donors. Transplant Proc 2006; 38:1456–1458.

19. Carnevale FC, Borges MV, de Paula Pinto RA, et al. Endovascular treatment of stenosis between hepatic vein and inferior vena cava following liver transplantation in a child: A case report. Pediatr Transplant 2004; 8:576–580.

20. Markiewicz M, Kalicinski P, Kaminski A, et al. Acute coagulopathy after reperfusion of the liver graft in children correction with recombinant activated factor VII. Transplant Proc 2003; 35(6):2318–2319.

21. Lorenz JM, Funaki B, Leef JA, et al. Percutaneous transhepatic cholangiography and biliary drainage in pediatric liver transplant patients. Am J Radiol 2001; 176:761–765.

22. Egawa H, Uemoto S, Inomata Y, et al. Biliary complications in pediatric living related liver transplantation. Surgery 1998; 124:901–910.

23. Salvalaggio PR, Whitington PF, Alonso EM, et al. Presence of multiple bile ducts in the liver graft increases the incidence of biliary complications in pediatric liver transplantation. Liver Transpl 2005; 11:161–166.

24. Karakayali H, Boyvat F, Sevmis S, et al. Biliary complications and their management in pediatric liver transplantations: One center's experience. Transplant Proc 2005; 37:3174–3176.

25. Schindel D, Dunn S, Casas A, et al. Characterization and treatment of biliary anastomtic stricture after segmental liver transplantation. J Pediatr Surg 2000; 35(6):940–942.

26. Kling K, Lau H, Colombani P. Biliary complications of living related pediatric liver transplant patients. Pediatr Transplant 2004; 8:178–184.

27. El-Husseini AA, Foda MA, Shokeir AA, et al. Determinants of graft survival in pediatric and adolescent live donor kidney transplant recipients: A single center experience. Pediatr Transplant 2005; 9:763–769.

28. Lapointe SP, Charbit M, Jan D, et al. Urologic complications after renal transplantation using ureteroureteral anastomosis in children. J Urol 2001; 166:1046–1048.

29. Shokeir AA, Osman Y, Eli-El-Dein B, et al. Surgical complications in live-donor pediatric and adolescent renal transplantation: Study of risk factors. Pediatr Transplant 2005; 9(1):33–38.

30. Sheldon C, Churchill BM, Khoury AE, et al. Complications of surgical significance in pediatric renal transplantation. J Pediatr Surg 1992; 27(4):485–490.

31. Nelson EW, Kessler R, Holman JM. Surgical complications in pediatric renal transplantation. Transplant Proc 1989; 21(1):2006–2007.

32. Kalicinski P, Kaminski A, Prokurat A, et al. Surgical complications after kidney transplantation in children. Transplant Proc 1994; 26(1):42–43.

33. Rawn JD, Tilney NL. The early course of a patient with a kidney transplant. Kidney Transplantation: Principles and Practice, Chapter 12. 4th ed. 167–178.

34. McDonald SP, Craig JC. Long-term survival of children with end-stage renal disease. N Engl J Med 2004; 350(26):2654–2662.

35. Tanabe K, Takahashi K, Kawaguchi H, et al. Surgical complications of pediatric kidney transplantation: A single center experience with the extraperitoneal technique. J Urol 1998; 160:1212–1215.

36. Shokeir AA, Osman Y, Ali-El-Dein B, et al. Surgical complications in live-donor pediatric and adolescent renal transplantation: Study of risk factors. Pediatr Transplant 2005; 9:33–38.

24 | Complications in Pediatric Urology

Jennifer K. Yates, M.D. and Anthony A. Caldamone, M.D.

Pediatric urology encompasses a wide variety of surgical cases, ranging from open oncologic and reconstructive surgeries to minimally invasive procedures. Unique to pediatric urology are genital reconstruction procedures that, while similar to adult reconstructive cases, have a different set of considerations when performed in the pediatric population.

While complications are expected in any surgical field, there are certain principles that may be applied to pediatric urology to minimize the risk of complications. These principles will be reviewed in detail with each section. Acknowledging that the urinary tract as a continuous system from renal pelvis to urethral meatus is critical. Taking care to preserve this continuity by performing watertight repairs and avoiding obstruction prevents many complications. Attempts to protect the sterility of the urinary tract helps prevent infection and associated tissue and suture line breakdown. The genitourinary system is supported by unique vascular networks. Meticulous dissection to preserve vascular pedicles is a critical principle in genital reconstruction. Attention to the vascular supply of the ureter, medially based proximally and laterally based distally, is important to prevent stricture and reconstructive failure.

This chapter will review the common complications, strategies to avoid complications, and techniques to repair or salvage complications of pediatric urology. Some of the most commonly performed procedures such as hypospadias repair, ureteral reimplantation, circumcision, nephrectomy, pyeloplasty, and endoscopic management of vesicoureteral reflux are included.

HYPOSPADIAS

The approach to the patient with hypospadias has changed over the past few decades with the development of new techniques and a better comprehension of the basic science of the formation and repair of hypospadias. The most commonly encountered complications of hypospadias repair include urethrocutaneous fistula, urethral diverticulum, meatal stenosis, meatal regression, stricture, persistent chordee, hairy urethra, and undesirable cosmetic outcome.

Choosing the most appropriate technique of repair based on anatomical features of the defect, such as chordee, the quality of skin coverage, the shape of the glans, and the quality of the urethral plate, is essential for a successful outcome.

Basic principles of tissue handling and surgical technique reduce the incidence of complications during the repair of hypospadias. Gentle tissue handling with appropriate instruments minimizes tissue trauma. Intermittent use of a tourniquet and the judicious use of pinpoint electrocautery are useful for the prevention of postoperative hemorrhage. Injection of glanular and subcutaneous tissues with local anesthetic and epinephrine (diluted 1:100000 to 1:200000) also assists in hemostasis and the development of tissue planes. Overlapping suture lines should be avoided when possible. The technique for hypospadias repair is based in large part on the position of the meatus, the presence of ventral chordee, the quality of the urethral plate, the coverage over the urethra, and available tissues for reconstruction. If chordee is present, the penis is first degloved to determine whether simply degloving the ventral shaft corrects the chordee. If there is persistent chordee after degloving, various techniques may be employed to release the chordee, which can be divided into those techniques which shorten the dorsal side and those which lengthen the ventral side.

Factors Affecting Rates and Types of Complications

The type and rate of complications vary by technique employed for hypospadias repair. There is a higher rate of complication associated with repair of proximal hypospadias. Early techniques used a two-stage approach with the belief that one-stage techniques, especially in the setting of more proximal hypospadias defects, were associated with an unacceptable complication rate. Kass et al. described single-stage hypospadias repair using a second layer of neourethral coverage in 206 patients (1). Only 4.4% of the patients required a secondary surgical procedure. The authors attribute their high success rate to the use of a second layer of coverage from nearby tissue beds. They also noted no difference in complication rates between the three age groups studied (6 to 18 months, 18 months to 5 years, and older than 6 years of age).

Several authors have examined the rate of complications that occurs with an onlay flap versus tubularized island flaps. These two techniques are often used with a more proximal defect, or in the case of a tubularized flap, when the urethral plate cannot be used. Wiener et al. compared these two techniques in patients with a proximal defect (2). They noted a similar incidence in the complication rate in general, as well as the rate of fistula formation. However, they found a significant difference in fistula size between the two groups, with all onlay fistulas pinpoint in size and repaired easily, while in 6 of the 10 tubularized group fistulas were large and required a complex repair. They also found that megalourethra or diverticula developed in 12% of the tubularized group while none formed in the onlay group. The authors suggest that the onlay graft receives support from the urethral plate and is fixed on either side of the plate, while the tubularized graft lacks this support. These findings are important to consider during a tubularized graft repair, and attempts to adequately tailor the graft and provide support with a second layer may help decrease this complication.

Powell et al. compared the use of flaps and grafts in the repair of proximal hypospadias (3). The majority of these patients demonstrated defects at the penoscrotal junction after excision of unhealthy urethral plate. They found that there was no difference in complication rates between those patients repaired with a flap versus a graft. However, the free onlay graft had fewer strictures than the free-tubed graft.

Meatal Stenosis and Meatal Regression

Meatal stenosis and regression are most commonly associated with the procedures that reposition the meatus at the tip of the glans in the setting of a distal hypospadias. Meatal stenosis can result from a tight closure of the glans wings or ischemia at the meatus. While meatal stenosis itself can be troublesome, it can also contribute to the pathogenesis of additional complications, such as urethral diverticulum and urethrocutaneous fistula (Fig. 1). Meatal stenosis may be amenable to simple dilation at home. If the stenosis is refractory to gentle dilation, a meatoplasty may be required. Cases that recur after meatoplasty may require more extensive reconstruction, often using an onlay flap or tubularized incised urethroplasty (4).

Palmer et al. described use of an island pedicle graft for repair of meatal stenosis (5). The meatus is incised along the ventral midline. The distance from the apex of the urethral incision to the original meatus is measured and mapped on normal adjacent penile skin. The skin incision is extended and an island of skin is created, preserving a vascular pedicle. The island pedicle is then mobilized until it reaches the meatal defect. The authors describe three patients in whom this technique was applied, and in all three meatal stenosis resolved and the patients had excellent postoperative flow rates.

Meatal regression occurs when the glanuloplasty is not performed adequately such that there is tension on the glanuloplasty from inadequate mobilization of the glans wings. Teague et al. described the use of a meatal-based flap (modified Mathieu) to repair retraction with excellent results (6). The advantages of island pedicled grafts include placement of normal skin with good vascularity, avoidance of suturing into scar tissue, and prevention of future contractures.

Persistent Chordee

The incidence of persistent chordee has diminished due to the intra-operative use of the artificial erection following degloving of the penis and after techniques to correct chordee is undertaken. If chordee is noted, it may be addressed and the appropriate hypospadias repair may then be undertaken. Techniques to repair chordee that is present after penile degloving include excision of fibrous spongiosal tissue vertically, dorsal plication as described by Nesbit (7), mobilization of

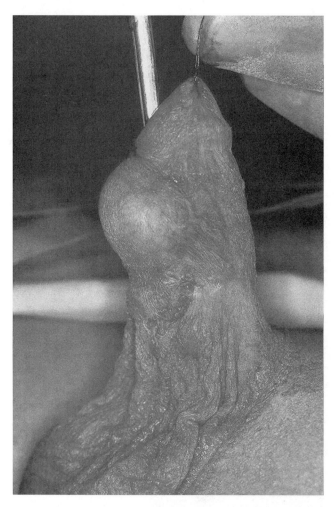

Figure 1 Megalourethra after hypospadias repair. Note the ballooning of ventral tissue.

the urethra from the corporal bodies, and dermal, tunica vaginalis, or progressed tissue grafts. Occasionally the urethral plate is incised to release chordee. In this situation, a tubularized urethroplasty technique or a two-stage repair would be required.

In reviewing the management of complications of hypospadias repair, Secrest et al. described 71 patients with residual chordee (8). Techniques used to repair the residual chordee include resection of residual chordee tissue and scar from the prior surgery, incision of the tunica albuginea with dermal graft, Nesbit tunica plication, penoscrotal Z-plasty, and excision of the scarred urethra. The reparative procedure was definitive in 63 patients, while 8 required additional surgery.

Urethral Diverticulum

Signs and symptoms suggesting a urethral diverticulum include post-void dribbling, ballooning of the ventral aspect of the urethra with voiding (Fig. 2), and stone formation. Factors implicated in formation of a diverticulum include distal obstruction and creation of a neourethra that is too wide.

In describing their experience with transverse preputial island flap urethroplasty (TPIF), Aigen et al. reported four patients with "megalourethra" (9). Of these four patients, one had concurrent meatal stenosis. They suggested this complication could be attributed to use of a graft that is too wide or of tissue that is inadequate to support the urethra. To prevent megalourethra, the authors recommend tailoring the width of the neourethra, and covering the neourethra with a tight second layer to provide support. Careful glanular tunneling in a free graft pedicled

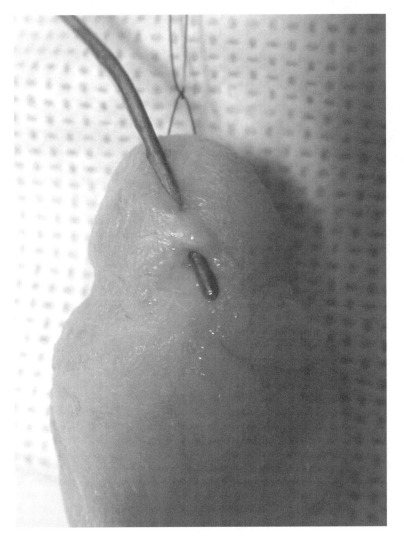

Figure 2 Meatal stenosis and urethral fistula after hypospadias repair. Note the lacrimal duct probe in urethral meatus. The meatus could not be sounded larger than the probe.

tubed repair and distal meatal anastomosis could prevent distal narrowing that can contribute to urethral diverticulum formation.

The rate of diverticulum formation varies among repairs. As previously mentioned, Wiener et al. (2) compared the complication rates of the onlay flap and tubularized island flap and found the rate of diverticulum formation to be higher in the tubularized group. This finding may be due to the tacking of the onlay graft on both sides of the urethral plate, which provides more support and creates a smaller neourethral lumen.

Repair of the diverticulum is usually performed by incising and trimming the excess tissue, and then closing the neourethra and overlying tissue. Zaontz et al. described a technique to repair anterior urethral diverticula with reinforced suture lines in a "pants over vest" technique (10).

Urethrocutaneous Fistulas

Fistulas are the most common complication following hypospadias repair. Signs and symptoms of fistula formation include an area of inflammation or infection on the ventral skin, wound breakdown, and leakage during spontaneous voiding. Several factors implicated in fistula formation include infection and tissue ischemia. To avoid infection, most patients are maintained on broad-spectrum antibiotics. There are no data proving that perioperative antibiotics decrease the fistula rate; however, many surgeons use these empirically. Tissue ischemia can be minimized with gentle tissue manipulation and ensuring an adequately vascularized bed for the repair, especially with the use of flaps.

Urethrocutaneous fistulas may be associated with distal obstruction or meatal stenosis. One must always be mindful of a possible distal stenosis or diverticulum as a contributing factor to the fistula. Therefore, evaluation of the urethra distal to the fistula is essential at the time of repair.

Management of fistulas begins with prolongation of the urinary diversion duration, as long as the catheter is still in place. If the catheter has been removed, we do not advocate replacement as it may result in further trauma to the repair. Repair of a fistula is best undertaken when the tissues have regained their suppleness. This is generally not before 6 months postoperatively. Small fistulas may be repaired with simple excision and closure. Inherent to the success of primary repair is adequate coverage, ideally with a well-vascularized second layer. The Durham–Smith technique employs de-epithelialized flaps of tissue found lateral to the fistula (4). This technique avoids overlapping suture lines.

Similarly, Geltzeiler et al. described the use of de-epithelialized tissue and skin advancement techniques for repair of fistulas (11). For coronal fistulas, a second layer of subcutaneous tissue from the shaft is used for coverage, followed by a freed skin edge from the proximal shaft, which is brought to a small area of de-epithelialized glans. For shaft fistulas, a "pants over vest" technique is used, involving creation of a subcutaneous lateral flap. This flap is brought over the repair and a skin flap from the opposite side is brought over the deep epithelialized subcutaneous flap, thus avoiding crossing the suture lines.

Santangelo et al. reviewed the outcomes of 94 fistula repairs (12). Simple fistula repairs were those requiring a single technique to gain coverage. Similar to the techniques described above, de-epithelialized flaps or skin advancement flaps were used for coverage in coronal and shaft fistulas. Complex repairs involved larger fistulas and those associated with other defects. These repairs often consisted of tubularized or onlay pedicled graft for repair of the fistula (Fig. 3). The overall failure rate was 6.4%, with a rate of 4.3% for simple repairs.

Urethral Strictures

Symptoms associated with postoperative strictures include straining to void, inadequate urinary stream, dysuria, urinary retention, and urinary tract infections (UTIs). As mentioned previously, a stricture may be associated with a urethrocutaneous fistula. Factors implicated in stricture formation include infection, trauma from instrumentation, tissue ischemia, and errors in technique. The rate of stricture formation varies depending on the type of repair.

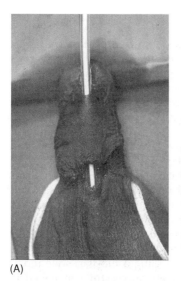 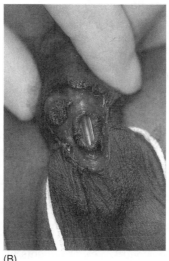 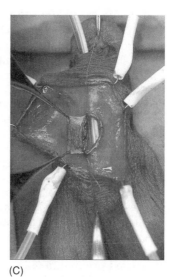

(A)   (B)   (C)

Figure 3 (**A**) Proximal fistula after hypospadias repair. (**B**) Island onlay graft harvested and fistula isolated. (**C**) Island onlay graft used to repair fistula.

Options for the treatment of strictures include serial urethral dilations, internal urethrotomy, and open urethroplasty. One limitation of internal urethrotomy is scar formation. Multiple internal urethrotomies can lead to propagation of scar tissue and the development of spongiofibrosis and ultimately a more difficult open urethroplasty. Techniques for open urethroplasty will be reviewed in the next section, as these techniques are also applied to those patients with extensive or refractory urethrocutaneous fistulas and failure of hypospadias repair.

With the advent of the tubularized incised plate (TIP) procedure described by Snodgrass, there was concern that the technique would have a high rate of stricture formation (13,14). The TIP involves a longitudinal incision in the urethral plate to allow enough tissue mobilization for tubularization. Intuitively, such an incision would seem to predispose for stricture, especially when considering that such incision in the adult urethra (during internal urethrotomy) results in scar formation. Snodgrass reviewed his initial 72 patients who underwent the procedure (15). In all of the patients, the urethra could be calibrated to at least 10 French. Urethroscopy was undertaken in seven patients who were undergoing anesthesia for another reason. In all of these patients, a normal caliber urethra was observed.

Complications Associated with Buccal Mucosal Grafts

Free grafts are employed when there is inadequate local tissue available for repair in the setting of either a severe hypospadias or during reoperative hypospadias repair. With the development of techniques that allow more versatile use of local tissues, the need for free grafts has diminished. Buccal mucosa is the most commonly used free graft for creation of the neourethra. Other free graft sources include bladder mucosa and skin, but these are often associated with a higher rate of complications, as well as the need for a second incision for harvest of the bladder mucosa. Duckett et al. examined free buccal grafts histologically and compared them to penile skin and urothelium (16). They found buccal mucosa had thinner lamina propria and thicker epithelium, as well as increased vascularity. This may explain the superior results found with buccal mucosal grafts compared to other free grafts.

The complication rate associated with buccal mucosal grafts ranges from 13% to 72% (17). The most common complications are stricture and meatal stenosis (16–18). Other complications include graft contracture, sloughing, fistula, and complications associated with the donor site. The majority of complications are noted within the first year after repair and seem to decrease with experience (16,18).

Caldamone et al. reported their experience with 22 urethral reconstructions using buccal mucosal graft; 11 of these patients were children (19). Six onlay grafts and 16 tubularized grafts were used. Nine complications were noted, eight in the tubularized graft group and one in the onlay group. The complications included two meatal stenoses, four fistulas, and three strictures.

Techniques for Salvage Hypospadias

The treatment of hypospadias in the setting of multiple failed procedures and repair of urethral strictures after hypospadias draws on many of the techniques used for urethrocutaneous fistula repair. The principles are similar, in that adequate tissue for a neourethra, multiple layers of vascularized coverage, and finally skin coverage can be challenging. Challenges of using local tissue include lack of available tissue, scarring of remaining penile skin, poor vascularity, and distortion of tissue planes. Figure 4 demonstrates complete loss of the penile urethra after an island onlay urethroplasty; subsequent repair is challenging when local tissue has been used for the original repair.

If local tissue is available, techniques such as meatal-based flaps and preputial flaps can be used. Jayanthi et al. (20) reported the results of 44 pedicle flaps for salvage repairs (20). Of these, 20 (71%) were Mathieu urethroplasties and required no further surgery. Sixteen patients underwent salvage island flap procedures, and 43% required no further procedures. Based on these results, they advocated the use of local skin flaps, with an appropriate period of time between the last repair and the salvage procedure (mean interval 3 years). Secrest et al. reported outcomes in patients requiring complete urethral reconstruction; of these, 65 patients presented with stricture, 57 had persistent hypospadias, 22 had urethral diverticuli, and 10 had an ablated neourethra (8). Of this cohort, 53% of patients undergoing a flip-flap style repair and 71% of those undergoing salvage island flap procedures were successfully managed in a single-stage repair. Simmons et al. similarly advocated preservation of the urethral plate in salvage procedures (20,21). Correction with a single procedure was possible in 83% of patients.

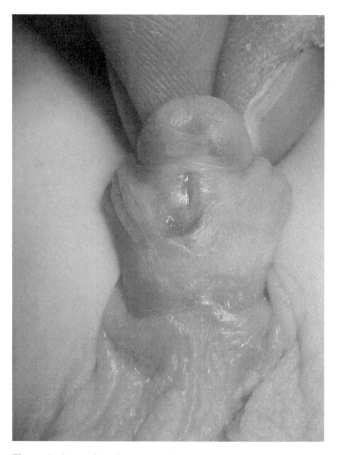

Figure 4   Loss of penile urethra after island onlay urethroplasty.

Of patients undergoing Mathieu repair, 76% of repairs were successful, while 86% of patients managed with an onlay flap had a successful outcome with a single procedure.

Utilization of the urethral plate during salvage hypospadias can also be accomplished using the TIP urethroplasty, provided that the urethral plate is not scarred. The advantages of this technique in repeat procedures include a well-vascularized native urethral plate and a urethroplasty that does not require additional skin flaps. Borer et al. reviewed 25 reoperations using this method and found a complication rate of 24% (22). Nguyen and Snodgrass (23) reported their experience with 31 patients who underwent reoperative repair using the TIP technique (23). Of these patients, a urethral plate incision had been made at a prior repair in 18 (58%). The authors included only those patients with a healthy appearing urethral plate in the TIP repair group. If the urethral plate did not have adequate mobility or was obviously scarred, a staged buccal mucosal repair was utilized. Ninety percent of patients had a successful outcome and had a functional neourethra and vertical slit meatus. The overall complication rate was 23%, with a higher fistula rate in those patients who had a second layer coverage derived from tissues lateral to the neourethra as opposed to those with a dartos barrier flap. The results of these studies suggest that TIP urethroplasty is a viable option for salvage hypospadias repair. When the urethral plate cannot be used, or when there is inadequate local tissue for neourethral repair or second layer coverage, free grafts and staged procedures are employed. Figures 5 and 6 demonstrate the use of buccal mucosal graft for salvage repairs.

Conclusion

Many complications associated with hypospadias repair can be prevented with meticulous surgical technique and appropriate technique selection based on individual anatomy. As the technical options for repair of hypospadias repair expand, success rates with both primary repairs and salvage procedures are improving.

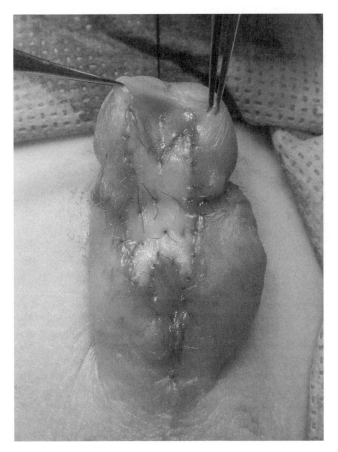

Figure 5   Salvage buccal mucosal graft. Buccal mucosa has been harvested and 'quilted' into place over the urethral plate.

URETERAL REIMPLANTATION

Vesicoureteral reflux (VUR) is associated with an increased risk of pyelonephritis and renal scarring. Recurrent episodes of upper UTI can lead to renal scarring. This may result in renal insufficiency, hypertension, complications during pregnancy, and end-stage renal disease.

The relationship between VUR and pyelonephritis with subsequent renal scarring was first reported by Hutch, who described the phenomenon in adult patients with neurogenic bladders (24). Since that time multiple surgical techniques have evolved for the correction of VUR. Most recently, endoscopic techniques have been explored for minimally invasive management of VUR. While the development of surgical and endoscopic techniques has made the surgical treatment of VUR safer and technically more successful, there is still debate as to which children would benefit from surgery versus medical management. The most recent "VUR guidelines panel summary report" helps to guide the clinician in determining the best course of management (25), although these recommendations preceded the FDA approval of endoscopic correction. A new guidelines panel summary report is currently in progress.

Reimplantation techniques can be divided into intravesical, extravesical, laparoscopic reimplantations, and robotic. This chapter will address the first two techniques. Each technique has unique attributes and potential complications.

Intravesical Reimplantation of the Ureter

The Politano–Leadbetter reimplantation technique creates a new internal hiatus. Following the creation of a new location of bladder entry, the ureter is passed in a retrovesical fashion to enter this new hiatus. This technique allows creation of a tunnel of varying length and the ureteral orifice remains in a typical anatomic position. This repositioning allows for future retrograde

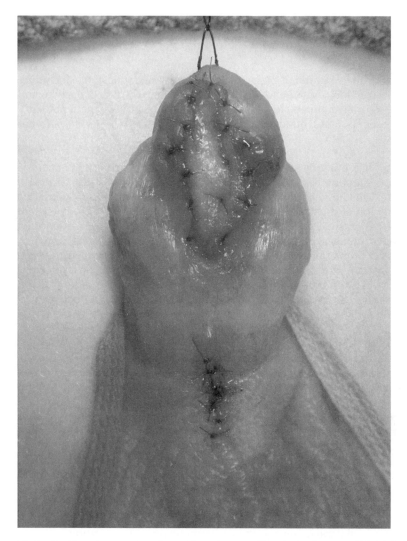

Figure 6 Buccal mucosal graft used for salvage urethroplasty of a more distal defect.

catheterization. Complications have been reported with blind passage of the ureter behind the bladder during creation of the neohiatus and mobilization of the ureter.

The Glenn–Anderson reimplantation technique is a ureteral advancement strategy, involving intravesical mobilization of the ureter and creation of a submucosal tunnel from the original hiatus toward the bladder neck. The advantage of this procedure is that there is no need for extravesical dissection. The main disadvantage is the limited tunnel length that can be created depending on the configuration of the bladder, more specifically the distance between the original orifice position and the bladder neck.

The Cohen reimplantation technique is a cross-trigonal advancement. The advantage of this technique is the ability to create a long submucosal tunnel and avoidance of complications related to creating a neohiatus. The tunnel is created along a fixed portion of the posterior bladder wall, which results in a solid muscular backing. The disadvantage of the Cohen reimplant is the displacement of the ureteral orifices out of their usual anatomic positions, theoretically making retrograde access difficult.

Extravesical Reimplantation of the Ureter

One of the main advantages of the Lich–Gregoir technique is that it does not require cystotomy. When first described, this technique was avoided in the United States due to high failure rate. Modifications to the Lich–Gregoir reimplant, with the distal advancement of the ureter, have made the technique more desirable (26). Advantages include reduced bladder spasms, hematuria, and ease of postoperative ureteral catheterization.

Early Complications
All reimplantation techniques share several of the early postoperative complications, including UTI, early postoperative obstruction, and wound infection. In a review of 322 patients who had undergone reimplantation, Mor et al. noted bleeding in six patients, fever in six patients, early postoperative UTI in five patients, and wound infection in two patients (27).

Persistent Reflux
In general, surgical repair of VUR is highly successful. Overall success rates in one meta-analysis were 95.9%, with success rates reported as 99% in Grade I, 99.1% in Grade II, 98.3% in Grade III, 98.5% in Grade IV, and 80.7% in Grade V (28). Lavine et al. reviewed 273 patients (534 ureters) who underwent reimplantation at multiple institutions over an 8-year period (29). Persistent reflux was noted in 4% of patients (2.2% of renal units). The risk factors that were identified for persistent reflux included preoperative and postoperative hydronephrosis, renal scarring, and reimplantations requiring ureteral tapering. There was no correlation between the type of reimplantation and persistent VUR. Persistent VUR may be best managed conservatively, as Siegelbaum and Rabinovitch reported four children with persistent high-grade VUR on postoperative voiding cystourethrograms (VCUG), who spontaneously resolved between 19 and 55 months postoperatively (30).

De novo Contralateral Reflux
As troubling as persistent reflux is the development of contralateral reflux which occurs de novo. The overall rate of new onset contralateral VUR as reported in the guidelines panel report was 9.1%, with no difference among the various reimplantation techniques (25). There are several theories to explain the onset of contralateral VUR, including a "pop-off" mechanism, distortion of the trigone after unilateral reimplantation, and undiagnosed preexisting contralateral VUR.

Diamond et al. compared outcomes between patients undergoing the Glenn–Anderson, Cohen, and extravesical ureteral reimplantation techniques (31). None of the contralateral orifices appeared abnormal on cystoscopy. There was an equivalent incidence in the development of contralateral reflux when comparing techniques. There was a significant trend toward an increased rate of contralateral VUR in patients with a higher grade of VUR upon presentation. The authors noted that extensive dissection of the trigone (as in the Cohen reimplantation) had similar rates of contralateral reflux when compared to the Glenn–Anderson procedure, which confine their dissection to the ipsilateral hemitrigone. Furthermore, patients undergoing extravesical reimplantation, which eliminates trigonal distortion, also had similar rates of contralateral VUR. This data does support the pop-off theory, as patients with higher initial grades of ipsilateral VUR were at greater risk for contralateral VUR. From this study, the authors concluded that patients at high risk for contralateral VUR were those with unilateral Grade V VUR and unilateral reimplantation of a duplex system.

Minevich et al. reported different results for a group of patients undergoing extravesical reimplantation (32). The rate of contralateral reflux was 5.6%, and the contralateral reflux had resolved in all patients by 31 months postoperatively. Of the four patients with contralateral VUR, two had only undergone one preoperative VCUG, and only 1 of 13 patients with high-grade VUR developed contralateral VUR. Of three patients with resolved contralateral VUR, one developed postoperative contralateral VUR. The authors suggest more accurate cyclic VCUGs to identify those at risk, as well as bilateral reimplantation for patients with a history of resolved contralateral VUR.

The presence of preoperative contralateral VUR plays an important role in the development of postoperative contralateral VUR (31–36). In the absence of complicating factors, these resolution rates favor initial conservative management.

Liu et al. evaluated the incidence of renal scarring with 99 m-dimercaptosuccinic acid (DMSA) renal scans in both ipsilateral and contralateral kidneys with reflux (35). They found that the association between scarring and contralateral VUR was more pronounced when the contralateral scarring was high grade. Based on these findings, the authors recommended bilateral ureteral reimplantation in patients with prior contralateral VUR or DMSA evidence of contralateral renal parenchymal scarring.

Postoperative Voiding Dysfunction

When the extravesical reimplantation technique was introduced, it was praised for the afore-mentioned attributes, but many urologists in the United States avoided the technique due to high rates of postoperative urinary retention with bilateral reimplantation. Follow-up data did confirm the increased risk of voiding dysfunction, but higher risk groups can be identified preoperatively. Usually the voiding dysfunction is short term. Currently, the reported rate of postoperative voiding dysfunction is between 4% and 15% (37).

Fung et al. characterized the voiding dysfunction in children after intravesical and extrav-esical repairs by evaluating post-void residuals (38). They found that the rate of voiding dysfunc-tion was similar after intravesical and unilateral extravesical repair. Those patients undergoing bilateral extravesical repair had a significantly higher rate of voiding dysfunction than the other two groups. This group also required bladder drainage for a longer postoperative period. Long-term follow-up revealed that all patients in this cohort ultimately regained normal voiding function.

Barrieras et al. proposed that dissection distal to the ureteral orifice plays a role in voiding dysfunction. They evaluated two modifications of the Lich–Gregoir extravesical reimplantation technique (39). The advancing suture modification involves a myotomy extending circumfer-entially around the ureteral orifice, thus freeing it completely from trigonal attachments. The inverted Y myotomy limits dissection distal to the ureter while preserving the ureterotrigonal unit. They found that both methods were equally effective in resolving reflux. There was a trend toward increased urinary retention in the advancing suture technique (15.2%) when compared to the Y detrusorrhaphy group (8.4%), although it did not reach statistical significance. They did identify a significantly higher rate of urinary retention in boys, patients with higher grades of reflux, and children younger than 3 years of age. In contrast, Lipski et al. did not find age or grade of reflux to be a significant predictor of postoperative dysfunction (37).

There has been some concern raised for the development of bladder dysfunction following ureteral reimplantation in young infants. Upadhyay et al. evaluated the outcome of reimplan-tation in a group of patients with a mean age of 5.4 months at the time of surgery (40). In this study, reimplantation technique included unilateral extravesical, Cohen, and modified Politano–Leadbetter reimplantation and bilateral extravesical reimplantation was not employed. Of 20 patients available for long-term follow-up, 19 had normal voided urinary volume, urinary flow, and post-void residual measurements. One patient with normal urinary flow had incomplete bladder emptying.

Diverticulum and Obstruction

Diverticuli at the ureteral hiatus can form when the neohiatus is constructed too large or if abnormal bladder pressure is present. Obstruction can occur when either the hiatus is too tight or in the face of a thick-walled bladder from previous outlet obstruction and/or elevated intravesical pressure. When closing the hiatus during an intravesical reimplant, passage of a small instrument with some ease into the hiatus provides assurance that the neohiatus will not obstruct or form a diverticulum (Fig. 7). The significance of diverticuli may be related to their association with UTIs. Ahmed et al. described 28 patients who underwent Cohen cross-trigonal reimplantation, all of whom had at least one postoperative VCUG (41). They found that 17% of patients developed diverticula, with a 2% rate of large (more than 1 cm) diverticuli formation. The large diverticuli were associated with a higher rate of UTI in female patients.

A meta-analysis by Elder et al. found the rate of ureteral obstruction to range from 0% to 9.1%, with a combined rate of 2% in those studies published after 1986 (41). This analysis found no differences between surgical techniques. As previously mentioned, closure of the ureteral hiatus must be undertaken with care to prevent obstruction. Early postoperative obstruction may occur due to edema and should be followed with serial ultrasounds or percutaneous supravesical diversion if symptomatic. A Lasix renogram should be performed to identify the degree of reduced urinary flow. If postoperative obstruction is persistently documented, revision of the reimplantation may be necessary. Weiss et al. reported on two patients who developed obstruction several years after reimplantation, presumably due to scarring (42). As a result of this experience, the suspicion for late obstruction must be maintained in the patient who presents after reimplantation with symptoms of pain, UTI, increased and persistent postoperative hydronephrosis or loss of renal function.

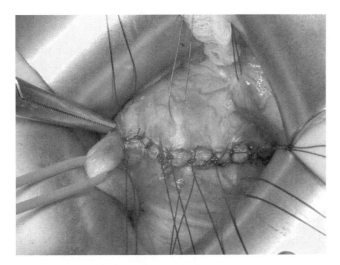

Figure 7   Easy passage of an instrument through the new ureteral hiatus helps prevent obstruction.

Laparoscopic Reimplantation

Several techniques for laparoscopic reimplantation have been described. The Gil–Vernet medial advancement was the first laparoscopic technique employed, but the technique did not gain popularity due to the high rate of failure (43). The laparoscopic adaptation of the Cohen cross-trigonal technique has also been described, with higher success rates than the Gil–Vernet technique. Yeung et al. described the procedure in 16 children (44). The reported success rate was 96%, with only one cystotomy required when a port became displaced. There were no major complications. Laparoscopic extravesical reimplantation reported by Lakshmanan and Fung had a 100% success rate without significant voiding dysfunction, but was complicated by three ureteral injuries requiring open surgical revision (45). Laparoscopic reimplantation, regardless of the success rate, is limited by the technically challenging nature of the procedure. Expansion of robotic applications in urology is being applied to reimplantation.

Conclusion

Ureteral reimplantation, whether performed intravesically or extravesically, is a well-tolerated procedure with a high success rate. Refinements in the technique have improved outcomes. The most important tenets to minimize complications are attention to operative technique, maintenance of a level of suspicion for postoperative complications, and the choice of the appropriate technique for the patient.

ENDOSCOPIC TREATMENT OF VUR

Endoscopic treatment for vesicoureteral reflux was introduced almost 20 years ago. Until recently, little data have supported the safety and efficacy of endoscopic subureteral injections, and thus the American Urologic Association guidelines for the treatment of VUR did not include this option. Polytetrafluoroethylene paste, cross-linked collagen, chondrocytes, and dextranomer/hyaluronic acid copolymer (Dx/HA) have all been used for subureteral injection. The only agent approved by the Federal Drug Administration for the endoscopic correction of VUR is Dx/HA. While the risk of complications associated with this procedure is low, the rates of failure are higher when compared to open reimplantation. Several recent studies have sought to identify the factors associated with failure.

In a meta-analysis, Elder et al. reviewed patients undergoing endoscopic treatment for VUR. The agents used for injection included polytetrafluoroethylene, collagen, Dx/HA, polydimethylsiloxane, chondrocytes, and blood (46). The analysis included 63 articles with a total of 5527 patients. They found a resolution rate by ureter of 85%; this represented an overall resolution rate that included one or more injections per ureter. Success varied by grade, with 78.5% for Grades I and II, 72% for Grade III, 63% for Grade IV, and 34% for Grade V. The success rate

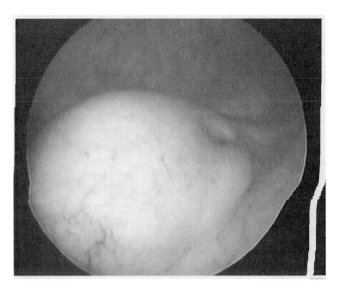

Figure 8 Endoscopic view of mound shift in a patient after failed subureteral deflux injection.

was lower in patients with duplicated collecting systems, voiding dysfunction, and neuropathic bladder. The rates of febrile UTIs and cystitis postoperatively were 6.0% and 0.75%, respectively.

To determine whether the appearance of the subureteral mound (see figures 8 and 9) could predict failure, Higham-Kessler et al. reviewed the appearance of the mound in Dx/HA treatment failures at the time of retreatment (47). The Dx/HA mound was inspected either cystoscopically or on gross inspection during cystotomy. After reviewing 80 patients with failed subureteral injections, all but 13 demonstrated mound abnormalities. These included shifted mound (49%), absent mound (21%), and loss of volume (11%). Children with dysfunctional voiding did not exhibit different mound characteristics, but did have a significantly higher chance of failure with a second injection. The authors concluded that while a perfect appearing mound does not necessarily predict success, most Dx/HA failures are associated with an abnormal mound, and the presence of dysfunctional voiding predicts failure after the second injection.

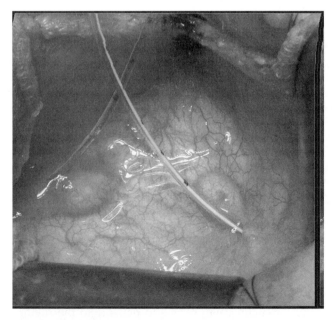

Figure 9 Illustration of mound shift in the same patient at the time of open ureteral reimplantation. Feeding tubes are placed in the ureteral orifices.

Endoscopic subureteral injection is associated with a very low risk of ureteral obstruction. Vandersteen et al. (48) performed a multi-institutional review and identified an obstruction rate requiring surgical treatment of 0.6%. Eighty percent of the obstructed patients presented in the early postoperative period with signs and symptoms. Only one patient presented more than 6 months postoperatively. The authors also identified a higher rate of neurogenic bladder and voiding dysfunction within this cohort of postoperative obstruction.

These series demonstrate that endoscopic subureteral therapy for VUR has a high success rate in well-selected patients. As more data become available, the ability to predict the ideal patient will improve, thus decreasing the rate of failure.

CIRCUMCISION

Circumcision is the fifth most commonly performed procedure in the United States. In 1992, 62% of newborn males in the United States were circumcised. It is estimated that one in six males in the world is circumcised (49). In the United States, circumcision is performed for religious, cultural, and medical reasons. Despite its wide prevalence, the practice of circumcision remains controversial. The most recent statement from the American Association of Pediatrics (AAP) neither supports nor condemns circumcision, but rather leaves the discussion and decision to the physician and family (50). Relative contraindications to circumcision include the prematurity, a bleeding disorder, and a penile abnormality such as hypospadias, penoscrotal webbing, or a buried penis.

The complications of circumcision can be divided into early and late complications. Early complications include bleeding, infection, and penile or urethral injury. Late complications include a trapped or buried penis, meatal stenosis, urethrocutaneous fistula, and persistence of redundant foreskin. Complication rates vary depending on where the procedure is performed, at what age, and which technique is employed. Ozdemir et al. examined trends of complications in Turkey, where circumcisions are frequently done for religious purposes, and found that 85% of circumcision complications occurred when performed by traditional nonmedical circumcisers (51). The complication rate dropped significantly when it was performed by medical personnel.

A variety of techniques are used to perform circumcision. When performed by medical personnel in the United States, newborn circumcision is most often done with a Gomco clamp or less commonly a plastibell. In older infants and children, a free-hand technique is generally employed under general anesthesia.

Early Complications
Bleeding is the most common early complication following circumcision. When a Gomco clamp is used for circumcision, the site of bleeding is most often at the frenulum. Horowitz and Gershbein found the incidence of bleeding to be higher when the Gomco clamp was used in children older than 3 months of age (52). There were no bleeding complications in patients younger than 30 days old. Thirty percent of older patients who had bleeding required either fulguration or sutures to stop the bleeding.

When circumcision is performed with a sleeve resection in older infants and children, the bleeding often arises from the dartos fascia. The bleeding vessels may not be identified during the procedure due to vasospasm. Meticulous hemostatis helps prevent bleeding postoperatively. Most bleeding complications respond to direct pressure or a compression dressing. In children with persistent bleeding, a hemostatic suture may occasionally be necessary. If the bleeding does not respond to standard management, a bleeding disorder such as von Willebrands disease should be considered.

Infection is another early, yet rare, complication of circumcision. Considering the anatomical location of the incision and proximity to stool, infection is surprisingly rare. Mucosal edema that normally develops postoperatively, especially on the ventral surface, can often be mistaken by the family and other health care providers as due to infection. The authors do not routinely use perioperative antibiotics due to the rarity of this complication. Postoperative infection should be managed with broad-spectrum antibiotics, and surgical drainage if necessary.

The most severe early complication of circumcision relates to damage to the urethra or glans. Amputation injuries can occur when the foreskin is removed without adequately protecting the glans (Figs. 10 and 11). In some cases of religious circumcisions, the foreskin is

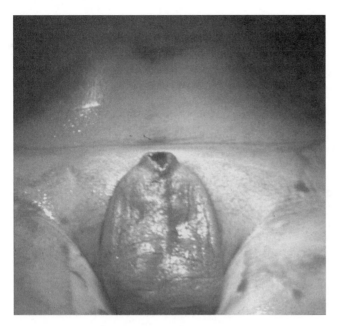

Figure 10 Amputation injury occurring during ritual circumcision.

pulled up and compressed between fingers. The ventral foreskin may be pulled excessively, tilting the frenulum and glans into the incision line. Injuries can also occur with clamp devices when the glans is not completely protected with the bell device. These complications are often related to failure to adequately lyse the normal physiologic adhesions from the glans to the foreskin, thus pulling the glans and urethra into the incision.

Multiple case reports in the literature of amputation injuries describe successful reattachment up to 8 hours after the injury. Amukele reported two successful glanular laceration repairs

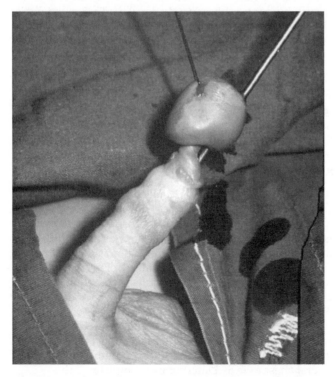

Figure 11 Circumcision partial amputation at the time of repair.

and one glanular amputation repair, while Gluckman reported a successful reattachment of distal glans 3 hours after the injury (53,54). Sherman described 7 neonates with amputation injuries, with successful reattachment between 30 minutes and 8 hours achieved in all patients (55).

Late Complications

Urethral Injury

One of the most significant late complications is a urethrocutaneous fistula. Urethrocutaneous fistulas can occur when the ventral urethra is injured from a crush, scalpel, or ischemia. The devitalized tissue ultimately breaks down and a fistula results. In his review of circumcision complications, Baskin reviewed the repair of 8 fistulas (56). All repairs were performed at least 6 months after the circumcision, and remained stented postoperatively for 7 to 10 days. Four were successfully repaired using a Mathieu style skin flap advancement with glanuloplasty. Four others were repaired using an onlay island flap from local penile skin. There were no fistula recurrences. Three patients presented with an iatrogenic hypospadias, in which the distal glans had been amputated. Baskin emphasizes the importance of surgical technique in these repairs and warns against excess urethral mobilization, which can result in distal ischemia and associated stenosis.

Trapped Penis

The trapped penis is another late complication of circumcision (Fig. 12). This occurs when a scar of penile skin forms over the glans, thus trapping the penis. It is usually related to inadequate foreskin removal where there is redundant tissue remaining that forms a concentric scar. Paradoxically, removal of excess foreskin, which pulls the penis into a buried configuration, may also result in a buried penis. It may also occur in cases when the penis is buried prior to the circumcision and removal of skin allows the penis to retract further into the suprapubic tissues with a band of scarred skin distally. The problems associated with trapped penis include infection, voiding difficulties, and appearance. Management of the trapped penis has traditionally involved surgical treatment of the scar and repair of the buried penis [Fig. 13 (A, B)]. Palmer et al. describe using betamethasone as a conservative means to manage the scar (57). In an evaluation of 14 patients who were circumcised as newborns and subsequently developed a trapped penis, 79% showed beneficial effects from the betamethasone application. Three patients ultimately required a formal penoplasty, but the rest were managed successfully with betamethasone.

Inadequate Foreskin Excision

Another late complication involves unsatisfactory post-circumcision appearance. This can occur for a number of reasons. Most commonly, inadequate foreskin is excised, leaving a collar of redundant tissue. This may be managed with revision of the circumcision if desired by the family and patient, or if it is related to secondary phimosis, skin bridges, or recurrent balantitis. Penile skin bridges may occasionally form (Fig. 14) and can be divided either in the office with topical anesthetia or in the operating room.

Circumcision of the Penis with a Preexisting Anomaly

Circumcision of the patient with hypospadias may result in technical challenges in obtaining skin coverage and in choosing an appropriate technique. Local skin flaps or skin grafts may be necessary for an acceptable functional and cosmetic outcome. Prevention is the best policy, and urologic consultation should be sought when there is an abnormality of the meatus. In the case of the megameatus intact prepuce hypospadias variant, the unsuspected abnormality is often noted after the circumcision has been completed (58). A recent review of 63 males with an intact prepuce and hypospadias by Snodgrass and Khavari (59) found that prior circumcision did not alter the outcome of subsequent hypospadias repair. The authors' result indicates that circumcision does not need to be interrupted once a suspected urethral anomaly is encountered. This recommendation could prevent the postponement of a circumcision with a mild meatal abnormality, which would require general anesthesia at a later time to complete.

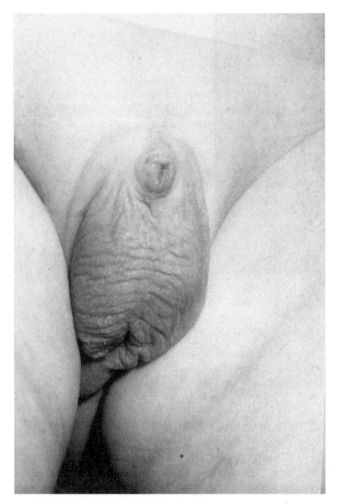

Figure 12   Trapped penis after circumcision.

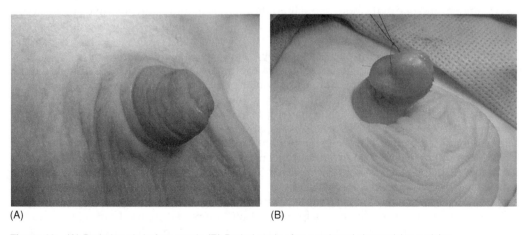

(A)   (B)

Figure 13   (**A**) Buried penis before repair. (**B**) Buried penis after repair and circumcision revision.

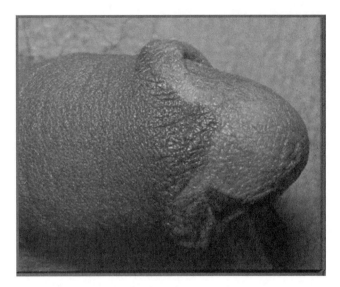

Figure 14   Skin bridge after circumcision.

Conclusion

While male circumcision remains controversial in the United States, it is a safe procedure with few serious complications. Most complications can be prevented by careful attention to the anatomy of the penis. Urologic consultation should be sought when there is any concern regarding the appropriateness of circumcision in a given patient.

NEPHRECTOMY, PARTIAL NEPHRECTOMY, AND LAPAROSCOPIC NEPHRECTOMY

The indications for nephrectomy, partial nephrectomy, and nephroureterectomy in children differ from those in adults. While in adults the main indication for nephrectomy is malignancy, in children a nonfunctioning kidney may be the reason for nephrectomy. In the pediatric population, the most frequent renal tumor is Wilms' tumor. With the changes in the management of Wilms' tumor brought about by the National Wilms' Tumor Study Group (NWTSG), the timing of surgical treatment as well as the approach has changed (60). The complication rates associated with nephrectomy and partial nephrectomy are related to the surgical approach and the indications for surgery. Within the last decade, the use of laparoscopy in pediatric urology has expanded, and one of its more popular applications is in minimally invasive nephrectomy. The addition of laparoscopy to this field has changed the profile of associated complications.

Open Nephrectomy and Partial Nephrectomy

The risks associated with open nephrectomy via a retroperitoneal approach are similar to those of adults. They include bleeding from the vascular pedicle or from the renal bed, damage to nearby structures, infection, injury to the other kidney, vascular injury, and incisional hernia. Other structures that are particularly vulnerable to injury during a retroperitoneal nephrectomy include the pancreas, bowel, the great vessels, and the pleural cavity. Intraoperative identification of injury and repair is the most important aspect of management. Elder et al. described a cohort of children who underwent outpatient nephrectomy for nonfunctioning or poorly functioning kidneys (61). One patient required laparotomy for bleeding. The remainder of the patients had no perioperative complications.

Partial nephrectomy carries the added risk of entry into the collecting system, and infusion of intravenous methylene blue can help rule out an unrepaired injury. If an injury is noted it should be repaired to avoid urinoma formation or stented (62). Cozzi et al. reported on their experience with nephron-sparing surgery with Wilms' tumor in 10 children. The only complication was gross hematuria in one child, which resolved spontaneously (63).

The transperitoneal approach to pediatric renal malignancy is associated with an expanded complication profile. The most recent report of the NWTSG-4 found that the rate of complications has decreased since the NWTSG-3 from 19.8% to 12.7%. The most common complication was bowel obstruction, which occurred in 5.1% of patients. Intraoperative hemorrhage was the second most common complication and occurred in 1.9% of patients. The risk of surgical complications was higher with increased tumor stage, tumor diameter (more than 10 cm), and intravascular extension in the inferior vena cava or atrium (60).

Laparoscopic Nephrectomy and Partial Nephrectomy

The first pediatric laparoscopic nephrectomy was reported in 1992 by Kavoussi and Koyle (64). Since that time the application of laparoscopic nephrectomy and partial nephrectomy has expanded. The advent of laparoscopic pediatric urologic surgery has introduced a new complication profile. Relatively soon after the introduction of pediatric laparoscopic nephrectomy, Peters reported on a survey of pediatric urologists regarding their complications associated with pediatric urologic laparoscopy. This report included a number of laparoscopic nephrectomies and partial nephrectomies, as well as other laparoscopic pediatric urologic procedures. The overall reported complication rate was 5.4%, and was adjusted to 1.18% when preperitoneal insufflation and subcutaneous emphysema were excluded. Forty-five percent of respondents used the Veress needle technique exclusively to initiate insufflation. Peters found that the method of initiating pneumoperitoneum was a predictor of complications, with a higher rate associated with the Veress technique. The complication rate for practitioners using laparoscopy exclusively for diagnostic purposes was 4.49%. This suggests that the greatest risk of complication during a laparoscopic urologic case occurs with trocar placement and insufflation. Peters also found that the strongest predictor of complications was the experience of the practitioner (65).

A number of published series of pediatric laparoscopy have documented complication rates equal to or lower than those reported by their adult counterparts. Yao and Poppas reported a series of 26 patients over 2 years, with no intraoperative complications or conversions to open procedures (66). Esposito et al. reviewed 701 laparoscopic pediatric urologic procedures, which included 38 laparoscopic nephrectomies and partial nephrectomies, and found a complication rate of 2.7% (67). This series included one patient with a peritoneal opening during a retroperitoneal nephrectomy, one renal parenchymal bleed during a partial nephrectomy and a vascular injury during trocar insertion. There were no postoperative complications. They found that the rate of complication was not related to the experience of the surgeon.

Waterman et al. reported four patients with pneumothorax, a complication that is known in the adult literature and is unique to laparoscopy (68). The procedures associated with pneumothorax included transperitoneal partial nephrectomy, partial nephroureterectomy, retroperitoneal nephrectomy, and extraperitoneal bilateral ureteral reimplantation for vesicoureteral reflux. Intraoperative findings suggesting pneumothorax included decreased oxygen saturation, subcutaneous emphysema, and decreased breath sounds. The pneumothorax was ipsilateral to the procedure in three patients and bilateral in one. Three patients were managed conservatively, whereas one required placement of a pigtail chest tube. Waterman proposed several etiologies for the development of pneumothorax, including increased CO_2 absorption, slightly higher insufflation pressures, unrecognized congenital defects, and pleural injury due to trocar placement. Regardless of the etiology, a high suspicion for pneumothorax should be maintained in the setting of changes in hemodynamic and respiratory parameters during pediatric laparoscopy. Shanberg et al. reported a tension pneumothorax during retroperitoneal laparoscopic upper pole nephrectomy. The authors suggested that the argon beam coagulator was the etiology. They indicate that the pneumothorax could have occurred due to barotrauma associated with a sudden increase in pressure during use of the argon beam, coupled with the decreased compliance associated with the retroperitoneal space. They recommend keeping the evacuation valves of the trocars open during argon beam use (69).

One of the touted advantages of laparoscopic partial nephrectomy is magnification of the parenchyma with the potential for improved visualization and less damage to the residual kidney. Several studies have compared the complication rates between laparoscopic and open partial nephrectomy. Robinson et al. compared 11 open procedures with 11 transperitoneal laparoscopic procedures. One patient undergoing laparoscopy required conversion to an open procedure due to transection of a lower pole ureter during an upper pole heminephrectomy. There was one complication in the open group in which a triplicated ureter was not identified intraoperatively. There was no difference in blood loss (70). Similarly, Piaggio et al. compared 14 transperitoneal laparoscopic nephrectomies with 20 open partial nephrectomies (71). There was one patient with significant bleeding in the open group necessitating reoperation. There was also one lower pole ureteral injury in the open group. Within the laparoscopic group, one urinoma required percutaneous draining, while one omental hernia was identified. Finally, Lee et al. (72) compared retroperitoneal laparoscopic partial nephrectomy with open surgery, one of the few studies evaluating the retroperitoneal approach (72). They found minimal blood loss in both groups, with the only complication being a urinoma that did not require treatment during a laparoscopic partial nephrectomy. This patient was followed for 4 years postoperatively without any adverse sequelae.

As a result of increased success with pediatric laparoscopy, many pediatric urologists have expanded this approach to younger patients. These experiences have been recently reviewed. Mulholland et al. described transperitoneal laparoscopic nephrectomy and heminephrectomy in 17 infants who weighed less than 10 kg. There were no conversions to open surgery. One diaphragmatic injury was repaired at the time of surgery without adverse outcome. One pneumothorax was noted on a postoperative chest film and it resolved without intervention (73). Similarly, Jesch et al. presented a series of 19 patients younger than one year of age. Two conversions to open surgery were necessary for poor visualization, and one suture dislocation required resuturing. There were no other complications (74). Finally, El-Ghoneimi et al. described a series of 12 patients with end-stage renal disease and ASA scores of three. Bilateral nephrectomy was performed in the same setting in three of these patients. There were no conversions to open, and the single complication was a postoperative hematoma which resolved spontaneously (75). Respiratory and hemodynamic parameters were measured during the procedure, and they noted increased systolic blood pressure and end-tidal carbon dioxide. However, there was no change in heart rate, peak airway pressure, or oxygen saturations. This series demonstrated that laparoscopic procedures can be safely carried out even in higher risk children.

While these three series are small, they help to demonstrate the safety of laparoscopic nephrectomy and partial nephrectomy in children. As more series are published, a more comprehensive complication profile will allow the practitioner to choose a technique with full awareness of the risks.

PYELOPLASTY

Ureteropelvic junction obstruction (UPJO) is a congenital disorder resulting from several possible etiologies. Among the various etiologies are intrinsic stenosis, an aperistaltic segment, insertional anomalies, crossing vessels, and extrinsic fibrous bands. Crossing vessels are less commonly seen in infants presenting with prenatal hydronephrosis. It is unclear whether crossing vessels cause intrinsic abnormalities within the UPJ or whether intrinsic stenosis or dysfunction distorts the UPJ such that the vessel appears to cause kinking. Extrinsic fibrous bands are more commonly found in the older child, or those with a history of distal obstruction or vesicoureteral reflux.

In prior decades, UPJO was diagnosed after the onset of sign and symptoms such as intermittent flank pain, flank mass, and UTI. With the advent of prenatal ultrasound, the finding of prenatal hydronephrosis has led to earlier diagnosis in infancy. The indications for intervention are symptoms from obstruction, impairment in renal function, and progressive loss of renal function. Treatment options include open surgical intervention, laparoscopic pyeloplasty, and endourologic techniques. This section will focus on the complications of open and laparoscopic pyeloplasty and not endourologic procedures as they are more commonly limited to the teenager.

The Anderson–Hynes dismembered pyeloplasty, the Foley Y–V pyeloplasty, and the spiral or vertical flap pyeloplasty are all options for repair of the obstructed ureteropelvic junction. The Anderson–Hynes technique is the most common procedure performed. It is appropriate for high or dependent insertions, and allows reduction of a large redundant pelvis. It also allows for anterior transposition of lower pole vessels if necessary. In this technique, the abnormal UPJ segment is completely excised. The Anderson–Hynes technique is not as useful in cases of a long segment of proximal ureteral obstruction and a small intrarenal pelvis. The Foley Y–V plasty can be used with high insertions, but cannot be used to transpose aberrant vessels or taper a redundant renal pelvis. The spiral or vertical flap technique is most appropriate for repair of long segments of narrowed ureter. Ureterocalicostomy is an option that can be used in cases of failed pyeloplasty or as a primary procedure when there is an intrarenal pelvis or inaccessible UPJ. The main complications associated with repair of UPJO are persistent UPJO (i.e., the failed pyeloplasty), urinary leakage, and UTI.

Obstruction and Failed Pyeloplasty

Early obstruction is usually diagnosed due to fever, persistent pain, or prolonged urinary leakage. The management of early obstruction differs from late obstruction. Late obstruction implies failed pyeloplasty. Early obstruction in the nonstented patient may be transient and respond to urinary diversion or stenting. In a review of 20 years of experience, Sutherland reported a 2.1% rate of failed pyeloplasty (76). Of the five patients (2.1%) with early obstruction, four were treated with percutaneous nephrostomy (PCN), and one with a ureteral stent. Three of these patients ultimately required reoperation. In the nonstented patient with symptomatic obstruction, treatment options include either retrograde or antegrade passage of a stent across the anastomosis, or placement of a temporary nephrostomy tube.

Delayed or persistent obstruction implies failed pyeloplasty. Success rates of open surgical repair range from 95% to 100%. Failed pyeloplasty is thought to be due to fibrosis and re-stenosis, and can be related to poor tissue handling, trauma, ischemia, and urinary extravasation. This emphasizes the need for the basic surgical principles of pyeloplasty, which include tension-free anastomosis, gentle handling of tissues, a watertight anastamosis, and preservation of vasculature to the ureter (77).

Surgical options for the failed pyeloplasty include repeat open pyeloplasty and minimally invasive endourologic techniques. Thomas et al. followed postoperative patients with ultrasound and evaluated patients with persistent or worsening hydronephrosis with renography (78). They reported on seven patients with failed initial procedures. Patients with initial failure of the procedure presented at a mean of 13.1 months postoperatively. Six patients presented with pain, and one with asymptomatic hydronephrosis. Retrograde pyelogram findings in these patients demonstrated a patent and dependent anastomosis in five of seven patients, with two showing a high ureteral insertion. Three patients underwent balloon dilation without success. Definitive management of the remaining patients involved open surgical management in six patients. Of the six patients, three underwent ureterocalicostomy and three underwent reoperative dismembered pyeloplasty. Intraoperative findings included dense scarring, redundant pelves with kinking, and unrecognized crossing vessels in two patients. Due to failure of minimally invasive methods, the authors recommended open repair for the management of failed initial pyeloplasty.

In a review of 127 primary pyeloplasties over a 10-year period, Lim et al. noted a failure rate of 2.4% (79). Failures were managed with repeat Anderson–Hynes (seven patients), Foley Y–V plasty (two patients), or spiral flap (one patient). Nephrectomy was required in three patients who failed the second procedure. From this study, the authors determined that failures in their patients were linked to young age at primary repair and prolonged urinary drainage postoperatively. Sutherland et al. noted five patients with persistent postoperative obstruction (failure rate 2.1%), four of whom were managed with PCN placement, and one with ureteral stenting (76). Three of the patients treated with PCN ultimately required reoperation. Based on their results, the authors advocated the placement of a stent across the anastomosis, stating that a failure to do so is more likely to result in obliteration of the ureteral lumen.

Figenshau and Clayman reviewed the success rates of endourologic techniques in the management of UPJO (80). They reviewed 8 series (86 patients) that used endopyelotomy to manage UPJO and of these patients 35 were treated for a failed primary procedure. The success rate for secondary procedures was 91% with a mean follow-up of 32 months. Successful results were related to older age of the patient, secondary UPJO compared to primary UPJO, low-grade hydronephrosis, and good renal function. Of four series of balloon dilation for UPJO, nine procedures were performed for a secondary UPJO and the overall success rate in this cohort was 66%. Based on these studies, no firm conclusions can be drawn regarding the best management of the failed pyeloplasty. As more experience is gained with endourologic techniques, perhaps the success rate and acceptance of this treatment option for the pediatric patient will improve.

Prolonged Urinary Leakage

Prolonged urinary leakage can be associated with pyeloplasty failure, as it induces periureteral inflammation and fibrosis. In the early postoperative period, prolonged drainage can also lead to reoperation, as reported by Sheu et al. (81). This group reported four patients with prolonged leakage from a penrose drain lasting more than 7 days. Two of these patients required repeat pyeloplasty for drainage for more than 400 mL per day.

The role of stents in preventing urinary leakage in the postoperative patient is controversial. The advantages of a "tubeless" repair include a lower risk of infection, lack of external tubing, and avoidance of an additional general anesthesia to remove an internal stent. Both Smith et al. and Tal et al. noted a trend that did not reach statistical significance correlating omission of stents and subsequent urinary leakage (82,83). Woo and Farnsworth reviewed infants younger than 12 months at the time of surgery, and found that all urinary leaks occurred in nonstented patients (84). Of six prolonged urinary leaks, two were also complicated by associated infection, and these two patients ultimately required repeat pyeloplasty. However, the patients in this study were a mean of 60 months of age at the time of surgery. Lim et al. (79) reviewed the management of pyeloplasty failures and noted that the postoperative course of the three patients who had undergone a tubeless repair all had prolonged urinary drainage (79). In contrast, in a review of pyeloplasty failures, Thomas et al. did not find that stenting played a role in subsequent failures (78).

In summary, there is a trend within the literature suggesting that urinary leakage is more often associated with a tubeless repair. The use of stents in operative repair is surgeon dependent, and must take into account the possibility that stents are associated with an increased rate of postoperative infection. Other considerations include renal function and the presence of a normal contralateral kidney. Ward et al. advocate stent placement in cases of poor renal function, repeat pyeloplasties, solitary kidney, and repairs requiring significant renal pelvis tailoring (85).

The management of persistent urinary leakage ranges from minimally invasive retrograde stent placement to open surgical drainage. Salem et al. successfully managed leaks with stents in three patients and reinsertion of the penrose drain in one patient (86). Sutherland et al. (76) treated three patients with a retrograde stent and one with PCN. In all four patients the urinary leak resolved. Based on these studies, it appears that urinary leaks can usually be managed with a minimally invasive approach by either retrograde ureteral stenting or PCN placement. Rarely, the patient will require open surgical drainage or pyeloplasty revision.

Urinary Tract Infection

The risk of UTI is present after any surgery on the urinary collecting system. After pyeloplasty, UTI may result in periureteral inflammation and subsequent fibrosis and failure. Therefore, infection should be treated aggressively and preoperative sterilization of urine should be the goal. In a comprehensive review of the literature, Smith et al. and Tal et al. found that the rate of infection associated with postoperative stent was slightly, but not significantly, higher compared to the nonstented group (82,83). However, Sutherland noted an increased rate of positive cultures in stented groups (76). Interestingly, Woo and Farnsworth noted four symptomatic UTIs in patients undergoing unstented repair, while stented patients had only one symptomatic UTI (84). These findings are in contrast to those previously mentioned that found a relationship between the presence of stents and UTI; this may be due to the number of bilateral repairs and young age of Woo's patients.

In summary, it appears that the use of stents may be associated with a higher incidence of positive urine cultures and UTI. This knowledge must be weighed against the apparent increased risk of urinary leakage associated with the tubeless repair, as well as surgeon preference.

Conclusion

Open pyeloplasty remains the gold standard treatment of UPJO in the pediatric population. The advent of laparoscopic repair and minimally invasive endourologic techniques may change the landscape of pediatric management as it becomes more accepted and fine-tuned in the adult population. The complications associated with open pyeloplasty can usually be managed with minimally invasive techniques, with a low incidence of repeat pyeloplasty reported in the literature.

Laparoscopic Pyeloplasty

The first laparoscopic pyeloplasty performed in the pediatric population was reported by Peters et al. in 1995 (87). Since that time there have been more reports of both retroperitoneal and transperitoneal laparoscopic approach for pyeloplasty. Tan et al. reported one of the earliest series of patients treated with transperitoneal pyeloplasty (88). There were two failures, both in infants 3 months old at the time of the procedure. This finding lead Tan to conclude that transperitoneal pediatric pyeloplasty is feasible in infants and children older than 6 months of age. Reddy et al. also reported their experience with the transperitoneal approach and noted that 2 of 16 patients developed postoperative ileus lasting more than 24 hours (89).

The retroperitoneal approach to the laparoscopic pediatric pyeloplasty has traditionally been considered more challenging due to the smaller working space. Yeung et al. presented their data on 13 patients with a mean age of 2.7 years old, treated with retroperitoneal laparoscopic pyeloplasty (90). Twelve of the cases were successful, and the one conversion to an open procedure was performed in a patient who had undergone prior percutaneous nephrostomy. In an unpublished report of their series, El-Ghoneimi et al. report that of 50 patients, only 4 were converted to open, with one failure requiring a repeat pyeloplasty (91). Additional complications included three misplaced stents. To prevent this problem the authors recommended filling the bladder with methylene blue, using fluoroscopy to place the stent, or inserting the stent by a retrograde approach at the end of the procedure.

These case series provide support for the efficacy and safety of pediatric laparoscopic pyeloplasty. With more experience, operative times will likely decrease, making the procedure even more attractive. Due to the burgeoning popularity of minimally invasive procedures in the adult population, undoubtedly many families will request information about minimally invasive options in the pediatric population. In experienced hands, laparoscopic pyeloplasty affords the same success rates as the open approach with low complication rates.

REFERENCES

1. Kass EJ, Bolong D. Single stage hypospadias reconstruction without fistula. J Urol 1990; 144(2):520–522.
2. Wiener JS, Sutherland RW, Roth DR, et al. Comparison of onlay and tubularized island flaps of inner preputial skin for the repair of proximal hypospadias. J Urol 1997; 158(3):1172–1174.
3. Powell CR, Mcaleer I, Alagiri M, et al. Comparison of flaps versus grafts in proximal hypospadias surgery. J Urol 2000; 163(4):1286–1289.
4. Retik AB, Atala A. Complications of hypospadias repair. Urol Clin North Am 2002; 29(2):329–339.
5. Palmer JS, Elder JS, Palmer LS. The use of betamethasone to manage the trapped penis following neonatal circumcision. J Urol 2005; 174(4):1577–1578.
6. Teague JL, Roth DR, Gonzales ET. Repair of hypospadias complications using the meatal based flap urethroplasty. J Urol 1994; 151(2):470–472.
7. Nesbit RM. Congenital curvature of the phallus: Report of three cases with description of corrective operation. J Urol 1965; 93:230–232.
8. Secrest CL, Jordan GH, Winslow BH, et al. Repair of the complications of hypospadias surgery. J Urol 1993; 150(5):1415–1418.
9. Aigen AB, Khawand N, Skoog SJ, et al. Acquired megalourethra: An uncommon complication of the transverse preputial island flap urethroplasty. J Urol 1987; 137(4):712–713.
10. Zaontz MR, Kaplan WE, Maizels M. Surgical correction of anterior urethral diverticula after hypospadias repair in children. Urology 1989; 33(1):40–42.
11. Geltzeiler J, Belman AB. Results of closure of urethrocutaneous fistulas in children. J Urol 1984; 132(4):734–736.
12. Santangelo K, Rushton HG, Belman AB. Outcome analysis of simple and complex urethrocutaneous fistula closure using a de-epithelialized or full thickness skin advancement flap for coverage. J Urol 2003; 170(4):1589–1592.
13. Snodgrass W. Tubularized incised plate urethroplasty for distal hypospadias. J Urol 1994; 151(2):464–465.
14. Snodgrass W, Koyle M, Manzoni G, et al. Tubularized incised plate hypospadias repair: Results of a multicenter experience. J Urol 1996; 156(2):839–841.
15. Snodgrass W. Does tubularized incised plate hypospadias repair create neourethral strictures? J Urol 1999; 162(3):1159–1161.
16. Duckett JW, Coplen D, Ewalt D, et al. Buccal mucosal urethral replacement. J Urol 1995; 153(3):1660–1663.

17. Hensle TW, Kearney MC, Bingham JB. Buccal mucosal grafts for hypospadias surgery: Long-term results. J Urol 2002; 168(4):1734–1737.
18. Metro MJ, Wu Hy, Snyder HM, et al. Buccal mucosal grafts: Lessons learned from an 8-year experience. J Urol 2001; 166:1459–1461.
19. Caldamone AA, Edstrom LE, Koyle MA, et al. Buccal mucosal grafts for urethral reconstruction. Urology 1998; 51(5 A):15–19.
20. Jayanthi VR, McLorie GA, Khoury AE, et al. Can previously relocated penile skin be successfully used for salvage hypospadias repair? J Urol 1994; 152(2):740–743.
21. Simmons GR, Cain MP, Casale AJ, et al. Repair of hypospadias complications using the previously utilized urethral plate. Urology 1999; 54(4):724–726.
22. Borer J, Bauer SB, Peters CA, et al. Tubularized incised plate urethroplasty: Expanded use in primary and repeat surgery for hypospadias. J Urol 2001; 165(2):581–585.
23. Nguyen MT, Snodgrass WT. Tubularized incised plate hypospadias reoperation. J Urol 2004; 171(6):2404–2406.
24. Hutch JA. Vesico-ureteral reflux in the paraplegic: Cause and correlation. J Urol 1952; 68(2):457–469.
25. Elder JS, Peters CA, Arant BS Jr, et al. Pediatric Vesicoureteral Reflux Guidelines Panel summary report on the management of primary vesicoureteral reflux in children. J Urol 1997; 157(5):1846–1851.
26. Zaontz MR, Maizels M, Sugar EC, et al. Detrusorrhaphy: Extravesical ureteral advancement to correct VUR in children. J Urol 1987; 138(4):947–949.
27. Mor Y, Leibovitch I, Zalts R, et al. Analysis of the long-term outcome of surgically corrected vesico-ureteral reflux. BJU Int 2003; 92(1):97–100.
28. Austin JC, Cooper CS. Vesicoureteral reflux: Surgical approaches. Urol Clin North Am 2004; 31(3):543–557.
29. Lavine MA, Siddiq FM, Cahn DJ, et al. Vesicoureteral reflux after ureteroneocystostomy: Indications for postoperative voiding cystography. Tech Urol 2001; 7(1):50–54.
30. Siegelbaum MH, Rabinovitch HH. Delayed spontaneous resolution of high grade vesicoureteral reflux after reimplantation. J Urol 1987; 138(5):1205–1206.
31. Diamond DA, Rabinowitz R, Hoenig D, et al. The mechanism of new onset contralateral reflux following unilateral ureteroneocystostomy. J Urol 1996; 156(2):665–667.
32. Minevich E, Wacksman J, Lewis AG, et al. Incidence of contralateral vesicoureteral reflux following unilateral extravesical detrusorrhaphy (ureteroneocystostomy). J Urol 1998; 159(6):2126–2128.
33. Burno DK, Glazier DB, Zaontz MR. Lessons learned about contralateral reflux after unilateral extravesical ureteral advancement in children. J Urol 1998; 160(3):995–997.
34. Ross JH, Kay R, Nasrallah P. Contralateral reflux after unilateral ureteral reimplantation in patients with a history of resolved contralateral reflux. J Urol 1995; 154(3):1171–1172.
35. Liu C, Chin T, Wei C. Contralateral reflux after unilateral ureteral reimplantation—Preexistent rather than new-onset reflux. J Pediatr Surg 1999; 34(11):1661–1664.
36. Hoenig DM, Diamond DA, Rabinowitz R, et al. Contralateral reflux after unilateral ureteral reimplantation. J Urol 1996; 156(1):196–197.
37. Lipski BA, Mitchell ME, Burns MW. Voiding dysfunction after bilateral extravesical ureteral reimplantation. J Urol 1998; 159(3):1019–1021.
38. Fung LC, McLorie GA, Jain U, et al. Voiding efficiency after ureteral reimplantation: A comparison of extravesical and intravesical techniques. J Urol 1995; 153(6):1972–1975.
39. Barrieras D, Lapointe S, Reddy PP, et al. Urinary retention after bilateral extravesical ureteral reimplantation: Does dissection distal to the ureteral orifice have a role? J Urol 1999; 162(3):1197–1200.
40. Upadhyay J, Shekarriz B, Fleming P, et al. Ureteral reimplantation in infancy: Evaluation of long-term voiding function. J Urol 1999; 162(3):1209–1212.
41. Ahmed S, Tan H. Complications of transverse advancement ureteral reimplantation. J Urol 1982; 127(5):970–973.
42. Weiss RM, Schiff M Jr, Lytton B. Late obstruction after ureteroneocystostomy. J Urol 1971; 106(1):144–148.
43. Cartwright PC, Snow BW, Mansfield JC, et al. Percutaneous endoscopic trigonoplasty: A minimally invasive approach to correct vesicoureteral reflux. J Urol 1996; 156(2):661–664.
44. Yeung CK, Sihoe JD, Borzi PA. Endoscopic cross-trigonal ureteral reimplantation under carbon dioxide bladder insufflation: A novel technique. J Endourol 2005; 19(3):295–299.
45. Lakshmanan Y, Fung LC. Laparoscopic extravesical ureteral reimplantation for vesicoureteral reflux: Recent technical advances. J Endourol 2000; 14(7):589–594.
46. Elder JS, Diaz M, Caldamone AA, et al. Endoscopic therapy for vesicoureteral reflux: A meta-analysis. I. Reflux resolution and urinary tract infection. J Urol 2006; 175:716–722.
47. Higham-Kessler J, Reinert SE, Snodgrass WT, et al. A review of failures of endoscopic treatment of vesicoureteral reflux with dextranomer microspheres. J Urol 2007; 177(2):710–715.
48. Vandersteen DR, Routh JC, Kirsch AJ, et al. Postoperative obstruction after subureteral injection of dextranomer/hyaluronic acid copolymer. J Urol 2006; 176(4):1593–1595.

49. Hutcheson JC. Male neonatal circumcision: Indications, controversies, and complications. Urol Clin North Am 2004; 31(3):461–467.

50. Lannon CM, et al. Circumcision policy statement. Task Force on Circumcision. Pediatrics 1999; 103(3):686–693.

51. Ozdemir E. Significantly increased complication risks with mass circumcisions. Br J Urol 1997; 80(1):136–139.

52. Horowitz M, Gershbein AB. Gomco circumcision: When is it safe? J Pediatr Surg 2001; 36(7):1047–1049.

53. Amukele SA, Lee GW, Stock JA, et al. 20-year experience with iatrogenic penile injury. J Urol 2003; 170(4):1691–1694.

54. Gluckman GR, Stoller ML, Jacobs MM, et al. Newborn penile glans amputation during circumcision and successful reattachment. J Urol 1995; 153(3):778–779.

55. Sherman J, Borer JG, Horowitz M, et al. Circumcision: Successful glanular reconstruction and survival following traumatic amputation. J Urol 1996; 156(2):842–844.

56. Baskin LS, Canning DA, Snyder HM 3rd, et al. Surgical repair of urethral circumcision injuries. J Urol 1997; 158(6):2269–2271.

57. Palmer JS, Elder JS, Palmer JS. The use of betamethasone to manage the trapped penis following neonatal circumcision. J Urol 2005; 174(4):1577–1578.

58. Duckett JW, Keating MA. Technical challenge of the megameatus intact prepuce hypospadias variant: The pyramid procedure. J Urol 1989; 141(6):1407–1409.

59. Snodgrass WT, Khavari R. Prior circumcision does not complicate repair of hypospadias with an intact prepuce. J Urol 2006; 176(1):296–298.

60. Ritchey ML, Shamberger RC, Haase G, et al. Surgical complications after primary nephrectomy for Wilms' tumor: Report from the National Wilms' Tumor Study Group. J Am Coll Surg 2001; 192(1):63–68.

61. Elder JS, Hladky D, Selzman AA. Outpatient nephrectomy for nonfunctioning kidneys. J Urol 1995; 154(2):712–715.

62. Ritchey ML, Shamberger RC. Pediatric urologic oncology. In: Wein AJ, Kavoussi LR, Novick AC, et al., eds. Campbell–Walsh Urology, Chapter 130. 9th ed. Vol. 4, Philadelphia, PA: Saunders, Elsevier, 2007:3870–3906.

63. Cozzi DA, Schiavetti A, Morini F, et al. Nephron-sparing surgery for unilateral primary renal tumors in children. J Pediatr Surg 2001; 36(2):362–365.

64. Koyle MA, Woo HH, Kavoussi LR. Laparoscopic nephrectomy in the first year of life. J Pediatr Surg 1993; 28(5):693–695.

65. Peters CA. Complications in pediatric urological laparoscopy: Results of a survey. J Urol 1996; 155(3):1070–1073.

66. Yao D, Poppas DP. A clinical series of laparoscopic nephrectomy, nephroureterectomy, and heminephrectomy in the pediatric population. J Urol 2000; 163(5):1531–1535.

67. Esposito C, Lima M, Mattioli G, et al. Complications of pediatric urological laparoscopy: Mistakes and risks. J Urol 2003; 169(4):1490–1492.

68. Waterman BJ, Robinson BC, Snow BW, et al. Pneumothorax in pediatric patients after urological laparoscopic surgery: Experience with 4 patients. J Urol 2004; 171(3):1256–1259.

69. Shanberg AM, Zagnoev M, Clougherty TP. Tension pneumothorax caused by the argon beam coagulator during laparoscopic partial nephrectomy. J Urol 2002; 168(5):2162.

70. Robinson BC, Snow BW, Cartwright PC, et al. Comparison of laparoscopic versus open partial nephrectomy in a pediatric series. J Urol 2003; 169(2):638–640.

71. Piaggio L, Franc-Guimond J, Figueroa TE, et al. Comparison of laparoscopic and open partial nephrectomy for duplication anomalies in children. J Urol 2006; 175(6):2269–2273.

72. Lee RS, Retik AB, Borer JG, et al. Pediatric retroperitoneal laparoscopic partial nephrectomy: Comparison with an age matched cohort of open surgery. J Urol 2005; 174(2):708–712.

73. Mulholland TL, Kropp BP, Wong C. Laparoscopic renal surgery in infants 10 kg or less. J Endourol 2005; 19(3):397–400.

74. Jesch NK, Metzelder ML, Kuebler JF, et al. Laparoscopic transperitoneal nephrectomy is feasible in the first year of life and is not affected by kidney size. J Urol 2006; 176(3):1177–1179.

75. El-Ghoneimi A, Sauty L, Maintenant J, et al. Laparoscopic retroperitoneal nephrectomy in high risk children. J Urol 2000; 164(3):1076–1079.

76. Sutherland RW, Chung SK, Roth DR, et al. Pediatric pyeloplasty: Outcome analysis based on patient age and surgical technique. Urology 1997; 50(6):963–966.

77. Kelalis P, King L, Belman B. Clinical pediatric urology. 4th ed. In: Leo F Yegappan L, eds. Chapter 20, Anomalies of the Renal Collecting System: Ureteropelvic Junction Obstruction (Pyelocalyectasis) and Infundibular Stenosis. London: Elsevier Science, 2001:609–612.

78. Thomas JC, DeMarco RT, Donohoe JM, et al. Management of the failed pyeloplasty: A contemporary review. J Urol 2005; 174(6):2363–2366.

79. Lim DJ, Walker RD 3rd. Management of the failed pyeloplasty. J Urol 1996; 156(2):738–740.

80. Figenshau RS, Clayman RV. Endourologic options for management of ureteropelvic junction obstruction in the pediatric patient. Urol Clin North Am 1998; 25(2):199–209.
81. Sheu JC, Koh CC, Chang PY, et al. Ureteropelvic junction obstruction in children: 10 years' experience in one institution. Pediatr Surg Int 2006; 22(6):519–523.
82. Smith KE, Holmes N, Lieb JI, et al. Stented versus nonstented pediatric pyeloplasty: A modern series and review of the literature. J Urol 2002; 168(3):1127–1130.
83. Tal R, Bar-Sever Z, Livne PM. Dismembered pyeloplasty in children: A review of 5 years single center experience. Int J Urol 2005; 12(12):1028–1031.
84. Woo HH, Farnsworth RH. Dismembered pyeloplasty in infants under the age of 12 months. Br J Urol 1996; 77(3):449–451.
85. Ward AM, Kay R, Ross JH. Ureteropelvic junction obstruction in children. Unique considerations for open operative intervention. Urol Clin North Am 1998; 25(2):211–217.
86. Salem YH, Majd M, Rushton HG, et al. Outcome analysis of pediatric pyeloplasty as a function of patient age, presentation, and differential renal function. J Urol 1995; 154(5):1889–1893.
87. Peters CA, Schlussel RN, Retik AB. Pediatric laparoscopic dismembered pyeloplasty. J Urol 1995; 153(6):1962–1965.
88. Tan HL. Laparoscopic Anderson-Hynes dismembered pyeloplasty in children. J Urol 1999; 162(3):1045–1048.
89. Reddy M, Nerli RB, Bashetty R, et al. Laparoscopic dismembered pyeloplasty in children. J Urol 2005; 174(2):700–702.
90. Yeung CK, Tam YH, Sihoe JD, et al. Retroperitoneoscopic dismembered pyeloplasty for pelvi-ureteric junction obstruction in infants and children. BJU Int 2000; 87(6):509–513.
91. El-Ghoneimi A, Farhat W, Bolduc S, et al. Laparoscopic dismembered pyeloplasty by a retroperitoneal approach in children. BJU Int 2003; 92(1):104–108.

Orchiopexy

Expert: Pierre Williot, M.D.

QUESTIONS

1. **What is the best technique to prevent recurrence of an undescended testicle?**
   The mobilization of the testicle and cord should be sufficient to allow the testicle to drop into the scrotum. No traction should be needed to keep the testicle in the scrotum. Traction on the testicle can result in testicular ascent and atrophy by vascular injury.

   It is extremely important to free the processus vaginalis from the cord and to tie the processus away from the cord, at the level of the internal inguinal ring.

   To achieve enough length to the cord, a retroperitoneal dissection of the spermatic vessels, Fowler–Stephens membrane and vas is frequently required. (The Fowler–Stephens membrane is the layer of tissue that is located between the spermatic vessels and the vas deferens. Vascular communications between the vas vessels and the spermatic vessels are present within this membrane.)

   The retroperitonal dissection involves the mobilization of the vas, Fowler–Stephens membrane, and vessels en-block from the posterior layer of the peritoneum and the incisions of the lateral bands to the spermatic vessels.

   Do not skeletonize the spermatic vessels. The retroperitoneal mobilization can go as high as the lower pole of the ipsilateral kidney. A short cord is almost always due to short spermatic vessels. On rare occasion, the vas is too short and becomes the limiting factor. The ligation and division of the ipsilateral obliterated umbilical artery can allow a more direct route to the vas.

   When facing a long looping vas, the portion of the vas between the ampulae of the vas and the testicle might be too short to allow proper mobilization of the testicle. In this rare circumstance, dissecting between the two limbs of the loop of vas (distal to the testicle) might provide the length needed. Be careful not to impair the blood supply during this dissection.

   Bringing the testicle through the floor of the inguinal canal can provide extra length. I have found that the gain in length with this technique is minimal, while increasing the risk of creating a direct inguinal hernia. This maneuver should be performed without ligating the inferior epigastric vessels.

When the testicle is intra-peritoneal, or high in the inguinal canal (especially in older children), it might be impossible to bring the testicle into the scrotum with the above described techniques. A Fowler–Stephens orchidopexy (ligation and transection of the spermatic vessels) is appropriate in these circumstances. The decision to do a Fowler–Stephens orchidopexy should be done early in the dissection to minimize the risk of testicular atrophy. To attempt a one stage Fowler–Stephens orchidopexy late in the dissection is not recommended.

A two stage Fowler–Stephens orchidopexy is recommended over a single stage procedure to decrease the risk of testicular atrophy. The first stage involves only the ligation of the spermatic vessels high above the testicle. During the second stage, the spermatic vessels are transected high above the testicle, the Fowler–Stephens membrane, distal spermatic vessels and the posterior peritoneum are mobilized en-block to bring the testicle down into the scrotum.

2. **When should laparoscopic mobilization be applied for the undescended testicle?**
   The main roles of laparoscopy are:
   1. evaluation/localization of non palpable testicle
   2. first stage Fowler–Stephens orchidopexy—controversy exists in determining if an intra-abdominal testicle needs a Fowler–Stephens orchidopexy. If the testicle can be pulled all the way to the controlateral internal inguinal ring, it is felt that enough length would be achieved without ligation/division of the spermatic vessels. This "trick" does not always work. In a young child (less than 2 years old), a "peeping" testicle should not require a Fowler–Stephens orchidopexy, but in a older child (more than 5 or 6 years old), especially a tall teenager, these testicles will require a two stage approach.
   3. The second stage Fowler–Stephens orchidopexy
   4. I do not use laparoscopy on palpable testicles.

3. **How should the premature infant with an asymptomatic hernia and an undescended testicle be managed?**
   In a premature infant, the full descent of the testicle could take up to one year from the date of birth. One should wait to do the orchidopexy until then, unless the hernia becomes symptomatic.

4. **How should the testicle be managed when it has been mobilized into the retroperitoneum and will not reach the scrotum?**
   Two options are described. Fixing the testicle in this new location and returning 4–6 months later to continue the mobilization. The second stage can be very difficult. Wrapping the testicle into a sheet of silicone has been described to facilitate the dissection during the second surgery.

   I prefer to perform a first stage Fowler–Stephens orchidopexy and leaving the testicle into the abdomen. This way, there is less risk of trauma to the testicle at the time of the second stage (4 to 6 months later).

5. **What are the most common complications of orchidopexy and how can they be avoided?**
   Main complications of orchidopexy:
   1. testicular atrophy—avoid: torsion of the cord, tension on the cord, pinching the cord with the forceps, skeletonization of the spermatic vessels, and preserve the Fowler–Stephens membrane. Do not include the cord in the suture during the reapproximation of the external oblique aponeurosis!
   2. testicular ascent—the testicle should drop down into the scrotum, not be pulled down.
   3. Injury to the vas—be careful. Avoid pinching the vas. The mobilization of a large hernia sac can be a challenge. The sac must be mobilized to the level of the internal inguinal ring and free from the vas, vessels, and Fowler–Stephens membrane at the time of the ligation.
   4. Persistent inguinal hernia—the hernia sac must be dissected free from the cord.
   5. Injury to the ilio-inguinal nerve. Again, careful dissection during the exploration and avoid trapping the nerve during the reapproximation of the external oblique aponeurosis.

6. **How would you approach a testicle which has reascended to the external ring postoperatively?**

This testicle will not descend spontaneously, but reoperation can be difficult.

Obtaining the initial operative report is recommended.

Some surgeons prefer using a different inguinal incision, but I normally use the same incision (for cosmetic reasons).

Take your time. The anatomy and aspect of the tissues can be misleading. The testicle is most likely not protected by the vaginalis.

A few key points to keep in mind:

a. The vas deferens is most likely medial to the testicle and vessels: avoid medial dissection until one has a clear understanding of the anatomy

b. A retroperitoneal dissection must be performed to obtain enough cord length. In my experience and by talking to colleagues, the retroperitoneal dissection was almost never performed during the initial surgery.

25 | Complications of Vascular Anomalies

Arin K. Greene, M.D., M.M.Sc. and Steven J. Fishman, M.D.

INTRODUCTION

Vascular anomalies are disorders of the endothelium that usually present during childhood. These lesions affect all parts of the vasculature: capillaries, veins, arteries, or lymphatics. Although benign, vascular anomalies can cause local destruction as well as systemic morbidity. While approximately 90% of these lesions do not require treatment, the remainder present challenging problems. The most conservative approach to minimize complications associated with vascular anomalies is to refer patients with problematic lesions to an interdisciplinary Vascular Anomalies Center with experienced medical and surgical specialists.

To facilitate the analysis of vascular anomalies complications presented in this chapter, we advocate the use of Ernest Amory Codman's (1869–1940) morbidity classification (1). Codman, the father of outcomes research, presented a classification of morbidity in 1914 so that the surgeon could critically assess the *reasons* for his failures to ensure that they are not repeated in the future (Table 1) (2). The simplicity of this system allows both the teacher and student to understand the reasons for errors so that they are less likely to be repeated. Surgeons who will not investigate why a poor result has occurred are likely to make the same mistakes again. In Codman's words, "The adoption of this system will at the same time render our work more scientific and our practice more honorable" (3).

PATIENT DISEASE (PD)

The most common cause of complications in the field of vascular anomalies are the lesions themselves. Significant progress in the understanding and treatment of these disorders has been made over the past quarter century. For example, imaging instead of biopsy is now standard for diagnostic confirmation, antiangiogenic drug treatment is available for problematic vascular tumors, sclerotherapy has replaced operative resection of malformations in many instances, and techniques for excision have been improved. In addition, interdisciplinary Vascular Anomalies Centers now serve as referral centers for patients with problematic lesions.

Despite improvements in the management of vascular anomalies, these disorders continue to cause significant morbidity and their etiopathogenesis remains poorly understood. The most common complication of vascular anomalies is psychological morbidity due to disfigurement; unfortunately, two-thirds of lesions affect the head and neck (Fig. 1). Vascular anomalies also may destroy local tissues and cause functional problems such as bleeding, ulceration, infection, obstruction, congestive heart failure, pulmonary embolism, or death. Even after treatment, these lesions often recur and can leave behind damaged structures requiring sophisticated reconstruction.

Tumors

Ten percent of hemangiomas cause significant deformity or severe complications (4). Like all vascular anomalies, disfigurement is the leading cause of morbidity. Five percent of cutaneous hemangiomas ulcerate, which is more common on the lips, anogenital region, or parotid area (Fig. 2) (5). Ulceration causes cutaneous scarring and may destroy important structures such as the eyelid, ear, nose, or lip. Treatment of ulceration includes hydrated petrolatum, topical lidocaine, antibiotic ointment, or dressing changes. In addition to esthetic concerns, hemangiomas

Table 1   Modern Translation of Ernest Amory Codman's
1914 Classification of Operative Morbidity

Type	Abbreviation
Error in diagnosis	ED
Error in technique	ET
Error in judgment	EJ
Error due to lack of care or equipment	EC
Patient disease	PD
Patient refusal of treatment	PR
Complications over which we have no control	C

may cause functional problems as well. For example, subglottic hemangiomas can obstruct
the airway, periorbital lesions may block the visual axis leading to amblyopia, gastrointestinal
hemangiomas may cause bleeding, and hepatic hemangiomas can result in congestive heart
failure, hypothyroidism, abdominal compartment syndrome, and death (6–8). Ultimately, 50%
of children will have residual skin changes after hemangioma involution, including redundant
skin, scarring, fibrofatty residuum, hypo or hyperpigmentation, alopecia, and telangiectasias
(9). Correction of residual deformities may range from simple excision of redundant skin to
complicated skin graft or flap reconstruction.

Other types of vascular tumors share a similar morbidity profile with hemangioma but
pose additional risks. For example, kaposiform hemangioendothelioma (KHE) can be associated with Kasabach-Merritt phenomenon (KMP) (thrombocytopenia, petechiae, bleeding) (10).
Children with KMP have severe thrombocytopenia (less than $10,000 \, mm^3$) and are at risk for
bleeding. Platelet transfusions should be avoided unless there is active bleeding or a planned
surgical procedure because exogenous platelets are trapped in the lesion causing swelling. In
addition, heparin should not be administered because it stimulates tumor growth and aggra-
vates platelet trapping, worsening bleeding (10).

Malformations

Capillary Malformation

Capillary malformation (CM) primarily causes psychological morbidity, especially when located
on the face. These lesions tend to worsen in appearance over time as they darken and develop
fibrovascular overgrowth. Functional problems are the result of soft tissue or bony hypertrophy.
For example, orthognathic treatment of malocclusion may be required to correct associated
maxillary or mandibular overgrowth. Pulse-dye laser (585 nm) is effective at lightening these
stains and may retard the progression of discoloration and cutaneous overgrowth.

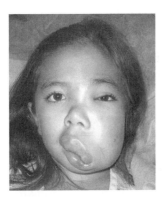 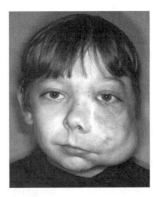

Figure 1   Most common complication of vascular anomalies is disfigurement and psychological morbidity due
to patient disease (PD). (*Left*) A nine-year-old female with a lymphatic malformation of her left face. (*Right*) An
eight-year-old male with an arteriovenous malformation of his left face. *Source*: Courtesy of John B. Mulliken, MD.

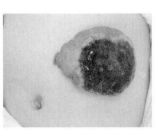
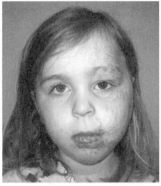

Figure 2   Complications of infantile hemangioma due to patient disease (PD). (*Left*) A six-month-old female with an ulcerated, bleeding, infected abdominal hemangioma requiring dressing changes, antibiotics, and resection. (*Right*) A five-year-old female with diffuse telangiectasias, scarring, and fibrofatty residuum of the left upper eyelid and lower lip after hemangioma involution. *Source*: Courtesy of John B. Mulliken, MD.

Lymphatic Malformation

Lymphatic malformation (LM) is most commonly located in the head and neck and like all vascular anomalies can cause psychological morbidity from disfigurement. LM is particularly susceptible to bleeding or infection. Intralesional bleeding occurs in up to 35% of lesions causing bluish discoloration, pain, or swelling (11). Infection complicates up to 71% of lesions and can progress rapidly to sepsis (11). Recurrent infections may necessitate prophylactic antibiotic treatment. Swelling due to bleeding, localized infection, or systemic illness can cause obstruction of important structures.

In addition to bleeding and infection, LM also can cause cutaneous vesicles leading to troublesome wounds. Secondary bony overgrowth is another complication of LM, often necessitating orthognathic surgery when located in the cervicofacial region (11). Upper airway LM often requires tracheostomy while thoracic LM may cause pleural, pericardial, or peritoneal chylous effusions (Fig. 3). Periorbital LM causes permanent reduction in vision in 40% of patients and blindness in 7% (12).

Treatment options for problematic LM include sclerotherapy or resection. Sclerotherapy is effective in shrinking macrocystic lesions with channels greater than 5 mm. Sclerosing agents include doxycycline, 100% ethanol, sodium tetradecyl sulfate, and OK-432 (killed group A Streptococcus pyogenes). The only treatment for microcystic LM is excision. Seventeen percent of LM recur due to reexpansion after sclerotherapy or excision (13).

Venous Malformation

Complications of venous malformation (VM), like all vascular anomalies, depend on the extent and location of the anomaly. Lesions located on the head or neck may cause progressive distortion or airway compromise. VM of the extremity may lead to leg-length discrepancy, pathologic fracture, or hemarthrosis causing degenerative arthritis. A large VM also can develop thrombosis leading to pulmonary embolism. Gastrointestinal VM can cause bleeding and chronic anemia (14). Stagnation within a large VM results in a localized intravascular coagulopathy and painful phlebothromboses. A coagulation profile should be obtained in patients with extensive lesions or who have a history of easy bruising. Aspirin or low-molecular weight heparin may be effective prevention and treatment of phlebothromboses. Like LM, symptomatic VM is treated by compression, sclerotherapy, or excision. Often, sclerotherapy is performed prior to excision to minimize bleeding and facilitate resection.

Arteriovenous Malformation

Arteriovenous malformation (AVM) is the most problematic vascular malformation due to its aggressive behavior and resistance to treatment. Although most are asymptomatic, an AVM typically worsens over time and may ultimately cause local ischemic changes, pain, bleeding, shunting, and heart failure. Treatment is reserved for symptomatic lesions because operative intervention can exacerbate its growth. Thus, if attempting to excise an AVM, complete

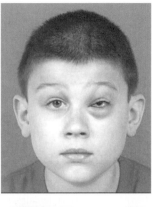
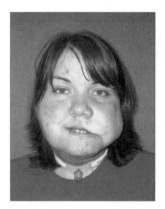
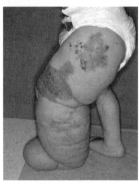
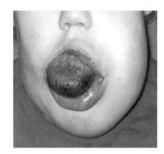

Figure 3 Functional complications of vascular anomalies due to patient disease (PD). (*Top, left*) A ten-year-old male with a lymphatic malformation of his left orbit causing infections, bleeding, glaucoma, amblyopia and reduced vision. (*Top, right*) A twenty-two-year-old female with cervicofacial lymphatic malformation necessitating permanent tracheostomy. (*Bottom, left*) A two-year-old female with Klippel-Trenaunay syndrome (capillary-lymphatic-venous malformation) showing cutaneous vesicles, a significant leg-length discrepancy, and preventing the use of regular footwear. (*Bottom, right*) A four-year-old female with lymphatic malformation of the tongue causing bleeding, infection, drainage from vesicles and inability to chew solid food. *Source*: Courtesy of John B. Mulliken, MD.

extirpation should be the goal, although this is usually not possible. Current management includes embolization, sclerotherapy, excision, or a combination of these modalities.

Combined Malformation

The most common combined malformation is Klippel-Trenaunay syndrome (KTS) which is an eponym denoting a slow flow, capillary-lymphatic-venous malformation (CLVM) associated with soft tissue or skeletal changes of a limb. It affects the lower extremity in 95% of patients, usually causing overgrowth of the affected extremity. Epiphysiodesis or partial foot amputation may be required for normal ambulation and the use of footwear. Thrombophlebitis occurs in 20% to 45% of patients with KTS and 4% to 25% suffer pulmonary embolism (9). Hemihypertrophy in these patients is a local process secondary to the vascular anomaly; children with KTS are not at risk for Wilms tumor and do not require ultrasound screening (15).

ERROR IN DIAGNOSIS (ED)

After patient disease the next most common cause of complications involving vascular anomalies is an error in diagnosis (Fig. 4). Diagnostic confusion is common in this field because 1) different vascular anomalies often look similar and 2) many practitioners use imprecise terminology, labeling lesions by descriptive, rather than histological names. Historically, vascular anomalies had been referred to by what food they resembled ("cherry", "strawberry", "port-wine") (9). After the development of histopathology in the 19th century, Virchow divided vascular anomalies into *angioma simplex*, *angioma* cavernosum, or *angioma racemosum*. His student, Wegener, separated LM into "lymphangioma" or "cystic hygroma" (9).

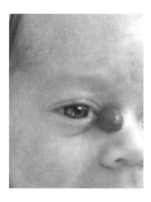
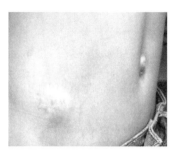
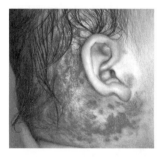
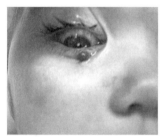

Figure 4 Errors in diagnosis (ED) of vascular anomalies. (*Top, left*) A seven-month-old male with proliferating infantile hemangioma. (*Top, right*) A six-year-old male with noninvoluting congenital hemangioma of the abdomen previously diagnosed as infantile hemangioma. (*Bottom, left*) A one-year-old male with KHE of the retroauricular area causing profound thrombocytopenia originally diagnosed as infantile hemangioma. (*Bottom, right*) A two-year-old female with pyogenic granuloma previously diagnosed as infantile hemangioma.

During the 20th century, "capillary" or "strawberry" hemangioma generally became associated with hemangioma affecting the dermis, which appears red (Table 2). Hemangioma located below the dermis is bluish and was often called "cavernous" hemangioma. Unfortunately, the terms "capillary" and "cavernous" also were used to describe CM and VM, respectively. In addition to "capillary hemangioma", "port-wine stain" also was used to describe CM. "Cystic hygroma" and "lymphangioma" became common terms for macrocystic LM and microcystic LM, respectively. To add to the confusing terminology, "hemangioma" continued to be used to

Table 2 Biological Classification of Vascular Anomalies

| | Malformations | |
| | Slow-flow | Fast-flow |
Tumors		
Infantile hemangioma	Capillary (CM) • Capillary-arteriovenous (CM-AVM)	Arterial malformation (AM)
Congenital hemangioma • Rapidly involuting congenital hemangioma (RICH) • Non-involuting congenital hemangioma (NICH) • Verrucous	Venous (VM) • Glomovenous	Arteriovenous fistula (AVF)
Kaposiform hemangioendothelioma (KHE)	Lymphatic (LM) • Microcystic • Macrocystic • Lymphedema	Arteriovenous malformation (AVM)
Pyogenic granuloma	Combined • Klippel Trenaunay (CLVM)	Combined • Parkes Weber (CLAVM)

Table 3 Common Incorrect Descriptions of Vascular Anomalies Leading to Errors in Diagnosis (ED)

Tumors		Malformations	
Correct biological name	**Incorrect description**	**Correct biological name**	**Incorrect description**
Hemangioma	"Capillary hemangioma" "Strawberry hemangioma"	Capillary (CM)	"Port-wine stain" "Hemangioma"
Kaposiform Hemangioendothelioma (KHE)	"Hemangioma"	Venous (VM)	"Cavernous hemangioma"
Pyogenic granuloma	"Lobular capillary hemangioma"	Lymphatic (LM)	"Lymphangioma" "Cystic hygroma"

describe any type of vascular anomaly. This imprecise nomenclature handicapped the field of vascular anomalies because physicians were unable to communicate with each other.

In 1982 a modern, biologic classification of vascular anomalies clarified the difference between vascular anomalies based on physical findings, natural history, and cellular characteristics (16). Vascular anomalies are broadly divided into two groups: tumors and malformations (Table 3). Vascular tumors are characterized by endothelial cell proliferation. Vascular malformations, in contrast, have normal endothelial cell turnover and arise from dysmorphogenesis. Malformations are further subdivided into slow-flow or fast-flow lesions. Combined vascular anomalies also exist which are often eponyms based on the physician responsible for the initial description. The suffix –oma, describing a lesion with proliferating cells (tumor), is not appropriate for malformations. Thus, terms such as "lymphangioma" (microcystic LM), "cystic hygroma" (macrocystic LM), and "cavernous hemangioma" (VM), which describe nonproliferating malformations, have been abandoned.

Unfortunately, descriptive terminology still exists today, which is the primary cause of errors in diagnosis (ED). Sixty percent of patients referred to our center have been given the wrong diagnosis and 90% of patients with an incorrectly diagnosed vascular anomaly receive improper treatment (17). Using the modern classification of vascular anomalies, a correct diagnosis can be made by history and physical exam in 90% of patients (18). In the remaining patients, a diagnosis usually can be obtained using radiological and immunohistochemical studies.

Tumors

The diagnosis of infantile hemangioma is most commonly confused with pyogenic granuloma, congenital hemangioma, or malignancy. Infantile hemangioma appears shortly after birth, undergoes rapid proliferation, and begins to involute at approximately 10 months of age. In contrast, pyogenic granuloma ("lobular capillary hemangioma") presents much later (mean age 6.7 years), remains small (less than 6.5 mm in diameter), frequently bleeds, and does not involute (19). Treatment of pyogenic granuloma includes curettage, laser therapy, or excision.

Unlike infantile hemangioma, congenital hemangioma is fully grown at birth. One type of congenital hemangioma, rapidly involuting congenital hemangioma (RICH), involutes after birth and has completed its regression by one year of age (20). The second type of congenital hemangioma, noninvoluting congenital hemangioma (NICH), does not undergo involution (21). Congenital hemangioma is managed differently than infantile hemangioma. Problematic infantile hemangioma is treated by corticosteroid to accelerate involution. In contrast, corticosteroid is not indicated for congenital hemangioma because RICH undergoes rapid postnatal involution and NICH does not respond to drug treatment. Instead, treatment of NICH is excision.

The diagnosis of infantile hemangioma is also commonly confused with KHE. Unlike infantile hemangioma, KHE does not completely regress and can cause Kasabach Merritt phenomenon (KMP) (thrombocytopenia, petechiae, bleeding). Patients with KHE are less likely than individuals with hemangioma to respond to corticosteroid. Vincristine is an effective treatment for patients with KHE who fail corticosteroid therapy.

In addition to KHE, more aggressive malignancies are also in the differential diagnosis of hemangioma. Like hemangioma, hemangioendotheliomas, tufted angioma, hemangiopericytoma, fibrosarcoma, and lymphoma are proliferating lesions present in childhood that can look similar to hemangioma. In the liver, hemangioma may be confused with hepatoblastoma or metastatic neuroblastoma. If the history and physical exam or radiographic imaging of a hemangioma is equivocal, then a biopsy of the lesion should be obtained to rule out malignancy.

Less commonly, hemangioma and arteriovenous malformation (AVM) can be confused because both lesions are fast-flow. Unlike AVM, though, infantile hemangioma grows rapidly and then involutes. Differentiating NICH from AVM is more difficult because NICH, like AVM, is a high-flow lesion that does not regress. Ultrasound or MRI may be required to differentiate infantile or congenital hemangioma from AVM.

Malformations

Vascular malformations are most commonly mistaken for hemangioma or for other malformations. Because many vascular lesions have a similar appearance, patients can be managed erroneously due to an incorrect diagnosis. For example, although drug therapy is indicated for problematic vascular tumors such as infantile hemangioma or KHE, patients with vascular malformations are often mistakenly given antiangiogenic regimens. Antiendothelial treatment (corticosteroid, interferon, vincristine) is not effective for malformations because these lesions lack significant cellular turnover. Patients are thus unnecessarily placed at risk for developing side effects from these drugs.

In addition to being confused with tumors, malformations also may be mistaken for other types of vascular malformations. LM and VM are most commonly confused because they are both slow-flow lesions that may look alike. When history and physical exam is equivocal, radiographic imaging or immunohistochemistry can differentiate between the two lesions. Errors in diagnosis between LM and VM may not be clinically significant because both are treated by compression, sclerotherapy, or excision. However, a correct diagnosis is important because LM and VM pose specific problems. For example, LM has a high risk of infection, potentially necessitating antibiotic prophylaxis, while VM often has painful phleboliths requiring aspirin therapy.

ERROR IN JUDGEMENT (EJ)

After patient disease and error in diagnosis, the next most common source of vascular anomalies complications is incorrect judgment after the correct diagnosis has been made.

Tumors

The most common error in judgment regarding infantile hemangioma is overaggressive treatment of the tumor. Most hemangiomas do not cause harm and involute without sequelea; only 10% require intervention (4). Pharmacological management of hemangioma should be judicious to avoid complications resulting from the treatment. For example, steroid injections can lead to ulceration while oral corticosteroid can cause temporary growth retardation, irritability, myopathy, hypertension, and gastric irritation (22).

A more problematic error in judgment than unnessecary drug treatment is the resection of a proliferating hemangioma. Excision of a proliferating hemangioma generally is not indicated because more destruction will be done than excising residual tissue after the tumor has involuted. Excision of a proliferating hemangioma can lead to significant blood loss, injury to vital structures, and even death (5). Ideally, resection should be postponed to the involuted phase when expanded skin and fibrofatty residuum is minimal. However, problematic small, pedunculated, or well-localized lesions may be excised if the resulting scar is no worse than would be expected after resection during involution.

Although overaggressive treatment of nonproblematic hemangiomas is common, incorrect management also occurs. For example, patients with problematic hemangioma are commonly treated with interferon-α, 2a or 2b (IFN) instead of corticosteroid. Interferon is reserved for patients who fail or have contraindications to corticosteroid or vincristine. IFN should not be used as primary therapy because it takes several weeks to work, requires subcutaneous injections, causes spastic diplegia (5%), and necessitates neurological monitoring (23,24).

Like hemangioma, KHE also can be treated incorrectly with drug therapy. Most often, patients with KHE are initially given corticosteroid. However, KHE has only a 10% response rate to corticosteroid, unlike infantile hemangioma (85% response rate) (5,10). Thus, first-line treatment of KHE is vincristine (87% response rate) followed by interferon (50% response rate) (25).

Another judgment error in the management of vascular tumors is the failure to recognize associated pathology. For example, children with five or more cutaneous hemangiomas are at risk for hemangiomas involving the internal organs (9). Cervicothoracic hemangioma has been associated with sternal nonunion or supraumbilical raphe while sacral hemangioma may signal an underlying spinal dysraphism (26–28). Hemangioma located in a trigeminal nerve dermatomal distribution should alert the surgeon to the possibility of PHACES syndrome (Posterior fossa malformations, Hemangiomas, Arterial anomalies, Coarctation of the aorta and cardiac defects, and Eye abnormalitieS) (28,29).

The presence of a diffuse hemangioma replacing hepatic parenchyma, causing hepatomegaly, should stimulate an investigation into thyroid function to prevent irreversible mental retardation. Hypothyroidism results from the expression of a deiodinase by the hemangioma which cleaves iodine from thyroid hormone. Massive intravenous thyroid replacement may be necessary until the hemangioma regresses (7). In contrast to diffuse hepatic hemangioma, a large single hemangioma in the liver is usually rapidly involuting congenital hemangioma (RICH). RICH does not require therapy unless it is associated with significant shunting. Similarly, multiple small hepatic hemangiomas also do not necessitate treatment unless large vascular shunts are present (8).

Malformations

Like hemangioma, a common judgment error in the management of vascular malformations is the treatment of lesions that do not require intervention. Many patients suffer unnessecary iatrogenic injury due to complications of treatment. For example, sclerotherapy is indicated only for problematic malformations, because it can cause ulceration, nerve injury, compartment syndrome, and inadvertent embolization (17). Similarly, surgical excision is associated with the same risks as excising hemangioma: bleeding, injury to vital structures, and even death. Intervention for malformations should be reserved for lesions causing severe disfigurement, bleeding, pain, infection, or functional problems.

In addition to overzealous treatment, incorrect management of vascular malformations is possible as well. For example, even after the correct diagnosis of a vascular malformation, patients may be given antiangiogenic drugs which not only do not help malformations, but place the patient at risk for side effects from the drugs. In addition, sclerotherapy may be erroneously used for microcystic LM, although it is only efficacious for macrocystic lesions.

Occasionally, the location of malformation should alert the surgeon to the possibility of an underlying structural abnormality. A midline occipital CM can be associated with an encephalocele, a CM over the spine may indicate a spinal dysraphism, and a CM on the posterior chest can signal an underlying AVM of the spinal canal (30). CM located in the ophthalmic (V1) trigeminal dermatome may be a component of Sturge–Weber syndrome which is associated with ipsilateral ocular and leptomeningeal vascular anomalies (31). Leptomeningeal anomalies can lead to seizures, contralateral hemiplegia, delayed motion, and cognition. Patients are at risk for retinal detachment and glaucoma and should be followed by an ophthalmologist biannually until age 2 and yearly thereafter (28).

ERROR IN TECHNIQUE (ET)

Errors in technique are less common causes of morbidity in the field of vascular anomalies compared to patient disease, errors in diagnosis, and errors in judgment (EJ). Most complications in technique involve incorrect delivery of drugs, sclerotherapy or embolization to properly diagnosed lesions.

Tumors

After making the correct diagnosis of a problematic hemangioma and initiating the correct first-line treatment, corticosteroid, errors in the technique of drug delivery can occur. Although the correct dose for oral prednisone is 2 to 3 mg/kg/day, patients can be undertreated or overtreated. If a lower dose or less frequent delivery of drug is given, then the tumor is unlikely to respond. On the other hand, higher doses of corticosteroid (5 mg/kg/day) can be equally troublesome, increasing the risk of steroid complications such as Cushingoid faces, slowed gain in height and weight, infection, myopathy, and bone resorption. Fortunately, after the cessation of corticosteroid, children return to their pretreatment growth curves by 24 months of age (22). Live vaccines (polio, measles, mumps, rubella, varicella) are not administered during corticosteroid treatment. Patients should be placed on an oral histamine receptor blocker to prevent corticosteroid-related gastritis (28). Corticosteroids and interferon should not be combined because increased efficacy has not been shown and patients have a greater risk of treatment-associated complications.

In addition to incorrect dosing, improper timing of drug delivery can be problematic as well. Because infantile hemangioma begins to involute at approximately 10 months of age, initiating corticosteroid treatment shortly before this time is usually not indicated. Also, children should not continue taking corticosteroids after 10 months of age, unless they are in the tapering phase of treatment. Tapering the corticosteroid too rapidly can increase the risk of rebound growth, thus necessitating another cycle of therapy. Injection of corticosteroid can cause morbidity as well; ulceration is not uncommon and blindness has been reported after injection of periorbital hemangioma (32).

Although flashlamp pulsed-dye laser treatment for proliferating hemangiomas has been advocated by some authors, almost all hemangiomas are beyond the reach of the laser. The laser penetrates only 0.75 to 1.2 mm into the dermis and thus only affects the superficial portion of the tumor, causing some lightening. The pulsed-dye laser has not been shown to decrease hemangioma bulk or accelerate involution (33). Instead, this laser can cause hypopigmentation and increased scarring by causing ulceration and partial thickness skin loss. The pulsed-dye laser is indicated, however, during the involuted phase to treat residual telangiectasias. Unlike the pulse-dye laser, a carbon dioxide laser may be useful for the treatment of a proliferating subglottic hemangioma (34).

For hemangiomas that require resection, lenticular excision results in a scar that may be as much as three times the length of the diameter of the lesion. Instead, we advocate circular excision of the lesion and purse-string closure to reduce the length of the scar in esthetically important areas, such as the face (35). Although this technique may require more than one stage, it ensures the smallest possible scar and minimizes the distortion of surrounding tissues.

Malformations

Errors in technique when treating malformations usually are related to either sclerotherapy (injecting irritant directly into a lesion) or embolization (occlusion of vessels by materials introduced through a remote catheter). Commonly used sclerosents include sodium tetradecyl sulfate (Sotradecol), doxycycline, and ethanol (28). All sclerosants can cause ulceration (10% incidence), swelling, venous thrombosis, thromboembolism, and renal toxicity (36). Ethanol typically produces the most swelling and pain and often requires general anesthesia. In addition, ethanol should not be used in proximity to important nerves (facial nerve) because of the potential for permanent nerve injury. Many malformations will reexpand and thus require multiple treatments.

Like sclerotherapy, embolization is also associated with complications such as ulceration, nerve injury, swelling, and thromboembolism. In addition, embolization can cause ischemic complications in areas not involved with vascular anomalies as well as cardiac arrythmias, pulmonary embolism when material passes through arteriovenous shunts, and death (17). Unsuccessful deployment of material may also cause occlusion in nontarget tissues. For example, stroke may occur after embolization of head and neck lesions. Procedures requiring catheterization may cause bleeding, thrombosis, or pseudoaneurysm of the catheterization site (17). Embolization of AVM is associated with a complication rate as high as 30% (17). Embolization should be directed toward the center of the AVM (nidus). Occlusion of proximal arteries to the AVM should not be performed because of tissue ischemia, development of collaterals, and inability to embolize the nidus of the lesion in the future (17).

Attempts at surgical excision should be planned carefully. When possible, the entire anomaly should be extirpated to prevent recurrence. However, complete resection is rarely possible and thus excision should be staged based on specific anatomic regions. Sclerotherapy of VM and embolization of AVM 24 to 36 hours before resection reduces bleeding and facilitates the removal of the malformation. Though patients may benefit from surgical debulking procedures, wound complications are common. Patients and families should be counseled that the tissue involving the malformation has abnormal vascularity and is predisposed to wound breakdown, infection, and the need for prolonged drainage.

CONCLUSIONS

Vascular anomalies are an exciting field combining several medical and surgical specialties. These lesions are particularly prone to complications because they are locally destructive, cause systemic problems, and are difficult to manage. In addition, vascular anomalies are often misdiagnosed, due to common clinical appearances and confusing terminology, leading to management errors. Practitioners must use correct biological terminology to describe these lesions so that communication, proper treatment, and research can be facilitated. To minimize complications in this field, patients with problematic vascular anomalies should be referred to an interdisciplinary Vascular Anomalies Center with specialists experienced with these lesions.

REFERENCES

1. Greene AK, May JW Jr. Ernest Amory Codman, MD (1869–1940): The influence of the end result idea on plastic and reconstructive surgery. Plast Reconstr Surg 2007; 119(5):1606–1609.
2. Codman EA. A Study in Hospital Efficiency as Demonstrated by the Case Report of the First Two Years of a Private Hospital. Boston, MA: Privately printed, 1914.
3. Codman EA. The Shoulder. Boston, MA: Privately printed, 1934.
4. Enjolras O, Gelbert F. Superficial hemangiomas: Associations and management. Pediatr Dermatol 1997; 14(3):173–179.
5. Greene AK, Rogers G, Mulliken JB. Management of parotid hemangioma in 100 children. Plast Reconstr Surg 2004; 113(1):53–60.
6. Boon LM, Burrows PE, Paltiel HJ, et al. Hepatic vascular anomalies in infancy: A twenty-seven-year experience. J Pediatr 1996; 129(3):346—354.
7. Huang SA, Tu HM, Harney JW, et al. Severe hypothyroidism caused by type 3 iodothyronine deiodinase in infantile hemangiomas. N Engl J Med 2000; 343(3):185–189.
8. Christison-Lagay ER, Burrows PE, Alomari A, et al. Hepatic hemangiomas: Subtype classification and development of a clinical practice algorithm and registry. J Pediatr Surg 2007; 42(1):62–67.
9. Mulliken JB, Fishman SJ, Burrows PE. Vascular anomalies. Curr Prob Surg 2000; 37(8):519–584.
10. Mulliken JB, Anupindi S, Ezekowitz RA, et al. Case records of the Massachusetts General Hospital. Weekly clinicopathological exercises. Case 13-2004. A newborn girl with a large cutaneous lesion, thrombocytopenia, and anemia. N Engl J Med 2004; 350(17):1764–1775.
11. Padwa BL, Hayward PG, Ferraro NF, et al. Cervicofacial lymphatic malformation: Clinical course, surgical intervention, and pathogenesis of skeletal hypertrophy. Plast Reconstr Surg 1995; 95(6):951–960.
12. Greene AK, Burrows PB, Smith L, et al. Periorbital lymphatic malformation: Clinical course and management in 42 patients. Plast Reconstr Surg 2005; 115(1):22–30.
13. Alqahtani A, Nguyen LT, Flageole H, et al. 25 years' experience with lymphangiomas in children. J Pediatr Surg 1999; 34(7):1164–1168.
14. Fishman SJ, Burrows PE, Leichtner AM, et al. Gastrointestinal manifestations of vascular anomalies in childhood: Varied etiologies require multiple therapeutic modalities. J Pediatr Surg 1998; 33(7):1163–1167.
15. Greene AK, Kieran M, Burrows PE, et al. Wilms tumor screening for Klippel-Trenaunay syndrome is unnecessary. Pediatrics 2004; 113(4):E326–E329.
16. Mulliken JB, Glowacki J. Hemangiomas and vascular malformations in infants and children: A classification based on endothelial characteristics. Plast Reconstr Surg 1982; 69(3):412–422.
17. Mulliken JB, Burrows PE. Vascular Malformations. In: Goldwyn RM, Cohen MN, eds. The Unfavorable Result in Plastic Surgery: Avoidance and Treatment, 3rd ed. Philadelphia, PA: Lippincott Williams and Wilkins, 2001:271–287.
18. Finn MC, Glowacki J, Mulliken JB. Congenital vascular lesions: Clinical application of a new classification. J Pediatr Surg 1983; 18(6):894–900.
19. Patrice SJ, Wiss K, Mulliken JB. Pyogenic granuloma (lobular capillary hemangioma): A clinicopathologic study of 178 cases. Pediatr Dermatol 1991; 8(4):267–276.
20. Berenguer B, Mulliken JB, Enjolras O, et al. Rapidly involuting congenital hemangioma: Clinical and histopathologic features. Pediatr Dev Pathol 2003; 6(6):495–510.

21. Enjolras O, Mulliken JB, Boon LM, et al. Noninvoluting congenital hemangioma: A rare cutaneous vascular anomaly. Plast Reconstr Surg 2001; 107(7):1647–1654.

22. Boon LM, MacDonald DM, Mulliken JB. Complications of systemic corticosteroid therapy for problematic hemangiomas. Plast Reconstr Surg 1999; 104(6):1616–1623.

23. Barlow CF, Priebe CJ, Mulliken JB, et al. Spastic diplegia as a complication of interferon alfa-2a treatment of hemangiomas of infancy. J Pediatr 1998; 132(3):527–530.

24. Dubois J, Hershon L, Carmant L, et al. Toxicity profile of interferon alfa-2b in children: A prospective evaluation. J Pediatr 1999; 135(6):782–785.

25. Haisley-Royster C, Enjolras O, Frieden IJ, et al. Kasabach-Merritt phenomenon: A retrospective study of treatment with vincristine. J Pediatr Hematol Oncol 2002; 24(6):459–462.

26. Hersh JH, Waterfill D, Rutledge J, et al. Sternal malformation/vascular dysplasia association. Am J Med Genet 1985; 21(1):177–186.

27. Albright AL, Gartner JC, Wiener ES. Lumbar cutaneous hemangiomas as indicators of tethered spinal cords. Pediatrics 1989;83(6):977–980.

28. Marler JJ, Mulliken JB. Current management of hemangiomas and vascular malformations. Clin Plast Surg 2005; 32(1):99–116.

29. Frieden IJ, Reese V, Cohen D. PHACE syndrome. The association of posterior fossa brain malformations, hemangiomas, arterial anomalies, coarctation of the aorta and cardiac defects, and eye abnormalities. Arch Dermatol 1996; 132(3):307–311.

30. Enjolras O, Mulliken JB. The current management of vascular birthmarks. Pediatr Dermatol 1993; 10(4)311–333.

31. Enjolras O, Riche MC, Merland JJ. Facial port-wine stains and Sturge-Weber syndrome. Pediatrics 1985; 76(1):48–51.

32. Ruttum MS, Abrams GW, Harris GJ, et al. Bilateral retinal embolization associated with intralesional steroid injection for capillary hemangioma of infancy. J Pediatr Ophthalmol Strabismus 1993; 30(1):4–7.

33. Batta K, Goodyear HM, Moss C, et al. Randomized controlled study of early pulsed dye laser treatment of uncomplicated childhood haemangiomas: Results of a 1-year analysis. Lancet 2002; 360(9332):521–527.

34. Sie KC, McGill T, Healy GB. Subglottic hemangioma: Ten years experience with carbon dioxide laser. An Otol Rhinol Laryngol 1994; 103(3):167–172.

35. Mulliken JB, Rogers GF, Marler JJ. Circular excision of hemangioma and purse-string closure: The smallest possible scar. Plast Reconstr Surg 2002 109(5):1544–1554.

36. Berenguer B, Burrows PE, Zurakowski D, et al. Sclerotherapy of craniofacial venous malformations: Complications and results. Plast Reconstr Surg 1999; 104(1):1–11.

Index